American Cancer Society
Atlas of Clinical Oncology

Published

Blumgart, Fong, Jarnagin	*Hepatobiliary Cancer (2001)*
Cameron	*Pancreatic Cancer (2001)*
Carroll, Grossfeld	*Prostate Cancer (2002)*
Char	*Tumors of the Eye and Ocular Adnexa (2001)*
Eifel, Levenback	*Cancer of the Female Lower Genital Tract (2001)*
Ginsberg	*Lung Cancer (2002)*
Grossbard	*Malignant Lymphomas (2001)*
Pollock	*Soft Tissue Sarcomas (2001)*
Posner, Vokes, Weichselbaum	*Cancer of the Upper Gastrointestinal Tract (2001)*
Prados	*Brain Cancer (2001)*
Shah	*Cancer of the Head and Neck (2001)*
Silverman	*Oral Cancer (1998)*
Sober, Haluska	*Skin Cancer (2001)*
Wiernik	*Adult Leukemias (2001)*
Willett	*Cancer of the Lower Gastrointestinal Tract (2001)*
Winchester, Winchester	*Breast Cancer (2000)*

Forthcoming

Clark, Duh, Jahan, Perrier	*Endocrine Tumors (2002)*
Droller	*Urothelial Cancer (2002)*
Fuller, Seiden, Young	*Uterine and Endometrial Cancer (2003)*
Ozols	*Ovarian Cancer (2002)*
Raghavan	*Germ Cell Tumors (2002)*
Richie, Steele	*Kidney Tumors (2003)*
Volberding	*Viral and Immunological Malignancies (2003)*
Yasko	*Bone Tumors (2002)*

American Cancer Society
Atlas of
Clinical Oncology

Editors

Glenn D. Steele Jr, MD
Geisinger Health System

Theodore L. Phillips, MD
University of California

Bruce A. Chabner, MD
Harvard Medical School

Managing Editor

Ted S. Gansler, MD, MBA
Director of Health Content, American Cancer Society

American Cancer Society

Atlas of

Clinical Oncology

Prostate Cancer

American Cancer Society

Atlas of

Clinical Oncology

Prostate Cancer

Peter R. Carroll, MD, FACS

Professor and Chair

Ken and Donna Derr-Chevron Chair in Prostate Cancer

Department of Urology

University of California

San Francisco, California

Gary D. Grossfeld, MD, FACS

Assistant Professor

Department of Urology

University of California

San Francisco, California

2002

BC Decker Inc

Hamilton • London

BC Decker Inc
P.O. Box 620, LCD 1
Hamilton, Ontario L8N 3K7
Tel: 905-522-7017; 1-800-568-7281
Fax: 905-522-7839; 1-888-311-4987
E-mail: info@bcdecker.com
www.bcdecker.com

02 03 04 05 / UTP / 9 8 7 6 5 4 3 2 1

ISBN 1–55009–130–1
Printed in Canada

Cover figure (top left and right) courtesy of Dr. Weidner, from Chapter 2, Pathology.
Cover figure (bottom left) courtesy of Drs. Carroll, Meng, Downs, and Grossfeld, from Chapter 12, Radical Retropubic Prostatectomy.
Cover figure (bottom right) courtesy of Drs. Rogers, Carroll, and Tanagho, from Chapter 6, Anatomy.

Sales and Distribution

United States
BC Decker Inc
P.O. Box 785
Lewiston, NY 14092-0785
Tel: 905-522-7017; 1-800-568-7281
Fax: 905-522-7839; 1-888-311-4987
E-mail: info@bcdecker.com
www.bcdecker.com

Canada
BC Decker Inc
20 Hughson Street South
P.O. Box 620, LCD 1
Hamilton, Ontario L8N 3K7
Tel: 905-522-7017; 1-800-568-7281
Fax: 905-522-7839; 1-888-311-4987
E-mail: info@bcdecker.com
www.bcdecker.com

Foreign Rights
John Scott & Company
International Publishers' Agency
P.O. Box 878
Kimberton, PA 19442
Tel: 610-827-1640
Fax: 610-827-1671
E-mail: jsco@voicenet.com

U.K., Europe, Scandinavia, Middle East
Elsevier Science
Customer Service Department
Foots Cray High Street
Sidcup, Kent
DA14 5HP, UK
Tel: 44 208 308 5760
Fax: 44 181 308 5702
E-mail: cservice@harcourt.com

Australia, New Zealand
Elsevier Science Australia
Customer Service Department
STM Division
Locked Bag 16
St. Peters, New South Wales, 2044
Australia
Tel: 61 02 9517-8999
Fax: 61 02 9517-2249
E-mail: stmp@harcourt.com.au
www.harcourt.com.au

Japan
Igaku-Shoin Ltd.
Foreign Publications Department
3-24-17 Hongo
Bunkyo-ku, Tokyo, Japan 113-8719
Tel: 81 3 3817 5680
Fax: 81 3 3815 6776
E-mail: fd@igaku-shoin.co.jp

Singapore, Malaysia, Thailand, Philippines, Indonesia, Vietnam, Pacific Rim, Korea
Elsevier Science Asia
583 Orchard Road, #09/01, Forum
Singapore 238884
Tel: 65-737-3593
Fax: 65-753-2145

Mexico and Central America
ETM SA de CV
Calle de Tula 59
Colonia Condesa
06140 Mexico DF, Mexico
Tel: 52-5-5553-6657
Fax: 52-5-5211-8468
E-mail: editoresdetextosmex@prodigy.net.mx

Argentina
CLM (Cuspide Libros Medicos)
Av. Córdoba 2067 – (1120)
Buenos Aires, Argentina
Tel: (5411) 4961-0042/(5411) 4964-0848
Fax: (5411) 4963-7988
E-mail: clm@cuspide.com

Brazil
Tecmedd
Av. Maurilio Biagi, 2850
Ribeirão Preto – SP – CEP: 14021-000
Tel: 0800 992236
Fax: (16) 3993-9000
E-mail: tecmedd@tecmedd.com.br

Contents

Preface

Prostate cancer is a major health care problem in the United States, where it is the most commonly diagnosed malignancy and second leading cause of cancer-related death in men. The economic, psychological, and physical burden associated with prostate cancer detection and treatment is significant and may be especially high for certain groups, such as African American men, who are approximately 1.5-fold more likely to be diagnosed with and 2.5-fold more likely to die from prostate cancer than their Caucasian-American counterparts. Despite its prevalence, there continues to be many unresolved issues regarding prostate cancer diagnosis and treatment, including uncertainty over the benefits of prostate cancer screening and a lack of consensus as to what constitutes the best form of treatment for any stage of disease.

The introduction and routine use of serum prostate-specific antigen (PSA) testing in the late 1980s in men at risk for prostate cancer has led to significant changes in the incidence, presentation, and treatment of the disease. Serum PSA testing initially led to a dramatic increase in the incidence of new prostate cancer cases in the United States, that reached a peak in the early 1990s. Along with the increased incidence, there was a marked migration to lower stage of disease at presentation and lower age at diagnosis. Such changes in the clinical presentation of prostate cancer patients have led to important differences in how the disease is managed. Earlier detection of prostate cancer in younger patients has resulted in the increased use of definitive local treatments such as radical prostatectomy and brachytherapy. In addition, there have been major changes in the use of imaging tests for initial prostate cancer staging. Increased awareness of prostate cancer recurrence following local therapy, as a result of serial PSA testing, has led to a new group of patients with "biochemical disease progression" and the use of androgen deprivation therapy earlier in the course of the disease for many patients. Perhaps reflecting the earlier disease stage at presentation, as well as more effective treatment for localized disease, 5-year cancer-specific survival rates have increased over the last decade. However, as of yet, there are no conclusive data to confirm that early detection and treatment will decrease disease-specific morbidity and mortality, and properly conducted trials are sorely needed to determine the benefits and risks of early prostate cancer detection and the accompanying treatment modalities.

To better define the relevant issues associated with prostate cancer diagnosis and treatment, this volume of the *Atlas of Clinical Oncology* brings together a talented group of urologic surgeons, medical oncologists, radiation oncologists, epidemiologists, health-services researchers, radiologists, pathologists, and basic scientists.

The editors are grateful for the commitment and passion of our colleagues in their treatment of patients with prostate cancer. We believe these qualities are reflected in their excellent contributions to this volume. We also would like to acknowledge Charmaine Sherlock, Kimmy Rolfe, and Brian Decker for their expert guidance and assistance in completing this excellent comprehensive text. Finally, we would like to express our gratitude to our patients and families who continue to inspire and guide us.

PRC
GDG
April 2002

Contributors

PETER R. CARROLL, MD, FACS
Department of Urology
University of California
San Francisco, California
Anatomy
Natural History
Radical Retropubic Prostatectomy
Laparoscopic Radical Prostatectomy
Local Therapy for Prostate-Specific Antigen Recurrence after Definitive Treatment
Complementary and Alternative Medicine

JUNE M. CHAN, SCD
Department of Epidemiology and Biostatistics and Urology
University of California
San Francisco, California
Epidemiology: Distribution and Determinants

MICHAEL L. CHER, MD
Department of Urology
Wayne State Unversity
Detroit, Michigan
The Bone Microenvironment

FERGUS V. COAKLEY, MD
Department of Radiology
University of California
San Francisco, California
Imaging

GERALD R. CUNHA, PHD
Department of Anatomy
University of California
San Francisco, California
Role of Stroma
In Vitro and In Vivo Models

RAJVIR DAHIYA, PHD
Department of Urology
University of California
San Francisco, California
Molecular Genetics
Role of Stroma

MARC A. DALL'ERA, MD
Department of Urology
University of Washington
Seattle, Washington
Tumor Markers

ANNEMARIE A. DONJACOUR, PHD
Department of Anatomy
University of California
San Francisco, California
Role of Stroma

TRACY M. DOWNS, MD
Department of Urology
University of California
San Francisco, California
Radical Retropubic Prostatectomy

CHRISTOPHER P. EVANS, MD, FACS
Department of Urology
University of California, Davis School of Medicine
University of California, David Medical Center
Sacramento, California
Tumor Markers

LAWRENCE FONG, MD
Department of Medicine
University of California
San Francisco, California
Novel Systemic Therapy

SHAHRAM GHOLAMI, MD
Department of Urology
University of California
San Francisco, California
Erectile Dysfunction after Treatment

ALEXANDER R. GOTTSCHALK, MD, PHD
Department of Radiation Oncology
University of California
San Francisco, California
Radiobiology: Old, Present, Future, and Practical Considerations

MICHAEL B. GOTWAY, MD
Department of Radiology
University of California
San Francisco General Hospital
San Francisco, California
Imaging

GARY D. GROSSFELD, MD, FACS
Department of Urology
University of California
San Francisco, California
Role of Stroma
Natural History
Radical Retropubic Prostatectomy
Laparoscopic Radical Prostatectomy
Local Therapy for Prostate-Specific Antigen Recurrence after Definitive Treatment
Complementary and Alternative Medicine

KATHERINE A. HARRIS, MD, PHD
Department of Medicine
Penn State Cancer Institute
Allentown, Pennsylvania
Androgen Deprivation Therapy: Timing and Type

SIMON W. HAYWARD, PHD
Department of Urology Surgery, Cancer Biology
Vanderbilt-Ingram Cancer Center
Vanderbilt University Medical Center
Nashville, Tennessee
Role of Stroma
In Vitro and In Vivo Models

I-CHOW J. HSU, MD
Department of Radiation Oncology
University of California
Mount Zion Cancer Center
San Francisco, California
Brachytherapy

CHRISTOPHER J. KANE, MD
Department of Urology
University of California
San Francisco, California
Laparoscopic Radical Prostatectomy

THERESA M. KOPPIE, MD
Department of Urology
University of California
San Francisco, California
Management of Bladder and Bowel Disorders after Treatment

WENDY LENG, MD
Department of Urology
University of Pittsburgh
Pittsburgh, Pennsylvania
Management of Bladder and Bowel Disorders after Treatment

DEBORAH P. LUBECK, PHD
Department of Urology
University of California
San Francisco, California
Complementary and Alternative Medicine

TOM LUE, MD
Department of Urology
University of California
San Francisco, California
Erectile Dysfunction after Treatment

PAUL C. MARKER, PHD
Department of Anatomy
University of California
San Francisco, California
Role of Stroma

MAXWELL V. MENG, MD
Department of Urology
University of California
San Francisco, California
Molecular Genetics
Radical Retropubic Prostatectomy
Local Therapy for Prostate-Specific Antigen Recurrence after Definitive Treatment

MAYA D. MEUX, MD
Department of Radiology
University of California
San Francisco, California
Imaging

JEFFREY A. NEMETH, PHD
Oncology Research
Centocor Company
Malvern, Pennsylvania
The Bone Microenvironment

JOSEPH C. PRESTI JR, MD
Department of Urology
Stanford University School of Medicine
Stanford, California
Detection: Evolving Role of Systematic Biopsy
Staging: Initial Risk Assessment

DAVID M. REESE, MD
Cancer International Research Group
Los Angeles, California
Role of Chemotherapy in the Treatment of Hormone-Refractory Prostate Cancer
Palliative Care

MACK ROACH III, MD
Department of Radiation Oncology
University of California
San Francisco, California
Radiobiology: Old, Present, Future, and Practical Considerations
External Beam Radiation Therapy
Brachytherapy

RODMAN S. ROGERS, MD
Department of Urology
California Pacific Medical Center
San Francisco, California
Anatomy
Erectile Dysfunction after Treatment

KATSUTO SHINOHARA, MD
Department of Urology
University of California
San Francisco, California
New Forms of Focal Therapy

ERIC J. SMALL, MD
Department of Medicine
University of California
San Francisco, California
Androgen Deprivation Therapy: Timing and Type
Novel Systemic Therapy

JOYCELYN L. SPEIGHT, MD, PHD
Department of Radiation Oncology
University of California San Francisco
Mount Zion Medical Center
San Francisco, California
External Beam Radiation Therapy

SANDY SRINIVAS, MD
Department of Medicine
Stanford University
Stanford, California
VA Medical Center/Stanford Medical Center
Palo-Alto, California
Second-Line Hormonal Therapy

MARSHALL L. STOLLER, MD
Department of Urology
University of California
San Francisco, California
Laparoscopic Radical Prostatectomy

EMIL TANAGHO, MD
Department of Urology
University of California
San Francisco, California
Anatomy

AXEL A. THOMSON, PHD
MRC Human Reproductive Sciences Unit
Edinburgh, United Kingdom
Role of Stroma

YUZHUO WANG, PHD
Department of Cancer Endocrinology
BC Cancer Agency
Vancouver, British Columbia
In Vitro and In Vivo Models

NOEL WEIDNER, MD
Department of Pathology
University of California
San Diego, California
Pathology

VERNON E. WELDON, MD
Department of Urology
University of California
San Francisco, California
Department of Surgery
Marin General Hospital
San Rafael, California
Radical Perineal Prostatectomy

DAVID S. WU, MD
Department of Urology
University of California
San Francisco, California
Complementary and Alternative Medicine

1

Epidemiology: Distribution and Determinants

JUNE M. CHAN, ScD

"Epidemiology is the study of the distribution and determinants of disease frequency in human populations."[1] Historically, the term epidemiology was reserved for the study of acute outbreaks of infectious disease. However, in the past several decades, the scope of epidemiology has broadened to address the study of numerous conditions of human health, including chronic ailments such as heart disease and cancer. To that end, this chapter outlines the basic characteristics of prostate cancer occurrence and describes the current state of knowledge regarding the risk factors for this disease, focusing on literature published in the past decade.

DISTRIBUTION OF PROSTATE CANCER BY GEOGRAPHY, RACE, AGE, AND TIME

The American Cancer Society predicts that in 2002, approximately 189,000 new cases of prostate cancer will be diagnosed and 30,200 men will die from this disease in the United States.[2] Globally, it is the ninth most common cancer, with the highest rates occurring in North America, Europe, and Australia and the lowest rates reported in Japan, India, Hong Kong, and China.[3]

Black Americans have the highest recorded age-standardized rates, estimated at 137 cases per 100,000 persons in 1997 according to Surveillance, Epidemiology, and End Results (SEER) data.[4] In contrast, the rates among Whites in the United States were 101 per 100,000. Europeans tended to have rates in the range of 20 to 50 cases per 100,000. Interestingly, Japanese living in Los Angeles had a rate of 47 per 100,000 as compared with 9 per 100,000 for Japanese in Miyagi, Japan, and Chinese living in Los Angeles had a rate of 20 per 100,000 as compared with 2 per 100,000 for Chinese in Shanghai, China. These contrasts may be explained in part by cultural differences in the discussion and reporting of cancers internationally. However, the dramatic difference also suggests the potential influence of environmental risk factors on prostate cancer.

The incidence of prostate cancer increases exponentially with age. The age-specific rate among men age 45 to 49 years was 11 per 100,000 during 1988 to 1992, whereas men age 75 to 79 years had an incidence of 1,400 per 100,000.[5] Between 1990 and 1995, the mean ages at diagnosis among Whites and Blacks in the United States were 70.6 and 68.7 years, respectively.[4] The mortality rates of prostate cancer also increase continuously with age. The mean age at death from prostate cancer between 1990 and 1995 was 77.6 years and 75.7 years for Whites and Blacks, respectively, in the United States.[4]

The age-adjusted incidence rates of prostate cancer have been increasing by approximately 3% annually worldwide over the past several decades.[6] Although the reasons for this constant rise remain unclear, in more developed nations, part of the increase can be attributed to widespread screening. Prostate-specific antigen (PSA) screening became more common in the United States beginning in the late 1980s, and data from SEER registries document an age-adjusted increase of 108% for white men between 1986 and 1992 and a 102% increase among black men between 1986 and 1993.[4]

In contrast to the exponential increase in incidence rates for prostate cancer in the United States, the mortality rates have been much more steady, with a slight increase between 1973 and 1991 (20.3/100,000 in 1973 versus 24.7/100,000 in 1991) and a decrease between 1991 and 1995 (22.9/100,000 in 1995).[4] The mortality rates of black and white Americans follow a similar pattern over time; however, the rates for Blacks have remained about twice that of Whites, at about 40 to 50 deaths per 100,000 over the past few decades.[4]

DETERMINANTS OF PROSTATE CANCER

Age, Race, and Family History/Genetics

Age, race, and family history have long been recognized as important nonmodifiable risk factors for prostate cancer. Other constitutional risk factors that have received growing attention in research years include androgens, the insulin-like growth factor (IGF) axis, and specific genetic polymorphisms. The term relative risk (RR) will be used to discuss possible determinants or predictors of prostate cancer and to quantify the magnitude of the associations between risk factors and prostate cancer occurrence and mortality. The RR is the ratio of the risk of disease among the exposed divided by the risk among the nonexposed (or reference group). An RR of 1.0 reflects no association between exposure and risk of disease, an RR > 1.0 implies a positive association, and an RR < 1.0 represents an inverse association. For example, being black as opposed to white in the United States was associated with an RR of approximately 2.0 for prostate cancer mortality, based on the statistics discussed above. Similarly, being age 75 years as opposed to age 45 years was associated with an RR of > 100. In this chapter, a weak to moderate elevation in risk will generally refer to RRs of 1.2 to 1.7, a moderate to strong positive association refers to RRs of 1.7 to 2.5, and a strong association reflects RRs > 2.5. The *p* values and 95% confidence intervals (CIs) reflect the precision of the risk estimates, and for this chapter, statistically significant results refer to those for which the 95% CI did not enclose the null value of 1.0 or the *p* value was less than .05.

Men with a first-degree relative (father, brother, or son) with prostate cancer are at higher risk than those without such a family history. A multiethnic study done among Whites, Blacks, and Asians in the United States estimated that a positive family history was associated with a two- to threefold increase in risk.[7] Other studies show that risk tends to rise with increasing number of relatives with a history of prostate cancer, especially if the relatives have cancer at a young age.[8]

A recent Scandinavian study examined the risk of cancers among monozygotic versus dizygotic twins, using data from over 44,000 twins in their twin registries.[9] Of the 28 anatomic sites investigated, the authors reported prostate cancer to have the largest genetic component. To the extent that the assumptions of this study were met, namely that there was random mating, no gene-environment interactions, and equivalent environments for monozygotic and dizygotic twins, the authors calculated that 42% of prostate cancer was attributable to genetic factors (95% CI 0.29–0.50).[9] Although it is likely that there will be important gene-environment interactions at play in the pathogenesis of prostate cancer, this estimate does emphasize the important role of genetics in cancer.

Although family history of prostate cancer definitely confers a greater risk for the disease, we have yet to identify and understand the specific genes involved in this process. A few genetic polymorphisms that modify androgen and vitamin D metabolism have been linked to prostate cancer and will be discussed below. Further advances in our understanding of the molecular genetics of prostate cancer will be addressed in Chapter 3.

Sex Hormones

Several lines of evidence support a role for sex hormones as initiators or promoters of prostate cancer.[10] The growth and maintenance of the normal prostate epithelium depend on both circulating testosterone (T) and the conversion of T to dihydrotestosterone (DHT) in the prostate.[10] Prostate cancer is often sex hormone dependent initially after diagnosis and can regress when androgen stimulation is removed. Men castrated at an early age rarely experience prostate cancer,[11] and prolonged administration of high levels of T can induce prostate cancer in rats.[12,13]

Although our understanding of physiology and experimental studies supports an association between androgens and prostate cancer, epidemiologic studies have had conflicting results.[14–21] A few prospective studies suggest that a high plasma T:DHT ratio, high circulating levels of T, low estrogen levels, or low levels of sex hormone–binding globulin (SHBG) may be associated with moderate to high elevations in prostate cancer risk.[17,18,21] In the Physicians Health Study, which had a large number of cases (N = 222), there was no association in the univariate models examining serum androgens, estrogen, and SHBG and the risk of prostate cancer.[18] However, when these hormonal components were considered simultaneously in a multivariate model, the individual effects of each were elucidated (RR = 2.6 for T, RR = 0.5 for SHBG, and RR = 0.6 for estrogen for comparisons of the fourth versus first quartiles, p value < .05 for each of these estimates).[18]

This contrast in results underscores the importance of considering the bioavailability and complete metabolic environment of androgen function in the prostate gland and not just the absolute levels in serum. Binding proteins, receptors, other metabolism modifiers, and genetic polymorphisms in these modifiers may all be crucial in determining the full effect of a single hormonal component on prostate cancer development.

To date, a few genetic polymorphisms that affect androgen metabolism have been identified and linked to prostate cancer risk. A missense substitution (A49T) in the 5α-reductase gene, *SRD5A2*, has been associated with very high elevations in prostate cancer risk among Blacks (RR = 7.2, p value < .001) and Hispanics (RR = 3.6, p value < .04).[22] The authors estimated that the population-attributable risk of prostate cancer owing to this polymorphism was approximately 8% for these ethnic groups.

Variable lengths in the CAG and GGN regions of exon 1 of the androgen receptor (AR) gene have been linked to prostate cancer risk. In general, shorter length of the CAG repeat sequence has been associated with an RR of 1.5 to 2.0,[23–28] although a large study among men with a family history of prostate cancer,[29] a study among British Caucasians,[30] and a study among French-Germans[31] did not observe an association. Shorter number of CAG repeats may also be positively correlated with Black race,[28,32,33] younger age,[25,34,35] and higher tumor stage and grade at diagnosis.[26,34] In one study, among men who had a low risk of recurrence based on a favorable Gleason score, PSA level, and stage at diagnosis, shorter CAG repeat length was associated with an eightfold increase in risk of recurrence (p value = .004).[36] Shorter number of GGC repeats in the GGN tract (GGT3GGG1GGT2GGCn) and a polymorphism in the androgen response element sequence of the PSA gene have also been associated with an elevated risk of prostate cancer.[23–25,28]

Insulin-Like Growth Factors

The IGF axis consists of two main hormones (IGF-I and IGF-II), the IGF-binding proteins (IGFBP-1 through 6), IGF receptors (types I and II), and IGFBP proteases.[37] Insulin-like growth factor I is a potent stimulator of normal and neoplastic cell growth and has antiapoptotic actions on prostate epithelial cells.[37–42] Insulin-like growth factor binding protein 3 is the major binding protein in the circulation, influences IGF-I bioavailability, and has demonstrated independent apoptotic characteristics in PC-3 prostate cancer cell lines.[37,38,41–43] Between-person variability in levels of plasma IGF-I and IGFBP-3 (the major circulating IGFBP)[44] is considerable,[45,46] and plasma IGF-I levels appear to reflect heterogeneity in tissue IGF-I bioactivity.[47–49]

In vitro and in vivo experiments demonstrate that IGF-I increases proliferation of both androgen-dependent and -independent prostate cancer cell lines,[40] and IGFBP-3 can decrease the growth stimulating effects of IGF-I.[37] Several recent epidemiologic studies support a strong statistically significant positive association between circulating IGF-I levels and prostate cancer risk, with RRs of approximately 2 to 4.[50–55] Insulin-like growth factor binding protein 3 has also been inversely linked to prostate cancer risk in two prospective studies,[50,54] but overall its association has been less consistently documented. Similar associations for IGF-I and IGFBP-3 have been found for breast cancer,[56] colon cancer,[57] and lung cancer,[58] underlining the importance of this hormonal system in carcinogenesis.

Smoking

Studies on the association between smoking and prostate cancer incidence have generally been null,[59–69] although a few studies report positive associations.[70–75] In contrast, there is more convincing evidence that smoking may be moderately related to prostate cancer death,[75–81] and some studies have found that smoking is positively related to worse tumor grade or stage at diagnosis.[76,82–84] One possible explanation is that smokers may delay diagnosis and treatment. Alternatively, tobacco may directly increase the virulence of prostate cancers by as yet unknown mechanisms. An interaction between smoking and a polymorphism in the glutathione S-transferase gene has been linked to a greater risk of prostate cancer.[85]

Body Size and Physical Activity

Height, weight, obesity, and body circumferences reflect hormonal profiles and growth patterns and have been studied as risk factors for prostate cancer. Height may be an indirect measure of growth factor levels, particularly early in life, and several studies report that taller men have a weak to moderate elevation in the risk of prostate cancer,[86–90] although other studies report no association.[59,91–94]

Obesity is associated with higher estrogen and lower T levels,[95–98] a hormonal profile that would be considered protective for prostate cancer.[10,18] However, studies on body mass index (BMI = kg/m^2) and prostate cancer have typically not been inverse but either positive[66,70,89,94,99] or null.[59,86,92,93,100,101] Intriguing inverse associations have been reported for childhood obesity and metastatic prostate cancer,[86] as well as obesity at diagnosis and prostate cancer mortality.[102] Part of this discrepancy may be because BMI also reflects lean body mass,[103] which may have a different association with prostate cancer risk. Interestingly, a study of lean (average BMI = 21.9 kg/m^2) Chinese men, a population typically at low risk of prostate cancer, reported that waist-to-hip ratio (a measure of abdominal obesity) was positively associated with prostate cancer risk, whereas greater hip circumference was statistically significant in protecting against prostate cancer risk.[92]

Studies on occupational or recreational physical activity[63,70,94,100,101,104–120] have also been conflicting but overall suggest a modest protective effect.[100,104,108–114,116–118] For example, in a large (N = 53,000) cohort study in Norway, those who walked at work and had high recreational levels of physical activity had a statistically significant 55% lower risk compared with sedentary men.[111] The Health Professionals Follow-up Study reported a nonlinear inverse association, with men who exercised for 3 or more hours per week experiencing a statistically significant 54% reduction in the risk of metastatic prostate cancer.[108]

Cardiorespiratory fitness, as measured by a treadmill test, was associated with a 74% reduction in prostate cancer risk, after adjusting for age, BMI, and smoking.[121] Higher pulse rate, as a reflection of lower fitness, has been positively linked to prostate cancer.[122,123] Overall, there is increasing evidence that some form of occupational or leisure-time physical activity may impart benefit against prostate cancer.

Occupational Exposures

A wide range of occupations and their incurred environmental exposures have been linked to greater risk of prostate cancer incidence or mortality. These include, but are not limited to the following: calcium carbonate,[124] metal working/metallic dust,[124,125] the agriculture industry/pesticides,[126–132] soaps/perfumes,[127] leather industry,[127] electrical industry/power plants,[125,129,133,134] diesel fumes,[135] fire fighting,[129] railroad industry,[129,134] polycyclic aromatic hydrocarbons,[125,129,134] brick masonry,[134] pilot industry,[125,134] wood dust,[136] chimney sweeping,[137] cadmium,[127,138] mining,[138] and the paper industry.[138] Taken together, these jobs/exposures are relatively rare, and the population-attributable risk associated with occupational environmental exposures is likely small. However, the risk associated with any individual occupation or exposure may be quite high and might provide insights into the etiology of prostate cancer.

Vasectomy

Eleven[139–149] of 19 studies suggest that vasectomy may be associated with a small to moderate increase in the risk of prostate cancer.[139–157] A few studies reported that time since vasectomy was positively related to prostate cancer,[143–146,148] and the lack of association in other studies may be attributable to insufficient follow-up. One hypothesis for this association is that vasectomized men have higher levels of circulating T and DHT, a higher ratio of DHT:T, and lower SHBG levels than nonvasectomized men.[149,158]

Diet

Nutritional epidemiology studies on prostate cancer, although varying widely in designs and dietary assessments, generally suggest that higher intakes of meat, animal fat, saturated fat, α-linolenic fatty acids, dairy products, and calcium may moderately to strongly elevate the risk of prostate cancer. In contrast, total and specific vegetables, tomatoes/lycopene, vitamin E, and selenium may impart some protection against the development of prostate cancer. One study estimated that 40% of prostate cancers in Greece could be reduced by increasing consumption of raw and cooked tomatoes, reducing dairy intake (including butter), and replacing seed oils with olive oil.[159] Thus, there is a great potential for diet to play an important role in prostate cancer risk reduction. (Further information on vitamin D, vitamin E, selenium, soy, and lycopene can be found in a later chapter 25, "Complementary and Alternative Medicine")

Meat and Fat

Total and specific fats[101,160–171] and meat (usually red meat)[170–181] have generally been associated with moderate to strong elevations in the risk of prostate cancer, although some studies reported no associations.[107,175,182–185] Saturated fat[101,162,164,166,170,186] and α-linolenic fatty acid,[160,161,170,171] in particular, were associated with greater risk, and associations tended to be stronger for advanced disease. At least one study reported an elevated risk of prostate cancer death associated with higher intakes of postdiagnostic saturated fat.[187]

A study among healthy men observed higher levels of circulating IGF-I among meat eaters versus non-meat eaters.[188] Another study compared sex hormone levels among men fed 150 g of lean meat versus 290 g of tofu on an isocaloric diet. The men on the meat diet had lower levels of SHBG and a higher ratio of T to estrogen.[189] Meat doneness has also been positively correlated with prostate cancer risk,[172] and free radical formation from fatty acid oxidation can damage DNA.[171]

Dairy, Calcium, and Vitamin D

Twelve[101,178,184,190–198] of 14 case-control studies[101,173,178,184,190–199] and 7[90,174,185,200–203] of 9 cohort studies[90,174,185,200–205] observed a positive association for some measure of dairy product intake and prostate cancer; in the majority of these studies, the associations were statistically significant.[90,174,178,184,185,190–194,200,201] This makes dairy intake one of the most consistent dietary predictors for prostate cancer in the published literature. In these studies, men with the highest dairy intakes had approximately double the risk of total prostate cancer and up to a fourfold increase in the risk of metastatic or fatal prostate cancer relative to low consumers.[200]

This association appears to be independent of fat consumption,[193,200,201] and recent studies suggest that the calcium in dairy foods might explain this association. Two cohort studies[200,201] and one large case-control study[193] reported moderate to strong statistically significant positive associations for calcium intake and prostate cancer risk; one cohort[174] and three case-control[197,206,207] studies observed no association, and one case-control study from Serbia observed a statistically significant inverse association.[208] An additional prospective investigation also reported a suggestive positive association; however, the trend was not statistically significant.[203]

The strongest evidence for an association between calcium intake and risk of prostate cancer comes from the Health Professionals Follow-up Study, which had a comprehensive dietary assessment of calcium from food as well as multivitamins, calcium supplements, and other sources (eg, antacids [TUMS]).[200] In this study, men who consumed greater than 2,000 mg of calcium daily had a multivariate RR of 4.6 (95% CI 1.9 to 11.1) for metastatic and fatal prostate cancer compared with men consuming less than 500 mg of calcium daily. This association was independent of age, BMI, total energy intake, fat, fructose, phosphorus, vitamin D, vitamin E, and lycopene intake. Independent associations were observed for calcium from supplements only and calcium from foods.

The following mechanism has been proposed to explain this association between calcium intake and prostate cancer risk: high calcium consumption increases serum calcium levels and high serum levels of calcium suppress production of 1,25-dihydroxyvitamin D_3 (1,25-D),[209] a hormone that is protective against prostate cancer growth in vivo and in vitro.[210–221] Higher consumption of calcium from dairy foods has been inversely correlated with serum levels of 1,25-D (r = approximately –.15, $p < .05$).[201,203] Direct studies of 1,25-D levels and prostate cancer risk have been less clear, with only one[222] of four[222–225] studies observing an inverse association. Variations in study design (eg, time/season of blood draw, sample size, ethnicity of the populations) may partially account for these discrepant results. Furthermore, it may be important to consider levels of vitamin D–binding proteins and polymorphisms in the vitamin D receptor gene; these polymorphisms have been linked to prostate cancer risk in other studies.[226–229]

In conclusion, dairy consumption, and possibly calcium intake specifically, is associated with moderate to strong elevations in the risk of prostate cancer, especially for more advanced disease. This might be attributable to the suppressive effects of calcium on 1,25-D levels, a hormone that potentially protects against prostate cancer.

Vegetables, Fruits, and Associated Micronutrients

A wide variety of vegetables have been investigated in relation to prostate cancer risk in diverse ethnic populations, and a review, "Food, Nutrition, and the Prevention of Cancer: a global perspective" conducted by the World Cancer Research Fund and the American Institute for Cancer Research,[3] concluded that diets high in vegetable intake could possibly decrease the risk of prostate cancer. Since the publication of that report in 1997, eight additional studies observed statistically significant inverse associations between specific and total vegetables and prostate cancer risk,[173,194,197,198,230–233] whereas eight other studies found no association.[90,101,181,190,192,199,203,234] Although the results have been mixed, it appears that beans, legumes, pulses and nuts,[194,204,230,231,233] carrots,[233,235] tomatoes and tomato products,[194,197,198,204,236] and green leafy[194,232,235] and possibly cruciferous vegetables[233,235] may offer some protection against prostate cancer.

In contrast, there is very little evidence that fruit consumption protects against prostate cancer,[3,90,101,162,198,203,233] and, if anything, it has been associated with a slight increase in risk.[192,194,230,231]

Carotenoids are found in fruits and vegetables and have provitamin A properties and antioxidant capabilities that could protect against free-radical damage to DNA.[237] Total carotenoids do not appear to be associated with prostate cancer risk, although several specific carotenoids warrant further study.[238] Higher intakes of lutein plus zeaxanthin[233] and lyocopene (found primarily in tomato products)[236,239,240] may help reduce the risk of prostate cancer. In one randomized trial, β-carotene supplementation protected against the occurrence of prostate cancer among men with low baseline plasma levels of β-carotene or lycopene.[241] However, in another randomized trial, β-carotene supplementation was associated with an overall increased risk of prostate cancer incidence.[242]

Vitamin E refers to several compounds: α-, β-, γ, and δ-tocopherol and the tocotrienols. Human diets contain predominantly α-tocopherol, which is the most potent tocopherol biologically.[243] However, recent evidence suggests a role for γ-tocopherol also to protect against prostate cancer.[244–247] Vitamin E has strong antioxidant properties and positive effects on immune function.[248,249] In vitro studies also demonstrate that vitamin E may decrease prostate cancer cell growth.[250,251]

Five observational studies report provocative inverse associations between dietary vitamin E and prostate cancer risk,[173,198,208,240,252] although not all of the results were statistically significant.[240,252] In contrast, seven studies found no association between dietary or supplemental vitamin E intake and prostate cancer risk.[194,231,253–257]

The most compelling evidence for a protective effect of vitamin E comes from the Alpha-Tocopherol Beta-Carotene Cancer Prevention Trial,[242] which observed statistically significant reductions of approximately 40% in both prostate cancer incidence and mortality among men receiving 50-IU supplements of α-tocopherol daily. All of the men in this trial had a long history of smoking. Interestingly, a large cohort study that observed no overall association for supplemental vitamin E intake and prostate cancer risk did observe a borderline statistically significant 50% reduction in the risk of metastatic and fatal prostate cancer among men with a recent smoking history. Consistent with this finding, other studies report statistically significant inverse associations between plasma levels of vitamin E and metastatic and fatal prostate cancer risk among smokers[239,258] but not overall.[239,254,258,259] One could speculate that vitamin E specifically counteracts the adverse promoting effect of smoking but is less beneficial among non-smokers.

There is growing interest in the potential protective effects of soy products for prostate cancer. Hypothesized anticancer mechanisms for soy include its role as a phytoestrogen, an antioxidant, an antiangiogenesis factor, a tyrosine-kinase inhibitor, and a proliferation inhibitor.[260] A few human epidemiologic studies reported inverse associations for greater soy or soy product intake and prostate cancer risk.[261–263] A statistically significant reduction in risk of approximately 40%was observed for total legumes, soy legumes, and non-soy legumes, suggesting a more general benefit of legumes.[262] There was a statistically significant 70% reduction in prostate cancer risk associated with frequent soy milk intake (more than once/day) in a study conducted among Adventist men,[263] and another study observed a nonstatistically significant inverse association for greater tofu consumption and risk of prostate cancer.[261]

Selenium

Laboratory studies,[264–266] observational investigations,[267–270] and a randomized trial[271] have demonstrated a potential anticarcinogenic effect of selenium. Selenium is a trace nutrient essential for the activity of glutathione peroxidase, which may reduce oxidative damage to DNA. Selenium is difficult to measure from dietary assessments because intake varies by the soil levels of selenium in which different foods are grown.[272] Thus, typically nail (representative of long-term intake) or serum (representative of short-term intake) levels of selenium or information on selenium supplementation is needed to quantify exposure.

Prospective investigations of serum selenium levels demonstrate an inverse association with prostate cancer risk.[267–269] Higher toenail selenium levels were also associated with a lower risk of prostate cancer in one study[270] but not another.[273] Provocative evidence comes from the Nutritional Prevention of Cancer Study Group, a randomized trial of selenium to reduce the recurrence of skin cancer. After 10 years of follow-up (mean time on treatment = 4.5 years), men taking daily supplements of 200-μg selenium experienced a 63 to 74% reduction in the risk of prostate cancer incidence ($p < .01$).[271] The observational studies also reported risk reductions in the range of 50 to 70%.[268–270] Thus, although the total number of studies is small, there is compelling evidence that selenium may impart substantial protection against prostate cancer occurrence.

CONCLUSION

Although the etiology of prostate cancer remains unknown, several modifiable dietary and lifestyle risk factors have been identified, and a wide range of genetic factors are under active investigation. In particular, future studies on genetics, ethnicity, sex hormones, growth factors, diet, and possible gene-environment interactions are likely to be important in furthering our understanding of this disease.

REFERENCES

1. MacMahon B, Trichopoulos D. Epidemiology principles and methods. 2nd ed. Boston: Little, Brown and Company; 1996.
2. American Cancer Society. Cancer facts and figures — 2002. Atlanta (GA): American Cancer Society; 2002.
3. World Cancer Research Fund and American Institution for Cancer Research. Food, nutrition and the prevention of cancer: a global perspective. Washington (DC): American Institute for Cancer Research; 1997.
4. Stanford JL, Stephenson RA, Coyle LM, et al. Prostate cancer trends 1973–1995. Bethesda (MD): SEER Program, National Cancer Institute; 1999.

5. National Institutes of Health and National Cancer Institute. SEER cancer statistics review: 1973–1992. Tables and graphs. Bethesda (MD): National Cancer Institute; 1995.
6. Boyle P, Maisonneuve P, Napalkov P. Geographical and temporal patterns of incidence and mortality from prostate cancer. Urology 1995;46:47–55.
7. Whittemore AS, Wu AH, Kolonel LN, et al. Family history and prostate cancer risk in black, white, and Asian men in the United States and Canada. Am J Epidemiol 1995;141:732–40.
8. Carter BS, S. B, Beaty H, et al. Hereditary prostate cancer: epidemiologic and clinical features. J Urol 1993;150:797–802.
9. Lichtenstein P, Holm NV, Verkasalo PK, et al. Environmental and heritable factors in the causation of cancer—analyses of cohorts of twins from Sweden, Denmark, and Finland. N Engl J Med 2000;343:78–85.
10. Wilding G. Endocrine control of prostate cancer. Cancer Surv 1995;23:43–62.
11. Hovenanian MS, Deming CL. The hetereologous growth of cancer of the human prostate. Surg Gynecol Obstet 1948; 86:29–35.
12. Noble RL. The development of prostatic adenocarcinoma in Nb rats following prolonged sex hormone administration. Cancer Res 1977;37:1929–33.
13. Pollard M, Luckert PH, Schmidt MA. Induction of prostate adenocarcinomas in Lobund Wistar rats by testosterone. Prostate 1982;4:563–8.
14. Nomura AM, Stemmermann GN, Chyou PH, et al. Serum androgens and prostate cancer. Cancer Epidemiol Biomarkers Prev 1996;5:621–5.
15. Vatten LJ, Ursin G, Ross RK, et al. Androgens in serum and the risk of prostate cancer: a nested case-control study from the Janus serum bank in Norway. Cancer Epidemiol Biomarkers Prev 1997;6:967–9.
16. Carter HB, Pearson JD, Metter EJ, et al. Longitudinal evaluation of serum androgen levels in men with and without prostate cancer. Prostate 1995;27:25–31.
17. Hsing AW, Comstock GW. Serological precursors of cancer: serum hormones and risk of subsequent prostate cancer. Cancer Epidemiol Biomarkers Prev 1993;2:27–32.
18. Gann PH, Hennekens Ch, Ma J, et al. Prospective study of sex hormone levels and risk of prostate cancer. J Natl Cancer Inst 1996;88:1118–26.
19. Dorgan JF, Albanes D, Virtamo J, et al. Relationships of serum androgens and estrogens to prostate cancer risk: results from a prospective study in Finland. Cancer Epidemiol Biomarkers Prev 1998;7:1069–74.
20. Demark-Wahnefried W, Lesko SM, Conaway MR, et al. Serum androgens: associations with prostate cancer risk and hair patterning. J Androl 1997;18:495–500.
21. Nomura A, Heilbrun LK, Stemmermann GN, et al. Prediagnostic serum hormones and the risk of prostate cancer. Cancer Res 1988;48:3515–7.
22. Makridakis NM, Ross RK, Pike MC, et al. Association of mis-sense substitution in SRD5A2 gene with prostate cancer in African-American and Hispanic men in Los Angeles, USA. Lancet 1999;354:975–8.
23. Hsing AW, Gao YT, Wu G, et al. Polymorphic CAG and GGN repeat lengths in the androgen receptor gene and prostate cancer risk: a population-based case-control study in China. Cancer Res 2000;60:5111–6.
24. Xue W, Irvine RA, Yu MC, et al. Susceptibility to prostate cancer: interaction between genotypes at the androgen receptor and prostate-specific antigen loci. Cancer Res 2000;60:839–41.
25. Stanford JL, Just JJ, Gibbs M, et al. Polymorphic repeats in the androgen receptor gene: molecular markers of prostate cancer risk. Cancer Res 1997;57:1194–8.
26. Giovannucci E, Stampfer MJ, Krithivas K, et al. The CAG repeat within the androgen receptor gene and its relationship to prostate cancer. Proc Natl Acad Sci U S A 1997;94:3320–3.
27. Schoenberg MP, Hakimi JM, Wang S, et al. Microsatellite mutation (CAG24—>18) in the androgen receptor gene in human prostate cancer. Biochem Biophys Res Commun 1994;198:74–80.
28. Irvine RA, Yu MC, Ross RK, et al. The CAG and GGC microsatellites of the androgen receptor gene are in linkage disequilibrium in men with prostate cancer. Cancer Res 1995;55:1937–40.
29. Lange EM, Chen H, Brierley K, et al. The polymorphic exon 1 androgen receptor CAG repeat in men with a potential inherited predisposition to prostate cancer. Cancer Epidemiol Biomarkers Prev 2000;9:439–42.
30. Edwards SM, Badzioch MD, Minter R, et al. Androgen receptor polymorphisms: association with prostate cancer risk, relapse and overall survival. Int J Cancer 1999;84:458–65.
31. Correa-Cerro L, Wohr G, Haussler J, et al. (CAG)nCAA and GGN repeats in the human androgen receptor gene are not associated with prostate cancer in a French-German population. Eur J Hum Genet 1999;7:357–62.
32. Platz EA, Rimm EB, Willett WC, et al. Racial variation in prostate cancer incidence and in hormonal system markers among male health professionals. J Natl Cancer Inst 2000;92:2009–17.
33. Sartor O, Zheng Q, Eastham JA. Androgen receptor gene CAG repeat length varies in a race-specific fashion in men without prostate cancer. Urology 1999;53:378–80.
34. Bratt O, Borg A, Kristoffersson U, et al. CAG repeat length in the androgen receptor gene is related to age at diagnosis of prostate cancer and response to endocrine therapy, but not to prostate cancer risk. Br J Cancer 1999;81:672–6.
35. Hardy DO, Scher HI, Bogenreider T, et al. Androgen receptor CAG repeat lengths in prostate cancer: correlation with age of onset. J Clin Endocrinol Metab 1996;81:4400–5.
36. Nam RK, Elhaji Y, Krahn MD, et al. Significance of the CAG repeat polymorphism of the androgen receptor gene in prostate cancer progression. J Urol 2000;164:567–72.
37. Cohen P, Peehl DM, Rosenfeld RG. The IGF axis in the prostate. Horm Metab Res 1994;26:81–4.
38. Cohen P, Peehl DM, Lamson G, Rosenfeld RG. Insulin-like growth factors (IGFs), IGF receptors, and IGF-binding proteins in primary cultures of prostate epithelial cells. J Clin Endocrinol Metab 1991;73:401–7.
39. LeRoith D, Baserga R, Helman L, Roberts CT Jr. Insulin-like growth factors and cancer. Ann Intern Med 1995;122:54–9.
40. Iwamura M, Sluss PM, Casamento JB, Cockett AT. Insulin-like growth factor I: action and receptor characterization in human prostate cancer cell lines. Prostate 1993;22:243–52.
41. Rajah R, Valentinis B, Cohen P. Insulin-like growth factor (IGF)-binding protein-3 induces apoptosis and mediates the effects of transforming growth factor-β1 on pro-

grammed cell death through a p53 and IGF-independent mechanism. J Biol Chem 1997;272:12181–8.

42. Yu H, Rohan T. Role of the insulin-like growth factor family in cancer development and progression. J Natl Cancer Inst 2000;92:1472–89.
43. LeRoith D. Insulin-like growth factor receptors and binding proteins. Baillieres Clin Endocrinol Metab 1996;10:49–73.
44. Jones J, Clemmons D. Insulin-like growth factors and their binding proteins-biological actions. Endocr Rev 1995; 16:3–34.
45. Juul A, Bang P, Hertel NT, et al. Serum insulin-like growth factor-I in 1030 healthy children, adolescents, and adults: relation to age, sex, stage of puberty, testicular size, and body mass index. J Clin Endocrinol Metab 1994;78:744–52.
46. Juul A, Dalgaard P, Blum WF, et al. Serum levels of insulin-like growth factor (IGF)-binding protein-3 (IGFBP-3) in healthy infants, children, and adolescents: the relation to IGF-I, IGF-II, IGFBP-1, IGFBP-2, age, sex, body mass index, and pubertal maturation. J Clin Endocrinol Metab 1995;80:2534–42.
47. Huynh H, Yang XF, Pollak M. A role for insulin-like growth factor binding protein 5 in the antiproliferative action of the antiestrogen ICI 182780. Cell Growth Differ 1996; 7:1501–6.
48. Huynh H, Yang X, Pollak M. Estradiol and antiestrogens regulate a growth inhibitory insulin-like growth factor binding protein 3 autocrine loop in human breast cancer cells. J Biol Chem 1996;271:1016–21.
49. Pollak M, Costantino J, Polychronakos C, et al. Effect of tamoxifen on serum insulinlike growth factor I levels in stage I breast cancer patients. J Natl Cancer Inst 1990;82:1693–7.
50. Chan JM, Stampfer MJ, Giovannucci E, et al. Plasma insulin-like growth factor-I and prostate cancer risk: a prospective study. Science 1998;279:563–6.
51. Wolk A, Mantzoros CS, Andersson S-D, et al. Insulin-like growth factor 1 and prostate cancer risk: a population-based, case-control study. J Natl Cancer Inst 1998;90:911–5.
52. Mantzoros CS, Tzonou A, Signorello LB, et al. Insulin-like growth factor 1 in relation to prostate cancer and benign prostatic hyperplasia. Br J Cancer 1997;76:1115–8.
53. Harman SM, Metter EJ, Blackman MR, et al. Serum levels of insulin-like growth factor I (IGF-I), IGF-II, IGF-binding protein-3, and prostate-specific antigen as predictors of clinical prostate cancer. J Clin Endocrinol Metab 2000; 85:4258–65.
54. Stattin P, Bylund A, Rinaldi S, et al. Plasma insulin-like growth factor-I, insulin-like growth factor-binding proteins, and prostate cancer risk: a prospective study. J Natl Cancer Inst 2000;92:1910–7.
55. Khosravi J, Diamandi A, Mistry J, Scorilas A. Insulin-like growth factor I (IGF-I) and IGF-binding protein-3 in benign prostatic hyperplasia and prostate cancer. J Clin Endocrinol Metab 2001;86:694–9.
56. Hankinson SE, Willett WC, Colditz GA, et al. Circulating concentrations of insulin-like growth factor-I and risk of breast cancer. Lancet 1998;351:1393–6.
57. Ma J, Pollak MN, Giovannucci E, et al. Prospective study of colorectal cancer risk in men and plasma levels of insulin-like growth factor (IGF)-1 and IGF-binding protein-3. J Natl Cancer Inst 1999;91:620–5.
58. Yu H, Spitz MR, Mistry J, et al. Plasma levels of insulin-like growth factor-I and lung cancer risk: a case-control analysis. J Natl Cancer Inst 1999;91:151–6.
59. Hsieh CC, Thanos A, Mitropoulos D, et al. Risk factors for prostate cancer: a case-control study in Greece. Int J Cancer 1999;80:699–703.
60. Furuya Y, Akimoto S, Akakura H, Ito H. Smoking and obesity in relation to the etiology and disease progression of prostate cancer in Japan. Int J Urol 1998;5:134–7.
61. Rohan TE, Hislop TG, Howe GR, et al. Cigarette smoking and risk of prostate cancer: a population-based case-control study in Ontario and British Columbia, Canada. Eur J Cancer Prev 1997;6:382–8.
62. Lumey LH, Pittman B, Zang EA, Wynder EL. Cigarette smoking and prostate cancer: no relation with six measures of lifetime smoking habits in a large case-control study among U.S. whites. Prostate 1997;33:195–200.
63. Ilic M, Vlajinac H, Marinkovic J. Case-control study of risk factors for prostate cancer. Br J Cancer 1996;74:1682–6.
64. Lumey LH. Prostate cancer and smoking: a review of case-control and cohort studies. Prostate 1996;29:249–60.
65. Engeland A, Andersen A, Haldorsen T, Tretli S. Smoking habits and risk of cancers other than lung cancer: 28 years' follow-up of 26,000 Norwegian men and women. Cancer Causes Control 1996;7:497–506.
66. Gronberg H, Damber L, Damber JE. Total food consumption and body mass index in relation to prostate cancer risk: a case-control study in Sweden with prospectively collected exposure data. J Urol 1996;155:969–74.
67. Slattery ML, West DW. Smoking, alcohol, coffee, tea, caffeine, and theobromine: risk of prostate cancer in Utah (United States). Cancer Causes Control 1993;4:559–63.
68. Fincham SM, Hill GB, Hanson J, Wijayasinghe C. Epidemiology of prostatic cancer: a case-control study. Prostate 1990;17:189–206.
69. Talamini R, Franceschi S, La Vecchia C, et al. Smoking habits and prostate cancer: a case-control study in Northern Italy. Prev Med 1993;22:400–8.
70. Cerhan JR, Torner JC, Lynch CF, et al. Association of smoking, body mass, and physical activity with risk of prostate cancer in the Iowa 65+ Rural Health Study (United States). Cancer Causes Control 1997;8:229–38.
71. Andersson SO, Baron J, Bergstrom R, et al. Lifestyle factors and prostate cancer risk: a case-control study in Sweden. Cancer Epidemiol Biomarkers Prev 1996;5:509–13.
72. Hayes RB, Pottern LM, Swanson GM, et al. Tobacco use and prostate cancer in blacks and whites in the United States. Cancer Causes Control 1994;5:221–6.
73. Hiatt RA, Armstrong MA, Klatsky AL, Sidney S. Alcohol consumption, smoking, and other risk factors and prostate cancer in a large health plan cohort in California (United States). Cancer Causes Control 1994;5:66–72.
74. van der Gulden JW, Verbeek AL, Kolk JJ. Smoking and drinking habits in relation to prostate cancer. Br J Urol 1994;73:382–9.
75. Lotufo PA, Lee IM, Ajani UA, et al. Cigarette smoking and risk of prostate cancer in the physicians' health study (United States). Int J Cancer 2000;87:141–4.
76. Giovannucci E, Rimm EB, Ascherio A, et al. Smoking and risk of total and fatal prostate cancer in United States health professionals. Cancer Epidemiol Biomarkers Prev 1999;8:277–82.

77. Yu GP, Ostroff JS, Zhang ZF, et al. Smoking history and cancer patient survival: a hospital cancer registry study. Cancer Detect Prev 1997;21:497–509.
78. Rodriguez C, Tatham LM, Thun MJ, et al. Smoking and fatal prostate cancer in a large cohort of adult men. Am J Epidemiol 1997;145:466–75.
79. Coughlin SS, Neaton JD, Sengupta A. Cigarette smoking as a predictor of death from prostate cancer in 348,874 men screened for the Multiple Risk Factor Intervention Trial. Am J Epidemiol 1996;143:1002–6.
80. Hsing AW, McLaughlin JK, Schuman LM, et al. Diet, tobacco use, and fatal prostate cancer: results from the Lutheran Brotherhood Cohort Study. Cancer Res 1990;50:6836–40.
81. Hsing AW, McLaughlin JK, Hrubec Z, et al. Tobacco use and prostate cancer: 26-year follow-up of US veterans. Am J Epidemiol 1991;133:437–41.
82. Daniell HW. A worse prognosis for smokers with prostate cancer. J Urol 1995;154:153–7.
83. Hussain F, Aziz H, Macchia R, et al. High grade adenocarcinoma of prostate in smokers of ethnic minority groups and Caribbean island immigrants. Int J Radiat Onocol Biol Phys 1992;24:451–61.
84. Spitz MR, Strom SS, Yamamura Y, et al. Epidemiologic determinants of clinically relevant prostate cancer. Int J Cancer 2000;89:259–64.
85. Kelada SN, Kardia SL, Walker AH, et al. The glutathione S-transferase-mu and -theta genotypes in the etiology of prostate cancer: genotype-environment interactions with smoking. Cancer Epidemiol Biomarkers Prev 2000;9: 1329–34.
86. Giovannucci E, Rimm EB, Stampfer MJ, et al. Height, body weight, and risk of prostate cancer. Cancer Epidemiol Biomarkers Prev 1997;6:557–63.
87. Hebert PR, Ajani U, Cook NR, et al. Adult height and incidence of cancer in male physicians (United States). Cancer Causes Control 1997;8:591–7.
88. Nilsen TI, Vatten LJ. Anthropometry and prostate cancer risk: a prospective study of 22,248 Norwegian men. Cancer Causes Control 1999;10:269–75.
89. Andersson SO, Wolk A, Bergstrom R, et al. Body size and prostate cancer: a 20-year follow-up study among 135,006 Swedish construction workers. J Natl Cancer Inst 1997; 89:385–9.
90. Le Marchand L, Kolonel KN, Wilkens LR, et al. Animal fat consumption and prostate cancer: a prospective study in Hawaii. Epidemiology 1994;5:276–82.
91. Freeman VL, Liao Y, Durazo-Arvizu R, Cooper RS. Height and risk of fatal prostate cancer: findings from the National Health Interview Survey (1986 to 1994). Ann Epidemiol 2001;11:22–7.
92. Hsing AW, Deng J, Sesterhenn IA, et al. Body size and prostate cancer: a population-based case-control study in China. Cancer Epidemiol Biomarkers Prev 2000;9:1335–41.
93. Schuurman AG, Goldbohm RA, Dorant E, van den Brandt PA. Anthropometry in relation to prostate cancer risk in the Netherlands Cohort Study. Am J Epidemiol 2000;151: 541–9.
94. Putnam SD, Cerhan JR, Parker AS, et al. Lifestyle and anthropometric risk factors for prostate cancer in a cohort of Iowa men. Ann Epidemiol 2000;10:361–9.
95. Amatrauda JM, Harman SM, Pourmotabbed G, Lockwood DH. Decreased plasma testosterone and fractional binding of testosterone in obese males. J Clin Endocrinol Metab 1978;47:268–71.
96. Pasquali R, Casimirri F, Cantobelli S, et al. Effect of obesity and body fat distribution on sex hormones and insulin in men. Metabolism 1991;40:101–4.
97. Field AE, Colditz GA, Willett WC, et al. The relation of smoking, age, relative weight, and dietary intake to serum adrenal steroids, sex hormones, and sex hormone-binding globulin in middle-aged men. J Clin Endocrinol Metab 1994;79:1310–6.
98. Wu AH, Whittemore AS, Kolonel LN, et al. Serum androgens and sex hormone-binding globulins in relation to lifestyle factors in older African-American, white, and Asian men in the United States and Canada. Cancer Epidemiol Biomarkers Prev 1995;4:735–41.
99. Sung JF, Lin RS, Pu YS, et al. Risk factors for prostate carcinoma in Taiwan: a case-control study in a Chinese population. Cancer 1999;86:484–91.
100. Clarke G, Whittemore AS. Prostate cancer risk in relation to anthropometry and physical activity: the National Health and Nutrition Examination Survey I Epidemiological Follow-Up Study. Cancer Epidemiol Biomarkers Prev 2000; 9:875–81.
101. Whittemore AS, Kolonel LN, Wu AH, et al. Prostate cancer in relation to diet, physical activity, and body size in blacks, whites, and Asians in the United States and Canada. J Natl Cancer Inst 1995;87:652–61.
102. Daniell HW. A better prognosis for obese men with prostate cancer. J Urol 1996;155:220–5.
103. Garn SM, Leonard WR, Hawthorne VM. Three limitations of the body mass index. Am J Clin Nutr 1986;44:996–7.
104. Lund Nilsen TI, Johnsen R, Vatten LJ. Socio-economic and lifestyle factors associated with the risk of prostate cancer. Br J Cancer 2000;82:1358–63.
105. Pu YS. Prostate cancer in Taiwan: epidemiology and risk factors. Int J Androl 2000;(6 Suppl 2):34–6.
106. Liu S, Lee IM, Linson P, et al. A prospective study of physical activity and risk of prostate cancer in US physicians. Int J Epidemiol 2000;29:29–35.
107. Villeneuve PJ, Johnson KC, Kreiger N, Mao Y. Risk factors for prostate cancer: results from the Canadian National Enhanced Cancer Surveillance System. The Canadian Cancer Registries Epidemiology Research Group. Cancer Causes Control 1999;10:355–67.
108. Giovannucci E, Leitzmann M, Spiegelman D, et al. A prospective study of physical activity and prostate cancer in male health professionals. Cancer Res 1998;58:5117–22.
109. Hartman TJ, Albanes D, Rautalahti M, et al. Physical activity and prostate cancer in the Alpha-Tocopherol, Beta-Carotene (ATBC) Cancer Prevention Study (Finland). Cancer Causes Control 1998;9:11–8.
110. Andersson SO, Baron J, Wolk A, et al. Early life risk factors for prostate cancer: a population-based case-control study in Sweden. Cancer Epidemiol Biomarkers Prev 1995;4: 187–92.
111. Thune I, Lund E. Physical activity and the risk of prostate and testicular cancer: a cohort study of 53,000 Norwegian men. Cancer Causes Control 1994;5:549–56.

112. Hsing AW, McLaughlin JK, Zheng W, et al. Occupation, physical activity, and risk of prostate cancer in Shanghai, People's Republic of China. Cancer Causes Control 1994; 5:136–40.
113. Dosemeci M, Hayes RB, Vetter R, et al. Occupational physical activity, socioeconomic status, and risks of 15 cancer sites in Turkey. Cancer Causes Control 1993;4:313–21.
114. Lee IM, Paffenbarger RS, Hsieh CC. Physical activity and risk of prostatic cancer among college alumni. Am J Epidemiol 1992;135:169–79.
115. Le Marchand L, Kolonel LN, Yoshizawa CN. Lifetime occupational physical activity and prostate cancer risk. Am J Epidemiol 1991;133:103–11.
116. Brownson RC, Chang JC, Davis JR, Smith CA. Physical activity on the job and cancer in Missouri. Am J Public Health 1991;81:639–42.
117. Albanes D, Blair A, Taylor PR. Physical activity and risk of cancer in the NHANES I population. Am J Public Health 1989;79:744–50.
118. Vena JE, Graham S, Zielezny M, et al. Occupational exercise and risk of cancer. Am J Clin Nutr 1987;45 Suppl:318–27.
119. Yu H, Harris RE, Wynder EL. Case-control study of prostate cancer and socioeconomic factors. Prostate 1988;13: 317–25.
120. Severson RK, Nomura AMY, Grove JS, Stemmermann GN. A prospective analysis of physical activity and cancer. Am J Epidemiol 1989;130:522–9.
121. Oliveria SA, Kohl HW III, Trichopoulos D, Blair SN. The association between cardiorespiratory fitness and prostate cancer. Med Sci Sports Exerc 1996;28:97–104.
122. Cerhan JR, Pavuk M, Wallace RB. Positive association between resting pulse and cancer incidence in current and former smokers. Ann Epidemiol 1999;9:34–44.
123. Steenland K, Nowlin S, Palu S. Cancer incidence in the National Health and Nutrition Survey I. Follow-up data: diabetes, cholesterol, pulse and physical activity. Cancer Epidemiol Biomarkers Prev 1995;4:807–11.
124. Weston TL, Aronson KJ, Siemiatycki J, et al. Cancer mortality among males in relation to exposures assessed through a job-exposure matrix. Int J Occup Environ Health 2000; 6:194–202.
125. Aronson KJ, Siemiatycki J, Dewar R, Gerin M. Occupational risk factors for prostate cancer: results from a case-control study in Montreal, Quebec, Canada. Am J Epidemiol 1996;143:363–73.
126. Mills PK. Correlation analysis of pesticide use data and cancer incidence rates in California counties. Arch Environ Health 1998;53:410–3.
127. Sharma-Wagner S, Chokkalingam AP, Malker HS, et al. Occupation and prostate cancer risk in Sweden. J Occup Environ Med 2000;42:517–25.
128. Parker AS, Cerham JR, Putnam SD, et al. A cohort study of farming and risk of prostate cancer in Iowa. Epidemiology 1999;10:452–5.
129. Krstev S, Baris D, Stewart P, et al. Occupational risk factors and prostate cancer in U.S. blacks and whites. Am J Ind Med 1998;34:421–30.
130. Cerhan JR, Cantor KP, Williamson K, et al. Cancer mortality among Iowa farmers: recent results, time trends, and lifestyle factors (United States). Cancer Causes Control 1998;9:311–9.
131. Morrison H, Savitz D, Sememciw R, et al. Farming and prostate cancer mortality. Am J Epidemiol 1993;137: 270–80.
132. Giovannucci E. Epidemiologic characteristics of prostate cancer. Cancer 1995;75 Suppl:1766–77.
133. Robinson CF, Petersen M, Palu S. Mortality patterns among electrical workers employed in the U.S. construction industry 1982–1987. Am J Ind Med 1999;36:630–7.
134. Krstev S, Baris D, Stewart PA, et al. Risk for prostate cancer by occupation and industry: a 24-state death certificate study. Am J Ind Med 1998;34:413–20.
135. Seidler A, Heiskel H, Bickeboller R, Elsner G. Association between diesel exposure at work and prostate cancer. Scand J Work Environ Health 1998;24:486–94.
136. Stellman SD, Demers PA, Colin D, Boffetta P. Cancer mortality and wood dust exposure among participants in the American Cancer Society Cancer Prevention Study-II (CPS-II). Am J Ind Med 1998;34:229–37.
137. Evanoff BA, Gustavsson P, Hogstedt C. Mortality and incidence of cancer in a cohort of Swedish chimney sweeps: an extended follow up study. Br J Ind Med 1993;50:450–9.
138. Elghany NA, Schumacher MC, Slattery ML, et al. Occupation, cadmium exposure, and prostate cancer. Epidemiology 1990;1:107–15.
139. Lightfoot N, Kreigr N, Sass-Kortsak A, et al. Prostate cancer risk. Medical history, sexual, and hormonal factors. Ann Epidemiol 2000;10:470.
140. Bernal-Delgado E, Latour-Perez J, Pradas-Arnal F, Gomez-Lopez LI. The association between vasectomy and prostate cancer: a systematic review of the literature. Fertil Steril 1998;70:191–200.
141. Platz EA, Yeole BB, Cho E, et al. Vasectomy and prostate cancer: a case-control study in India. Int J Epidemiol 1997;26:933–8.
142. Hsing AW, Wang RT, Gu FL, et al. Vasectomy and prostate cancer risk in China. Cancer Epidemiol Biomarkers Prev 1994;3:285–8.
143. Giovannucci E, Ascherio A, Rimm EB, et al. A prospective cohort study of vasectomy and prostate cancer in US men. JAMA 1993;269:873–7.
144. Giovannucci E, Tosteson TD, Speizer FE, et al. A retrospective cohort study of vasectomy and prostate cancer in US men. JAMA 1993;269:878–82.
145. Hayes RB, Pottern LM, Greenberg R, et al. Vasectomy and prostate cancer in US blacks and whites. Am J Epidemiol 1993;137:263–9.
146. Mettlin C, Natarajan N, Huben R. Vasectomy and prostate cancer risk. Am J Epidemiol 1990;132:1056–65.
147. Rosenberg L, Palmer JR, Zauber AG, et al. Vasectomy and the risk of prostate cancer. Am J Epidemiol 1990;132:1051–5; discussion 1062–5.
148. Honda GD, Bernstein L, Ross RK, et al. Vasectomy, cigarette smoking, and age at first sexual intercourse as risk factors for prostate cancer in middle-aged men. Br J Cancer 1988;57:326–31.
149. John EM, Whittemore AS, Wu AH, et al. Vasectomy and prostate cancer: results from a multiethnic case-control study. J Natl Cancer Inst 1995;87:662–9.
150. Stanford JL, Wicklund KG, McKnight B, et al. Vasectomy

and risk of prostate cancer. Cancer Epidemiol Biomarkers Prev 1999;8:881–6.
151. Lesko SM, Louik C, Vezina R, et al. Vasectomy and prostate cancer. J Urol 1999;161:1848–53.
152. Magnani RJ, Haws JM, Morgan GT, et al. Vasectomy in the United States 1991 and 1995. Am J Public Health 1999;89:92–4.
153. Zhu K, Stanford JL, Daling JR, et al. Vasectomy and prostate cancer: a case-control study in a health maintenance organization. Am J Epidemiol 1996;144:717–22.
154. Sidney S, Quesenberry CP, Sadler MC, et al. Vasectomy and the risk of prostate cancer in a cohort of multiphasic health-checkup examinees: second report. Cancer Causes Control 1991;2:113–6.
155. Sidney S. Vasectomy and the risk of prostatic cancer and benign prostatic hypertrophy. J Urol 1987;138:795–7.
156. Rosenberg L, Palmer JR, Zauber AG, et al. The relation of vasectomy to the risk of cancer. Am J Epidemiol 1994; 140:431–8.
157. Nienhuis H, Goldacre M, Seagroatt V, et al. Incidence of disease after vasectomy: a record linkage retrospective cohort study. BMJ 1992;304:743–6.
158. Mo ZN, Huang X, Zhang SC, Yang JR. Early and late long-term effects of vasectomy on serum testosterone, dihydrotestosterone, luteinizing hormone and follicle-stimulating hormone levels. J Urol 1995;154:2065–9.
159. Bosetti C, Tzonou A, Lagiou P, et al. Fraction of prostate cancer incidence attributed to diet in Athens, Greece. Eur J Cancer Prev 2000;9:119–23.
160. De Stefani E, Deneo-Pellegrini H, Boffetta P, et al. Alpha-linolenic acid and risk of prostate cancer: a case-control study in Uruguay. Cancer Epidemiol Biomarkers Prev 2000;9:335–8.
161. Ramon JM, Bou R, Romea S, et al. Dietary fat intake and prostate cancer risk: a case-control study in Spain. Cancer Causes Control 2000;11:679–85.
162. Lee MM, Wang R-T, Hsing AW, et al. Case-control study of diet and prostate cancer in China. Cancer Causes Control 1998;9:545–52.
163. Tzonou A, Signorello LB, Lagiou P, et al. Diet and cancer of the prostate: a case-control study in Greece. Int J Cancer 1999;80:704–8.
164. Harvei S, Bjerve KS, Tretli S, et al. Prediagnostic level of fatty acids in serum phospholipids: omega-3 and omega-6 fatty acids and the risk of prostate cancer. Int J Cancer 1997;71:545–51.
165. Godley PA, Campbell MK, Gallagher P, et al. Biomarkers of essential fatty acid consumption and risk of prostatic carcinoma. Cancer Epidemiol Biomarkers Prev 1996;5:889–95.
166. West DW, Slattery ML, Robison LM, et al. Adult dietary intake and prostate cancer risk in Utah: a case-control study with special emphasis on aggressive tumors. Cancer Causes Control 1991;2:85–94.
167. Hursting SD, Thornquist M, Henderson MM. Types of dietary fat and the incidence of cancer at five sites. Prev Med 1990;19:242–53.
168. Kolonel LN, Yoshizawa CN, Hankin JH. Diet and prostatic cancer: a case-control study in Hawaii. Am J Epidemiol 1988;127:999–1012.
169. Kolonel LN, Nomura AM, Hinds MW, et al. Role of diet in cancer incidence in Hawaii. Cancer Res 1983;43 Suppl: 2397s–402s.
170. Giovannucci E, Rimm EB, Colditz GA, et al. A prospective study of dietary fat and risk of prostate cancer. J Natl Cancer Inst 1993;85:1571–9.
171. Gann PH, Hennekens CH, Sacks FM, et al. Prospective study of plasma fatty acids and risk of prostate cancer. J Natl Cancer Inst 1994;86:281–6.
172. Norrish AE, Ferguson LR, Knize MG, et al. Heterocyclic amine content of cooked meat and risk of prostate cancer. J Natl Cancer Inst 1999;91:2038–44.
173. Deneo-Pellegrini H, De Stefani E, Ronco A, Mendilaharsu M. Foods, nutrients and prostate cancer: a case-control study in Uruguay. Br J Cancer 1999;80:591–7.
174. Schuurman AG, van den Brandt PA, Dorant E, Goldbohm RA. Animal products, calcium, and protein and prostate cancer risk in the Netherlands Cohort Study. Br J Cancer 1999;80:1107–13.
175. Veierod MB, Laake P, Thelle DS. Dietary fat intake and risk of prostate cancer: a prospective study of 25,708 Norwegian men. Int J Cancer 1997;73:634–8.
176. Ewings P, Bowie C. A case-control study of cancer of the prostate in Somerset and east Devon. Br J Cancer 1996; 74:661–6.
177. De Stefani E, Fierro L, Barrios E, Ronco A. Tobacco, alcohol, diet and risk of prostate cancer. Tumori 1995;81:315–20.
178. Talamini R, Franceschi S, La Vecchia C, et al. Diet and prostatic cancer: a case-control study in Northern Italy. Nutr Cancer 1992;18:277–86.
179. Bravo MP, Castellanos E, del Rey Calero J. Dietary factors and prostatic cancer. Urol Int 1991;46:163–6.
180. Le Marchand L, Kolonel LN, Wilkens LR, et al. Animal fat consumption and prostate cancer: a prospective study in Hawaii. Epidemiology 1994;5:276–82.
181. Graham S, Haughey B, Marshall J, et al. Diet in the epidemiology of carcinoma of the prostate gland. J Natl Cancer Inst 1983;70:687–92.
182. La Vecchia C, Negri E, D'Avanzo B, et al. Dairy products and the risk of prostatic cancer. Oncology 1991;48:406–10.
183. Key TJ, Silcocks PB, Davey GK, et al. A case-control study of diet and prostate cancer. Br J Cancer 1997;76:678–87.
184. Mettlin C, Selenskas S, Natarajan NS, Huben R. Beta-carotene and animal fats and their relationship to prostate cancer risk: a case-control study. Cancer 1989;64:605–12.
185. Severson RK, Nomura AMY, Grove JS, Stemmermann GN. A prospective study of demographics, diet, and prostate cancer among men of Japanese ancestry in Hawaii. Cancer Res 1989;49:1857–60.
186. Slattery ML, Schumacher MC, West DW, et al. Food-consumption trends between adolescent and adult years and subsequent risk of prostate cancer. Am J Clin Nutr 1990; 52:752–7.
187. Meyer F, Bairati I, Shadmani R, et al. Dietary fat and prostate cancer survival. Cancer Causes Control 1999;10:245–51.
188. Allen NE, Appleby PN, Davey GK, Key TJ. Hormones and diet: low insulin-like growth factor-I but normal bioavailable androgens in vegan men. Br J Cancer 2000;83:95–7.
189. Habito RC, Montalto J, Leslie E, Ball MJ, et al. Effects of replacing meat with soyabean in the diet on sex hormone concentrations in healthy adult males. Br J Nutr 2000;84: 557–63.

190. Talamini R, La Vecchia C, Decarli A, et al. Nutrition, social factors, and prostatic cancer in a Northern Italian population. Br J Cancer 1986;53:817–21.
191. La Vecchia C, Negri E, D'Avanzo B, et al. Dairy products and the risk of prostatic cancer. Oncology 1991;48:406–10.
192. De Stefani E, Fierro L, Barrios E, Ronco A. Tobacco, alcohol, diet and risk of prostate cancer. Tumori 1995;81:315–20.
193. Chan JM, Giovannucci E, Andersson S-D, et al. Dairy products, calcium, phosphorous, vitamin D, and risk of prostate cancer. Cancer Causes Control 1998;9:559–66.
194. Jain MG, Hislop GT, Howe GR, Ghadirian P. Plant foods, antioxidants, and prostate cancer risk: findings from case-control studies in Canada. Nutr Cancer 1999;34:173–84.
195. Rotkin ID. Studies in the epidemiology of prostatic cancer: expanded sampling. Cancer Treat Rep 1977;61:173–80.
196. Schuman LM, Mandel JS, Radke A, et al. Some selected features of the epidemiology of prostatic cancer: Minneapolis-St. Paul, Minnesota case-control study 1976–1979. In: Magnus K, editor. Trends in cancer incidence: causes and practical implications. Washington (DC): Hemisphere Publishing Corp; 1982. p. 345–54.
197. Hayes RB, Ziegler RG, Gridley G, et al. Dietary factors and risk for prostate cancer among blacks and whites in the United States. Cancer Epidemiol Biomarkers Prev 1999;8:25–34.
198. Tzonou A, Signorello LB, Lagiou P, et al. Diet and cancer of the prostate: a case-control study in Greece. Int J Cancer 1999;80:704–8.
199. Ewings P, Bowie C. Case-control study of cancer of the prostate in Somerset and East Devon. Br J Cancer 1996;74:661–6.
200. Giovannucci E, Rimm EB, Wolk A, et al. Calcium and fructose intake in relation to risk of prostate cancer. Cancer Res 1998;58:442–7.
201. Chan JM, Stampfer MJ, Ma, J, et al. Dairy products, calcium, and prostate cancer in the Physicians' Health Study. Am J Clin Nutr 2001;74:549–54.
202. Snowdon DA, Phillips RL, Choi W. Diet, obesity, and risk of fatal prostate cancer. Am J Epidemiol 1984;120:244–50.
203. Chan JM, Pietinen P, Virtanen M, et al. Diet and prostate cancer risk in a cohort of smokers, with a specific focus on calcium and phosphorous. Cancer Causes Control 2000; 11:859–67.
204. Mills PK, Beeson WL, Phillips RL, Fraser GE. Cohort study of diet, lifestyle, and prostate cancer in Adventist men. Cancer 1989;64:598–604.
205. Hsing AW, McLaughlin JK, Schuman LM, et al. Diet, tobacco use, and fatal prostate cancer: results from the Lutheran Brotherhood Cohort Study. Cancer Res 1990;50:6836–40.
206. Ohno Y, Yoshida O, Oishi K, et al. Dietary beta-carotene and cancer of the prostate: a case-control study in Kyoto, Japan. Cancer Res 1988;48:1331–6.
207. Kristal AR, Stanford JL, Cohen JH, et al. Vitamin and mineral supplement use is associated with reduced risk of prostate cancer. Cancer Epidemiol Biomarkers Prev 1999;8:887–92.
208. Vlajinac HD, Marinkovic JM, Ilic MD, Kocev NI. Diet and prostate cancer: a case-control study. Eur J Cancer 1997; 33:101–7.
209. Holick MF. Vitamin D. In: Shils ME, Olson JA, Shike M, Ross AC, editors. Modern nutrition in health and disease. Baltimore: Wiliams & Wilkins; 1999. p. 329–45.
210. Feldman D, Skowronski RJ, Peehl DM. Vitamin D and prostate cancer. In: American Institute for Cancer Research, editor. Diet and cancer: molecular mechanisms of interactions. New York: Plenum Press; 1995. p. 53–63.
211. Schwartz GG, Oeler TA, Uskokovic MR, Bahnson RR. Human prostate cancer cells: inhibition of proliferation by vitamin D analogs. Anticancer Res 1994;14:1077–81.
212. Skowronski RJ, Peehl DM, Feldman D. Vitamin D and prostate cancer: 1,25 dihydroxyvitamin D_3 receptors and actions in human prostate cancer cell lines. Endocrinology 1993;132:1952–60.
213. Esquenet M, Swinnen JV, Heyns W, Verhoeven G. Control of LNCaP proliferation and differentiation: actions and interactions of androgens 1alpha,25-dihydroxycholecalciferol,all-trans retinoic acid, 9-cis retinoic acid, and phenylacetate. Prostate 1996;28:182–94.
214. Peehl DM, Skowronski RJ, Leung GK, et al. Antiproliferative effects of 1,25-dihydroxyvitamin D_3 on primary cultures of human prostatic cells. Cancer Res 1994;54:805–10.
215. Miller GJ, Stapleton GE, Hedlund TE, Moffatt KA. Vitamin D receptor expression 24—hydroxylase activity, and inhibition of growth by 1α,25– dihydroxyvitamin D_3 in seven human prostatic carcinoma cell lines. Clin Cancer Res 1995;1:997–1003.
216. Hsieh T-C, Ng C-Y, Mallouh C, et al. Regulation of growth, PSA/PAP and androgen receptor expression by 1α,25-dihydroxyvitamin D_3 in androgen-dependent LNCaP cells. Biochem Biophys Res Commun 1996;223:141–6.
217. Skowronski RJ, Peehl DM, Feldman D. Actions of vitamin D3 analogs on human prostate cancer cell lines: comparison with 1,25-dihydroxyvitamin D3. Endocrinology 1995;136:20–6.
218. Schwartz GG, Wang M-H, Zhang M, et al. 1α,25-dihydroxyvitamin D (calcitriol) inhibits the invasiveness of human prostate cancer cells. Cancer Epidemiol Biomarkers Prev 1997;6:727–32.
219. Bahnson RR, Oeler T, Trump D, et al. Inhibition of human prostatic carcinoma cell lines by 1,25-dihydroxyvitamin D_3 and vitamin D analogs [abstract]. J Urol 1993;149 Suppl: 471a.
220. Schwartz GG, Hill CC, Oeler TA, et al. 1,25-dihydroxy-16-ene-23-yne-vitamin D_3 and prostate cancer cell proliferation in vivo. Urology 1995;46:365–9.
221. Lokeshwar BL, Schwartz GG, Selzer MG, et al. Inhibition of prostate cancer metastases in vivo: a comparison of 1,25-dihydroxyvitamin D (Calcitriol) and EB 1089. Cancer Epidemiol Biomarkers Prev 1999;8:241–8.
222. Corder EH, Guess HA, Hulka BS, et al. Vitamin D and prostate cancer: a prediagnostic study with stored sera. Cancer Epidemiol Biomarkers Prev 1993;2:467–72.
223. Braun MM, Helzlsouer KJ, Hollis BW, Comstock GW. Prostate cancer and prediagnostic levels of serum vitamin D metabolites (Maryland, United States). Cancer Causes Control 1995;6:235–9.
224. Nomura AMY, Stemmermann GN, Lee J, et al. Serum vitamin D metabolite levels and the subsequent development of prostate cancer. Cancer Causes Control 1998;9:425–32.
225. Gann PH, Ma J, Hennekens CH, et al. Circulating vitamin D metabolites in relation to subsequent development of prostate cancer. Cancer Epidemiol Biomarkers Prev 1996; 5:121–6.

226. Ingles SA, Ross RK, Yu MC, et al. Association of prostate cancer risk with genetic polymorphisms in vitamin D receptor and androgen receptor. J Natl Cancer Inst 1997;89:166–70.
227. Taylor JA, Hirvonen A, Watson M, et al. Association of prostate cancer with vitamin D receptor gene polymorphism. Cancer Res 1996;56:4108–10.
228. Ma J, Stampfer MJ, Gann PH, et al. Vitamin D receptor polymorphisms, circulating vitamin D metabolites, and risk of prostate cancer in United States physicians. Cancer Epidemiol Biomarkers Prev 1998;7:385–90.
229. Habuchi T, Suzuki T, Sasaki R, et al. Association of vitamin D receptor gene polymorphism with prostate cancer and benign prostatic hyperplasia in a Japanese population. Cancer Res 2000;15:305–8.
230. Shuurman AG, Goldbohm RA, Dorant E, van den Brandt PA. Vegetable and fruit consumption and prostate cancer risk: a cohort study in the Netherlands. Cancer Epidemiol Biomarkers Prev 1998;7:673–80.
231. Key TJA, Silcocks PB, Davey GK, et al. A case-control study of diet and prostate cancer. Br J Cancer 1997;76:678–87.
232. Ross RK, Shimizu H, Paganini-Hill A, et al. Case-control studies of prostate cancer in Blacks and Whites in Southern California. J Natl Cancer Inst 1987;78:869–74.
233. Cohen JH, Kristal AR, Stanford JL. Fruit and vegetable intake and prostate cancer risk. J Natl Cancer Inst 2000;92:61–8.
234. Norrish AE, Jackson RT, Sharpe SJ, Skeaff CM. Prostate cancer and dietary carotenoids. Am J Epidemiol 2000;151: 119–23.
235. Walker ARP, Walker BF, Tsotetsi NG, et al. Case-control study of prostate cancer in black patients in Soweto, South Africa. Br J Cancer 1992;65:438–41.
236. Giovannucci E, Ascherio A, Rimm EB, et al. Intake of carotenoids and retinol in relation to risk of prostate cancer. J Natl Cancer Inst 1995;87:1767–76.
237. Brody T. Vitamin A. In: Nutritional biochemistry. Boston: Academic Press; 1999. p. 554–65.
238. Chan JM, Giovannucci E. Vegetables, fruits, and associated micronutrients. Epidemiol Rev 2001;23:82–6.
239. Gann PH, Ma J, Giovannucci E, et al. Lower prostate cancer risk in men with elevated plasma lycopene levels: results of a prospective analysis. Cancer Res 1999;59:1225–30.
240. Hsing AW, Comstock GW, Abbey H, Polk BF. Serologic precursors of cancer. Retinol, carotenoids, and tocopherol and risk of prostate cancer. J Natl Cancer Inst 1990;82:941–6.
241. Cook NR, Stampfer MJ, Ma J, et al. Beta-carotene supplementation for patients with low baseline levels and decreased risks of total and prostate carcinoma. Cancer 1999;86:1783–92.
242. Heinonen OP, Albanes D, Virtamo J, et al. Prostate cancer and supplementation with alpha-tocopherol and beta-carotene: incidence and mortality in a controlled trial. J Natl Cancer Inst 1998;90:440–6.
243. Brody T. Vitamin E. In: Nutritional biochemistry. Boston: Academic Press; 1999. p. 628–37.
244. Kapoor N, Degroff VL, Cornwell DG, et al. Anti-proliferative and pro-apoptotic effects of gamma-tocopheryl quinone in human prostate cancer cell lines in vitro. American Association for Cancer Research 91st Annual Meeting—Proceedings 2000;41:339.
245. Huang H-Y, Alberg AJ, Hoffman SC, et al. Association of blood concentrations of antioxidant micronutrients and the risk of prostate cancer. In: American Association for Cancer Research 91st Annual Meeting—Proceedings 2000;41:809.
246. Christen S, Woodall AA, Shigenaga MK, et al. Gamma-tocopherol traps mutagenic electrophiles such as NOx and complements alpha-tocopherol: physiologic implications. Med Sci 1997;94:3217–22.
247. Helzlsouer KJ, Huang H-Y, Alberg AJ, et al. Association between α-tocopherol, γ-tocopherol, selenium, and subsequent prostate cancer. J Natl Cancer Inst 2000;92:2018–23
248. Packer L. Protective role of vitamin E in biological systems. Am J Clin Nutr 1991;53:1050S–5S.
249. Grimble RF. Effect of antioxidative vitamins on immune function with clinical applications. Int J Vitam Nutr Res 1997;67:312–20.
250. Shklar G, Oh S-K. Experimental basis for cancer prevention by vitamin E. Cancer Invest 2000;18:214–22.
251. Israel K, Yu W, Sanders BG, Kline K. Vitamin E succinate induces apoptosis in human prostate cancer cells: role for Fas in vitamin E succinate-triggered apoptosis. Nutr Cancer 2000;36:90–100.
252. Hayes RB, Bogdanovicz JFAT, Schroeder FH, et al. Serum retinol and prostate cancer. Cancer 1988;62:2021–6.
253. Rohan TE, Howe GR, Burch JD, Jain M, et al. Dietary factors and risk of prostate cancer: a case-control study in Ontario, Canada. Cancer Causes Control 1995;6:145–54.
254. Hartman T, Albanes D, Pietinen P, et al. The association between baseline vitamin E, selenium, and prostate cancer in the Alpha-Tocoperol, Beta-Carotene Cancer Prevention Study. Cancer Epidemiol Biomarkers Prev 1998;7:335–40.
255. Chan JM, Stampfer MJ, Ma J, et al. Supplemental vitamin E intake and prostate cancer risk in a large cohort of men in the United States. Cancer Epidemiol Biomarkers Prev 1999;8:893–9.
256. Andersson S-O, Wolk A, Bergström R, et al. Energy, nutrient intake and prostate cancer risk: a population-based case-control study in Sweden. Int J Cancer 1996;68:716–22.
257. Meyer F, Bairati I, Fradet Y, Moore L. Dietary energy and nutrients in relation to preclinical prostate cancer. Nutr Cancer 1997;29:120–6.
258. Eichholzer M, Stahelin HB, Gey KF, et al. Prediction of male cancer mortality by plasma levels of interacting vitamins: 17-year follow-up of the prospective Basel study. Int J Cancer 1996;66:145–50.
259. Nomura AMY, Stemmermann GN, Lee J, Craft NE. Serum micronutrients and prostate cancer in Japanese Americans in Hawaii. Cancer Epidemiol Biomarkers Prev 1997; 6:487–91.
260. Messina MJ. Legumes and soybeans: overview of their nutritional profiles and health effects. Am J Clin Nutr 1999;70 (3 Suppl):439S–50S.
261. Severson RK, Nomura AM, Grove JS, Stemmermann GN. A prospective study of demographics, diet, and prostate cancer among men of Japanese ancestry in Hawaii. Cancer Res 1989;49:1857–60.
262. Kolonel LN, Hankin JH, Whittemore AS, et al. Vegetables, fruits, legumes and prostate cancer: a multiethnic case-control study. Cancer Epidemiol Biomarkers Prev 2000; 9:795–804.
263. Jacobsen BK, Knutsen SF, Fraser GE. Does high soy milk

intake reduce prostate cancer incidence? The Adventist Health Study (United States). Cancer Causes Control 1998;9:553–7.

264. Redman C, Scott JA, Baines AT, et al. Inhibitory effect of selenomethionine on the growth of three selected human tumor cell lines. Cancer Lett 1998;125:103–10.
265. Webber MM. Selenium prevents the growth stimulatory effects of cadmium on human prostatic epithelium. Biochem Biophys Res Commun 1985;127:871–7.
266. Webber MM, Perez-Ripoll EA, James GT. Inhibitory effects of selenium on the growth of DU-145 human prostate carcinoma cells in vitro. Biochem Biophys Res Commun 1985;130:603–9.
267. Helzlsouer KJ, Huang HY, Alberg AJ, et al. Association between alpha-tocopherol, gamma-tocopherol, selenium, and subsequent prostate cancer. J Natl Cancer Inst 2000; 92:2018–23.
268. Nomura AM, Lee J, Stemmermann GN, Combs GF. Serum selenium and subsequent risk of prostate cancer. Cancer Epidemiol Biomarkers Prev 2000;9:883–7.
269. Hardell L, Degerman A, Tomic R, et al. Levels of selenium in plasma and glutathione peroxidase in erythrocytes in patients with prostate cancer or benign hyperplasia. Eur J Cancer Prev 1995;4:91–5.
270. Yoshizawa K, Willett WC, Morris SJ, et al. Study of prediagnostic selenium level in toenails and the risk of advanced prostate cancer. J Natl Cancer Inst 1998;90:1219–24.
271. Clark LC, Dalkin B, Krongrad A, et al. Decreased incidence of prostate cancer with selenium supplementation: results of a double-blind cancer prevention trial. Br J Urol 1998;81:730–4.
272. Brody T. Selenium and glutathione. In: Nutritional biochemistry. Boston: Academic Press; 1999. p. 825–78.
273. Ghadirian P, Maisonneuve P, Perret C, et al. A case-control study of toenail selenium and cancer of the breast, colon, and prostate. Cancer Detect Prev 2000;24:305–13.

2

Pathology

NOEL WEIDNER, MD

This chapter reviews the pathology of prostate adenocarcinoma and emphasize the features critical for light microscopic diagnosis and proper patient management. Prostate carcinoma is currently the most common cancer in American men (~189,000 cases per year or ~25% of male malignancies).[1] Up to 1992, it appeared to be increasing in incidence, but since then, it has declined. Moreover, the fact that only approximately 35,000 American men die of prostate adenocarcinoma annually (~15% of the cancer-related deaths in men and second only to lung cancer)[1] indicates that the majority of prostate cancers do not progress.[2] Moreover, thousands of latent cases are discovered in prostatectomy specimens removed for benign prostatic hyperplasia.[3] The incidence of prostate adenocarcinoma increases progressively with age and in autopsy studies varies from a 0% incidence in men less than 30 years old to an approximately 70% incidence in men between 80 and 89 years old.[4] Children, however, can also develop prostate adenocarcinoma, and one report discussed five patients under 10 years of age.[5] Although the survival rates for young and old men with prostate adenocarcinoma are about the same, "young" men (< 50 years old) often present with more advanced disease and do more poorly. Prostate adenocarcinoma appears to be more common in Blacks than in Whites and often presents at a more advanced stage.[2,6] The reasons for these differences remain unknown, and much remains to be learned about the cytogenetics and pathobiology of prostate adenocarcinoma, especially about those factors that cause aggressive tumor behavior. Thus, development of accurate prognostic indicators, which correlate with outcome, would help identify those patients who may require aggressive therapies because they are at higher risk for recurrence and death.

Many prostate adenocarcinomas are found either at autopsy or in transurethral resection (TUR) specimens. Also, approximately 50% of clinically nodular prostates will prove to have adenocarcinoma at biopsy,[7,8] and approximately 20% of prostate specimens submitted with a clinical diagnosis of "benign hyperplasia" will have foci of adenocarcinoma.[9] Less commonly, prostate adenocarcinomas may present as bony metastases, in left-sided cervical or supradiaphragmatic lymph nodes, or as a rectal mass closely mimicking primary rectal adenocarcinoma (Table 2–1).[10–12]

Before the introduction of screening serum for prostate-specific antigen (PSA), some reports indicated that approximately 55% of prostate adenocarcinomas were first diagnosed in TUR specimens. With the recent development of screening techniques (eg, transrectal ultrasonography [TRUS], elevations in serum PSA levels), more and more cases of prostate

Table 2–1. UNUSUAL PRESENTATIONS OF PROSTATE ADENOCARCINOMA

I. Metastases to left-sided cervical and/or supradiaphragmatic lymph nodes
  - May have normal serum PAP or PSA, normal rectal examination, and no bone metastases
  - Usually poorly differentiated tumors
  - PAP and/or PSA positive in almost all

II. Presentation as a rectal mass
  - From anal verge to 20 cm above
  - Can grow as a stenosing annular tumor
  - Intramucosal tumor present in 20%
  - Usually poorly differentiated tumors
  - PSA and/or PAP positive in almost all
  - Carcinoids may be PAP positive but PSA negative

PAP = prostatic acid phosphatase; PSA = prostate-specific antigen.

adenocarcinoma are being diagnosed on needle biopsy.[13–15] This biopsy technique, especially when employing an 18-gauge biopsy gun,[10] is well tolerated by patients, and multiple biopsies can be taken, usually transrectally. Although transperineal biopsy of the prostate has a lower infection rate, it is less sensitive than transrectal biopsy. Adequate biopsy specimens will contain stromal or glandular elements. Transrectal ultrasonography has an approximately 60% sensitivity rate for detecting invasive tumors over 0.5 cm; inflammation, prior TUR, cystic prostate glands, prostatic intraepithelial neoplasia (PIN), and atrophy may result in false-positive diagnoses.[16,17] Transperineal magnetic resonance imaging (MRI)-guided prostate biopsy is a technique that may be useful in detecting prostate cancer in patients with an increased serum PSA who are not candidates for TRUS-guided biopsy.[18] Normal serum PSA levels can be found in as many as 50% of organ-confined prostate adenocarcinomas and in approximately 33% when the tumor penetrates the capsule.[10,19–21] Serum PSA levels in cases in which there is benign hyperplasia, a history of prior biopsy, or inflammation may mimic those in adenocarcinomas. On a volume basis, adenocarcinomas release more PSA than benign hyperplastic tissue and produce more rapidly rising serum PSA levels than benign hyperplastic tissue. Biopsy is clearly indicated when PSA is over 10 ng/mL and there is a positive digital rectal examination.[22] A serum PSA of 60 ng/mL or more has a positive predictive value of 98% for the presence of prostate carcinoma and can be used as a surrogate for histologic diagnosis where facilities for obtaining prostate biopsies are not readily available.[23]

Fine-needle aspiration (FNA) biopsy can also be used to diagnose prostate adenocarcinoma.[24] It can be performed as an outpatient procedure without anesthesia and may induce fewer complications than biopsies with 14-gauge, Tru-CUT, or core needles. However, 18-gauge needles provide thin histologic cores with the same advantages as FNA. Although FNA may be as sensitive as core needle biopsy, it requires considerable training and practice before a sufficient level of expertise is reached to justify its use. Moreover, FNA will result in more borderline or indeterminate diagnoses, which will require repeat FNA and/or follow-up core needle biopsy. Moreover, two recent studies have shown that the 18-gauge biopsy gun is superior to FNA.[25,26] At many centers, FNA appears to be waning in popularity.[10,27]

STAGING

Prognosis and therapy are clearly dependent on the extent or stage of the carcinoma. A careful determination of the extent of the tumor in the pathologic specimen is critical for proper patient management. Some of the important features for the pathologist to look for are outlined in various staging systems such as the International Union Against Cancer (UICC) system, the tumor-nodes-metastasis (TNM) staging system (Table 2–2). The pathologic stage should be determined and included in all signouts of resection specimens for adenocarcinoma.

Grossly, some prostate adenocarcinomas are pale yellow, firm, and easily detected and measured. But many prostate adenocarcinomas cannot be reliably

Table 2–2. AJCC OR UICC TNM AND AMERICAN UROLOGICAL SYSTEMS

Tx		Primary tumor cannot be assessed
T0		No evidence of primary tumor
T1		Tumor is an incidental histologic finding (ie, not palpated or imaged)
	T1a	5% or less of specimen involved by tumor
	T1b	More than 5% of specimen involved by tumor
	T1c	Tumor found in needle biopsy (ie, after elevated serum PSA)
T2		Tumor present clinically or grossly but limited to gland
	T2a	Tumor involves one lobe only
	T2b	Tumor in more than one lobe
T3		Tumor invades beyond the prostate capsule but is not fixed
	T3a	Extracapsular extension (unilateral or bilateral)
	T3b	Tumor invades seminal vesicles
T4		Tumor fixed to or invades adjacent structures other than seminal vesicles (ie, bladder neck, external sphincter, rectum, levator muscles, and/or pelvic wall). *Invasion into the prostatic apex or into (but not beyond) the prostatic capsule is not classified as T3 but as T2*
Nx		Regional lymph nodes cannot be assessed
N0		No regional lymph node metastases
N1		Metastasis in a single or multiple lymph node(s)
Mx		Distant metastasis cannot be assessed
M0		No distant metastasis
M1		Distant metastasis
	M1a	Nonregional lymph node(s)
	M1b	Bone metastases
	M1c	Other site(s). *If more than one site of metastasis is present, the most most advanced category is used. M1c is most advanced*

AJCC = American Joint Committee on Cancer; UICC = Internatonal Union Against Cancer; TNM = tumor-nodes-metastasis; PSA = prostate-specific antigen.

outlined or differentiated from benign tissues on gross examination. Thus, accurate staging requires both careful gross dissection and microscopic examination of the prostatectomy specimen. Resection margins should be inked, clearly labeled on cassettes, and, if necessary, color-coded to identify specific margins. After inking, dipping the specimen in Bouin's solution or acetic acid acts as a mordant and fixes the ink in place, thus minimizing smearing. Also, multiple representative sections should be taken from right and left lobes, in continuity with lateral, anterior, posterior, basal, and apical resection margins, and from both seminal vesicles, where they merge with the prostate gland. A detailed diagrammatic record of the location of each section and the distribution of invasive adenocarcinoma within the sections should be completed and included with the final written report (Figure 2–1).

The prostatic apex can be particularly difficult to evaluate. Nonetheless, amputating the distal apex and making multiple longitudinal cross-sections similar to the manner in which cervical cone biopsies are handled usually yields good results. A semiconical specimen is removed from the apex at a point 2 to 4 mm from the urethral margin. This specimen is placed flat on its surface (inked surgical margin side up) and multiply cross-sectioned at right angles. All cross-sections are embedded; the inked apical margins should be clear at light microscopic examination. Other authors prefer an en face "shave" section of the apex margin. These shave sections should be considered positive for tumor if they contain tumor material only and no benign glands or if they have high-grade or extensive low- to intermediate-grade tumor tissue (even when admixed with benign glands).[10] Except with extensive or high-grade adenocarcinoma, the finding of tumor material and benign glands indicates that the tumor remains within the prostate, a finding associated with a low rate of local recurrence.[10]

In over 70% of cases, carcinoma arises along the periphery of the gland and secondarily invades the central portion. Since prostate adenocarcinomas are frequently multifocal, representative sections of

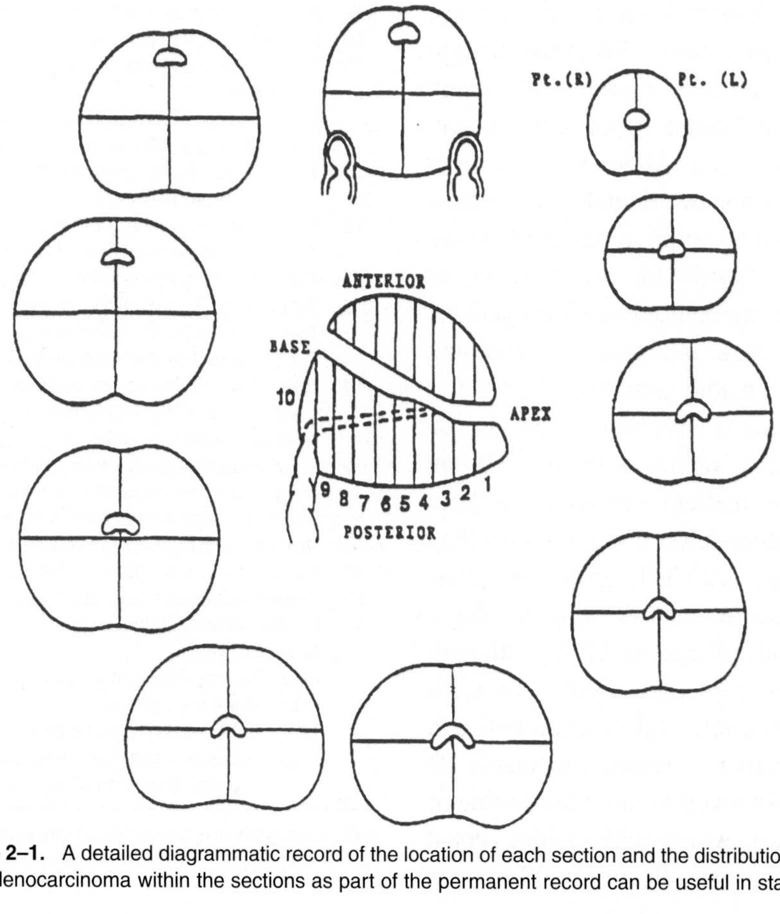

Figure 2–1. A detailed diagrammatic record of the location of each section and the distribution of invasive adenocarcinoma within the sections as part of the permanent record can be useful in staging.

both right and left prostate lobes are needed for accurate staging. Some data suggest tumor size is important in predicting metastasis.[28]

In fact, the College of American Pathologists (CAP) recommends that in subtotal and radical prostatectomy specimens, the percentage of tissue involved by tumor can be "eyeballed." In these latter specimens it may be possible to measure a dominant tumor nodule in at least two dimensions and to indicate the number of blocks involved by tumor over the total number of prostate blocks submitted. Moreover, it is recommended that at the very least, the proportion (percentage) of prostatic tissue involved by tumor be included for all specimens, including core needle biopsies and prostate chips positive for cancer (number of positive chips divided by total number of chips).

True prostatic capsular penetration by adenocarcinoma (ie, tumor growing through the capsule into periprostatic tissue[9]) has been associated with higher progression rates, but this may not be an independent prognostic indicator after tumor grade and surgical margins are included in multivariate analyses.[10] The prostatic capsule is not a well-defined histologic structure, which makes the determination of true capsular penetration problematic. Nonetheless, invasion of the capsule (ie, tumor infiltrating into but not passing through the capsule) is distinct from true capsular penetration. On resected specimens, the appearance of a smooth, rounded inked margin indicates that the tumor has not penetrated the capsule. This type of margin is considered by some as negative for tumor.[10] In contrast, an adenocarcinoma that extends to a rough and irregular inked margin, which results from infiltration of periprostatic neurovascular tissues with or without a desmoplastic stromal reaction, indicates that true capsular penetration has occurred. Clearly, this type of margin should be considered positive for tumor. Extraprostatic extension (EPE) is the preferred term for the presence of tumor beyond the confines of the prostate gland. EPE is present when tumor cells are admixed with fat, involve perineural spaces in the neurovascular bundles, or extend beyond the confines of normal glandular prostate where there is a paucity of fat such as the anterior prostate and bladder neck regions. At the apex, tumor admixed with skeletal muscle elements does not constitute extraprostatic extension. Curiously, some studies have indicated that perineural invasion by tumor cells has no impact on prognosis,[29] although the perineural space would appear to provide a clear pathway for spread beyond the prostate (ie, true capsular penetration). In fact, the finding of perineural invasion in a needle biopsy has a 95% association with capsular penetration in the subsequent radical prostatectomy specimen.[30] However, the value of perineural invasion as an independent prognostic factor has been questioned after multivariate analysis.[31] Capsular penetration most commonly occurs along the posterior and posterolateral margins of resection, and increasing histologic grade is associated with increasing incidence of capsular penetration, positive surgical margins, and metastases.[10] Currently, urologists perform six (or more), site-designated biopsies, but much variation persists in prostate biopsy sampling and reporting. Should each biopsy be submitted separately and diagnosed separately, or should those from the left side be lumped together and those from the right side lumped together and "diagnosed" in aggregate? Yet, positive sextant biopsy location (apex to base) does not appear to predict the size of positive surgical margins at radical prostatectomy. However, ipsilateral positive surgical margins are more likely as the number of positive sextant biopsies on that side increases. Thus, while pathologic processing of biopsy specimens according to longitudinal prostate location (base, mid, apex) is probably unnecessary, the number of positive biopsies on a given side may be useful preoperative information.[32,33] Seminal vesicle invasion most likely results from capsular penetration through the base of the gland and subsequently into the seminal vesicles. Seminal vesicle invasion appears to have a particularly dire prognosis, with 80% of patients having tumor progression within 5 years.[10] In the individual patient, the serum PSA level does not facilitate precise pathologic staging, although advanced stage tends to correlate with relatively high serum PSA levels.[34] Nonetheless, the value of surgical margin evaluation is diminished by the knowledge that after radical prostatectomy, the serum PSA level is exquisitely sensitive to recurrent or residual disease.[34] Also, serum PSA levels that decrease to the reference range, following radiation or androgen deprivation therapy, have a favorable prognosis.[34]

Because metastases (even micrometastases) to pelvic lymph nodes decrease the value of radical surgery, frozen sections of pelvic lymph nodes are taken before surgery is performed (some urologists may proceed with radical proctectomy anyway). Frozen sections will detect about two-thirds of the patients with micrometastases to lymph nodes.[35] Because small lymph nodes can be hard to dissect, the entire lymphadenectomy specimen should be submitted for permanent sections. Even micrometastases to tiny lymph nodes are significant.[35]

Although counting microscopic foci of adenocarcinoma in TUR specimens is the commonly used technique for separating stage T1a from T1b lesions, some believe that the best predictor of prognosis in this group is estimating the percentage of the area of the specimen involved by tumor.[36,37] When less than 5% of the TUR specimen is involved by tumor (stage T1a), 2% of patients show tumor progression at 4 years following diagnosis, whereas 32% progress in patients who have specimens with greater than 5% tumor by area (stage T1b).[36,37] About 16% of TUR specimens will contain invasive prostate adenocarcinoma.[7,9]

Recent studies show that up to 100% of stage T1b adenocarcinomas and approximately 90% of stage T1a adenocarcinomas will be detected by submitting 8 blocks of TUR chips (about 12 g).[7,9] Submitting the entire TUR specimen will reveal all of the stage T1a adenocarcinomas, yet many pathologists believe that this practice is excessive, especially those who believe that stage T1a disease is clinically insignificant. However, poorly differentiated prostate adenocarcinoma can be focal,[38] and repeat TUR for stage T1a disease has resulted in upstaging to T1b disease in up to 26% of cases.[39] Also, significant progression of untreated stage T1a adenocarcinoma was found in 16 to 25% of patients observed for 8 to 10 years.[40–42] Thus, missing a stage T1a lesion because of inadequate sampling in a "young" man may be dangerous. The author believes that all TUR tissues from men under 65 years of age should be submitted for histologic examination. However, definitive surgery may not be performed in some institutions for stage T1a disease, and according to some studies, survival among patients (all ages) with stage T1a disease does not differ from that of the general population.[43,44] Stage T2a cancers (ie, tumor 1.5 cm or less in diameter) appear less aggressive than stage T1b cancers; in fact, patients with stage T2a disease may have survival rates similar to that of the general population.[43,44] Patients with stage T2b cancer (ie, tumor more than 1.5 cm in diameter or in more than one lobe) have low survival rates with progression rates of over 50%, and most patients with tumor into the seminal vesicle, bladder neck, and/or beyond the prostatic "capsule" but not metastatic and presence of metastatic tumor will eventually die from them.[43,44] Clearly, the pathologist is indispensable in determin-

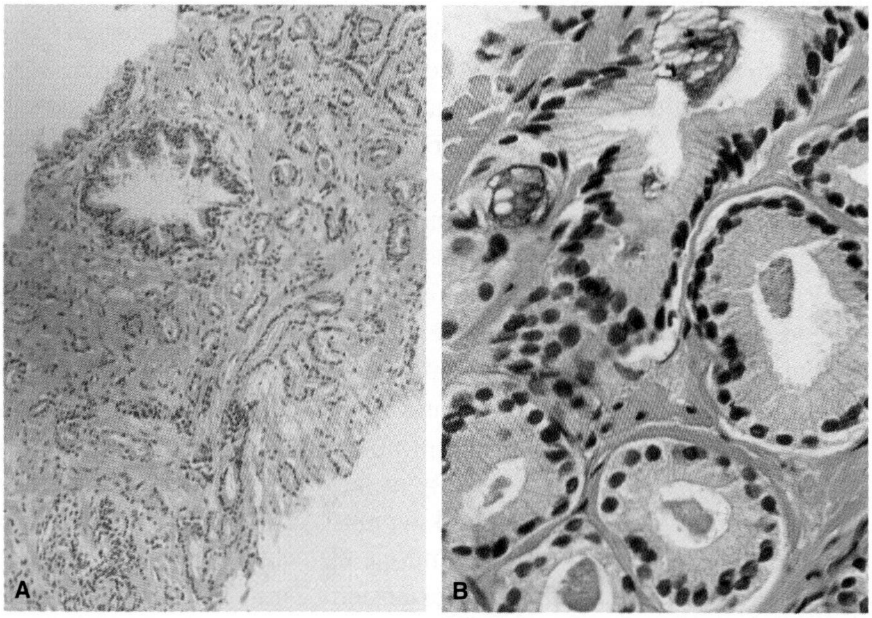

Figure 2–2. *A*, Moderately differentiated prostate carcinoma (Gleason patterns 3 + 3). Note small acinar pattern of glands infiltrating around benign gland (*upper center*) (hematoxylin and eosin; × 25 original magnification. *B*, Note uniform basilar-oriented nuclei and cuboidal to columnar epithelial differentiation with formation of sharp-edged lumen. Also note dense eosinophilic secretion and intraluminal blue mucin (hematoxylin and eosin; × 100 original magnification).

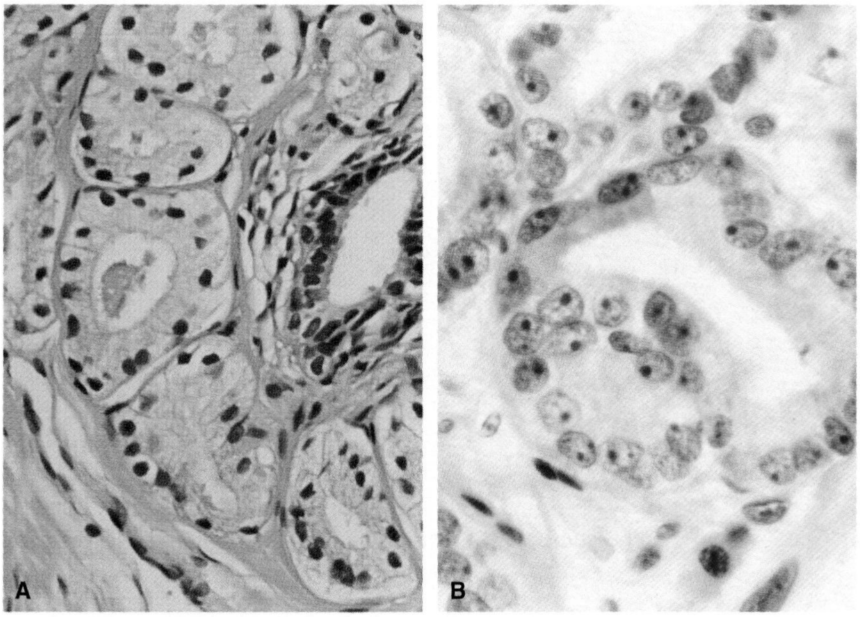

Figure 2–3. *A*, Moderately differentiated prostate carcinoma (Gleason pattern 3 + 3). Note rigid, small acinar pattern of malignant glands surrounding a single benign gland. Nuclei are monotonous but do not show prominent nucleoli, which are usually but not always prominent in prostate carcinoma (hematoxylin and eosin; × 100 original magnification). *B*, Moderately differentiated prostate carcinoma. Note prominent nucleoli (hematoxylin and eosin; × 100 original magnification).

ing the prognosis and proper therapy for patients with prostate adenocarcinoma.

CLASSIFICATION OF PROSTATE CARCINOMA

Carcinoma accounts for the vast majority of prostate tumors; the remaining types account for less than 2%.[43,44] Types of prostate carcinoma include the following:

- Adenocarcinoma (small acinar and large duct types)
- Small-cell carcinoma
- Carcinosarcoma (sarcomatoid carcinoma)
- Transitional cell carcinoma
- Squamous cell carcinoma
- Mucinous (colloid) adenocarcinoma
- "Adenoid cystic or basaloid carcinoma"
- Lymphoepithelioma-like carcinoma
- Signet-ring cell carcinoma
- Adenosquamous carcinoma
- Undifferentiated carcinoma
- Metastatic carcinoma

Whereas the vast majority of prostate adenocarcinomas exhibit acinar differentiation (Figures 2–2, and 2–3), rare adenocarcinomas show true papillary and/or complex cribriform glandular patterns composed of tall pseudostratified epithelium.[45] This so-called prostatic duct or "large duct" pattern (Figure 2–4) can be mixed with acinar adenocarcinoma (~5% of cases) or pure (~1% of cases). Large duct adenocarcinomas of the prostate are thought to arise from or differentiate toward the larger, central prostate ducts. They often arise near the verumontanum. Because the verumontanum is considered a müllerian remnant and the large duct type of adenocarcinoma resembles those of endometrial origin, "large duct" adenocarcinomas of the prostate have wrongly been called endometrioid adenocarcinoma of the prostate.[45] However they are PSA and prostatic acid phosphatase (PAP) positive, and about one-third of large duct adenocarcinomas respond to estrogen therapy.[45] Most behave in an aggressive fashion with patients showing mean survivals of approximately 37 months.[46] Because of this aggressiveness, this author grades duct carcinoma as Gleason score 7 (3 + 4). Large duct adenocarcinomas with a cribriform pattern may be mistaken for cribriforming PIN; however, in contrast to cribriforming PIN, large duct adenocarcinomas have true papillae with fibrovascular cores, greater nuclear atypia, comedonecrosis, and/or slitlike rather than rounded lumens. Both lesions may have a preserved basal cell layer, as does benign clear cell cribriforming hyperplasia, which can mimic the cribriform variant of PIN and prostate carcinoma.[10] Unlike these latter lesions, benign clear cell cribriforming hyperplasia (Figure 2–5) has a distinctive clear cytoplasm and

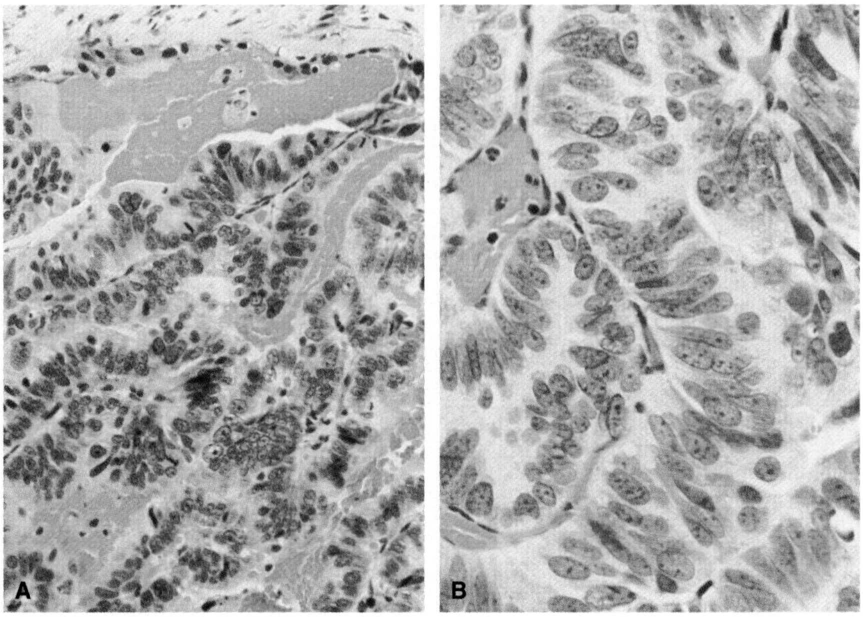

Figure 2–4. *A*, Large duct-type prostate carcinoma. Note delicate fibrous papillae lined by stratified malignant cells (hematoxylin and eosin; × 50 original magnification). *B*, Large duct-type prostate carcinoma. Note fibrous papillae lined by stratified malignant cells (hematoxylin and eosin; × 100 original magnification).

benign nuclei with inconspicuous nucleoli throughout, including next to the basal cell layer.

Small cell carcinoma of the prostate (Figure 2–6) has the same histology as small cell carcinomas of the lung, yet 50% are mixed with typical prostate acinar-type adenocarcinoma.[47,48] The small cell component may be PAP and PSA negative and contain neuroendocrine features (ie, neurosecretory granules by electron microscopy or reactivity with neuron-specific enolase).[47,48] Small cell carcinomas of the prostate are aggressive tumors; the average patient survival length is less than 1 year. The concomitant presence of a small acinar-type prostate adenocarcinoma does not alter the poor prognosis. Up to 47% of typical small acinar-type prostate adenocarcinomas will reveal neuroendocrine differentiation when studied with immunohistochemical techniques, and some may have a carcinoid-like appearance.[49] However, this neuroendocrine differentiation has not been found to have distinct clinicopathologic significance, and such tumors are best called prostate adenocarcinoma with neuroendocrine differentiation.[10]

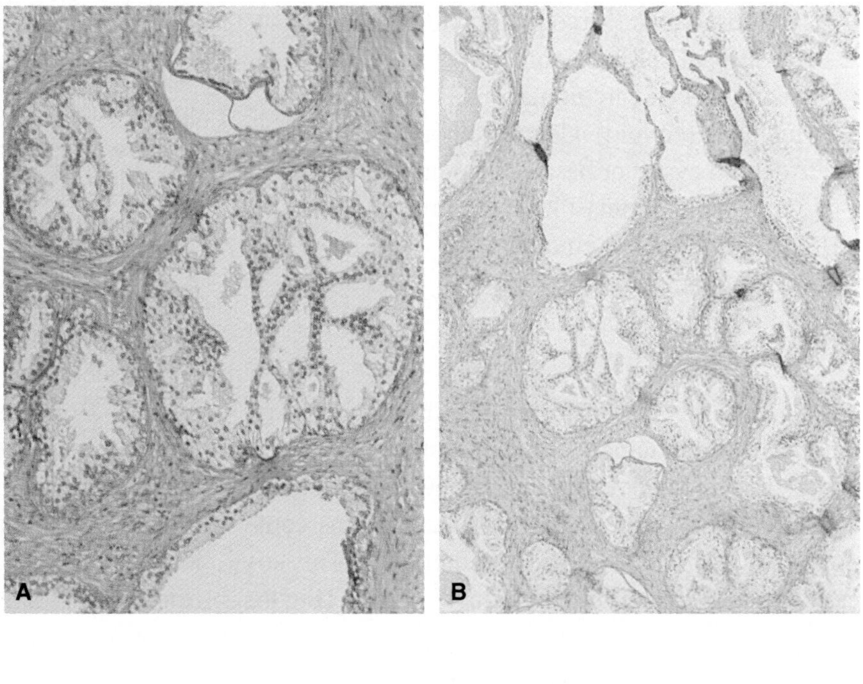

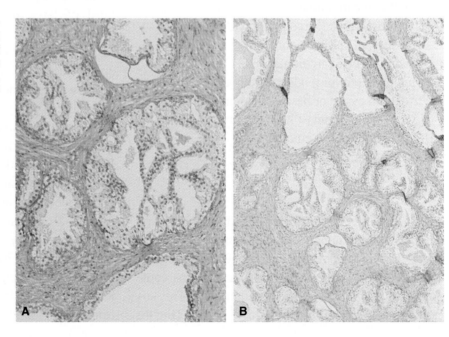

Figure 2–5. *A*, Clear cell cribriform hyperplasia. (hematoxylin and eosin; × 25 original magnification). *B*, Higher magnification of clear cell cribriform hyperplasia. Note the even rounded contours, cleared cytoplasm, and bland nuclear features (hematoxylin and eosin; × 50 original magnification).

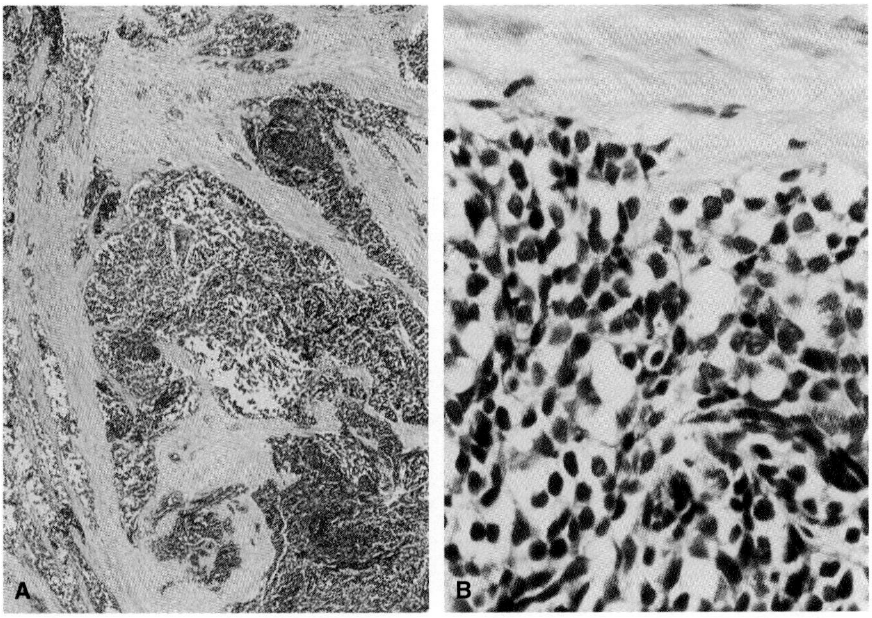

Figure 2–6. *A*, Shown are sheets of small cell undifferentiated prostate carcinoma. Note the intense dark blue staining cells (hematoxylin and eosin; × 25 original magnification). *B*, Small cell prostate carcinoma. Note that the cells are almost all nucleus with scant cytoplasm (hematoxylin and eosin; × 100 original magnification).

Carcinosarcoma is a rare tumor that exhibits both carcinomatous and sarcomatous differentiation (so-called sarcomatoid carcinoma).[43,44,50,51] The latter may be chondrosarcoma, osteosarcoma, myosarcoma, liposarcoma, and/or angiosarcoma. The clinicopathologic features of carcinosarcoma are similar to very poorly differentiated, acinar-type adenocarcinoma of the prostate. Mean survival is about 2 years.[43,44,51] These tumors most probably arise from metaplastic differentiation of a high-grade adenocarcinoma.[50] The carcinomatous components are PAP and PSA positive, whereas the sarcomatous components are negative for these markers.[50] Carcinosarcoma or sarcomatoid carcinoma need to be differentiated from primary prostatic stromal sarcomas and related phyllodis-like atypical stromal proliferations.[52–54]

Transitional cell carcinomas can arise within the periurethral region of the prostate.[55,56] They often present with obstruction, spread as transitional cell carcinoma in situ (Figure 2–7) along prostate ducts, metastasize early after invasion, and are associated with a poor prognosis.[44] More commonly, transitional cell

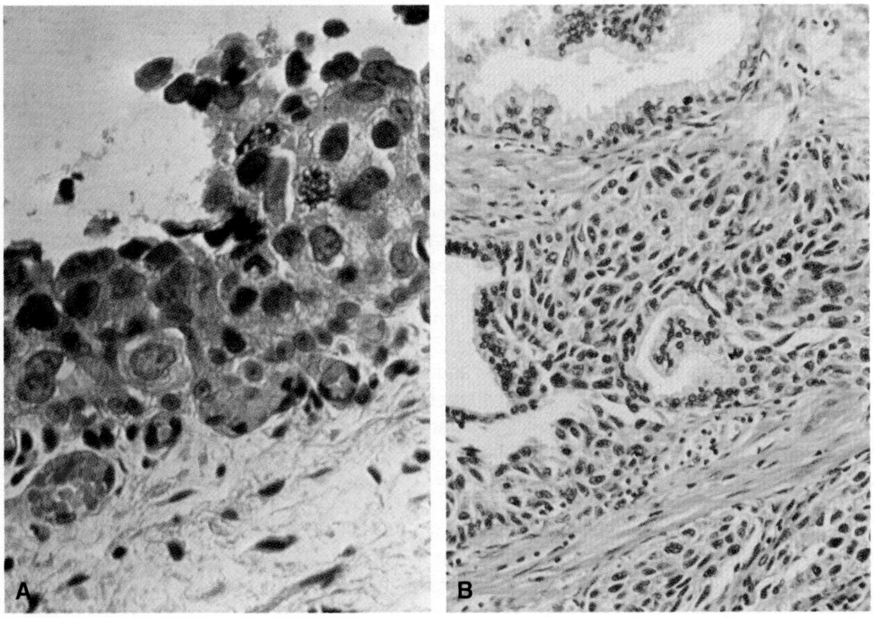

Figure 2–7. *A*, Transitional cell carcinoma in situ extending into the bladder neck from the bladder (hematoxylin and eosin; × 100 original magnification). *B*, Transitional cell carcinoma in situ is shown extending under and replacing benign prostate epithelium (hematoxylin and eosin; × 100 original magnification).

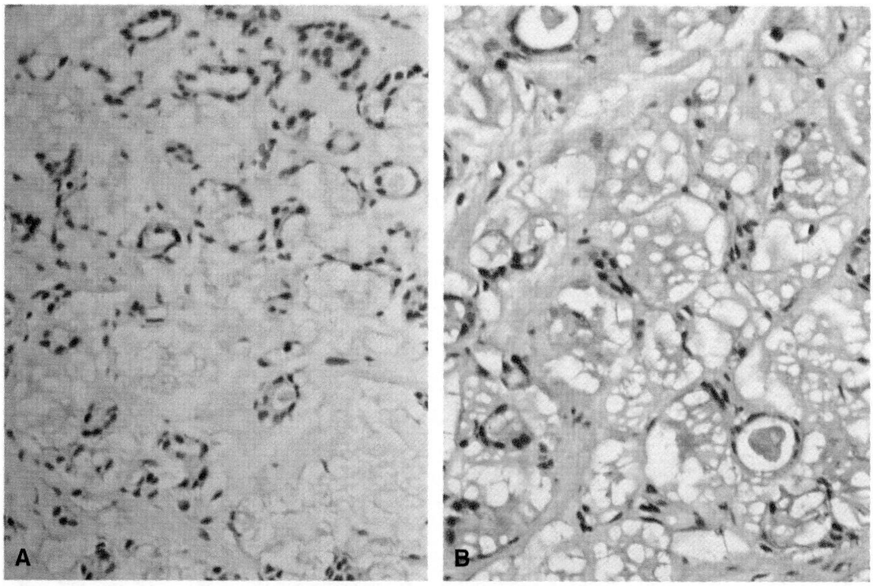

Figure 2–8. *A*, Mucin-producing prostate carcinoma is shown with small glands floating within a "sea" of mucin (hematoxylin and eosin; × 50 original magnification). *B*, Same mucin-producing prostate carcinoma is shown with mucicarminophilic mucin (mucicarmine stain; × 50 original magnification).

carcinoma of the prostate occurs with concomitant or prior bladder transitional cell carcinoma.[43] Some data indicate at least a 20% incidence of prostate involvement in primary bladder carcinoma,[5,56] an association which makes assessment of the prostate-bladder neck margin important in determining the completeness of the resection for bladder carcinoma.

Primary squamous cell carcinoma of the prostate is very rare and is associated with poor survival.[57,58] These tumors do not respond to estrogens or react with antibodies to PAP or PSA.[57,58] They should not be confused with estrogen-treated prostate adenocarcinomas, which may develop squamous metaplasia following therapy. Rarely, some prostate carcinomas will show combined squamous and glandular differentiation; a combination referred to as adenosquamous carcinoma.

Mucinous adenocarcinoma of the prostate (Figure 2–8) is uncommon and should not be diagnosed unless malignant glands appear to "float in a sea" of mucin,[59] a pattern that must be diffuse and comprise at least 25% of the tumor area.[10] From 60 to 90% of small acinar-type adenocarcinoma of the prostate secrete intraluminal epithelial mucin. This can be seen in a standard hematoxylin and eosin stain (see Figure 2–2), but it is best determined by alcian-blue staining at pH = 2.5 or with mucicarmine. This finding can help in making a definitive diagnosis of malignancy since benign prostate epithelium uncommonly produces intraluminal mucin.[60] Mucinous adenocarcinomas of the prostate tend not to respond to hormonal therapy and follow an aggressive course. Rare signet-ring adenocarcinomas occur in the prostate and are epithelial-mucin negative and positive for PSA and PAP.[61]

So-called adenoid cystic carcinomas of the prostate show some resemblance to the same tumors

Table 2–3. HISTOPATHOLOGIC FEATURES SUGGESTING PROSTATE ADENOCARCINOMA

- Small glands (relatively uniform) infiltrating between benign glands
- Cytoarchitectural features of malignant glands contrast sharply with benign glands and do not show admixed glands having transitional or intermediate features
- Prominent nucleoli (but may be absent) within relatively enlarged, rounded nuclei (but may be small)
- Well-developed amphophilic cytoplasm (but may be clear, granular, or eosinophilic)
- Some adenocarcinomas have voluminous, xanthomatous cytoplasm with small, round, and bland nuclei and pink luminal secretions
- Adenocarcinoma lumens may be prominent and have even straight intraluminal edges without epithelial enfoldings
- Dense, pink intraluminal secretions and/or crystalloids suggest adenocarcinoma
- Intraluminal basophilic secretions, which are mucicarminophilic and/or alcian blue positive, suggest adenocarcinoma and are found in approximately 70% of cases. But both intercellular and/or intracellular mucin may be focal in benign glands (the latter also known as mucinous metaplasia)
- Mitotic figures and perineural invasion are highly suggestive of adenocarcinoma
- Caution is always indicated when atrophy and/or inflammation are present
- The final diagnosis of prostate adenocarcinoma should be based on finding a number of mutually supportive histopathologic features rather than a single feature

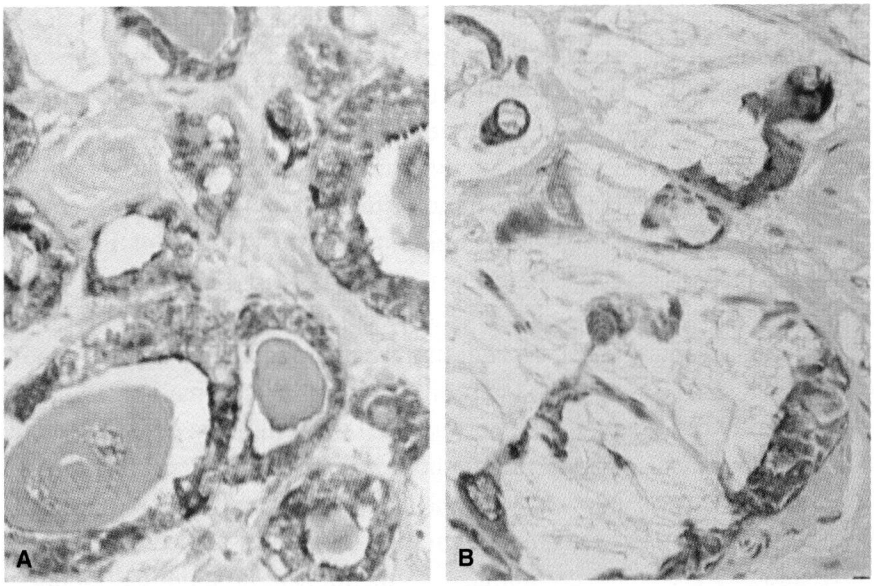

Figure 2–9. *A*, Prostate carcinoma glands are shown immunostaining for prostate-specific antigen (hematoxylin and eosin; × 50 original magnification). *B*, Prostate carcinoma cells are shown immunostaining for prostatic acid phosphatase (hematoxylin and eosin; × 50 original magnification).

of the salivary glands. They do not express PAP or PSA and have a very good prognosis since no metastases have thus far been reported.[62–67] Adenoid cystic carcinoma of the prostate is extraordinarily rare.[67] It has also been called basaloid carcinoma of the prostate, and in this author's view, adenoid cystic or basaloid carcinoma of the prostate is likely an atypical, floridly proliferative, and/or cribriforming example of benign basal cell hyperplasia.[62–67] Yet, others believe that a true basaloid carcinoma exists.[68]

Metastatic carcinoma to the prostate is uncommon; most cases have been from primary lung carcinomas.[43,44] Leukemia/lymphoma infiltrates (ie, usually chronic lymphocytic leukemia) and metastatic melanoma are more common secondary tumors of the prostate.[43,44] Many pathologists have had the experience of finding chronic lymphocytic leukemia in prostate specimens.

HISTOLOGIC DIAGNOSIS OF PROSTATIC ADENOCARCINOMA

The majority of invasive prostate adenocarcinomas are multifocal lesions within peripheral lobules. They

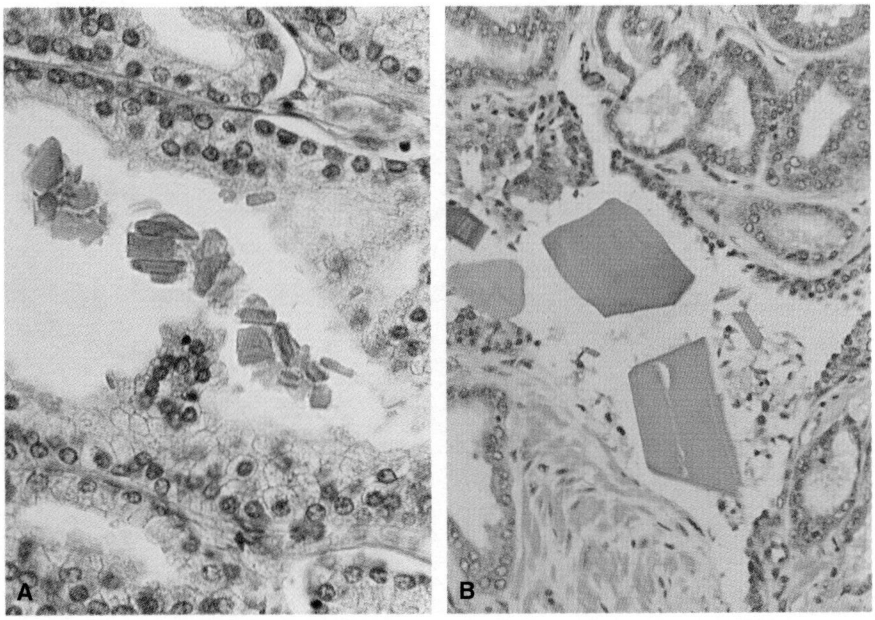

Figure 2–10. *A* and *B*, Prostate carcinoma. Note eosinophilic crystalloids within the glandular lumens. They show sharp angulated borders (hematoxylin and eosin; × 50 original magnification).

are infiltrating adenocarcinomas that lack a lobular pattern; they grow in sheets, cords, or small rounded to irregular glands (see Figures 2–2 and 2–3; and Table 2–3). These tumors (especially those poorly differentiated) have enlarged, rounded nuclei with prominent nucleoli. Tumor cell cytoplasm is variably granular and usually amphophilic but may be either eosinophilic, basophilic, xanthomatous, and/or vacuolated. Mixed patterns are frequent. Very poorly differentiated tumors are usually easily diagnosed but may be mistaken for granulomatous prostatitis in some cases; likewise, granulomatous prostatitis can mimic poorly differentiated adenocarcinoma. The latter distinction can be made with immunohistochemical stains for cytokeratin, PAP, and/or PSA.[69] Tumor cells are positive for keratin, PAP, and/or PSA (Figure 2–9), whereas epithelioid histiocytes are negative for these same markers.

The typical small acinar adenocarcinoma of the prostate is composed of small acini lined by a single layer of tall columnar or cuboidal cells with well-developed cytoplasm[10,43,44] (see Figures 2–2 and 2–3 and Table 2–3). In the better differentiated examples, there is marked uniformity of gland patterns within a microscopic area. Malignant glands have a rigid structure, and their luminal borders are uniform or sharply outlined. There is little tendency for them to be convoluted or to have branched luminal patterns. Nuclei are usually located in a single row next to the basement membrane, and they are different from those of adjacent benign nuclei. Nucleoli are usually, but not always, prominent; there is no apparent connection to benign glands, and corpora amylacea are almost never present within acini; and the growth pattern is random or haphazard (ie, invasive). Prostate adenocarcinomas contain eosinophilic, luminal crystalloids in 25 to 60% of cases (especially lower-grade tumors) (Figure 2–10), but they may also be present in about 10% of glands lined by PIN and in about 4% of benign hyperplastic glands.[10,43,44] When crystalloids are found in benign glands, a thorough and careful search for nearby malignant glands should be performed. If no malignant cells are found, consideration should be given to a repeat biospy. In one study, repeat biopsy after initially finding crystaloids in benign prostate glands, proved to have adenocarcinoma.[70] As mentioned, intraluminal mucin is found in 60 to 90% of cases of prostate adenocarcinoma, but PIN may be associated with luminal mucin; benign prostate glands rarely show luminal mucin (especially in some ectatic atrophic glands). Benign intraepithelial mucinous metaplasia can occur focally and should not be confused with invasive prostate adenocarcinoma or PIN.[10,43,44] Positive immunohistochemical staining of basal cells for high-molecular-weight keratin (HMWK) around suspicious glands almost always rules out invasive adenocarcinoma (Figure 2–11). However, negative staining for HMWK around suspicious glands does not always indicate that adenocarcinoma is present because HMWK staining in benign glands can be patchy and absent in a small, benign biopsy speci-

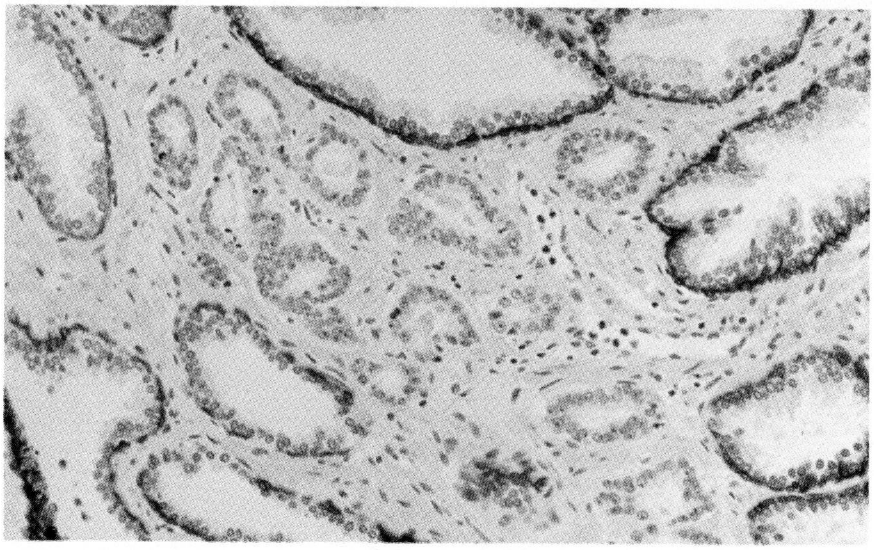

Figure 2–11. Shown are benign prostate glands rimmed by brown-staining basal cells, which have immunoreacted with antibody to high molecular weight keratin. Centrally, small acinar carcinoma cells are shown without a corresponding rim of basal cells (peroxidase antiperoxidase immunohistochemistry technique with diaminobenzidine as substrate; × 25 original magnification).

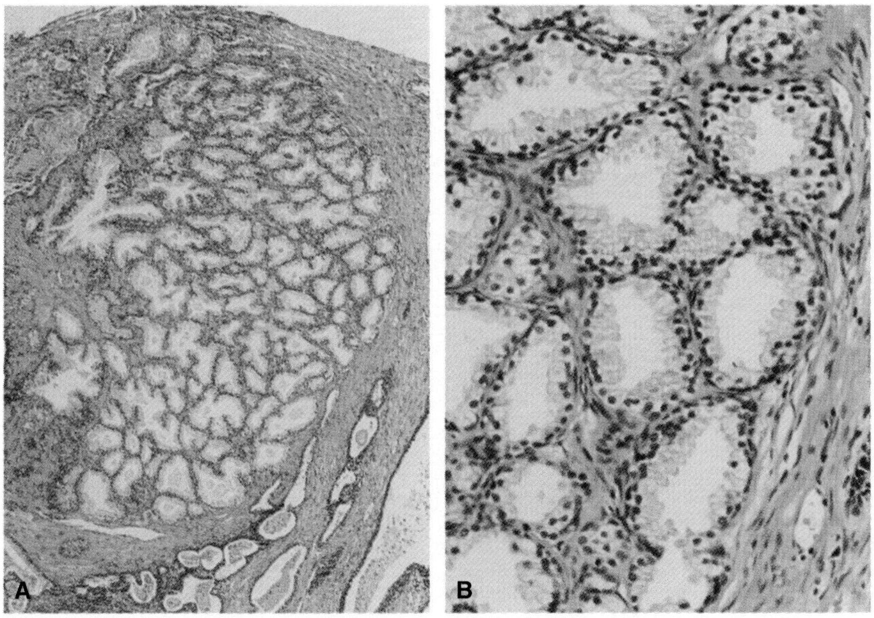

Figure 2–12. *A*, Adenosis or atypical adenomatous hyperplasia. Note the compact grouping of benign-appearing prostate glands (hematoxylin and eosin; × 10 original magnification). *B*, Shown are the details of benign-appearing adenosis glands (hematoxylin and eosin; × 100 original magnification).

men.[10,43,44] Indeed, the final diagnosis of prostate adenocarcinoma should always be based on finding a number of mutually supportive histopathologic features rather than on just a single feature.

The criteria for diagnosing prostate carcinoma in small-needle biopsy specimens are no different than the criteria for diagnosing carcinoma in large specimens, except that the diagnostic process is performed on smaller tissue samples, wherein invasive patterns, which are best appreciated in larger samples at lower magnification, are more difficult to appreciate. Thus, cytologic features of prostate carcinoma assume greater diagnostic importance in needle biopsies, and tiny foci of carcinoma of the prostate should not be diagnosed unless the cytologic criteria of malignancy are clearly met. Yet atypical foci should be noted as suspicious but not diagnostic of adenocarcinoma and additional biopsies recommended. These atypical foci can be diagnosed as "atypical small acinar proliferations (ASAP), suspicious but not diagnostic for malignancy." The high predictive value of ASAP for sub-

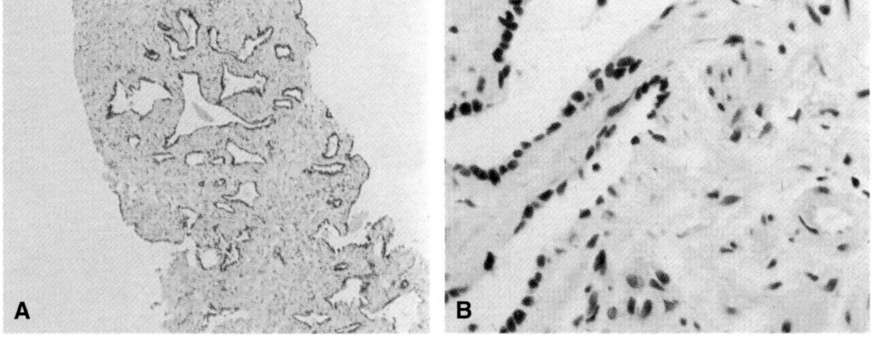

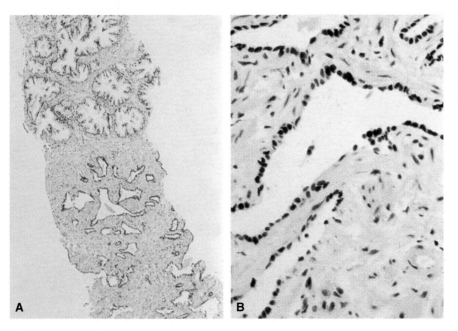

Figure 2–13. *A*, Shown is a patch of glandular atrophy covering the bottom half of the needle prostate biopsy (hematoxylin and eosin; × 10 original magnification). *B*, Note the flattened or attenuated epithelium of glandular atrophy (hematoxylin and eosin; × 100 original magnification).

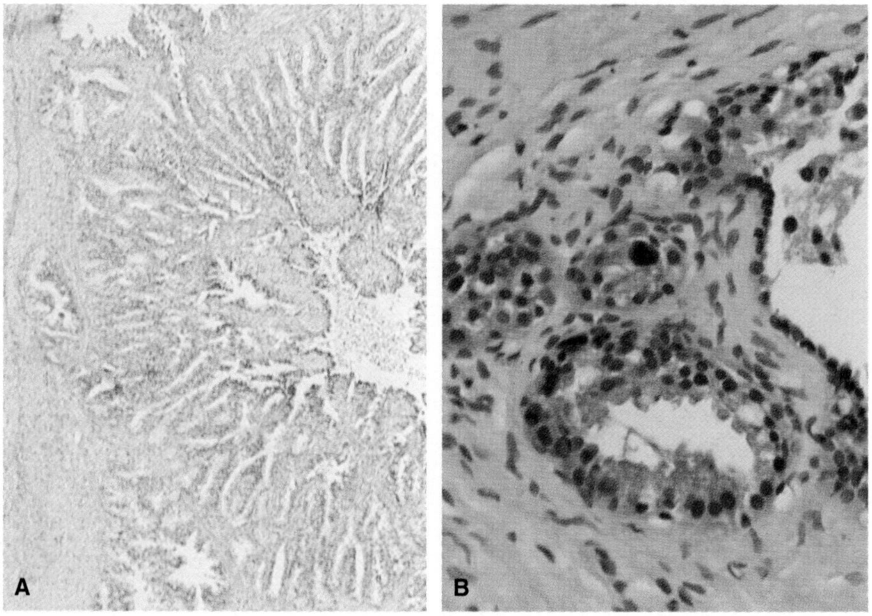

Figure 2–14. *A*, Seminal vesicle is shown (hematoxylin and eosin; × 5 original magnification). *B*, Seminal vesicle epithelium. Note enlarged dark nuclei and golden-brown pigment within cytoplasm (hematoxylin and eosin; × 100 original magnification).

sequent carcinoma warrants repeat biopsy. The problem is confounded by some clear-cut prostate adenocarcinomas having areas resembling benign hyperplasia. Immunohistochemistry with antibodies against high molecular weight cytokeratins are helpful in this difficult case.[71–74] If these additional biopsies fail to reveal clear-cut carcinoma, then continued clinical surveillance is indicated. If a carcinoma has been missed after multiple biopsies, it is likely small, well differentiated, and less likely to cause serious harm to the patient.

DIFFERENTIAL DIAGNOSIS OF PROSTATIC ADENOCARCINOMA

The differential diagnosis of small acinar-type adenocarcinoma includes nodular adenosis (also known as atypical adenomatous hyperplasia [AAH]), sclerosing adenosis, glandular atrophy, seminal vesicle epithelium, basal cell hyperplasia, verumontanum mucosal gland hyperplasia, mesonephric remnant hyperplasia, nephrogenic metaplasia or adenoma, benign clear cell hyperplasia with cribriforming,

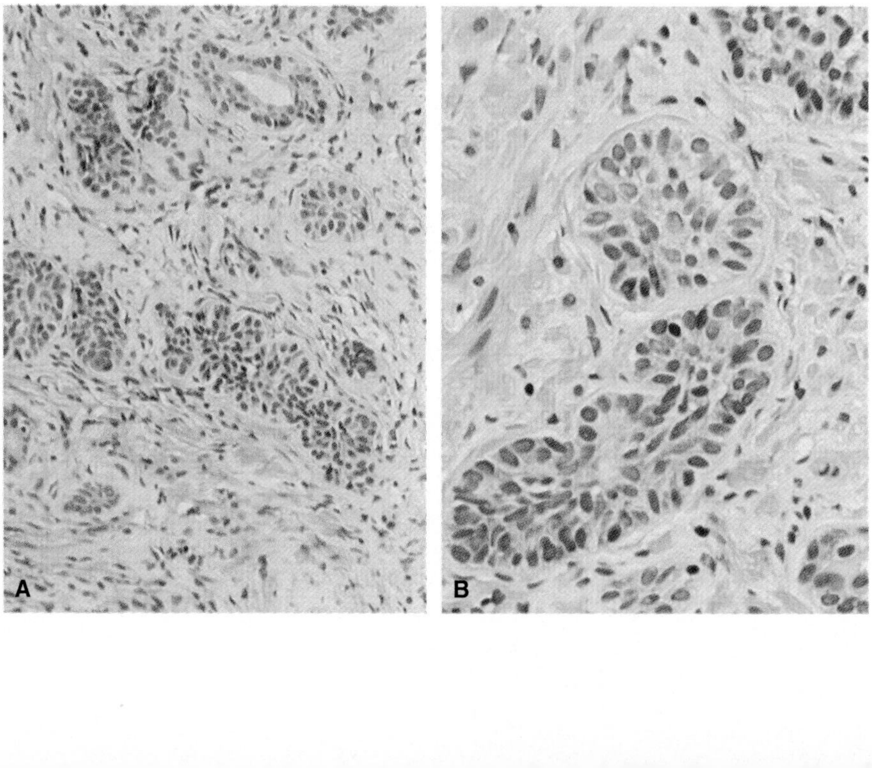

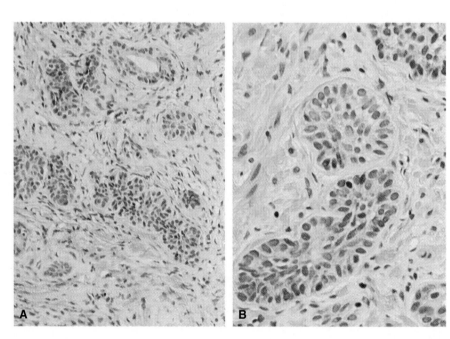

Figure 2–15. *A*, Basal-cell hyperplasia. Note prostate glands replaced by proliferation of relatively dark epithelial cells (hematoxylin and eosin; × 25 original magnification). *B*, Basal cell hyperplasia of prostate glands (hematoxylin and eosin; × 100 original magnification).

radiation-induced atypia, PIN, and other carcinoma types.[10,43,44,62–67,75,76] Nodular adenosis or AAH (Figure 2–12) consists of a lobulocentric growth of crowded, relatively small glands, which are focally admixed with more typically sized and branching benign glands. Like the typical benign glands, the adenosis glands often have irregular or branching luminal borders with papillary enfoldments, pale-clear cytoplasm, small nuclei with inconspicuous nucleoli, and focally identifiable, yet patchy, basal cells. Nodular adenosis tends to occur centrally and appears in TUR specimens rather than in needle biopsy specimens. The relationship of adenosis or atypical adenomatous hyperplasia with adenocarcinoma remains controversial. Yet, there are morphologic and some cytogenetic data suggesting a relationship to low-grade (Gleason patterns 1 and 2) adenocarcinoma arising in the transition zone.[77–80] Sclerosing adenosis is a rare variant wherein lobulocentric and closely packed small glands are separated by spindled epithelial cells or by a thick hyaline basement membrane-like material.[75,81] Sclerosing adenosis of the prostate shows a pseudoinfiltrative pattern and superficially resembles the so-called adenomatoid tumor. The spindled cells of sclerosing adenosis tend toward myoepithelial differentiation (ie, HMWK, muscle actin, and S-100 protein positive), a combination that is not seen in normal human prostatic basal cells.[82] Nevertheless, in a small number of cases this differential diagnosis remains impossible even after immunohistochemical stains are attempted. Also, at present there appears to be no relationship between sclerosing adenosis and increased risk of carcinoma.[83] Glandular atrophy (Figure 2–13) is composed of patches, discrete areas, and/or lobulocentric groups of branching glands lined by low epithelial cells containing small dark nuclei without atypia. Postatrophic hyperplasia of the prostate often has overlapping histologic features with prostate adenocarcinoma, including small acinar growth and enlarged nuclei with prominent nucleoli. Indeed, some data suggest a relationship. Moreover, cases of clear-cut prostate carcinoma reported within areas resembling atrophy have been described.[84–86] Seminal vesicle epithelium (Figure 2–14) contains crowded small glands situated adjacent to a large open central lumen lined by identical cells. Seminal vesicle glandular cells are negative for PSA and PAP; contain deposits of chunky, golden-brown lipofuscin pigment; and display large, variably sized, atypical nuclei with dark chromatin that appears degenerative and obscures nuclear detail. Ironically, nuclei of acinar adenocarcinoma cells tend not to be as large, as hyperchromatic, or as variable as those found in seminal vesicle glands. Remember that prostate glands can also have granular lipofuscin pigment and red brown-staining lysosomal granules.[10] Basal cell hyperplasia may be a

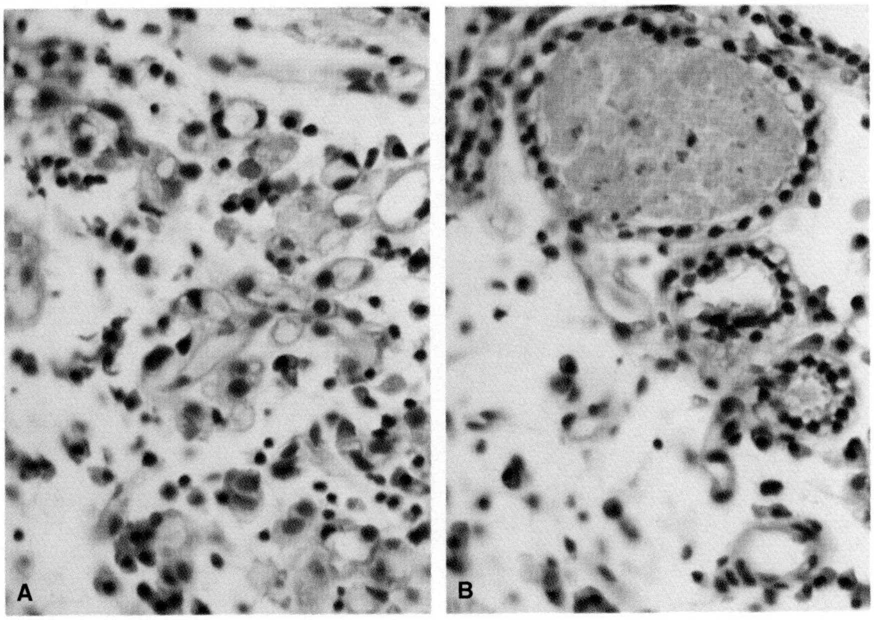

Figure 2–16. *A*, Mesonephric metaplasia. Note small vacuolated cells (hematoxylin and eosin; × 100 original magnification). *B*, Mesonephric metaplasia. Note ectactic gland composed of low cuboidal cells (hematoxylin and eosin; × 100 original magnification).

focal microscopic finding, form a nodule with fibrotic stroma, or have a diffusely infiltrative character.[64–66] Basal cell hyperplasia (Figure 2–15) is characterized by prostate glands variably replaced by multiple layers of basal cells (ie, HMWK positive), which have increased nuclear-to-cytoplasmic ratios and show peripheral palisading. Cytoplasm is usually scant, but it can also be abundant and clear, and nuclei can be enlarged, contain nucleoli, and show mitotic figures (ie, atypical basal cell hyperplasia).[67] The replacement of normal prostatic glands is variable, extending from those with retained lumens to solid nests or cribriform patterns of basaloid cells. When these lesions have been associated with prominent stromal fibrosis, atypical nuclei, and a diffusely infiltrative pattern, the author suspects that at least some of them were reported as being adenoid cystic carcinoma[67] or basaloid carcinoma. No metastases have been reported.[62–65] Florid hyperplasia of mesonephric remnants occurs very rarely at the prostate base and in periprostatic tissues[67,75] (Figure 2–16). As in the female urogenital tract, mesonephric remnants present as a proliferation of lobulocentric tubules lined by a single layer of epithelium with prominent nucleoli and containing the characteristic colloid-like material. Mesonephric remnants are negative for PAP and PSA. These mesonephric tubules may infiltrate perineural spaces. Nephrogenic metaplasia or adenoma most often presents as an exophytic lesion protruding into the urethral lumen or confined to the immediate suburethral connective tissues. But, rarely, the glands of nephrogenic metaplasia will extend to involve the central prostate. Like sclerosing adenosis, the glands of nephrogenic metaplasia have an adenomatoid tumor look; indeed, this change has been called adenomatoid metaplasia of the urethra. Nephrogenic metaplasia glands are lined by cells showing varying combinations of cuboidal, hobnail, and endothelial-like morphologies. Nucleoli are usually not conspicuous, but if doubt remains, nephrogenic metaplasia is negative for PAP and PSA.[67]

Radiation-induced atypia and PIN will be covered below; benign clear cell, cribriforming hyperplasia has already been mentioned. The diagnosis of small cell carcinoma, carcinosarcoma, transitional cell carcinoma, prostatic large duct adenocarcinoma, squamous cell carcinoma, and mucinous adenocarcinoma depends on familiarity with the histopathology of these tumors as they present in the prostate and/or in other organs, where some occur more commonly. They should not present major difficulties if they are considered in a differential diagnosis of an unusual tumor in the prostate.

IMMUNOLOGIC MARKERS

Immunohistochemical staining of prostate adenocarcinoma with PAP and/or PSA is a highly sensitive (99%) and reliable method of showing prostate epithelial differentiation[75] (see Figure 2–9). Both are strongly expressed in benign and malignant prostate epithelium. Whereas PSA tends to be more specific,

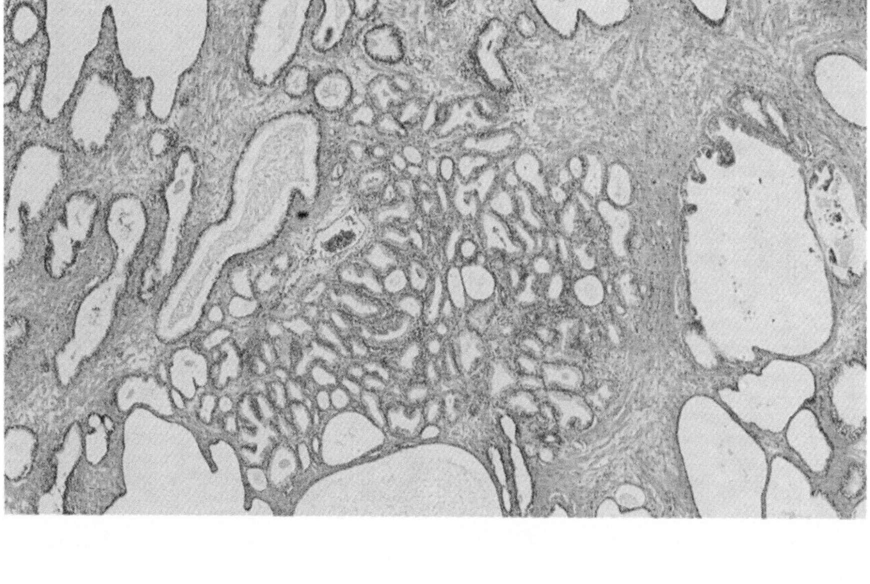

Figure 2–17. Invasive prostate carcinoma, Gleason pattern 1. A circumscribed nodule of uniform, single, separate, closely packed glands (hematoxylin and eosin; × 5 original magnification).

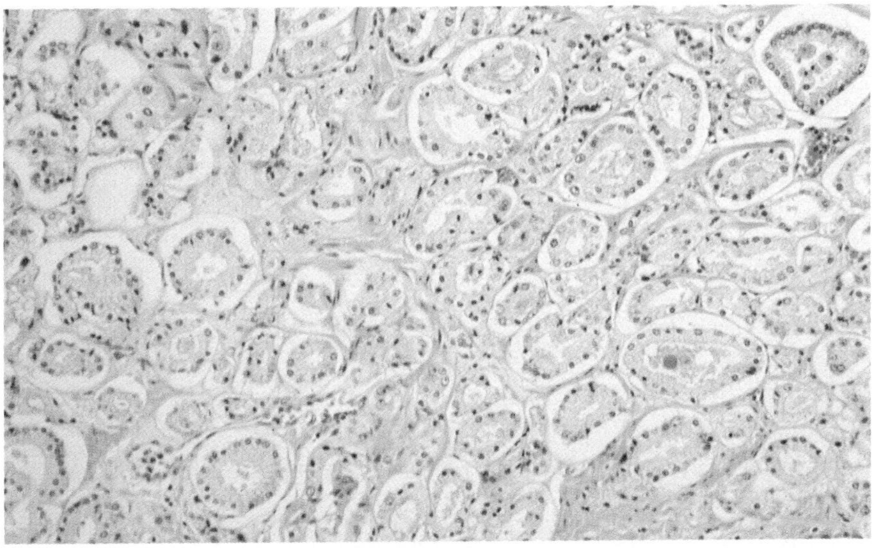

Figure 2–18. Invasive prostate carcinoma, Gleason pattern 2. Fairly circumscribed nodule with minimal extension of tumor glands into benign prostate tissues. Glands are single and separated by stroma and more loosely arranged than in pattern 1 (hematoxylin and eosin; × 25 original magnification).

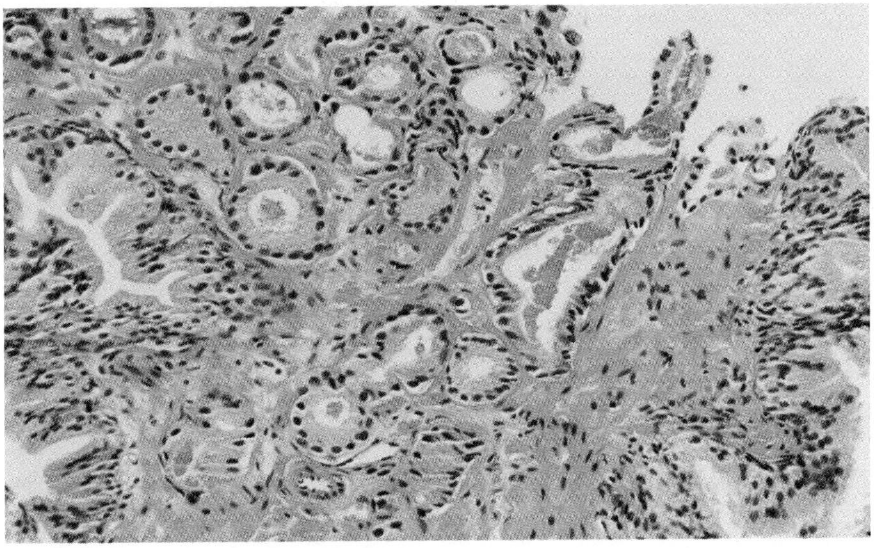

Figure 2–19. Invasive prostate carcinoma, Gleason pattern 3. Tumor glands infiltrate in and among the benign prostate glands, with the glands having marked variation in size and shape. Many glands are smaller than those of patterns 1 and 2 (hematoxylin and eosin; × 25 original magnification).

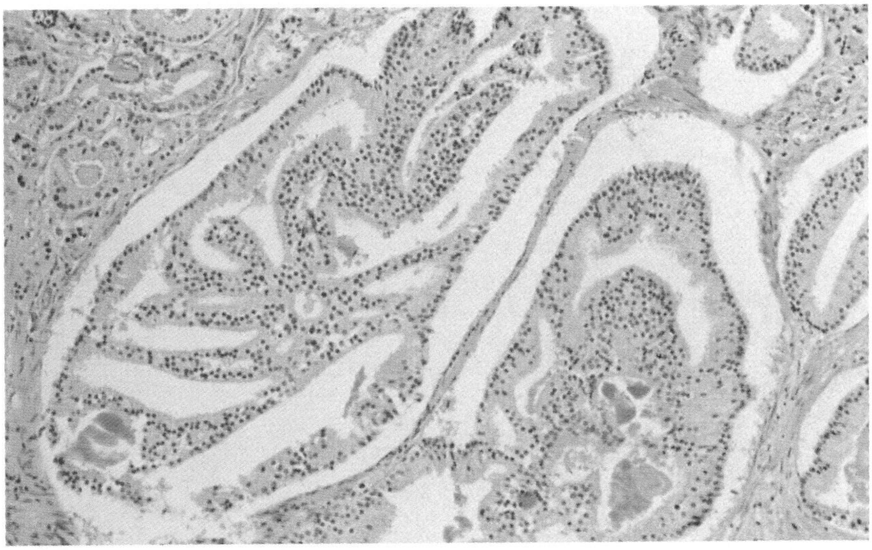

Figure 2–20. Invasive prostate carcinoma, Gleason pattern 3. Smoothly circumscribed cribriform nodules are consistent with pattern 3 (hematoxylin and eosin; × 25 original magnification).

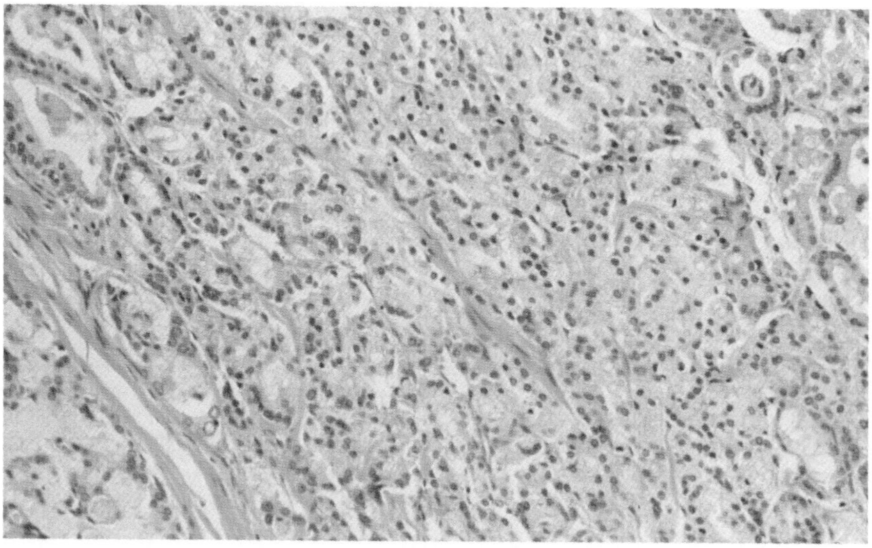

Figure 2–21. Invasive prostate carcinoma, Gleason pattern 4. Tumor glands are fused (ie, glands are no longer separate as in patterns 1, 2, and 3 (hematoxylin and eosin; × 25 original magnification).

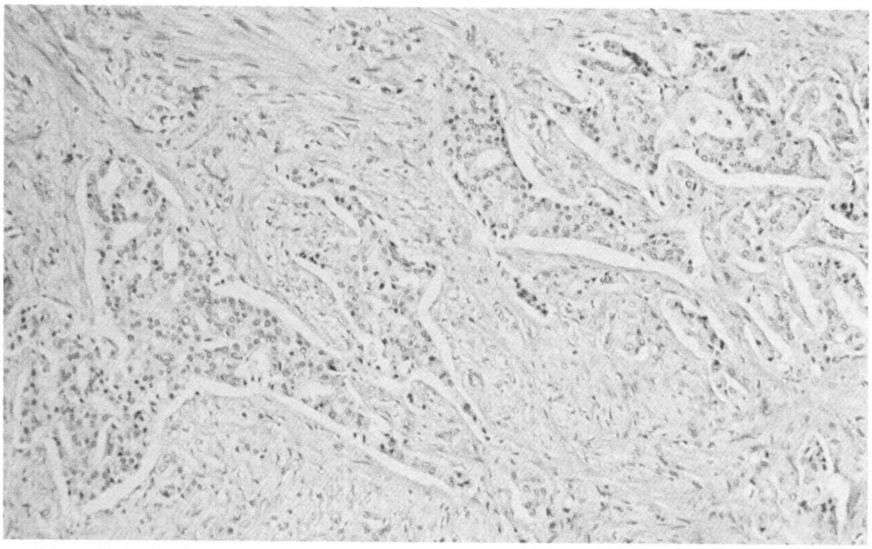

Figure 2–22. Invasive prostate carcinoma, Gleason pattern 4. Ragged infiltrating edges (hematoxylin and eosin; × 25 original magnification).

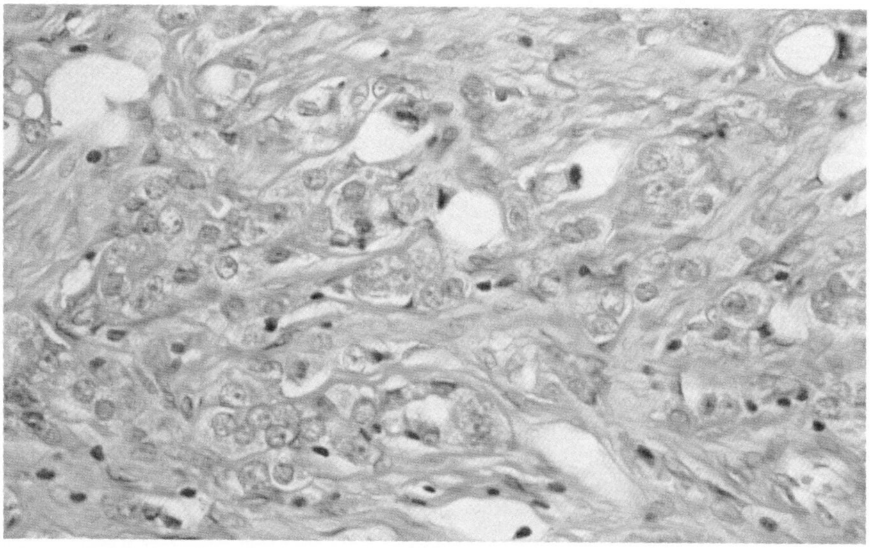

Figure 2–23. Invasive prostate carcinoma, Gleason pattern 5. Tumor shows no glandular differentiation with solid masses of cells (hematoxylin and eosin; × 25 original magnification).

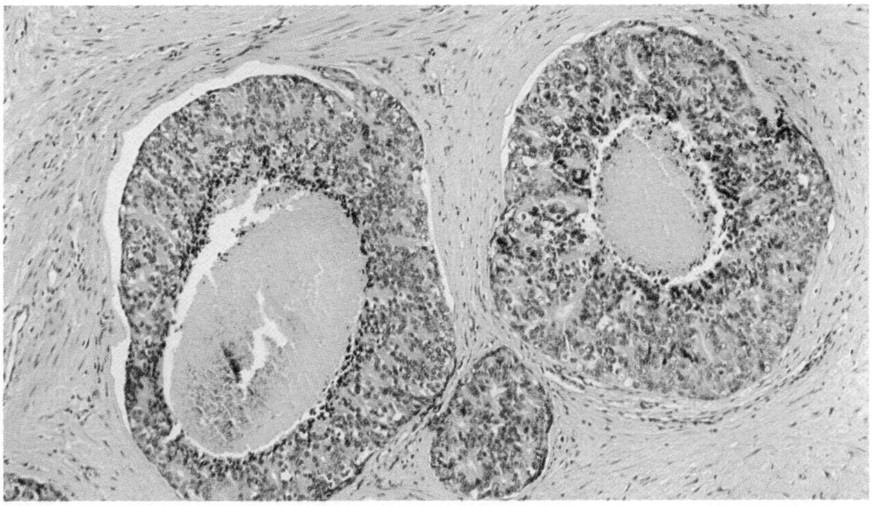

Figure 2–24. Invasive prostate carcinoma, Gleason pattern 5 with infiltrating tumor nests showing a central comedolike necrosis pattern (hematoxylin and eosin; × 25 original magnification).

PAP is slightly more sensitive.[10,43,44] Virtually all properly fixed and immunostained, low- to intermediate-grade prostate adenocarcinomas will stain with both PAP or PSA, but 5 to 10% of poorly differentiated prostate adenocarcinomas that lack glandular differentiation will show no immunoreactivity with one of the two antibodies; hence, the best results occur when both are used concomitantly.[10,43,44] Also, poorly differentiated tumors may contain only foci of reactivity (as few as 1% of cells positive). As a result, small biopsies may lead to a false negative diagnosis.[10,43,44] Besides prostate adenocarcinoma, PAP has been reported to react weakly with breast adenocarcinoma and renal cell adenocarcinoma and strongly with bladder adenocarcinomas and intestinal carcinoids. Some antibodies for PAP will also react with granulocytes, islet cells, gastric parietal cells, and hepatocytes.[10,43,44] Nonspecific PSA staining with nonprostatic adenocarcinomas is rare and anecdotal, yet weak focal immunostaining with either PAP or PSA should be interpreted with caution.[10,43,44] Currently, PSA appears to be the superior reagent, but it is fortunate that prostate adenocarcinoma only very rarely metastasizes to salivary glands because salivary gland tumors can immunoreact with antibodies to PSA and PAP.[87] Finally, PSA and PAP immunoreactivity has also been variably noted in cystitis cystica et glandularis, periurethral glands, perianal glands, and urachal remnants.[10]

Table 2–4. GLEASON GRADING SYSTEM

Pattern 1	A circumscribed nodule of uniform, single, separate, closely packed glands
Pattern 2	Fairly circumscribed nodule with minimal extension of tumor glands into benign prostate tissues. Glands are single and separated by stroma and more loosely arranged than in pattern 1
Pattern 3	Tumor glands infiltrate in and among the benign prostate glands, with the glands having marked variation in size and shape. Many glands are smaller than those of patterns 1 and 2. Smoothly circumscribed cribriform nodules are consistent with pattern 3*
Pattern 4	Tumor glands are fused with ragged infiltrating edges (ie, glands are no longer separate as in patterns 1, 2, and 3)
Pattern 5	Tumor shows no glandular differentiation with either solid masses of cells or individually infiltrating cells or tumor nests with central comedolike necrosis

*If on needle biopsy the tumor glands are seen infiltrating between benign prostate glands, the tumor is scored 3 + 3 = 6, even though only a few glands are present. If the glands are more open, larger, and uniform than a core of 6 would justify, yet still infiltrative between benign glands, then a score of 5 is given. If the same infiltrative pattern is present, but there is some loss of discrete glandular differentiation, then a score of 7 is given.[9]

Poorly differentiated transitional cell carcinoma of the bladder involving the prostate may be mistaken for poorly differentiated prostate adenocarcinoma. Immunohistochemical studies can be very helpful in making a clear distinction. Prostate adenocarcinomas show immunoreactivity for PSA, PAP, and low-molecular-weight keratin (LMWKC)

Table 2–5. INCIDENCE OF LYMPH NODE METASTASES AS PREDICTED BY GLEASON SCORE

Gleason Score	Range (%)	Mean (%)
2–4	0–27	12
5–7	10–54	35
8–10	26–93	61

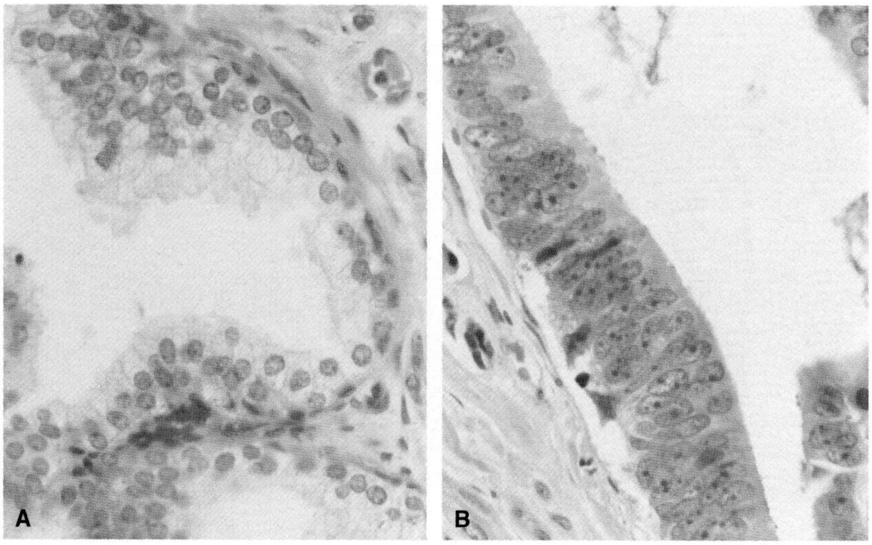

Figure 2–25. *A*, Normal hyperplastic prostate epithelium is shown (hematoxylin and eosin; × 100 original magnification). *B*, Prostatic intraepithelial neoplasia is present. Note "darker" epithelium and nuclear crowding (hematoxylin and eosin; × 100 original magnification).

reagents; they are negative for carcinoembryonic antigen (CEA) (especially when using the monoclonal antibodies) and HMWKs. In contrast, transitional cell carcinomas immunoreact with CEA (~90%) and both LMWK and HMWK reagents; they are negative for PSA and PAP. Additional studies have shown that prostate carcinomas are less likely to stain for cytokeratins 7 and 20; whereas, urothelial carcinomas are much more likely to stain consistently and strongly for cytokeratins 7 and 20.[88]

HISTOLOGIC GRADING

Prostate adenocarcinomas project a spectrum of differentiation that allows relatively accurate grading, which is helpful in predicting prognosis and optimizing therapy.[89] Although arguments persist over which method is best, several grading schemes have been developed, and all appear to work when applied by an experienced pathologist.[89] Yet, the Gleason protocol is by far the most widely used and accepted.[10,43,44,90]

The Gleason system is the most widely accepted grading system. Many studies in the literature have attested to this system's reproducibility, reliability, and prognostic value.[10,43,44,90] The Gleason system recognizes five growth patterns of invasive adenocarcinoma representing a progressive scale of decreasing glandular differentiation and more undifferentiated, disorganized growth (Figures 2–17 through 2–24 and Table 2–4). Traditionally, Gleason scores of 2 to 4 have been equivalent to well-differentiated (low—grade 1) adenocarcinomas; 5 to 7, moderately differentiated (intermediate—grade 2) adenocarcinomas; and 8 to 10, poorly differentiated (high—grade 3) adenocarcinomas. However, Epstein presents evidence that a Gleason score of 7 should be considered a moderate to poorly differentiated (high-grade) prostate adenocarcinoma.[10] This becomes very important in accurate staging, wherein all high-grade adenocarcinomas are considered by some to be at least stage T1b, regardless of tumor volume.

A variety of histologic patterns within an individual tumor are frequently seen in prostate adeno-

Table 2–6. HISTOLOGIC GRADING OF PROSTATE INTRAEPITHELIAL NEOPLASIA

PIN Grade	Architecture	Nuclei	Nucleoli
I—low grade	Crowding, stratification, intact basal layer	Variable size	Rare
II—high grade	Similar to PIN I; increased crowding; may have basal cell layer disruption	Variable size, prominent	Present; may be large
III—high grade	Similar to PIN II; may be cribriform; frequent basal cell layer disruption	Enlarged, prominent	Frequent, large

PIN = prostate intraepithelial neoplasia.

carcinoma. This variability is incorporated in the final grade by adding the pattern number of the major and minor patterns. The major pattern by area is listed first and then the minor pattern (eg, Gleason 5 + 4 or a total score of 9). In contrast to other systems, the Gleason system is based on invasive patterns and examination at low magnification. It does not include an assessment of cytologic atypia, although increasing cytologic atypia correlates very well with increasing Gleason grade. The Gleason system can also be applied to needle biopsies of the prostate, but there is a tendency to undergrade compared with the final grade determined from examining the radical prostatectomy specimen.[91]

The Gleason system can be used to predict the presence of pelvic lymph node metastases (Table 2–5). For Gleason scores 2 to 4 (well differentiated), there is an approximately 12% incidence of nodal metastases; for scores 5 to 7 (moderately differentiated), there is about a 35% incidence; and for scores 8 to 10 (poorly differentiated), there is about a 61% incidence.[10,43,44,90] Gleason grading has also been shown to correlate with capsular and seminal vesicle invasion.[10,43,44,90] Gleason score can be combined with serum PSA at diagnosis, clinical tumor stage, and the percentage of positive biopsies to predict pathologic tumor stage and outcome after local therapy (see Chapters 7 and 10).

Screening programs have increased the number of prostate adenocarcinomas diagnosed by needle biopsy, and many are relatively low-grade, low-volume adenocarcinomas that may not need aggressive surgery but rather close follow-up,[92] particularly for those with grade 1 or 2, clinically localized carcinoma and who have an average life expectancy of 10 years or less.[92] Thus, accurate grading of prostate adenocarcinomas in needle biopsies can prove to be a valuable tool in patient management, and the criteria are worthy of review[10, 92a–92d] (see Table 2–5).

PROSTATIC INTRAEPITHELIAL NEOPLASIA

Prostatic intraepithelial neoplasia (or intraductal dysplasia) is a proliferation of atypical epithelial cells lining ducts and acini[93] (Figure 2–25). Cytologically, the atypical epithelial cells resemble prostatic adenocarcinoma cells and are thought to be the precursor cells of invasive tumor.[93] Both low- (PIN grade I) and high-grade (PIN grades II and III) varieties occur. The hallmark of high-grade PIN is the presence of prominent nucleoli, and high-grade PIN has been considered prostate adenocarcinoma in situ by some authors.[93] Low-grade PIN is a difficult diagnosis to reproduce between pathologists. Foci of PIN are found in 82 to 100% of prostates containing invasive prostate adenocarcinoma and in up to 43% of prostates without adenocarcinoma.[94] The severity (grade) and extent of PIN are greater in the prostates with invasive adenocarcinoma. High-grade PIN was found in 33% of prostates with invasive adenocarcinoma but in only 4% of the benign prostates.[94] Because there is no current proof that PIN is a direct precursor of invasive adenocarcinoma,[95,96] a diagnosis of PIN (any grade) should not prompt definitive therapy, but continued close surveillance is clearly indicated.

The Departments of Pathology and Urology at the University of California at San Francisco investigated the relationship between the detection of PIN on initial prostate biopsy and subsequent invasive prostatic adenocarcinoma in 36 patients. Prostatic intraepithelial neoplasia was diagnosed and graded according to the criteria shown in Table 2–6. All had digital rectal examination (DRE), PSA measurement, and TRUS before initial biopsy and documentation of PIN. They were then followed closely with serial PSA, TRUS, and repeat biopsy every 6 months until either invasive adenocarcinoma was identified or 2 years had elapsed. The results revealed that 58% had evidence of invasive adenocarcinoma on repeat biopsy (group I patients), whereas 42% showed persistence of PIN (group II patients). Ninety percent of group I patients had high-grade PIN on initial biopsy compared with 5% in group II. Age and DRE findings were not significantly different between groups. Transrectal ultrasonography revealed a hypoecholic lesion in 70% of patients in group I compared with 46% in group II. Increased PSA levels were seen in 85% of group I patients (from 8.4 to 11.6 ng/mL). The conclusion was that there is a close association of PIN with invasive adenocarcinoma and that the likelihood for coexistence is higher in patients with high-grade PIN, increased PSA levels, or a positive TRUS. It is recommended that all patients with biopsy-evident high-grade PIN be followed very closely with serial PSA measurements and repeat biopsies from both the area of PIN and other areas of the prostate.

Another lesion generally considered to be benign, yet possibly premalignant, is AAH or nodular adenosis[93] (see Figure 2–11). Others believe that AAH is totally benign and just mimics adenocarcinoma, especially in needle biopsy fragments. In either event, AAH resembles well-differentiated prostate adenocarcinoma architecturally, but the cells of AAH are identical to those of normal prostate, have inconspicuous nucleoli and infrequent crystalloids, usually lack luminal mucin, and show a fragmented basal cell layer.[93,97] The association of AAH with invasive prostate adenocarcinoma is weaker than with PIN. Yet there is an increased frequency of AAH with invasive adenocarcinoma, suggesting an association, but this association remains of uncertain significance.[93] Because some authors believe that AAH is at the benign end of a spectrum of small acinar lesions culminating in adenocarcinoma, where the line is drawn between AAH and small acinar-type adenocarcinoma becomes problematic and subjective. This has led some investigators to subdivide AAH into low- and high-grade types.[97] Indeed, sometimes a diagnosis of AAH or adenosis is made when the histopathologic findings are indeterminant for adenocarcinoma. Yet the nature of AAH or adenosis remains uncertain, and the more appropriate terminology for these latter situations is "findings suspicious for adenocarcinoma but not diagnostic," and a repeat biopsy should be recommended.

Currently, when the pathologist finds either PIN or AAH, additional level sections of the suspicious areas should be ordered and the entire specimen should be submitted for light microscopic examination.[93] The clinician should also perform TRUS with guided biopsy and order a serum PSA, especially for patients with high-grade PIN. If the biopsy fails to reveal invasive adenocarcinoma, TRUS, biopsy, and a serum PSA assay should be repeated at 6-month intervals for 2 years and, after that, at 12-month intervals.

FLOW CYTOMETRY AND PROSTATE ADENOCARCINOMA

Predicting the progression of occult prostate adenocarcinoma to overt clinical cancer is not a simple matter, and not all of the important variables are currently known. Some investigators have advocated that determining tumor DNA content by flow cytometry is a useful means of predicting the biologic behavior of prostate adenocarcinomas. Among all prostate adenocarcinomas, about 10% are flow DNA aneuploid, 25 to 50% flow DNA tetraploid, and the remainder flow DNA diploid.[98] Some data indicate that prostate adenocarcinomas with DNA content in the diploid range have a better clinical course than those with DNA content in the aneuploid or tetraploid range.[97] About 80% of prostate adenocarcinomas still confined to the prostate are in the diploid range, whereas those that have spread beyond the prostate are mostly tetraploid and/or aneuploid.[99] Furthermore, most prostate adenocarcinomas of stage T1 or T2 have a diploid DNA pattern (diploid-to-aneuploid ratio of 4:1), whereas most adenocarcinomas of stage T3 or metastatic are nondiploid (diploid-to-aneuploid ratio 1:4).[99]

Other studies have indicated that flow ploidy analysis weakly correlates with pathologic stage, once Gleason grading has been included in multivariate analysis, and there is no further prognostic information provided by ploidy.[100,101] Epstein concluded that there is little rationale for assessing ploidy on needle biopsy in patients who are undergoing radical prostatectomy.[10] The one exception may be stage D1 disease, wherein patients with diploid tumors who have had radical prostatectomy fare significantly better than those with nondiploid tumors and respond favorably to early hormonal therapy.[10,102] Another confounding factor of flow ploidy determination in prostate adenocarcinoma is the significant degree of DNA heterogeneity that exists within individual tumors.[103]

PROGNOSTIC INDICATORS

An ideal prognostic indicator should have the following features: (1) the factor should be an expression of a biologic phenomenon related to tumor growth, invasion, and/or metastasis; (2) its measurement should be technically feasible, reproducible, and sensitive; (3) it should have a highly significant predictive value for the outcome in question, as shown by univariate analysis; (4) it should be independent of other known clinicopathologic indicators, as shown by multivariate analysis; (5) it should

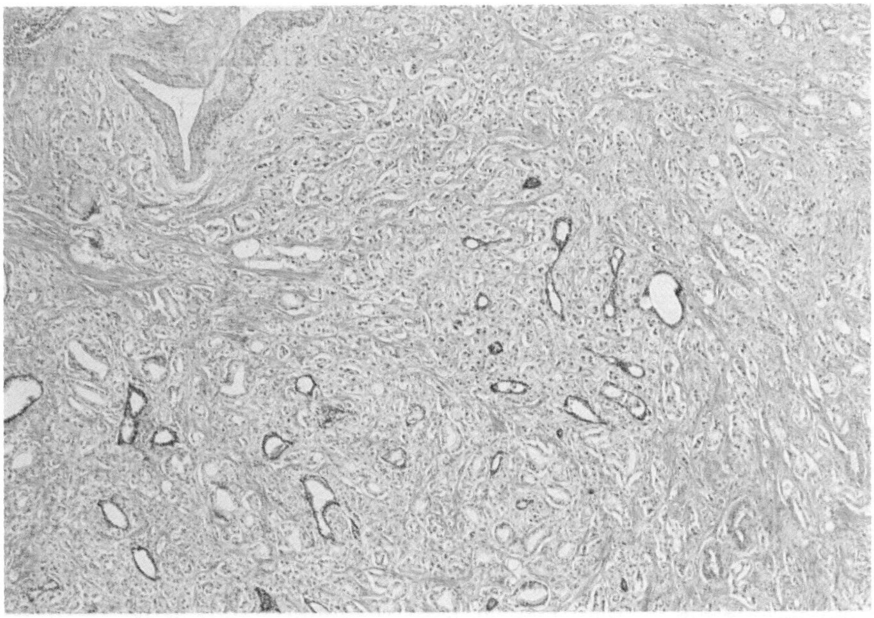

Figure 2–26. Invasive prostate carcinoma is shown following antiandrogen therapy. The field is quite eosinophilic, and benign glands are lined by low epithelium. The prostate carcinoma cells are difficult to find (hematoxylin and eosin; × 5 original magnification).

identify a distinct subgroup of prostate cancer patients destined to have recurrence and/or die of cancer; (6) it should be easily interpretable; (7) it should be proven in prospective studies to improve the overall outcome when used to select a subgroup for therapy when compared with existing conventional methods; and (8) these findings should be reproduced in multiple studies performed by different medical centers on different patient databases. Unfortunately, very few ideal prognosticators that meet all of these criteria are known for prostate carcinoma. However, pathologic stage or lymph node status would likely satisfy most of these criteria, with histologic grade coming close to meeting these criteria. Moreover, many newly discovered prognosticators show promise but have not been completely studied to establish whether the above criteria are all satisfied. Until these studies are completed and reproduced at multiple centers, many of these new prognosticators should be considered experimental.

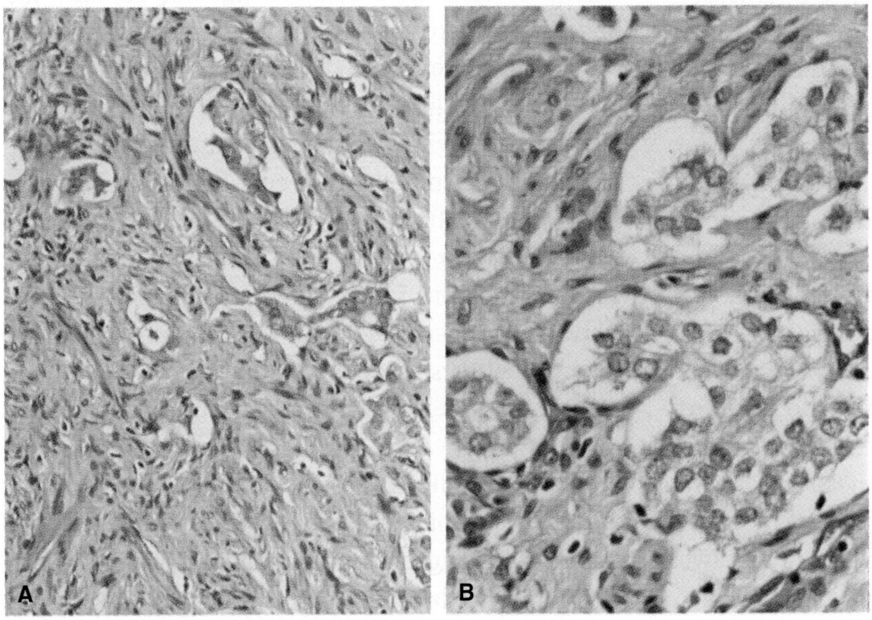

Figure 2–27. *A* and *B*, Invasive prostate carcinoma is shown following antiandrogen therapy. Note marked diminished cytoplasm and retraction artifact. Sometimes antikeratin antibody immunostains are needed to find residual carcinoma. Current grading schemes cannot be applied to prostate carcinomas following antiandrogen therapies (hematoxylin and eosin; ×50 and ×100 original magnification, respectively).

Yet, an accurate and simple method for predicting the outcome of early-stage prostate adenocarcinomas is needed, especially for those tumors of intermediate grade. Many tests have been tried, including standard pathologic grading systems and a variety of morphometric, cytophotometric, flow cytometric, and immunohistochemical techniques.[104] Determination of the random sample absolute and relative nuclear roundness factors (NRFs) has shown promise as a good prognosticator in prostate cancer, yet "the tedious and time-consuming nature of NRF measurement continues to provide the primary obstacle to wide-scale use of nuclear shape analysis for outcome measurement."[104] Markers of tumor cell proliferation, such as 5-bromodeoxyuridine incorporation or Ki-67 protein expression, may prove valuable and deserve further study.[105,106]

Tumor growth and metastasis require angiogenesis; microvessel density, a measure of tumor angiogenesis, correlates with metastasis in breast, lung, and squamous carcinomas.[107] To determine how microvessel density correlated with metastasis in prostate adenocarcinoma, we counted microvessels within the initial invasive adenocarcinomas of 74 patients (29 with metastasis, 45 without). Microvessels were highlighted by immunostaining endothelial cells for factor VIII–related antigen. Without knowledge of outcome, microvessels were counted in a times 200 field (0.739 mm^2) in the most active areas of neovascularization. The mean microvessel count in tumors from patients with metastases was 76.8 microvessels per times 200 field (median = 66, SD = 44.6). The counts within adenocarcinomas from patients without metastasis were significantly lower, 39.2 (median = 36, SD = 18.6) ($p < .0001$). Microvessel counts increased with increasing Gleason score ($p < .0001$), but this increase was present predominantly in the poorly differentiated tumors. Although Gleason score also correlated with metastasis ($p = .01$), multivariate analysis showed that Gleason score added no additional information to that provided by microvessel count alone. Assay of microvessel density within invasive tumors may prove valuable in selecting patients for aggressive adjuvant therapies in early prostate adenocarcinoma.[108] Brawer and colleagues[109] have reported similar findings.

HISTOLOGIC EFFECTS OF HORMONAL OR RADIATION OR ABLATION THERAPY

Antiandrogen therapy causes adenocarcinoma cells to atrophy (ie, they appear small, show vacuolated cytoplasm, and have pyknotic-appearing nuclei)[110,111] (Figures 2–26 and 2–27). Normal glands will also appear atrophic and stroma somewhat more fibrotic. The net effect is that the affected adenocarcinoma appears to be more high grade by Gleason pattern grading, yet the nuclei appear more benign. Estrogen therapy causes the same cytologic changes plus squamous metaplasia. Radiation decreases the numbers of adenocarcinoma glands but without significant cytologic effects on the cancer cells.[112] Moreover, the effects of radiation on adenocarcinoma may take at least 6 months, and up to 12 to 18 months, to become apparent. Thus, biopsies should be performed after this interval.[113] Benign prostate glands may show considerable radiation-induced atypia superimposed over atrophied cells and squamous metaplasia, which can make their distinction from persistent or recurrent adenocarcinoma difficult. Looking for the lobulocentric and branching growth pattern of benign glands should resolve most of the difficult cases, but HMWK immunohistochemistry can also be used effectively.

Knowledge of the histopathologic patterns induced by cryoablation therapy is important. The histopathologic findings indicate that cryosurgery results in distinctive changes in both tumoral and non-tumoral prostate tissue; and, the information provides the clinicians with information on treatment efficacy or failure. The histologic findings in the prostate following cryotherapy are in decreasing order of frequency: (1) full core fibrosis; (2) necrosis; (3) granulation tissue; (4) basal cell hyperplasia; (5) cell swelling; (6) hemosiderin deposits; (7) chronic inflammation; (8) thick nerves; and (9) prostatic hyperplasia. Necrosis was of the coagulative type, sometimes associated with nuclear debris, and seen at relatively short interval from cryotherapy. Fibrosis with hyaline qualities was seen especially at the 12–18 months interval. The presence of necrosis, as well as granulation tissue, hemosiderin deposits and cell swelling, strongly correlate to intervals from cryosurgical ablation. Residual tumor tissue was focal and recognizable in 9 cores from 4 patients sampled especially from the prostatic apex. Incipient tumor necrosis was seen in 11 cores, without particular distribution.[114]

REFERENCES

1. Jemal A, Thomas A, Murray T, Thun M. Cancer Statistics, 2002. Ca Cancer J Clin 2002;52:23–47.
2. Sakr WA, Partin AW. Histological markers of risk and the role of high-grade prostatic intraepithelial neoplasia. Urology 2001;57(4 Suppl 1):115–20.
3. Sheldon CA, Williams RD, Fraley EE. Incidental carcinoma of the prostate: a review of the literature and critical reappraisal of classification. J Urol 1980;124:626–31.
4. Franks LM. Latent carcinoma of the prostate. J Pathol Bacteriol 1954;68:603–14.
5. Shimada H, Misugi K, Sasaki Y, et al. Carcinoma of the prostate in childhood and adolescence: report of a case and review of the literature. Cancer 1980;46:2534–42.
6. Hutchison GB. Incidence and etiology of prostate cancer. Urology 1981;17 Suppl:4–10.
7. Murphey WM, Dean PJ, Brasfield JA, Tatum L. Incidental carcinoma of the prostate. How much sampling is adequate? Am J Surg Pathol 1986;10:170–4.
8. Hudson PB, Stout AP. Prostate cancer: comparison of physical examination and biopsy for detection of curable lesions. N Y State J Med 1966;66:351–5.
9. Vollmer RT. Prostate cancer and chip specimens: complete versus partial sampling. Hum Pathol 1986;17:285–90.
10. Epstein JE. The prostate and seminal vesicles. In: Sternberg SS, editor. Diagnostic surgical pathology. New York: Raven Press; 1994. p. 1807–53.
11. Cho DR, Epstein JI. Metastatic prostate carcinoma to supradiaphragmatic lymph nodes: a clinicopathologic and immunohistochemical study. Am J Surg Pathol 1987;11:457–63.
12. Fry DE, Amin M, Harbrecht PJ. Rectal obstruction secondary to carcinoma of the prostate. Ann Surg 1979;189:488–92.
13. Lee F, Torp-Pedersen ST, Siders DB. The role of transrectal ultrasound in the early detection of prostate cancer. Cancer 1989;39:337–60.
14. Hinman F. Screening for prostate carcinoma. J Urol 1991; 145:126–30.
15. Oesterling JE. Prostate specific antigen: a critical assessment of the most useful tumor marker for adenocarcinoma of the prostate. J Urol 1991;145:907–23.
16. Rifkin MD, Zerhouni EA, Gatsonis CA, et al. Comparison of magnetic resonance imaging and ultrasonography in staging early prostate cancer: results of a multi-institutional cooperative trial. N Engl J Med 1990;323:621–6.
17. Sheth S, Hamper UM, Walsh PC, Epstein JI. Stage A adenocarcinoma of the prostate: transrectal US and sonographic-pathologic correlation. Radiology 1991;179:35–9.
18. D'Amico AV, Tempany CM, Cormack R, et al. Transperineal magnetic resonance image guided prostate biopsy. J Urol 2000;164:385–7.
19. Oesterline JE, Chan DW, Epstein JI, et al. Prostate-specific antigen in the pre- and post-operative evaluation of localized prostatic cancer treated with radical prostatectomy. J Urol 1988;139:766–72.
20. Carter HB, Pearson JD, Metter EJ, et al. Longitudinal evaluation of prostate-specific antigen levels in men with and without prostate disease. JAMA 1992;267:2215–20.
21. Ruckle HC, Klee GG, Oesterling JE. Prostate-specific antigen: critical issues for the practicing physician. Mayo Clin Proc 1994;69:59–68.
22. Schmid HP, Ravery V, Toublanc M, Boccon-Gibod L. [Early diagnosis of prostate carcinoma with reference to the density of prostate-specific antigen.] Schweiz Med Wochenschr 1996;126:1530–5.
23. Heyns CF, Naude AM, Ahmed G, et al. Serum prostate-specific antigen as surrogate for the histological diagnosis of prostate cancer. S Afr Med J 2001;91:685–9.
24. Ljung B, Cherrie R, Kaufmann JJ. Fine needle aspiration biopsy of the prostate gland: a study of 103 cases with histological follow-up. J Urol 1986;135:955–8.
25. Narayan P, Jajodia P, Stein R. Core biopsy instrument in the diagnosis of prostate cancer: superior accuracy to FNA. J Urol 1991;145:795–7.
26. Renfer LB, Kieslinn VJ Jr, Kelley J, et al. Digitally directed transrectal biopsy using biopsy gun versus transrectal needle aspiration: comparison of diagnostic yield and comfort. Urology 1991;38:108–12.
27. Bocking A. [Cytopathology of the prostate.] Pathologe 1998;19:53–8.
28. McNeal JE, Bostwick DG, Kindrachuk RA, et al. Patterns of progression in prostate cancer. Lancet 1986;1:60–3.
29. Hassan MO, Maksen J. The prostate perineural space and its relation to tumor spread. Am J Surg Pathol 1980;4:143–8.
30. Bastacky SI, Walsh PC, Epstein JI. Relationship between perineural tumor invasion on needle biopsy and radical prostatectomy capsular penetration in clinical stage B adenocarcinoma of the prostate. Am J Surg Pathol 1993;17:336–41.
31. Egan AJM, Bostwick DG. Prediction of extraprostatic extension of prostate cancer on needle biopsy findings: perineural invasion lacks significance on multivariate analysis. Am J Surg Pathol 1998;21:1496–500.
32. Borboroglu PG, Amling CL. Correlation of positive prostate sextant biopsy locations to sites of positive surgical margins in radical prostatectomy specimens. Eur Urol 2001; 39:648–53, discussion 654.
33. Iczkowski KA, Bostwick DG. Sampling, submission, and report format for multiple prostate biopsies: a 1999 survey. Urology 2000;55:568–71.
34. Prostate-specific antigen: concepts for staging prostate cancer and monitoring response to therapy. Mayo Clin Proc 1994;69:69–79.
35. Epstein JI, Oesterling JE, Eggleston JC, Walsh PC. Frozen section detection of lymph node metastases in prostatic carcinoma: accuracy in grossly uninvolved pelvic lymphadenectomy specimens. J Urol 1986;136:1234–7.
36. Cantrell BB, DeKlerk DP, Eggleston JC, et al. Pathologic factors that influence prognosis in stage A prostatic cancer. The influence of extent versus grade. J Urol 1981;125:516–20.
37. Byar DP, Mostofi FK, Veterans Administrative Cooperative Urologic Research Groups. Carcinoma of the prostate: prognostic evaluation of certain pathologic features in 208 radical prostatectomies. Cancer 1972;30:5–13.
38. Moore GH, Lawshe B, Murphey J. Diagnosis of adenocarcinoma in transurethral resections of the prostate gland. Am J Surg Pathol 1986;10:165–9.
39. McMillen SM, Wettlaufer JN. The role of repeat transurethral biopsy in stage A carcinoma of the prostate. J Urol 1986; 136:840–3.

40. Blute ML, Zincke H, Farrow GM. Long-term follow-up of young patients with stage A adenocarcinoma of the prostate. J Urol 1986;136:840–3.
41. Epstein JI, Paul G, Eggleston JC, Walsh PC. Prognosis of untreated stage A1 prostate carcinoma: a study of 94 cases with extended followup. J Urol 1986;136:837–9.
42. Roy CR II, Horne D, Raife M, Pienkos E. Incidental carcinoma of the prostate. Long term followup. Urology 1990; 36:210–3.
43. Petersen RO. Prostate. In: Urologic pathology. Philadelphia: JB Lippincott; 1986. p. 147–218.
44. Murphey WM, Gaeta JF. Diseases of the prostate gland and seminal vesicles. In: Urologic pathology. Philadelphia: WB Saunders; 1989. p. 147–218.
45. Epstein JI, Woodruff JM. Adenocarcinoma of the prostate with endometrioid features. Cancer 1986;57:111–9.
46. Bostwick DG, Kindrachuk RW, Rouse RV. Prostatic adenocarcinoma with endometrioid features. Am J Surg Pathol 1985;9:595–609.
47. Tetu B, Ro JY, Ayala AG, et al. Small cell carcinoma of the prostate. I. A clinicopathologic study of 20 cases. Cancer 1987;59:1803–9.
48. Ro JY, Tetu B, Ayala AG, Ordonez NG. Small cell carcinoma of the prostate. II. Immunohistochemical and electron microscopic studies of 18 case. Cancer 1987;59:977–82.
49. di Santagnese PA, de Mesy Jensen KL. Neuroendocrine differentiation in prostatic carcinoma. Hum Pathol 1987;18:849–56.
50. Weidner N. Sarcomatoid carcinoma of the upper aerodigestive tract. Semin Diagn Pathol 1987;4:157–68.
51. Wick MR, Young RH, Malvesta R, et al. Prostatic carcinosarcomas. Am J Clin Pathol 1963;92:131–9.
52. Humphrey PA, Kaleem Z, Swanson PE, Vollmer RT. Pseudohyperplastic prostatic adenocarcinoma. Am J Surg Pathol 1998;22:1239–46.
53. Gaudin PB, Rosai J, Epstein JI. Sarcomas and related proliferative lesions of specialized prostatic stroma: a clinicopathologic study of 22 cases. Am J Surg Pathol 1998;22: 148–62.
54. Tijare JR, Shrikhande AV, Shrikhande VV. Phyllodes type of atypical prostatic hyperplasia. J Urol 1999;162(3 Pt 1): 803–4.
55. Ende N, Woods LP, Shelley HS. Carcinoma originating in ducts surrounding the prostatic urethra. Am J Clin Pathol 1963;40:183–90.
56. Schellhammer PF, Bean MA Whitmore WF Jr. Prostatic involvement by transitional cell carcinoma: pathogenesis, patterns, and prognosis. J Urol 1977;118:399–403.
57. Mott LJM. Squamous cell carcinoma of the prostate: report of 2 cases and review of the literature. J Urol 1979;121:833–5.
58. Accetta PA, Gardner WA. Adenosquamous carcinoma of the prostate. Urology 1983;22:73–5.
59. Epstein JI, Lieberman PH. Mucinous adenocarcinoma of the prostate gland. Am J Surg Pathol 1985;9:299–308.
60. Ro JY, Grignon DJ, Tronoso P, Ayala AG. Mucin in prostatic adenocarcinoma. Semin Diagn Pathol 1988;5:273–83.
61. Ro JY, el-Naggar A, Ayala AG, et al. Signet-ring-cell carcinoma of the prostate. Electron microscopic and immunohistochemical studies of eight cases. Am J Surg Pathol 1988;12:453–60.
62. Kuhajda FP, Mann RB. Adenoid cystic carcinoma of the prostate. A case report with immunoperoxidase staining for prostate-specific acid phosphatase and prostate-specific antigen. Am J Clin Pathol 1984;81:257–60.
63. Grignon DJ, Ro JY, Ordonez NG, et al. Basal cell hyperplasia, adenoid basal cell tumor, and adenoid cystic carcinoma of the prostate gland: an immunohistochemical study. Hum Pathol 1988;19:1425–33.
64. Epstein JI, Armas OA. Atypical basal cell hyperplasia of the prostate. Am J Surg Pathol 1992;16:1205–14.
65. Denholm SW, Webb JN, Howard GC, Chisholm GD. Basaloid carcinoma of the prostate gland: histogenesis and review of the literature. Histopathology 1992;20:151–5.
66. Young RH, Frierson HF Jr, Mills SE, et al. Adenoid cystic-like tumor of the prostate gland. A report of two cases and review of the literature on "adenoid cystic carcinoma" of the prostate. Am J Clin Pathol 1988;89:49–56.
67. Jones EC, Young RH. The differential diagnosis of prostatic carcinoma. Its distinction from premalignant and pseudocarcinomatous lesions of the prostate gland. Am J Clin Pathol 1994;101:48–64.
68. Yang XJ, McEntee M, Epstein JI. Distinction of basaloid carcinoma of the prostate form benign basal cell lesions by using immunohistochemistry for bcl-2 and Ki-67. Hum Pathol 1998;29:1447–50.
69. Presti B, Weidner N. Granulomatous prostatitis and poorly differentiated prostate carcinoma. Their distinction with the use of immunohistochemical methods. Am J Clin Pathol 1991;95:330–4.
70. Henneberry JM, Kahane H, Humphrey PA, et al. The significance of intraluminal crystalloids in benign prostatic glands on needle biopsy. Am J Surg Pathol 1997;21:725–8.
71. Iczkowski KA, MacLennan GT, Bostwick DG. Atypical small acinar proliferation suspicious for malignancy in prostate needle biopsies: clinical significance in 33 cases. Am J Surg Pathol 1997;21:1489–95.
72. Helpap B, Kollermann J, Oehler U. Limiting the diagnosis of atypical small glandular proliferations in needle biopsies of the prostate by the use of immunochemistry. J Pathol 2001;193:350–3.
73. Levi AW, Epstein JI. Pseudohyperplastic prostatic adenocarcinoma on needle biopsy and simple prostatectomy. Am J Surg Pathol 2000;24:1039–46.
74. Yamanaka Y, Ishida H, Okada K, Nemoto N. [Immunohistochemical analysis with ani-cytokeratin antibody in the prostatic epithelium.] Nippon Hinyokika Gakkai Zasshi 2001;92:545–53.
75. Gikas PW, Del Buono EA, Epstein JI. Florid hyperplasia of mesonephric remnants involving prostate and periprostatic tissue. Possible confusion with adenocarcinoma. Am J Surg Pathol 1993;17:454–60.
76. Muezzinoglu B, Erdamar S, Chakraborty S, Wheeler TM. Verumontanum mucosal gland hyperplasia is associated with atypical adenomatous hyperplasia of the prostate. Arch Pathol Lab Med 2001;125:358–60.
77. Helpap B, Bonkhoff H, Cockett A, et al. Relationship between atypical adenomatous hyperplasia (AAH), prostatic intraepithelial neoplasia (PIN) and prostatic adenocarcinoma. Pathologica 1997;89:288–300.
78. Grignon DJ, Sakr WA. Atypical adenomatous hyperplasia of the prostate: a critical review. Eur Urol 1996;30:206–11.
79. Cheng L, Shan A, Cheville JC, et al. Atypical adenomatous hyperplasia of the prostate: a premalignant lesion? Cancer Res 1998;58:389–91.
80. Ruska KM, Sauvageot J, Epstein JI. Histology and cellular kinetics of prostatic atrophy. Am J Surg Pathol 1998; 22:1073–7.

81. Ronnett BM, Epstein JI. A case showing sclerosing adenosis and basal cell hyperplasia of the prostate. Am J Surg Pathol 1989;13:866–72.
82. Srigley JR, Dardick I, Warren R, et al. Basal epithelial cells of human prostate gland are not myoepithelial cells. A comparative immunohistochemical and ultrastructural study with the human salivary gland. Am J Pathol 1990; 136:957–66.
83. Meister P. [Sclerosing adenosis of the prostate. Carcinoma simulation.] Pathologe 1996;17:157–62.
84. Shah R, Mucci NR, Amin A, et al. Postatrophic hyperplasia of the prostate gland: neoplastic precursor or innocent bystander? Am J Pathol 2001;158:1767–73.
85. Billis A, Magna LA. Prostate elastosis: a microscopic feature useful for the diagnosis of postatrophic hyperplasia. Arch Pathol Lab Med 2000;200:1306–9.
86. Egan AJ, Lopez-Beltran A, Bostwick DG. Prostatic adenocarcinoma with atrophic features: malignancy mimicking a benign process. Am J Surg Pathol 1997;21:931–5.
87. Johan van Krieken JHJM. Prostate marker immunoreactivity in salivary gland neoplasms. A rare pitfall in immunohistochemistry. Am J Surg Pathol 1993;17:410–4.
88. Lindeman N, Weidner N. Immunohisto-chemical profile of prostate and urothelial carcinoma. Appl Immunohistochem 1996;4:264–75.
89. Brawn PN, Ayala AG, Von Eschenbach AC, et al. Histologic grading study of prostate adenocarcinoma. The development of a new system and comparison with other methods—preliminary study. Cancer 1982;49:525–32.
90. Gleason DF, Mellinger GT, The Veterans Administration Cooperative Urologic Research Group. The prediction of prognosis for prostate adenocarcinoma by combined histologic grading and clinical staging. J Urol 1974;111:58–64.
91. Mills SE, Fowler JE. Gleason histologic grading of prostate carcinoma. Correlations between biopsy and prostatectomy specimens. Cancer 1986;57:346–9.
92. Chodak GW, Thisted RA, Gerber GS, et al. N Engl J Med 1994;330:242–8.
92a. Cookson MS, Fleshner NE, Soloway SM, Fair WR. Correlation between Gleason score of needle biopsy and radical prostatectomy specimen: accuracy and clinical implications. J Urol 1997;157:563–4.
92b. Kronz JD, Silberman MA, Allsbrook WC, et al. Pathology residents' use of a Web-based tutorial to improve Gleason grading of prostate carcinoma on needle biopsies. Hum Pathol 2000;31:1044–50.
92c. Djavan B, Kadesky K, Klopukh B, et al. Gleason scores from prostate biopsies obtained with 18-gauge biopsy needles poorly predict Gleason scores of radical prostatectomy specimens. Eur Urol 1998;33:261–70.
92d. Carlson GD, Calvanese CB, Kahane H, Epstein JI. Accuracy of biopsy Gleason scores from a large uropathology laboratory: use of a diagnostic protocol to minimize observer variability. Urology 1998;51:525–9.
93. Bostwick DG. The pathology of early prostate cancer. Cancer 1989;39:376–93.
94. McNeal JE, Bostwick DG. Intraductal dysplasia: a premalignant lesion of the prostate. Hum Pathol 1986;17:64–71.
95. Weinberg DS, Weidner N. Concordance of DNA content between prostatic intra-epithelial neoplasia and concomitant invasive carcinoma: evidence that prostatic intraepithelial neoplasia is a precursor of invasive prostatic carcinoma. Arch Pathol Lab Med 1993;117:1132–7.
96. Deschenes JL, Weidner N. Nucleolar organizer regions (NORs) in hyperplastic and neoplastic prostate disease. Am J Surg Pathol 1991;14:1148–55.
97. Bostwick DG, Srigley J, Grignon D, et al. Atypical adenomatous hyperplasia (AAH) of the prostate [abstract]. Mod Pathol 1991;44A.
98. Klein FA, Ratcliff JE, White FKH. DNA distribution pattern of prostatic tissue obtained at the time of transurethral resection. Urology 1988;33:260–5.
99. Koss LG. The puzzle of prostatic carcinoma. Mayo Clin Proc 1988;63:193–7.
100. Badalament RA, O'Toole RV, Young DC, Drago JR. DNA ploidy and prostate-specific antigen as prognostic factors in clinically resectable prostate cancer. Cancer 1991; 67:3014–23.
101. Epstein JI, Pizov G, Steinberg GC, et al. Correlation of prostate cancer nuclear deoxyribonucleic acid, size, shape and Gleason grade with pathologic stage at radical prostatectomy. J Urol 1992;148:87–91.
102. Winkler HZ, Rainwater LM, Myers RP, et al. Stage D1 prostatic adenocarcinoma: significance of nuclear DNA ploidy patterns studied by flow cytometry. Mayo Clin Proc 1988;63:103–12.
103. O'Malley FP, Grignon DJ, Keeney M, et al. DNA heterogeneity in prostate adenocarcinoma. A DNA flow cytometric mapping study with whole organ sections of prostate. Cancer 1993;71:2797–802.
104. Mohler JL, Partin AW, Epstein JI, et al. Prediction of prognosis in untreated stage A2 prostate carcinoma. Cancer 1992;69:511–9.37.
105. Carroll PR, Waldman FM, Rosenau W, et al. Cell proliferation in prostatic adenocarcinoma: in vitro measurement by 5-bromodeoxyuridine incorporation and proliferating cell nuclear antigen expression. J Urol 1993; 149:403–7.
106. Lloyd SN, Brown IL, Leake RE. Ki-67 antibody immunostaining in benign and malignant human prostatic disease. Int J Biol Markers 1992;7:256–9.
107. Weidner N. Tumor angiogenesis: basic concepts and review of current applications in tumor prognostication. Semin Diagn Pathol 1993;10:302–13.
108. Weidner N, Carroll PR, Flax J, et al. Tumor angiogenesis: correlation with metastases in invasive prostate carcinoma. Am J Pathol 1993;143:401–9.
109. Brawer MK, Deering RE, Brown M, et al. Predictors of pathologic stage in prostate carcinoma: the role of neovascularity. Cancer 1994;73:678–87.
110. Tetu B, Srigley JR, Boivin JC, et al. Effect of combination endocrine therapy (LHRH agonist and flutamide) on normal prostate and prostatic adenocarcinoma. A histopathologic and immunohistochemical study. Am J Surg Pathol 1991;15:111–20.
111. Franks LM. Estrogen–treated prostatic cancer: the variation in responsiveness of tumor cells. Cancer 1960;13:490–501.
112. Bostwick DG, Egbert BM, Fajardo LF. Radiation injury of the normal and neoplastic prostate. Am J Surg Pathol 1982;6:541–51.
113. Scardino PT, Frankel JM, Wheeler TM, et al. The prognostic significance of post-irradiation biopsy results in patients with prostatic cancer. J Urol 1986;135:510–6.
114. Falconieri G, Lugnani F, Zanconati F, et al. Histopathology of the frozen prostate. The microscopic bases of prostatic carcinoma cryoablation. Pathol Res Pract 1996;192:579–87.

3

Molecular Genetics

MAXWELL V. MENG, MD
RAJVIR DAHIYA, PHD

Adenocarcinoma of the prostate is one of the most common cancers in men worldwide and is the second leading cause of cancer-specific death in the United States.[1] Over the past 15 years, significant advances have been made in the treatment of prostate cancer, largely owing to earlier diagnosis and the evolution of surgical techniques and improvements in radiation therapy. Nevertheless, tremendous uncertainty and controversy exist regarding the appropriate clinical management of prostate cancer in many patients. Similarly, despite the magnitude of the problem, understanding of the pathogenesis, biology, and natural history of human prostate cancer remains incomplete and unclear. Progress has been made in the past decade in elucidating the molecular and genetic changes involved in prostate cancer development and progression. A better understanding of the underlying disease mechanisms will allow rational treatment strategies and improved outcomes.

The classic model of tumor development describes a multistep process in which a series of genetic alterations leads to aberrant, uncontrolled cell growth. This is best characterized in the case of colon cancer, for which specific genetic changes have been correlated with clinical and pathologic disease progression.[2] These genetic alterations can be both hereditary (germline mutation) and acquired (somatic mutation). The paradigm is less well established in prostate cancer (Figure 3–1). We discuss the current understanding of the molecular genetics and biology of prostate cancer development, including genetic predispositions, early changes associated with prostatic intraepithelial neoplasia (PIN), and the traditional classes of genes involved in promoting and repressing cancer development (proto-oncogenes/oncogenes and tumor suppressor genes, respectively). In addition, we describe recent studies on the role of genetic instability, telomerases, growth factors, cell-adhesion molecules, DNA methylation, and the androgen receptor (AR) in prostate cancer.

HEREDITARY FACTORS

Multiple etiologies have been proposed to contribute to the development of prostate cancer. Environmental factors likely play the major role in most cases; however, inherited genetic factors are clearly important in some men. Epidemiologic analysis of almost 3,000 men in the Utah cancer registry demonstrated familial clustering of prostate cancer patients, even greater than that for both breast and colon cancer, for which a hereditary component has already been demonstrated.[3] The risks of developing disease are dependent on both the number of affected first-degree relatives and early age of disease onset. Carter and colleagues, using segregation analysis in 691 families, proposed a model of a rare autosomal dominant susceptibility gene with an allele frequency of 0.006 and penetrance of 89% at 85 years of age.[4,5] Overall, this gene may account for approximately 9% of all prostate cancer cases but an increased proportion in those patients diagnosed at earlier ages.[6] The criteria for hereditary prostate cancer include a cluster of at least three first-degree relatives with disease, at least two relatives with prostate cancer diagnosed under the age of 55 years, or prostate cancer in each of three generations in the paternal or maternal lineage.

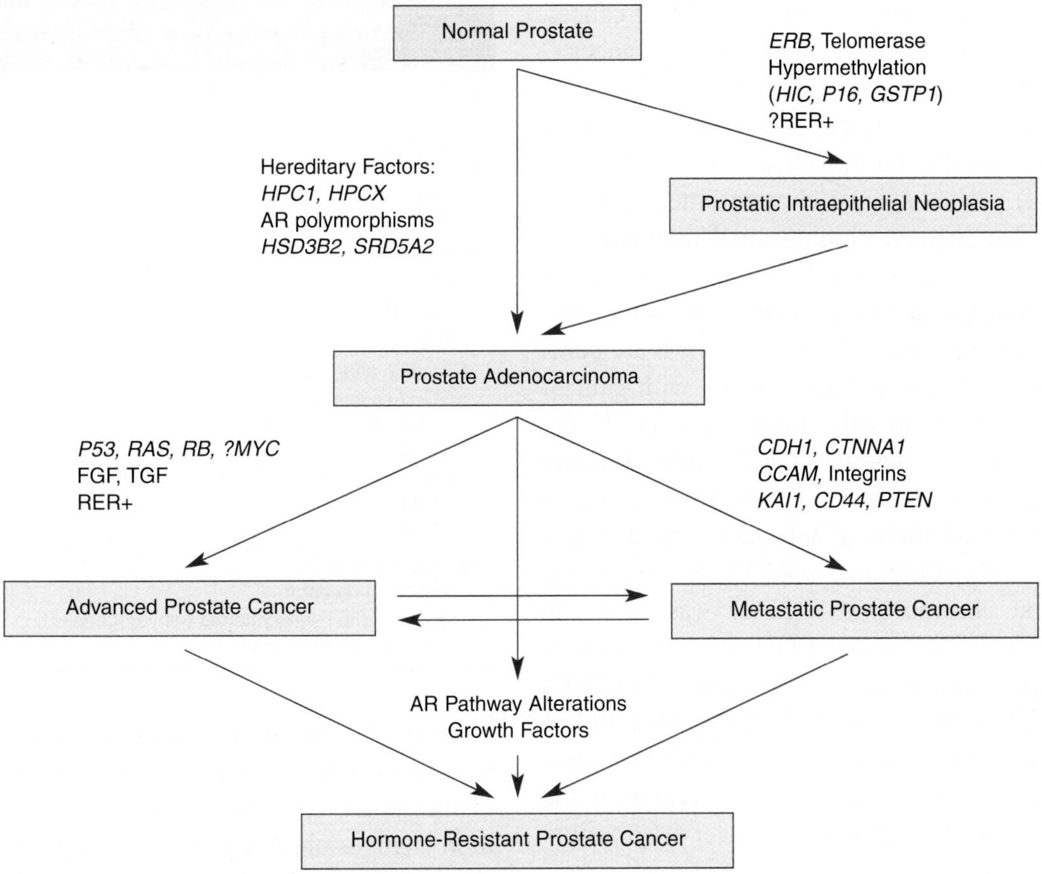

Figure 3–1. Schematic illustrating the potential factors in the development of prostatic intraepithelial neoplasia and prostate cancer and the subsequent progression of prostate cancer. AR = androgen receptor; FGF = fibroblast growth factor; TGF = transforming growth factor; RER = replication error.

Genome-wide analysis in 66 high-risk prostate cancer families suggested evidence of linkage to a locus on the long arm of chromosome 1 (1q24-25).[7] This hereditary prostate cancer locus (*HPC1*) demonstrated linkage in an additional 25 North American and Swedish families studied. The gene has not yet been cloned, but candidate genes in the region include *SKI*, *ABL2*, *TRK*, and *LAMC2*.[8] Other reports, however, have shown no evidence of linkage and no significant loss of heterozygosity (LOH) at the *HPC1* locus.[9,10] Narod and colleagues suggested a recessive or X-linked gene in hereditary prostate cancer.[11,12] A second prostate cancer susceptibility gene (*HPCX*) has recently been identified, accounting for approximately 16% of hereditary prostate cancer cases. A total of 360 prostate cancer families in North America, Finland, and Sweden were analyzed, and linkage to chromosome Xq27-28 was observed.[13] This finding was confirmed in a study of another 153 families by Lange and colleagues.[14]

Thus, there is strong evidence for genetic factors in the potential for development of prostate cancer. The *HPC1* gene may play a role in up to a third of hereditary prostate cancer cases. Further work should identify the *HPC1* and *HPCX* gene products and their functions, as well as other potential prostate cancer susceptibility genes.

GENETIC ALTERATIONS IN PRECURSOR LESIONS

Histopathologic features of PIN have provided evidence that it represents a precursor lesion of prostate cancer. Changes noted in both high-grade PIN and early invasive prostate cancer include disruption of the basal cell layer, alterations in markers of secretory differentiation, nuclear and nucleolar enlargement, and increased cell proliferation.[15] Identification of similar molecular changes in PIN and prostate cancer further strengthens this hypothesis. Sequential magnification of the abnormalities in

PIN is seen in the progression to localized cancer, metastatic cancer, and hormone-refractory cancer.

Allelic loss is common in both PIN and prostate cancer (Table 3–1). Qian and colleagues used centromere-specific fluorescence in situ hybridization (FISH) probes against chromosomes 7, 8, 10, and Y to demonstrate chromosomal anomalies in 50% of PIN and carcinoma foci. Foci of metaststic cancer demonstrated increased chromosomal anomalies.[16] Other alterations of chromosome 8 are common in both PIN and prostate cancer, with gain of chromosome 8q being the most frequent. Using polymerase chain reaction (PCR) and a novel microdissection technique, Emmert-Buck and colleagues described allelic imbalance of chromosome 8p12-21 in 64% of PIN foci and 91% of cancer foci; no LOH at chromosome 8p12-21 was found in benign tissue.[17] Additional LOH at chromosomes 8p, 10q, and 16q has been identified in 29% of PIN and 42% of primary tumors.[18] Taken together, PIN is a precursor of prostate cancer and exhibits abnormalities in biomarkers, which likely represent the early genetic changes in prostate cancer progression.

GENETIC ALTERATIONS IN PROSTATE CANCER

Evolution in techniques has allowed more refined analysis of somatic genetic changes in prostate cancer cells. Methods that have been used include cytogenetic analysis, FISH, and comparative genomic hybridization (CGH). More recently, molecular analysis has focused on specific oncogenes and tumor suppressor genes (Table 3–2), growth factors and their receptors, and the AR.

Whereas cytogenetic analysis has yielded important information regarding hematologic malignancies, interpretation of solid tumor karyotypes is more difficult. In addition, prostate cancer is characterized by low mitotic rates, tumor heterogeneity, significant stromal elements, and poor morphology of metaphase spreads. Nevertheless, the most common changes observed are nonrandom loss of the Y chromosome and gain of chromosome 7.[19,20] Others have observed deletions of chromosomes 7q, 8p, and 10q, as well as structural aberrations of chromosomes 8p22, 10q24, and 1.[21,22] These chromosomal abnormalities were observed more frequently in poorly differentiated, locally extensive tumors with poor clinical outcomes. Identification of double minutes and homogeneously staining regions, features associated with oncogene amplification, have been rare in prostate cancer specimens.[22,23]

Table 3–1. GENETIC ALTERATIONS IN PROSTATE CANCER

	Gains	Losses
Prostatic intraepithelial neoplasia	7, 8q, 10	8p, 10q, 16q, Y
Prostate adenocarcinoma	7, 8q, 10, X	2q, 5q, 6q, 7q, 8p, 9p 10q 13q, 15q, 16q, 16p 17p, 17q, 18q, 20q 22q, Y

Table 3–2. GENES POTENTIALLY INVOLVED IN PROSTATE CARCINOGENESIS

Tumor suppressor genes
- *N33*
- *MXI1*
- *P53*
- *RB1*
- *DCC*

Oncogenes
- *MYC*
- *ERBB2*
- *RAS*

Metastatic genes
- *CDH1* (E-cadherin)
- *CTNNA1* (α-catenin)
- *CCAM*
- *KAI1*
- *CD44*
- *PTEN*

Androgen cascade
- Androgen receptor
- *HSD3B2* (3β-hydroxysteroid dehydrogenase)
- SRD5A2 (5α-reductase)

Fluorescence in situ hybridization and CGH data have confirmed cytogenetic findings and enabled detection of additional areas of change in prostate cancer cells. Aneuploidy occurs in 66 to 100% of prostate cancers.[24] The most common alterations include chromosome 8 (23%) and chromosome 7 (20%), with involvement of chromosomes 10, 12, X, and Y occurring less frequently.[25] Aneuploid tumors demonstrated more frequent disease progression, most notably with chromosomes 8 and Y, and may have use as prognostic markers for locally advanced prostate cancer.[26,27] Chromosome 7 trisomy was noted more often in tumors of higher stage and Gleason grade. Others have postulated that S-phase fraction, like DNA ploidy, correlates with both pathologic features and clinical outcomes. However, the importance of both DNA ploidy and S-phase fraction over standard clinical and pathologic information remains unclear.

Comparative genomic hybridization allows genome-wide survey for regions of amplification or loss by hybridizing DNA from normal and tumor tissues with normal metaphase chromosomes. Alterations as detected by CGH are present in up to 70% of prostate cancer cases, with losses five times more common than gains.[28–31] Areas of loss involve chromosomes 2q, 5q, 10q, 13q, 15q, 16q, 16p, 17p, 17q, 18q, 9p, 20q, and Y, whereas gains involve chromosomes 11p, 1q, 3q, 9q, 20, 23, and 2p. New alterations revealed by CGH include loss at chromosomes 6q, 9p, and 22q and amplifications at chromosome 8q24.[28,32] Fluorescence in situ hybridization and molecular methods of restriction fragment length polymorphism and PCR have generally confirmed these regions of change detected by CGH. The more frequent finding of DNA loss suggests that inactivation of tumor suppressor genes in these areas may play an important role in prostate cancer development.

More recent studies have specifically examined alterations in Y chromosome number. Multani and colleagues found that prostate cancer cell lines were able to consistently induce an increase in the number of copies of the Y chromosome in three murine tumor cell lines in vivo.[33] Fluorescence in situ hybridization demonstrated that the majority of cells had two to three copies of the Y chromosome and that the amplification was specific, without other chromosomes being involved. Tricoli, however, did not find significant changes in Y chromosome number.[34] Using touch preparations from prostate tumors, 42 specimens were analyzed by whole Y chromosome paint FISH. Only a single case of Y chromosome gain, and no evidence of loss of the entire Y chromosome, was found.

TUMOR SUPPRESSOR GENES

Cancer development relies on alterations in normal homeostatic mechanisms exhibiting precise control on cellular proliferation. The genes involved in negative regulation of cell growth can be disrupted, thus allowing tumorigenesis. These tumor suppressor genes are recessive and typically require inactivation of both alleles.

As mentioned, sites of chromosomal deletion from LOH studies may suggest the presence and location of tumor suppressor genes. Loss of part, or all, of the short arm of chromosome 8 (8p) is the most common genetic defect in prostate cancer and has been confirmed by several studies.[18,31,35] Loss of heterozygosity studies in other cancers such as lung, colon, and breast also demonstrate frequent chromosome 8p loss, further suggesting the presence of a potential tumor suppressor gene that may be fundamental in tumor development. Smaller regions of deletion, chromosomes 8p11-12 and 8p22, have been reported.[36,37] Only recently has a candidate tumor suppressor gene been identified from the chromosome 8p22 region.[38] This *N33* gene, expressed in most tissues, is downregulated in colon cancer cell lines; however, studies in prostate cancer cell lines have not revealed mutations in *N33* or evidence of down-regulation. No other candidate tumor suppressor genes have been reported in these regions.

Another frequent site of loss, initially described by classic cytogenetic analysis, is the terminal region of chromosome 10q (10q24-25).[18,39] A potential tumor suppressor gene, *MXI1*, has been mapped to this chromosomal region.[40] The protein acts as a negative regulator of the *MYC* oncogene, and its inactivation may potentially result in increased activity of the MYC protein. Eagle and colleagues however, found that mutations of the *MXI1* gene are rare, whereas Gray and colleagues demonstrated that the allelic losses of chromosomes 10q24-25 occur near the chromosome 10q23-24 boundary and not at the *MXI1* locus.[40,41]

P53 is one of the most widely studied tumor proteins, and abnormalities of the *P53* tumor suppressor gene are the most common genetic alterations associated with human malignancy. P53 plays a key role in the regulation of the cell cycle, ensuring DNA integrity by negatively affecting cell growth after DNA damage (Figure 3–2). Overall, the incidence of LOH and mutations at the *P53* locus (chromosome 17p13.1) in prostate cancer is less than in other malignancies, ranging between 10 and 30%.[42,43] Evidence suggests that changes in P53 are important in the subset of patients with advanced disease and thus may be a late event. Studies of cell lines derived from metastatic deposits demonstrated frequent *P53* mutations, and transfection of wild-type P53

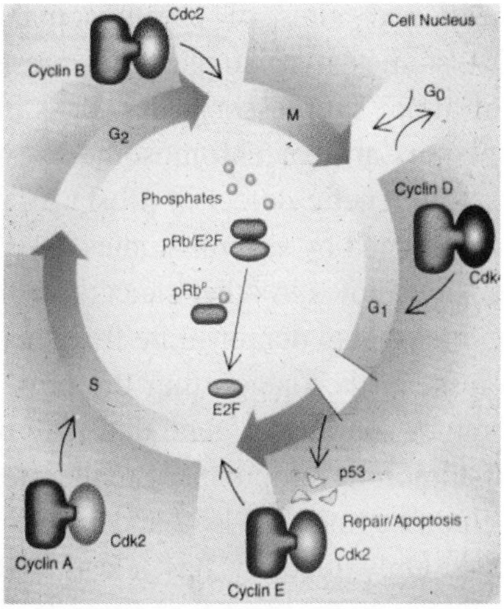

Figure 3–2. Overview of the role of P53, RB, and related proteins in the cell cycle and regulation of apoptosis.

resulted in suppression of growth. Ability to detect P53 by immunohistochemisty often accompanies mutations in the gene caused by increases in the protein half-life, thus allowing study of paraffin-embedded specimens. Nuclear accumulation of P53 correlated with metastatic disease or androgen independence.[44,45] In addition, P53-positive tumors were found to have a greater frequency of *P53* mutations.[46,47] These mutations are primarily localized to exon 7.[48] An association between P53 expression and poor clinical outcome has been reported. Moreover, alterations in P53 may affect and therefore predict response to radiation therapy.[49–52] Several regulatory genes, including *P53*, *BCL2*, *CMYC*, and *RAS*, have been implicated in the apoptotic process. It is postulated that defects in these genes may limit the ability of cells to induce apoptosis; thus, partial resistance to agents that act through programmed cell death may be imparted with P53 alterations.[49] Several studies demonstrate an attenuated response to ionizing radiation in cells harboring *P53* mutations. Similarly, *P53* mutations adversely predict overall survival in patients with locally advanced disease treated with androgen deprivation after radiotherapy.[53] Impaired apoptosis, after either radiotherapy or androgen ablation, may be important in tumors with *P53* mutations. Variations in studies of P53 may result from many factors. First, commercially available antibodies recognizing P53 differ in sensitivity and specificity. Second, quantification of P53 staining is subject to interobserver variability. Third, ability to detect *P53* mutations is dependent on the technique used, such as temperature or denaturing gradient gel electrophoresis or single-stranded conformation polymorphisms. In addition, heterogeneity in the distribution of *P53* alterations can result in variations, depending on which regions of the tumors are examined.

The retinoblastoma tumor suppressor gene (*RB1*) is associated with the development of retinoblastoma in the immature retina as well as tumors of the breast and lung. Because of the frequent LOH of chromosome 13q (30 to 35%) and the location of *RB1* at chromosome 13q14, *RB1* has been postulated to be a tumor suppressor gene involved in prostate tumorigenesis.[54–56] The phosphoprotein likely interacts with transcription factors, such as the E2F family, and negatively regulates cell growth. Although decreased or absent RB protein expression was found in a third of tumors with LOH, few mutations of the *RB1* gene have been identified.[56] The DU145 cell line possesses a mutated *RB1* gene, and reintroduction of wild-type *RB1* is able to reduce tumorigenicity.[57] Using single-stranded conformation polymorphism analysis of ribonucleic acid (RNA), Kubota and colleagues revealed that 4 of 25 primary cancers (16%) had *RB* alterations.[58] Interestingly, LOH at *RB* has been found not only in cancer specimens but also in benign prostatic hyperplasia (BPH) samples. More recent data do not demonstrate prognostic significance of altered RB protein expression.[59] The true importance of *RB1* and exact nature of LOH at 13q remain to be determined.

In prostate cancer, chromosome 18q locus LOH has been reported in up to 45% of primary tumors.[60,61] The deleted in colorectal carcinoma (*DCC*) gene is a candidate tumor suppressor gene located in this region and possesses homology with neural cell adhesion molecules. Although mutations of the gene have not been reported, decreased expression of the *DCC* gene, as well as allelic loss, suggest a role in prostate cancers.[62] Alternative tumor suppressor genes may be located at chromosome 18q21, as suggested by Ueda and colleagues.[63]

ONCOGENES

The second major class of genes implicated in tumor development is the so-called oncogenes. Initially recognized in cells transformed by retroviruses, oncogenes are derived from normal cellular genes, or proto-oncogenes, that contribute to tumorigenesis once activated by mutation or increased expression. The typical functions of these proto-oncogenes in normal cells include control of differentiation and proliferation. The critical role of oncogenes has been well documented in many malignancies. Unlike other cancers, though, prostate cancer initiation and progression do not predominantly rely on oncogenes.

As discussed above, genetic losses are much more common than DNA amplification. Nevertheless, region 8q, specifically 8q24, is the only region to demonstrate significant gain or amplification (5 to 16%).[31,32,64] *MYC*, located at chromosome 8q24, is a member of the *MYC* proto-oncogene family. *MYC* encodes a nuclear DNA-binding phosphoprotein involved in transcriptional regulation and is frequently amplified in breast, lung, and cervical cancers. Amplification, rearrangement, and overexpression of *MYC* has been documented in the LNCaP cell line but not in primary tumor specimens.[65–68] Elevated *MYC* expression has been shown in prostate cancer, compared to BPH, by Northern blot analysis.[69–71] Others have suggested that higher *MYC* levels, seen with higher grades and lymph node metastases, correlate with biologic aggressiveness. Conflicting data from in situ hybridization do not confirm a role of *MYC* in prostate cancer, and additional studies are required.

Another oncogene, *ERBB2* or *HER2/NEU* located at chromosome 17p21, has been studied in prostate cancer. The proteins in the *ERBB* family are transmembrane receptors with tyrosine kinase activity, including the *ERBB1* gene encoding the epidermal growth factor (EGF) receptor.[72] *ERBB2* is implicated in cancers of the breast and ovaries and is typically overexpressed as a result of gene amplification or transcriptional and post-transcriptional processing. The results do not clearly show increased ERBB2 expression in prostate cancer; some have found higher protein expression in prostate cancer, whereas others demonstrate overexpression in BPH.[73–76] Similarly, the prognostic value of *ERBB2* amplification and P185*NEU* protein expression is controversial.[77,78] The finding of P185*NEU* in PIN and carcinoma by immunohistochemistry suggests that *ERB* oncogenes may be an early event in prostate transformation and provide further evidence for PIN as a preneoplastic state.[14] Molecular studies do agree that *ERBB2* amplification is not the mechanism of activation in prostate cancer. As with P53 studies, technical factors, such as method of antigen retrieval and type of antibody used, may significantly influence the results of immunohistochemical staining. It has recently been demonstrated that FISH is more sensitive in the detection of *HER2/NEU* abnormalities, and further studies should investigate the use of this method.[79]

The *RAS* oncogene family is involved in a wide variety of human cancers. The three proteins (H-RAS, K-RAS, and N-RAS) are guanosine triphosphate–binding proteins essential for signal transduction.[80] Point mutations within codons 12, 13, and 61 are the most common activating changes found that lead to uncontrolled cell growth.[80] Immunohistochemistry has suggested high levels of RAS expression in prostate cancer; overexpression correlates with progression and metastatic disease rather than tumor initiation and has limited value in diagnosis and staging.[81–83] *RAS* mutations, detected by molecular techniques, are rare in Western populations (< 5%) and almost absent in localized prostate cancer.[84,85] In Japan, however, mutations in the *RAS* gene have been found in up to 25% of cases.[86,87] These data suggest that different mechanisms of prostate cancer initiation and progression may exist within different ethnic or geographic groups.

DNA REPAIR

The classic paradigm of tumor development involves oncogenes and tumor suppressor genes. More recent research describes a third class of genes that lead to tumorigenesis, those involved in DNA repair. Maintenance of genomic integrity is essential to prevent the acquisition of mutations; thus, genetic instability allows accumulation of changes, which may lead to tumor formation. It has been estimated that mutation in up to 100 genes can result in genomic instability.[88] Efforts have focused primarily on microsatellite instability, originally described in hereditary nonpolyposis colorectal cancer (HNPCC).[89,90] Mutations, either inherited or acquired, in DNA mismatch repair genes lead to the replication error phenotype (RER). Several of these genes have been identified in humans (*MSH2*, *MLH1*, *PMS1*, *PMS2*) and are homologous to the same genes in yeast.[91,92] Defects are manifested by variations in the lengths of noncoding mono-, di-, tri-, and tetranucleotide repeats, the so-called microsatellites.

Whereas microsatellite instability is found in HNPCC as well as sporadic colorectal, endometrial, stomach, and pancreatic cancers, the frequency in prostate cancer ranges from 5 to 70% .[93–96] Two studies reported high frequency of alterations at specific microsatellite loci, although microsatellite instability at multiple loci is rare in prostate cancer.[95,97,98] We found frequent microsatellite instability (45%) in prostate cancer using normal and tumor cells of 40 microdissected prostate cancer specimens.[99] It is essential to use pure epithelial cells isolated by microdissection from 5-micron sections of prostate tissue. Variations in results may be the product of differences in PCR primer and tissue selection as well as definitions of RER. Recent reports have not found the RER phenotype in prostate cancer, with the more common finding of focal instability and the lack of widespread microsatellite instability. Crundwell and colleagues found evidence of microsatellite instability in 19% of cancers, with no difference between clinically apparent tumors and incidentally discovered cancers at transurethral prostatectomy.[100] Miet and colleagues analyzed 10 loci in 60 prostate cancers.[101] RER was found in both areas of cancer and PIN but rarely in areas of glandular hyperplasia. Egawa and colleagues noted racial differences in the frequency of microsatellite instability.[102] Another report suggested that the frequency of RER is much higher in the United States when compared with Japan. The DU145 cell line demonstrates microsatellite instability and mutations in *MLH1* and *PMS2*.[103] Overall, RER is not predominant in most prostate cancers but may be associated with high-grade and advanced tumors, although this remains controversial.[104,105]

TELOMERASE

Telomeres are repetitive, noncoding DNA sequences found at the ends of all eukaryotic chromosomes that play a role in protection and replication of the chromosomes, as well as prevent loss of genetic coding regions. In humans, hundreds of TTAGGG tandem repeats compose the telomeres.[106] Normal cells lose between 50 and 200 of these nucleotides at each mitosis and, after 50 to 100 cell doublings, a critical amount of sequence is lost and the cells senesce. Thus, telomeres and their shortening serve as a mitotic clock. Telomerase, a ribonucleoprotein enzyme, is able to add telomeric sequences to the ends of newly replicating DNA and can compensate for telomere shortening.[107] Germline cells and fetal cells typically have high telomerase activity, whereas normal somatic cells have undetectable telomerase activity. It is postulated that increased telomerase activity allows unlimited cell division and therefore is associated with cellular immortalization, an important phenotypic feature in the progression of normal cells to malignant.[108]

Normal prostate tissue does not exhibit telomerase activity. Sommerfeld and colleagues assayed benign and malignant tissue for telomerase activity using a sensitive PCR technique.[109] A large number (84%) of cancers were strongly positive, as well as all lymph nodes with metastases. All human prostate cancer cell lines tested (DU145, LNCaP, PC3, PPC1, TSU) demonstrated telomerase activity. In contrast, no normal tissue from the cancer specimens or BPH samples from patients without evidence of cancer demonstrated telomerase activity. Benign prostatic hyperplasia tissue adjacent to areas of cancer demonstrated weak telomerase activity in 12% of cases. Paradoxically, telomere length from cancer tissue was significantly and consistently shorter than that detected in either adjacent normal or BPH tissue. Other studies have confirmed the high incidence of telomerase activity in prostate cancer, and some data suggest a correlation with Gleason grade.[110,111] Interestingly, telomerase activity has been found frequently in adjacent areas of PIN (74%).[111,112] These findings lead to several conclusions. First, telomerase activity in a majority of PIN and cancer further supports the hypothesis than PIN is a precursor of cancer and harbors early genetic changes. Second, telomerase activity is nearly ubiquitous in prostate cancer, and expression occurs early in prostate carcinogenesis. Third, the finding of telomerase activity in associated areas that appear histologically normal suggests that telomerase activity may be useful as a sensitive diagnositc marker for malignant tissue prior to visible, microscopic changes.

GROWTH FACTORS

Growth factors in the prostate have been studied in two settings: the production of factors within the tissue and the effects of exogenous factors on prostate cells in culture. It should be noted that virtually all studies relating to growth factor expression have been performed in normal adult prostates, which are either growth quiescent or only slowly growing. Only the report of Mansson and colleagues used prostates from young rats (6 to 8 weeks) to characterize expression of heparin-binding growth factors.[113] Most studies in human tissue have used BPH specimens from older men, in whom growth is exceedingly slow. Thus, the function of growth factors in the adult prostate, as determined by current data, is likely more homeostatic than stimulatory. Further description of growth factor expression in the growing prostate is required to clarify these issues and inconsistencies.

Polypeptide growth factors and their receptors play a role in both normal prostate growth and prostate cancer development. These growth factors act in either an autocrine or paracrine fashion and play a role in stimulating or inhibiting proliferation, differentiation, development, chemotaxis, and tissue repair. They are divided into four major families: EGF, fibroblast growth factor (FGF), insulin-like growth factor (IGF), and transforming growth factor-β (TGF-β).

The EGF family includes EGF, TGF-α, amphiregulin, heparin-binding EGF, and *cripto*. Both EGF and TGF-α have been implicated in prostate cancer and act on the EGF receptor in a paracine manner.[114–116] Autocrine stimulation of the EGF receptor may also be important in the regulation of prostate epithelial proliferation and differentiation, although this remains controversial. Transforming growth factor-α, whose overexpression in transgenic mice results in hyperplasia and dysplasia of the anterior prostate, has been found in tumor cells but not in normal prostatic cells.

The FGF family has at least nine members; only FGF1, 2, 3, 7, and 8 have been found in prostate tissue. Moreover, their role in prostate cancer is currently unclear. Increased expression of both FGF7 and FGF8 has been reported in adenocarcinoma and was associated with hormone-refractory disease and higher grade, respectively.[117,118] Interestingly, the stroma produces FGF7 exclusively and is the site of most FGF messenger RNA (mRNA) expression.[119] This further confirms the vital role of the prostatic stoma and fibroblasts in affecting epithelial cell behavior and carcinogenesis. Fibroblast growth factor, also known as keratinocyte growth factor, is expressed only by epithelial cells, and studies in the developing mouse seminal vesicle have shown it to be an important paracrine mediator of androgen action. Similar effects may be important in prostate cancer and epithelial cell proliferation and morphology.

The IGF family, comprised of IGF-I, IGF-II, and relaxin, is involved in cell growth, cell division, and apoptosis. Insulin-like growth factor-II is an autocrine and paracrine regulator of cell proliferation in the adult prostate. In androgen-insensitive prostate cancer, the IGF-I receptor is overexpressed, and IGF-II autocrine stimulation results in uncontrolled proliferation. Typically, the IGF2 gene demonstrates imprinting, in which one allele is inactivated and silent. Jarrard and colleagues reported bi-allelic expression in cases of cancer and suggested that loss of imprinting may be involved in abnormal growth in prostatic tissue.[120] The Physician's Health Study prospectively examined a matched population of 152 men for IGF-I. The study concluded that higher plasma IGF-I levels were associated with higher rates of prostate cancer; men in the highest quartile were 4.3 times more likely to develop prostate cancer. These findings were independent of prostate-specific antigen (PSA) level, stage, and grade.[121]

The TGF-β family has three isoforms in humans and regulates cell cycle kinetics by acting on RB, MYC, and cyclin-dependent kinase inhibitor activity.[122] Transforming growth factor-β, detected in normal and neoplastic prostate tissue, is an inhibitor of normal prostate epithelial cell growth, and its activity is modulated by other growth factors, androgens, and the extracellular matrix.[123,124] Conversely, TGF-β can also stimulate cell growth and contribute to tumor aggressiveness. Immunohistochemistry revealed increasing levels of TGF-β1 in tumors with metastatic and nodal involvement.[125] Plasma TGF-β1 levels may have use as a tumor marker or predictor of clinical prognosis.[126] The TGF-β effects are mediated through the heteromeric complex of the type I and II receptors. Thus, loss of function of either receptor results in resistance to TGF-β inhibitory signals. Decreased levels of type I and II receptors are correlated with higher grade and advanced disease.[127–129]

Other growth factors implicated include hepatocyte growth factor, platelet-derived growth factor, nerve growth factor, and interleukin-6.[130] Further investigation is required to elucidate their exact roles in prostate carcinogenesis.

METASTASIS SUPPRESSOR GENES

The invasive nature of prostate cancer is dependent on the loss of usual cell-cell and cell-matrix interactions. Several candidate genes involved in this process have been identified in prostate cancer that typically act as tumor suppressor genes. Ultimately, a metastatic phenotype may be acquired after inactivation of one or many of these genes.

As discussed above, loss at chromosome 16q, as detected by all methods, is frequent in prostate cancer and led to a search for a tumor suppressor gene. E-cadherin, located at chromosome 16q22.1, has been studied thoroughly. The protein is a calcium-dependent, epithelial cell-cell adhesion molecule and plays a vital role in the invasive potential of cancer cells[131] (Figure 3–3). Decreased E-cadherin expression is found in prostate cancer and associated with higher grade and worse clinical outcome. In addition, metastases express less E-cadherin than primary tumors.[132–134] Blocking E-cadherin function using antibodies or antisense transcripts increases invasive behavior.[135–137] Conversely, re-expression of E-cadherin in epithelial cells can induce a reversion to a noninvasive phenotype[136–138] (Figure 3–4). Newer techniques in immunohistochemistry may reduce the inconsistencies from formalin fixation and autolytic artifacts that characterized prior studies. Ruijter and colleagues have described an alterative approach for fixing prostatectomy specimens that yields samples amenable to E-cadherin immunohistochemistry as well as extraction of longer DNA fragments.[139]

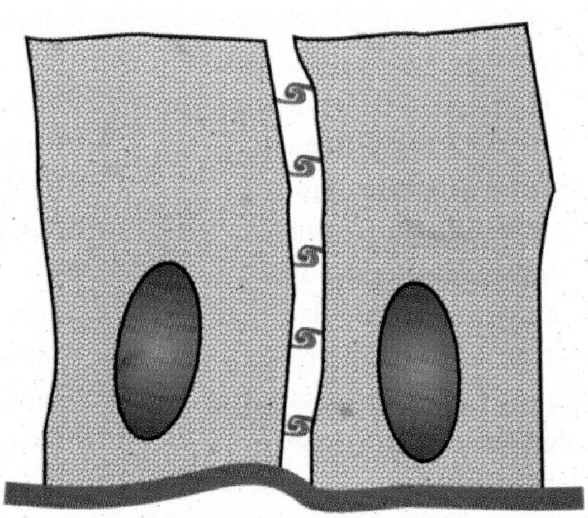

Figure 3–3. Illustration depicting the role of E-cadherin. The surface molecule interacts with other E-cadherin molecules, contributing to epithelial cell adhesion. The cytoplasmic domain, not shown, normally interacts with the intracellular catenin proteins.

Mutations in the E-cadherin gene (*CDH1*) are rare, suggesting other mechanisms of regulation and inactivation.[140,141] Hypermethylation of the 5'-CpG islands of *CDH1* may silence the gene, and this has been found in E-cadherin–negative cell lines. After treatment with demethylating agents, E-cadherin RNA and protein levels were partially restored.[142] E-cadherin function is also dependent on sex steroids, which increase expression, and interaction with cytoskeletal and other adhesion molecules such as the catenins.[143]

The catenins are a family of three (α-, β-, γ-) proteins involved in intercellular adhesion and signal transduction. They associate with the cytoplasmic domain of E-cadherin to allow coupling to the microfilament cytoskeleton. Because of frequent chromosome 5q losses and mapping of α-catenin (*CTNNA1*) to chromosome 5q21-q22, it is of particular interest.[144] The PC-3 cell line expresses E-cadherin; however, α-catenin is absent owing to homozygous deletion of the gene. Re-expression of α-catenin by either transfection with α-catenin complementary DNA or transfer of chromosome 5 was associated with a return of cell-cell contact and decreased tumorigenicity in mice.[145,146] Thus, both E-cadherin and α-catenin function is required in reducing invasive potential. Like E-cadherin, loss of α-catenin expression, as determined by immunohistochemistry, predicts invasiveness and poor prognosis.[147,148] Further study is needed of β- and γ-catenin. Voeller and colleagues found only 5 β-catenin mutations in 104 specimens.[149] In addition, the adenomatous polyposis gene product (APC) interacts with β-catenin. APC is also located at chromosome 5q21, and inactivation may lead to altered cell-cell function.

Other epithelial cell adhesion molecules may act as repressors of growth and invasion. One that has been evaluated is CCAM, a member of the immunoglobulin gene superfamily. CCAM expression in human prostate cancer cells reduces anchorage-independent growth and tumor invasion in vitro and in vivo, respectively.[150,151] Antisense CCAM expression in less tumorigenic cell lines was able to increase tumorigenicity. Studies in human tissue reveal absence of CCAM in prostate cancer and decreased staining in BPH and high-grade PIN.

Members of the integrin family mediate interactions between cells and extracellular matrix proteins, affecting cell migration, proliferation, and invasion. These heterodimeric cell surface receptors are composed of noncovalently associated α and β subunits. Overall, down-regulation of the various integrin subunits occurs in prostate cancer development. These include α2, α4, α5, αv, and β4.[152–154] Conversely, increased expression of integrin α6 is associated with more invasive activity.[155] An increased invasive phenotype in prostate cancer is associated with α3β1, α4β1, and α6β1. More recently, Zheng and colleagues found that αvβ3 integrin expression in prostate cancer generates a migratory phenotype, which is modulated by a focal adhesion kinase signaling pathway.[156] Other integrins, α6β4 and α2β1, attach the cells to the basement membrane and bone matrix, respectively.

The *KAI1* metastasis suppressor gene is found on chromosome 11p11.2.[157] It belongs to a family of membrane glycoproteins and is thought to participate in cell-cell interaction and cell migration. KAI1 is expressed in normal human prostate epithelial cells but absent in cell lines derived from metastases, such as DU145, PC-3, and LNCaP. Re-introduction of the *KAI1* gene into the Dunning rat AT6.1 cell line suppressed the metastatic potential.[157] Down-regulation of KAI1 is found in the progression of prostate cancer, with decreased protein expression in 70% of primary cancer specimens and in almost all patients with lymph node metastases or hormone-refractory disease.[158] Allelic loss or mutations do not appear to be the mechanism of KAI1 decrease.

Located near *KAI1*, CD44 is a transmembrane protien associated with cell-cell and cell-extracellular matrix interactions. Conflicting data exist regarding CD44's function in prostate cancer. Loss of expression of CD44 standard isoform (CD44s) correlated with poor prognosis in several studies, whereas others demonstrate increased CD44 expression associated with high-grade and metastatic potential.[159–162] Neutralizing antibodies to CD44 inhibited cell proliferation and basement membrane invasion.[162] In another report, transfection-enhanced expression suppressed metastatic ability in the AT3.1 cell line without affecting in vivo growth or tumorigenicity.[159]

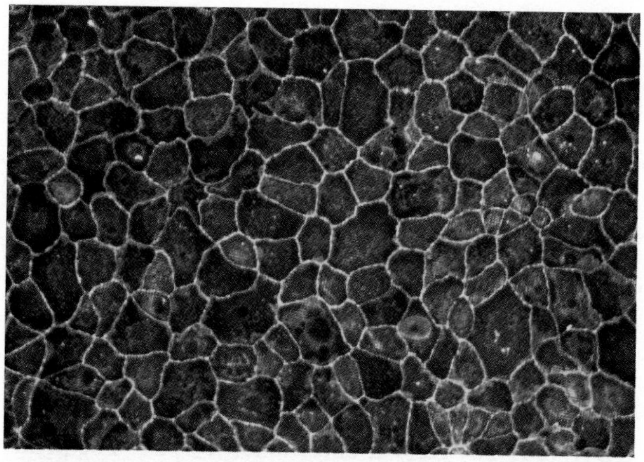

Figure 3–4. Immunocytochemistry after staining using an antibody to E-cadherin. The immortalized, but non-tumorigenic, prostate epithelial cells demonstrate strong staining for E-cadherin in the areas of cell-cell adhesion.

Pentaerythritol tetranitrate (PTEN) is a tyrosine phosphatase, mapping to chromosome 10q23, that negatively regulates cell migration and cell survival. In addition, its homology to a protein that interacts with actin filaments at focal adhesions suggests that PTEN may regulate cell invasion and metastasis.[163] Loss of *PTEN* may occur in 13 to 37% of primary prostate cancers. Increased frequency of mutations and LOH is found in cases with metastases.[164–167] Recent immunohistochemistry confirms these observations. Total absence of PTEN expression correlated significantly with Gleason score and advanced pathologic stage.[168] Pentaerythritol tetranitrate, along with CD44 and KAI1, has potential as a marker to evaluate the metastatic ability of prostate cancer, and further studies are warranted.

DNA METHYLATION

Abnormal patterns of DNA methylation often characterize human cancer cells. These include hypermethylation, redistribution of methylation, and demethylation of normally methylated regions. Although hypomethylation has been reported in prostate cancer, its significance is unclear.[169] More recently, hypermethylation of particular areas has been noted and characterized. The most important sites of hypermethylation are the CpG islands, with a high density of C-G dinucleotide sequences, found in the 5' regions of genes.

Methylation of CpG-rich islands may be associated with transcriptional inactivation of the associated gene. This has been demonstrated for the CDKN2 (*P16*) gene at chromosome 9p21. The product, a cyclin-dependent kinase inhibitory protein, controls passage through the G_1 phase of the cell cycle.[170] Inactivation by homozygous deletion, found in 20% of prostate specimens studied, may induce progression through the cell cycle in tumors.[171] Analysis of the CpG-rich promoter region in exon 1 of *P16* in the prostate cancer cell lines PC-3, PPC1, and TSU revealed dense methylation in these areas. In addition, this hypermethylation correlated with lack of mRNA expression as determined by reverse transcriptase PCR. In vitro treatment with the demethylation agent 5-aza-2'-deoxycytidine induced re-expression of CDKN2 transcripts.[172] Jarrard and colleagues found promoter methylation in 13 and 8% of primary and metastatic tumor samples, respectively, whereas no normal prostate tissues were methylated at the CDKN2 gene promoter.[173] Gu and colleagues were unable to demonstrate intragenic alterations in methylation pattern in early-stage cancers, suggesting that *P16* methylation may be involved in disease progression rather than initiation.[174]

The π-class glutathione-S-transferase (*GSTP1*) gene at 11q13 is important in the pathway, preventing damage from electrophilic metabolites of carcinogens and reactive oxygen species. Decreased GSTP1 expression was found to accompany human prostate carcinogenesis.[175] Analysis of a CpG island in the promoter region of the *GSTP1* gene revealed hypermethylation in all prostate cancer specimens examined but no aberrant methylation in 12 nonmalignant tissues, including BPH. Further immunohistochemistry in 91 cases of cancer was unable to detect GSTP1 expression in almost all samples (97%). These findings were confirmed in vitro, with protein expression limited to prostatic cell lines with *GSTP1* alleles hypomethylated at the promoter sequences. Additional work has substantiated that CpG island hypermethylation is abnormal in both alleles in most prostate cancers; in normal tissue, the entire CpG island is unmethylated with extensive methylation outside the *GSTP1* gene.[176–178] *GSTP1* hypermethylation and associated reduction in GSTP1 expression have also been demonstrated in areas of PIN. The high frequency of *GSTP1* CpG hypermethylation may serve as a biomarker in prostate cancer detection and staging.[179]

Another locus of hypermethylation in the prostate has been found at the hypermethylated in cancer (*HIC1*) gene on chromosome 17p13.3.[180] The methylation of NotI restriction sites at D17S5 is a common occurrence in prostate cancer and is thus postulated to be an important step in carcinogenesis. However, nonmalignant prostate, but not seminal vesicle, tissues also demonstrated *HIC1* hypermethylation, suggesting that the locus, and its tissue-specific methylation, may be important in the organ's susceptibility to uncontrolled growth. The CpG island in the *CD44* transcriptional regulatory region is also often hypermethylated. This leads to transcriptional inactivation of the gene, as with *GSTP1*, and a resultant decrease in CD44 expression.[181] CD44-negative cell lines, such as LNCaP, demonstrate hypermethylation of the promoter, whereas CD44-expressing cells do not exhibit this methylation. Examination of primary prostate cancer specimens confirms the increased presence of CpG hypermethylation when compared to normal tissues. Aberrant methylation has also been found at the endothelin B (*ETB*) receptor gene. Endothelin B is not expressed in human prostate cancer cell lines and shows decreased binding to endothelin-1 in prostate cancer tissues. Nelson and colleagues correlated the low ETB expression in prostate cancer with methylation of the CpG island sequences in the *ETB* gene.[182] Normal tissues were unmethylated at the *ETB* transcriptional regulatory region, whereas treatment of cancer cell lines with a demethylating agent induced *ETB* mRNA expression. Thus, CpG island methylation and transcriptional silencing appear to be important in many genes involved in prostate cancer.

ANDROGEN RECEPTOR

The AR mediates the actions of androgens in both the normal and abnormal prostate cell. This, combined with the necessity of androgens in prostate carcinogenesis and the inevitable development of androgen insensitivity with continued androgen deprivation, has focused much effort into examining the role of AR in early and late prostate cancer.

Inherited susceptibility to prostate cancer may be transmitted by AR polymorphisms. Two microsatellite repeats, CAG and GGN, are located within exon 1 of the *AR* gene. Whereas expansion of the CAG repeats to 40 to 62 is associated with spinal and bulbar muscular atrophy (Kennedy's syndrome), less than 19 CAG repeats are associated with a 1.52 relative risk for prostate cancer ($p = .04$).[183,184] In addition, men with shorter CAG microsatellites were at higher risk for metastatic disease. Stanford and colleagues noted a 3% decrease in prostate cancer risk with each additional CAG repeat, and other studies have found similar results.[185–187] However, variations in the lengths have not been consistently associated with altered AR function. Although patients with Kennedy's syndrome have been reported to possess reduced androgen binding capacity, other investigators have found normal hormone binding, transactivation, and transrepression potential in these men. The frequency of CAG repeat lengths differs among the ethnic groups. Shorter repeats are more common in black men, who have a higher incidence of prostate cancer. Conversely, more CAG repeats are found in populations at lower risk such as Asians and Whites.[185,188] This polymorphism could, in part, explain the ethnic differences in prostate cancer incidence. Length of the GGN repeat has been inconsistently associated with potential for prostate cancer development. Some have found any deviation from a repeat length of 16 to impart a higher risk (odds ratio 1.18), whereas others report lengths less than 16 to be a risk factor. Platz and colleagues found no significant differences between cancer cases and controls with respect to GGN repeat length.[189]

The observed gain of chromosome Xq in hormone-refractory prostate cancer suggested involvement of the AR, located at chromosome Xq12. Amplification of AR was detected in 30% of recurrent cancers, but none of the primary tumors, in patients receiving hormonal therapy.[190] *AR* gene amplification leads to increased mRNA levels, and high AR expression is seen in androgen-independent tumors. Almost all primary and metastatic lesions express AR, however, prior to endocrine treatment. Thus, mechanisms other than loss of AR are involved in progression to a metastatic or androgen-independent state. Indeed, prior androgen ablation may select for *AR* gene amplification. Koivisto and colleagues found significantly longer median survival in patients with *AR* amplification than those without.[191]

AR mutations are relatively infrequent, ranging from 0 to 41%.[192] This further suggests that the development of prostate cancer occurs in the presence of normal AR expression. Moreover, the AR pathway likely remains important in advanced and hormone-refractory cancers. Often, mutations are found in metastatic but not primary tumors. Taplin and colleagues found *AR* mutations in half of the hormone-independent, metastatic lesions, all of which were clustered in the steroid-binding domain (exons 4 to 8).[193] Changes in this area may lead to loss of repression of AR transactivation in the absence of androgen or increased affinity to steroids such as estrogen and progesterone. Over 50 *AR* mutations have been identified and can occur in the amino terminal domain (exon 1), DNA-binding domain (exons 2 to 3), and hinge region (exon 4).[194–196]

Mutations in the AR and overexpression may provide the cells with a means of continued growth despite low androgen conditions, a sensitization of the AR pathway. Other means of sensitizing the pathway include activation of AR in a ligand-independent manner by growth factors and cytokines or amplification of coactivators. Finally, some prostate cancer cells have bypassed the AR pathway altogether.[197]

Overall, the AR plays an important role in prostate cancer recurrence. *AR* amplification may lead to continued stimulation with low, residual androgens, whereas *AR* mutations can alter receptor specificity. New reports document an important role of AR coactivators in bypassing traditional methods of androgen ablation.[198] A better understanding of the mechanisms of AR-dependent and -independent growth will improve current and target future methods of androgen manipulation in prostate cancer.

Polymorphisms in other genes of the androgen-signaling cascade may contribute to the racial and ethnic differences in prostate cancer incidence and biologic behavior. 3β-Hydroxysteroid dehydrogenase (type 2) (*HSD3B2)* is involved in the catabolism of dihydrotestosterone. Twenty-five alleles of the $(TG)_n(TA)_n(CA)_n$ dinucleotide repeat in the *HSD3B2* gene have been identified, with the 289-bp form being the most common.[199] The shorter 275-bp allele was more common in Blacks, and longer alleles (281-bp, 302 to 340 bp) were more common in European-Americans and Asians. A similar polymorphism exists in the 3' untranslated region of the 5α-reductase type 2 gene (*SRD5A2*), whose product converts testosterone to dihydrotestosterone.[200] The most common allele is the $(TA)_0$ form, without TA repeats, found in the majority of men, whereas the two other alleles are less frequent ($(TA)_9$, $(TA)_{18}$).[201] Blacks possessed the $(TA)_{18}$ allele in 18% of cases studied; this allele was not found in Asian or White populations.[202] In addition to reporting the epidemologic finding of increased risk of cancer in Black and Hispanic men with the A49T missense substitution in *SRD5A2*, Makridakis and colleagues found high enzymatic activity of the A49T variant in an in vitro, mammalian system.[203] It is thought that the *HSD3B2* and *SRD5A2* polymorphisms result in increased prostatic levels of dihydrotestosterone and therefore increased risks of prostate cancer. Additional functional and in vivo studies are necessary to substantiate this hypothesis.

CONCLUSIONS

A wide variety of genetic alterations are potentially involved in prostate carcinogenesis. An improved understanding of the molecular basis will improve screening of patients at high risk for tumor, allow more accurate assessment of prognosis prior to and after initial therapy, and direct research toward novel and rational treatment strategies.

REFERENCES

1. Whittemore AS. Prostate cancer. Cancer Surv 1994;19:309–22.
2. Fearon ER, Vogelstein B. A genetic model for colorectal tumorigenesis. Cell 1990;16:759–67.
3. Cannon L, Bishop DT, Skolnick M, et al. Genetic epidemiology of prostate carcinoma in the Utah Mormon genealogy. Cancer Surv 1982;1:48–69.
4. Carter BS, Beaty TH, Steinberg GD, et al. Mendelian inheritance of familial prostate cancer. Proc Natl Acad Sci U S A 1992;89:3367–71.
5. Schaid DJ, McDonnell SK, Blute ML, Thibodeau SN. Evidence of autosomal dominant inheritance of prostate cancer. Am J Hum Genet 1998;62:1425–38.
6. Carter BS, Bova GS, Beaty TH, et al. Hereditary prostate cancer: epidemiologic and clinical features. J Urol 1993;150:797–802.
7. Smith JR, Freije D, Carpten JD, et al. Major susceptibility locus for prostate cancer on chromosome 1 suggested by genome-wide search. Science 1996;274:1371–4.
8. Latil A, Lidereau R. Genetic aspects of prostate cancer. Virchows Arch 1998;432:389–406.
9. McIndoe RA, Stanford JL, Gibbs M, et al. Linkage analysis of 49 high-risk families does not support a common familial prostate cancer-susceptibility gene at 1q24-25. Am J Hum Genet 1997;61:347–53.
10. Latil A, Cussenot O, Fournier G, Lidereau R. Infrequent allelic imbalance at the major susceptibility HPC1 locus in sporadic prostate tumors. Int J Cancer 1997;71:1118.
11. Narod SA, Dupont A, Cusan L, et al. The impact of family history on early detection of prostate cancer. Nat Med 1995;1:99–101.
12. Monroe KR, Yu MC, Kolonel MN, et al. Evidence of an X-linked or recessive genetic component to prostate cancer risk. Nat Med 1995;1:827–9.
13. Xu J, Meyers D, Freije D, et al. Evidence for a prostate cancer susceptibility locus on the X chromosome. Nat Genet 1998;20:175–9.
14. Lange EM, Chen H, Brierley K, et al. Linkage analysis of 153 prostate cancer families over a 30-cM region containing the putative susceptibility locus HPCX. Clin Cancer Res 1999;5:4013–20.
15. Bostwick DG, Pacelli A, Lopez-Beltran A. Molecular biology of prostate intraepithelial neoplasia. Prostate 1996;29:117–34.
16. Qian J, Bostwick DG, Takahashi S, et al. Chromosomal anomalies in prostatic intraepithelial neoplasia and carcinoma detected by fluorescence in situ hybridization. Cancer Res 1995;55:5408–14.
17. Emmert-Buck MR, Vocke CD, Pozzatti RO, et al. Allelic loss on chromosome 8p12–21 in microdissected prostatic intraepithelial neoplasia. Cancer Res 1995;55:2959–62.
18. Sakr WA, Macoska JA, Benson P, et al. Allelic loss in locally metastatic, multisampled prostate cancer. Cancer Res 1994;54:3273–7.
19. Brothman AR, Peehl DM, Patel AM, McNeal JE. Frequency and pattern of karyotypic abnormalities in human prostate cancer. Cancer Res 1990;50:3795–803.
20. Micale MA, Mohamed A, Sakr W, et al. Cytogenetics of primary prostatic adenocarcinoma. Clonality and chromosome instability. Cancer Genet Cytogenet 1992;61:165–73.
21. Avery A, Standberg MD. Chromosomal abnormalities and related events in prostate cancer. Hum Pathol 1992;23: 368–80.
22. Lundgren R, Manhad N, Heim S, et al. Cytogenetic analysis

of 57 primary prostatic adenocarcinomas. Genes Chromosomes Cancer 1992;4:16–24.
23. Limon J, Lundgren R, Elfving P, et al. Double minutes in two primary adenocarcinomas of prostate. Cancer Genet Cytogenet 1989;39:191–4.
24. Dong JT, Isaacs WB, Isaacs JT. Molecular advances in prostate cancer. Curr Opin Oncol 1997;9:101–7.
25. Brown JA, Alcaraz A, Takahashi S, et al. Chromosomal aneusomies detected by fluorescent in situ hybridization analysis in clinically localized prostate carcinoma. J Urol 1994;152:1157–62.
26. Takahashi S, Alcaraz A, Brown JA, et al. Aneusomies of chromosomes 8 and Y detected by fluorescence in situ hybridization are prognostic markers for pathological stage C (pT3N0M0) prostate carcinoma. Clin Cancer Res 1996;2:137–45.
27. Takahashi S, Qian J, Brown JA, et al. Potential markers of prostate cancer aggressiveness detected by fluorescence in situ hybridization in needle biopsies. Cancer Res 1994;54:3574–9.
28. Cher ML, MacGrogan D, Bookstein R, et al. Comparative genomic hybridization, allelic imbalance, and fluorescence in situ hybridization on chromosome 8 in prostate cancer. Genes Chromosomes Cancer 1994;11:153–62.
29. Cher ML, Bova GS, Moore DH, et al. Genetic alterations in untreated metastases and androgen-independent prostate cancer detected by comparative genomic hybridization and allelotyping. Cancer Res 1996;56:3091–102.
30. Joos S, Bergerheim USR, Pan Y, et al. Mapping of chromosomal gains and losses in prostate cancer by comparative genomic hybridization. Genes Chromosomes Cancer 1995;14:267–76.
31. Visakorpi T, Kallioniemi AH, Syvänen A-C, et al. Genetic changes in primary and recurrent prostate cancer by comparative genomic hybridization. Cancer Res 1995;55: 342–7.
32. VanDenBerg C, Guan X-Y, VonHoff D, et al. DNA sequence amplification in human prostate cancer identified by chromosome microdissection: potential prognostic implication. Clin Cancer Res 1995;1:11–8.
33. Multani AS, Ozen M, Agrawal A, et al. Amplification of the Y chromsome in three murine tumor cell lines transformed in vivo by different human prostate cancers. In Vitro Cell Dev Biol Anim 1999;35:236–9.
34. Tricoli JV. Y chromosome enumeration in touch preparations from 42 prostate tumors by interphase fluorescence in situ hybridization analysis. Cancer Genet Cytogenet 1999; 111:1–6.
35. Macoska JA, Trybus TM, Benson PD, et al. Evidence for three tumor suppressor gene loci on chromosome 8p in human prostate cancer. Cancer Res 1995;55:5390–5.
36. Bova GS, Carter BS, Bussemakers MJ, et al. Homozygous deletion and frequent allelic loss of chromosome 8p22 loci in human prostate cancer. Cancer Res 1993;53:3869–73.
37. Trapman J, Sleddens HF, van der Weiden MM, et al. Loss of heterozygosity of chromosome 8 microsatellite loci implicates a candidate tumor suppressor gene between loci D8S87 and D8S133 in human prostate cancer. Cancer Res 1994;54:6061–4.
38. MacGrogan D, Levy A, Bova GS, et al. Structure and methylation-associated silencing of a gene within a homozygously deleted region of human chromosome band 8p22. Genomics 1996;35:55–65.
39. Lacombe L, Orlow I, Reuter VE, et al. Microsatellite instability and deletion analysis of chromosome 10 in human cancer. Int J Cancer 1996;69:110–3.
40. Eagle LR, Yin X, Brothman AR, et al. Mutation of the MXI1 gene in prostate cancer. Nat Genet 1995;9:249–55.
41. Gray IC, Phillips SM, Lee SJ, et al. Loss of the chromosomal region 10q23-24 in prostate cancer. Cancer Res 1995;55: 4800–3.
42. Brooks JD, Bova GS, Ewing CM, et al. An uncertain role for p53 gene alterations in human prostate cancers. Cancer Res 1996;56:3814–22.
43. Kunimi K, Amano T, Uchibayashi T. Point mutation of the p53 gene is an infrequent event in untreated prostate cancer. Cancer Detect Prevent 1996;20:218–22.
44. Stapleton AMF, Timme TL, Gousse EA, et al. Primary human prostate cancer cells harboring p53 mutations are clonally expanded in metastases. Clin Cancer Res 1997;3:1389–97.
45. Heidenberg HB, Sesterhenn IA, Gaddipati JP, et al. Alteration of the tumor suppressor gene p53 in a high fraction of hormone refractory prostate cancer. J Urol 1995;154:414–21.
46. Bookstein R, MacGrogan D, Hilsenbeck SG, et al. p53 is mutated in a subset of advanced-stage prostate cancers. Cancer Res 1993;53:3369–73.
47. Wertz IE, Deitch AD, Gumerlock PH, et al. Correlation of genetic and immunodetection of TP53 mutations in malignant and benign prostate tissues. Hum Pathol 1996;27:573–80.
48. Dahiya R, Deng G, Chen KM, et al. P53 tumor-suppressor gene mutations are mainly localised on exon 7 in human primary and metastatic prostate cancer. Br J Cancer 1996;74:264–8.
49. Prendergast NJ, Atkins MR, Schatte EC, et al. p53 immunohistochemical and genetic alterations are associated at high incidence with post-irradiated locally persistent prostate carcinoma. J Urol 1996;155:1685–92.
50. Lee JM, Bernstein A. p53 mutations increase resistance to ionizing radiation. Proc Natl Acad Sci U S A 1993;90:5742–6.
51. O'Connor PM, Jackman J, Jondle D, et al. Role of the p53 tumor suppressor gene in cell cycle arrest and radiosensitivity of Burkitt's lymphoma cell lines. Cancer Res 1993;53:4776–80.
52. Lowe SW, Schmitt EM, Smith SW, et al. p53 is required for radiation-induced apoptosis in mouse thymocytes. Nature 1993;362:847–9.
53. Grignon DJ, Caplan R, Sarkar FH, et al. p53 status and prognosis of locally advanced prostatic adenocarcinoma: a study based on RTOG 8610. J Natl Cancer Inst 1997;89: 158–65.
54. Brooks JD, Bova GS, Isaacs WB. Allelic loss of the retinoblastoma gene in primary human prostatic adenocarcinomas. Prostate 1995;26:35–9.
55. Ittmann MM, Wieczorek R. Alterations of the retinoblastoma gene in clinically localized, stage B prostate adenocarcinomas. Hum Pathol 1996;27:28–34.
56. Konishi N, Hiasa Y, Tsuzuki T, et al. Detection of Rb, p16/cdkn2 and p15 (Ink4b) gene alterations with immunohistochemical studied in human prostate carcinomas. Int J Oncol 1996;8:107–12.

57. Bookstein R, Shew J-Y, Chen PL, et al. Suppression of tumorigenicity of human prostate carcinoma cells by replacing a mutated RB gene. Science 1990;247:712–5.
58. Kubota Y, Fujinami K, Uemura H, et al. Retinoblastoma gene mutations in primary human prostate cancer. Prostate 1995;27:314–20.
59. Vesalainen S, Lipponen P. Expression of retinoblastoma gene (Rb) protein in T1,2M0 prostatic adenocarcinoma. J Cancer Res Clin Oncol 1995;121:429–33.
60. Kunimi K, Bergerheim U, Larsson IL, et al. Allelotyping of human prostatic adenocarcinoma. Genomics 1991;11: 530–6.
61. Latil A, Baron J-C, Cussenot O, et al. Genetic alterations in localized prostate cancer identification of a common region of deletion on chromosome arm 18q. Genes Chromosomes Cancer 1994;11:119–25.
62. Gao X, Honn KV, Grignon D, et al. Frequent loss of expression and loss of heterozygosity of the putative tumor suppressor gene DCC in prostatic carcinomas. Cancer Res 1993;53:2723–7.
63. Ueda T, Komiya A, Emi M, et al. Allelic losses on 18q21 are associated with progression and metastasis in human prostate cancer. Genes Chromosomes Cancer 1997;20: 140–7.
64. Macoska JA, Trybus TM, Sakr WA, et al. Fluorescence in situ hybridization analysis of 8p allelic loss and chromosome 8 instability in human prostate cancer. Cancer Res 1994;54:3824–30.
65. Fournier G, Latil A, Amet Y, et al. Gene amplifications in advanced-stage human prostate cancer. Urol Res 1994;22:343–7.
66. Fukumoto M, Shevrin DH, Roninson IB. Analysis of gene amplification in human tumor cell line. Proc Natl Acad Sci U S A 1988;85:6846–50.
67. Latil A, Baron J-C, Cussenot O, et al. Oncogene amplifications in early-stage human prostate carcinomas. Int J Cancer 1994;59:637–8.
68. Nag A, Smith RG. Amplification, rearrangement, and elevated expression of c-myc in the human prostatic carcinoma cell line LNCaP. Prostate 1989;15:115–22.
69. Fleming WH, Hamel A, MacDonald R, et al. Expression of the c-myc protooncogene in human prostatic carcinoma and benign prostatic hyperplasia. Cancer Res 1986;46: 1535–8.
70. Buttyan R, Sawczuk IS, Benson MC, et al. Enhanced expression of the c-myc protooncogene in high-grade human prostate cancers. Prostate 1987;11:327–37.
71. Matusik RJ, Fleming WH, Hamel A, et al. Expression of the c-myc proto-oncogene in prostatic tissue. Prog Clin Biol Res 1987;239:91–112.
72. Thompson TC. Growth factors and oncogenes in prostate cancer. Cancer Cells 1990;2:345–54.
73. Natali PG, Nicotra MR, Bigotti A, et al. Expression of the p185 encoded by HER2 oncogene in normal and transformed human tissues. Int J Cancer 1990;45:457–61.
74. Mellon K, Thompson S, Charlton RG, et al. p53, c-erbB-2, and the epidermal growth factor receptor in the benign and malignant prostate. J Urol 1992;147:496–9.
75. Gu K, Mes Masson AM, Gauthier J, Saad F. Overexpression of her-2/neu in human prostate cancer and benign hyperplasia. Cancer Lett 1996;99:185–9.
76. Giri DK, Wadhwa SN, Upadhaya SN, Talwar GP. Expression of NEU/HER-2 oncoprotein (p185neu) in prostate tumors: an immunohistochemical study. Prostate 1993; 23:329–36.
77. Fox SB, Persad RA, Coleman N. Prognostic value of c-erbB-2 and epidermal growth factor receptor in stage A1 (T1a) prostatic adenocarcinoma. Br J Urol 1994;74:214.
78. Kuhn EJ, Kurnot RA, Sesterhenn IA, et al. Expression of the c–erbB-2 (HER-2/neu) oncoprotein in human prostatic carcinoma. J Urol 1993;150:1427–33.
79. Ross JS, Sheehan C, Hayner-Buchan AM, et al. HER-2/neu gene amplification status in prostate cancer by fluorescence in situ hybridization. Hum Pathol 1997;28:827–33.
80. Prendergast NJ, Walther PJ. Genetic alterations in prostate adenocarcinoma. Surg Oncol Clin N Am 1995;4:241–55.
81. Buchman EC, Nayak RN, Bushman W. Immunohistochemical staining of ras p21: staining in benign and malignant prostate tissue. J Urol 1995;153:233–7.
82. Hamdy SM, Aprikian AG, Begin LR, et al. ras p21 overexpression is a late event in prostate cancer. Int J Oncol 1994;4:627–31.
83. Viola MV, Fromovitz F, Oravez S, et al. Expression of ras oncogene p21 in prostate cancer. N Engl J Med 1986;314:133–7.
84. Moul JW, Friedrichs PA, Lance RS, et al. Infrequent Ras oncogene mutations in human prostate cancer. Prostate 1992;20:327–38.
85. Gumerlock PH, Poonamallee UR, Meyers FJ, de Vere White RW. Activated ras alleles in human carcinoma of the prostate are rare. Cancer Res 1991;51:1632–7.
86. Konishi N, Hiasa Y, Tsuzuki T, et al. Comparison of ras activation in prostate carcinoma in Japanese and American men. Prostate 1997;30:53–7.
87. Carter BS, Epstein JI, Isaacs WB. Ras gene mutations in human prostate carcinoma. Cancer Res 1990;50:6830–2.
88. Cheng KD, Loeb LA. Genomic instability and tumor progression: mechanistic considerations. Adv Cancer Res 1993;60:121–56.
89. Leach FS, Nicolaides NC, Papadopoulos N, et al. Mutations of a mutS homolog in hereditary nonpolyposis colorectal cancer. Cell 1993;75:1215–25.
90. Parsons R, Li GM, Longley MJ, et al. Hypermutability and mismatch repair deficiency in RER+ tumor cells. Cell 1993;75:1227–36.
91. Bronner CE, Baker SM, Morrison PT, et al. Mutation in the DNA mismatch repair gene homologue hMLH1 is associated with hereditary non-polyposis colon cancer. Nature 1994;368:258–61.
92. Loeb LA. Microsatellite instability: marker of a mutator phenotype in cancer. Cancer Res 1994;54:5059–63.
93. Gao X, Wu N, Grignon D, et al. High frequency of mutator phenotype in human prostate cancer. Oncogene 1995;9: 2999–3003.
94. Terrell RB, Willie AH, Cheville JC, et al. Microsatellite instability in adenocarcinoma of the prostate. Am J Pathol 1995;147:799–805.
95. Uchida T, Wada C, Wang C, et al. Microsatellite instability in prostate cancer. Oncogene 1995;10:1019–22.
96. Cunningham JM, Shan A, Wick MJ, et al. Allelic imbalance and microsatellite instability in prostatic adenocarcinoma. Cancer Res 1996;56:4475–82.

97. Suzuki H, Komiya A, Aida S, et al. Microsatellite instability and other molecular abnormalities in human prostate cancer. Jpn J Cancer Res 1995;86:956–61.
98. Isaacs WB, Bova GS, Morton RA, et al. Molecular biology of prostate cancer. Semin Oncol 1994;21:514–21.
99. Dahiya R, Lee C, McCarville J, et al. High frequency of genetic instability of microsatellites in prostatic adenocarcinoma. Int J Cancer 1997;72:762–7.
100. Crundwell MC, Morton DG, Arkell DG, Phillips SM. Genetic instability in incidentally discovered and advanced prostate cancer. BJU Int 1999;84:123–7.
101. Miet SM, Neyra M, Jaques R, et al. RER(+) phenotype in prostate intra-epithelial neoplasia associated with human prostate-carcinoma development. Int J Cancer 1999;82: 635–9.
102. Egawa S, Uchida T, Suyama K, et al. Genomic instability of microsatellite repeats in prostate cancer: relationship to clinicopathological variables. Cancer Res 1995;55:2418–21.
103. Boyer J, Umar A, Risinger J, et al. Microsatellite instability, mismatch repair deficiency, and genetic defects in human cancer cell lines. Cancer Res 1995;55:6063–70.
104. Watanabe M, Imai H, Kato H, et al. Microsatellite instability in latent prostate cancers. Int J Cancer 1996;69:394–7.
105. Suzuki H, Komiya A, Aida S, et al. Microsatellite instability and other molecular abnormalities in human prostate cancer. Jpn J Cancer Res 1995;86:956–61.
106. Blackburn EH. Structure and function of telomeres. Nature 1991;350:569–73.
107. Morin GB. The human telomere transferase is a ribonucleoprotein that synthesizes TTAGGG repeats. Cell 1989;59:521–9.
108. DeLange T. Activation of telomerase in a human tumor. Proc Natl Acad Sci U S A 1994;91:2882–5.
109. Sommerfeld H-J, Meeker AK, Piatyszek MA, et al. Telomerase activity: a prevalent marker of malignant human prostate tissue. Cancer Res 1996;56:218–22.
110. Lin Y, Uemura H, Fujinami K, et al. Telomerase activity in primary prostate cancer. J Urol 1997;157:1161–5.
111. Zhang W, Kapusta LR, Slingerland JM, Klotz LH. Telomerase activity in prostate cancer, prostatic intraepithelial neoplasia, and benign prostatic epithelium. Cancer Res 1998;58:619–21.
112. Paradis V, Dargere D, Laurendeau I, et al. Expression of the RNA component of human telomerase (hTR) in prostate cancer, prostatic intraepithelial neoplasia, and normal prostate tissue. J Pathol 1999;189:213–8.
113. Mansson PE, Adams P, Kan M, McKeehan WL. Heparin-binding growth factor gene expression and receptor characteristics in normal rat prostate and two transplantable rate prostate tumors. Cancer Res 1989;49:2485–94.
114. Ching KZ, Ramsey E, Pettigrew N, et al. Expression of mRNA for epidermal growth factor, transforming growth factor-alpha and their receptor in human prostate tissue and cell lines. Mol Cell Biochem 1993;126:151–8.
115. Fowler JE, Lau JT, Ghosh L, et al. Epidermal growth factor and prostatic carcinoma: an immunohistochemical study. J Urol 1988;139:857–61.
116. Turkeri LN, Sakr WA, Wykes SM, et al. Comparative analysis of epidermal growth factor receptor gene expression and protein product in benign, premalignant, and malignant prostate tissue. Prostate 1994;25:199–205.
117. Leung HY, Dickson C, Robson CN, Neal DE. Over-expression of fibroblast growth factor-8 in human prostate cancer. Oncogene 1996;12:1833–5.
118. Leung HY, Mehta P, Gray LB, et al. Keratinocyte growth factor expression in hormone insensitive prostate cancer. Oncogene 1997;15:1115–20.
119. Yan G, Fukabori Y, Nikolaropoulos S, et al. Heparin-binding keratinocyte growth factor is a candidate stromal to epithelial andromedin. Mol Endocrinol 1992;6:2123–8.
120. Jarrard DF, Bussemakers MJ, Bova GS, Isaacs WB. Regional loss of imprinting of the insulin-like growth factor II gene occurs in human prostate tissues. Clin Cancer Res 1995; 1:1471–8.
121. Chan JM, Stampfer MJ, Giovannucci E, et al. Plasma insulin-like growth factor-I and prostate cancer risk: a prospective study. Science 1998;279:563–6.
122. Alexandrow MG, Moses HL. Transforming growth factor β and cell cycle regulation. Cancer Res 1995;55:1452–7.
123. Kim IY, Kim JH, Zelner DJ, et al. Transforming growth factor-beta-1 is a mediator of androgen-regulated growth arrest in an androgen-responsive prostatic cancer cell line, LNCaP. Endocrinology 1996;137:991–9.
124. Morton DM, Barrack ER. Modulation of transforming growth factor beta 1 effects on prostate cancer cell proliferation by growth factors and extracellular matrix. Cancer Res 1995;55:2596–602.
125. Eastham JA, Truong LD, Rogers E, et al. Transforming growth factor-beta-1: comparative immunohistochemical localization in human primary and metastatic prostate cancer. Lab Invest 1995;73:628–35.
126. Ivanovic V, Melman A, David-Joseph B, et al. Elevated plasma levels of TGF-β1 in patients with invasive prostate cancer. Nat Med 1995;1:282–4.
127. Kim IY, Ahn HJ, Zelner DJ, et al. Loss of expression of transforming growth factor beta type I and type II receptors correlates with tumor grade in human prostate cancer tissues. Clin Cancer Res 1996;2:1255–61.
128. Williams RH, Stapleton AMF, Yang G, et al. Reduced levels of transforming growth factor beta receptor type II in human prostate cancer: an immunohistochemical study. Clin Cancer Res 1996;2:635–40.
129. Kim IY, Zelner DJ, Sensibar JA, et al. Modulation of sensitivity to transforming growth factor beta-1 (TGF-beta-1) and the level of type II TGF-beta receptor in LNCaP cells by dihydrotestosterone. Exp Cell Res 1996;222:103–10.
130. Steiner MS. Review of peptide growth factors in benign prostatic hyperplasia and urological malignancy. J Urol 1995;153:1085–96.
131. Takeichi M. Cadherin cell adhesion receptors as a morphogenetic regulator. Science 1991;251:1451–5.
132. Cheng L, Nagabhushan M, Pretlow TP, et al. Expression of E-cadherin in primary and metastatic prostate cancer. Am J Pathol 1996;148:1375–80.
133. Umbas R, Isaacs WB, Bringuier PP, et al. Decreased E-cadherin expression is associated with poor prognosis in patients with prostate cancer. Cancer Res 1994;54:3929–33.
134. Morton RA, Ewing CM, Watkins JJ, Isaacs WB. The E-cadherin cell-cell adhesion pathway in urologic malignancies. World J Urol 1995;13:364–8.
135. Behrens J, Mareel MM, VanRoy FM, Birchmeier W. Dissect-

ing tumor cell invasion: epithelial cells acquire invasive properties after loss of uvomorulin-mediated cell-cell adhesion. J Cell Biol 1989;108:2435–47.
136. Vleminckx K, Vakaet L Jr, Mareel M, et al. Genetic manipulation of E-cadherin expression by epithelial tumor cells reveals an invasion suppressor role. Cell 1991;66:107–19.
137. Frixen UH, Behrens J, Sachs M, et al. E-cadherin-mediated cell-cell adhesion prevents invasiveness of human carcinoma cells. J Cell Biol 1991;113:173–85.
138. Chen WC, Obrink B. Cell-cell contacts mediated by E-cadherin (uvomorulin) restrict invasive behavior of L-cells. J Cell Biol 1991;114:319–27.
139. Ruijter ET, Miller GJ, Aalders TW, et al. Rapid microwave-stimulated fixation of entire prostatectomy specimens. Biomed-II MPC Study Group. J Pathol 1997;183:369–75.
140. Schalken JA, Smit F, Bringuier PP, et al. The role of E-cadherin mutations in bladder and prostate cancer: is E-cadherin a classical tumor suppressor gene? Urol Res 1995;23:P57.
141. Suzuki H, Komiya A, Emi M, et al. Three distinct commonly deleted regions of chromosome arm 16q in human primary and metastatic prostate cancers. Genes Chromosomes Cancer 1996;17:225–33.
142. Graff JR, Herman JG, Lapidus RG, et al. E-cadherin expression is silenced by DNA hypermethylation in human breast and prostate carcinomas. Cancer Res 1995;55:5195–9.
143. Carruba G, Miceli D, D'Amico D, et al. Sex steroids up-regulate E-cadherin expression in hormone-responsive LNCaP human prostate cancer cells. Biochem Biophys Res Commun 1995;212:624–31.
144. McPherson JD, Morton RA, Ewing CM, et al. Assignment of the human α-catenin gene (CTNNA1) to chromosome 5q21-q22. Genomics 1994;19:188–90.
145. Giroldi LA, Bringuier PP, Schalken JA. Defective E-cadherin function in urological cancers: clinical implications and molecular mechanisms. Invasion Metastasis 1994;14: 71–81.
146. Ewing CM, Ru N, Morton RA, et al. Chromosome 5 suppresses tumorigenicity of PC3 prostate cancer cells: correlation with re-expression of alpha-catenin and restoration of E-cadherin function. Cancer Res 1995;55:4813–7.
147. Umbas R, Isaacs WB, Bringuier PP, et al. Relation between aberrant α-catenin expression and loss of E-cadherin function in prostate cancer. Int J Cancer 1997;74:374–7.
148. Richmond PJ, Karayiannakis AJ, Nagafuchi A, et al. Aberrant E-cadherin and α-catenin expression in prostate cancer: correlation with patient survival. Cancer Res 1997;57:3189–93.
149. Voeller HJ, Truica CI, Gelmann EP. β-catenin mutations in human prostate cancer. Cancer Res 1998;58:2520–3.
150. Hsieh JT, Luo W, Song W, et al. Tumor suppressive role of an androgen-regulated epithelial cell adhesion molecule (C-CAM) in prostate carcinoma cell revealed by sense and antisense approaches. Cancer Res 1995;55:190–7.
151. Kleinerman DI, Troncoso P, Lin SH, et al. Consistent expression of an epithelial cell adhesion molecule (C-CAM) during human prostate development and loss of expression in prostate cancer: implication as a tumor suppressor. Cancer Res 1995;5:1215–20.
152. Allen MV, Smith GJ, Juliano R, et al. Downregulation of the beta4 integrin subunit in prostatic carcinoma and prostatic intraepithelial neoplasia. Hum Pathol 1998;29:311–8.
153. Cress AE, Rabinovitz I, Zhu WG, Nagle RB. The alpha-6-beta-1 and alpha-6-beta-4 integrins in human prostate cancer progrssion. Cancer Metastasis Rev 1995;14:219–28.
154. Nagle RB, Hao JS, Knox JD, et al. Expression of hemidesmosomal and extracellular matrix proteins by normal and malignant human prostate tissue. Am J Pathol 1995;146: 1498–507.
155. Rabinovitz I, Nagle RB, Cress AE. Integrin alpha 6 expression in human prostate carcinoma cells is associated with a migratory and invasive phenotype *in vitro* and *in vivo*. Clin Exp Metastasis 1996;13:481–91.
156. Zheng DQ, Woodard AS, Fornaro M, et al. Prostatic carcinoma cell migration via alpha(v)beta3 integrin is modulated by a focal adhesion kinase pathway. Cancer Res 1999;59:1655–64.
157. Dong JT, Lamb PW, Rinker-Schaeffer CW, et al. KAI1, a metastasis suppressor gene for prostate cancer on human chromosome 11p11.2. Science 1995;268:884–6.
158. Dong JT, Suzuki H, Pin SS, et al. Down-regulation of the KAI1 metastasis suppressor gene during progression of human prostatic cancer infrequently involved gene mutation or allelic loss. Cancer Res 1996;56:4387–90.
159. Gao AC, Lou W, Dong JT, Isaacs JT. CD44 is a metastasis suppressor gene for prostatic cancer located on human chromosome 11p13. Cancer Res 1997;57:846–9.
160. Noordzij MA, vanSteenbrugge G-J, Verkaik NS, et al. The prognostic value of CD44 isoforms in prostate cancer patients treated by radical prostatectomy. Clin Cancer Res 1997;3:805–15.
161. Zhang XH, Sakamoto H, Takenaka I. Accumulation of p53 and expression of CD44 in human prostatic cancer and benign prostatic hyperplasia: an immunohistochemical study. Br J Urol 1996;77:441–4.
162. Lokeshwar BL, Lokeshwar VB, Block NL. Expression of CD44 in prostate cancer cells: association with cell proliferation and invasive potential. Anticancer Res 1995;15: 1191–8.
163. Li J, Yen C, Liaw D, et al. PTEN, a putative protein tyrosine phosphatase gene mutated in human brain, breast, and prostate cancer. Science 1997;275:1943–7.
164. Suzuki H, Freije D, Nusskern DR, et al. Interfocal heterogeneity of PTEN/MMAC1 gene alterations in multiple metastatic prostate cancer tissues. Cancer Res 1998;58:204–9.
165. Wang SI, Parsons R, Ittmann M. Homozygous deletions of the PTEN tumor suppressor gene in a subset of prostate adenocarcinomas. Clin Cancer Res 1998;4:811–5.
166. Cairns P, Okami K, Halachmi S, et al. Frequent inactivation of PTEN/MMAC1 in primary prostate cancer. Cancer Res 1997;57:4997–5000.
167. Feilotter HE, Nagai MA, Boag AH, et al. Analysis of PTEN and the 10q23 region in primary prostate carcinomas. Oncogene 1998;16:1743–8.
168. McMenamin ME, Soung P, Perera S, et al. Loss of PTEN expression in paraffin-embedded primary prostate cancer correlates with high Gleason score and advanced stage. Cancer Res 1999;59:4291–6.
169. Bedford MT, van Helden PD. Hypomethylation of DNA in pathological conditions of the human prostate. Cancer Res 1987;47:5274–6.

170. Serrano M, Hannon GJ, Beach D. A new regulatory motif in cell-cycle control causing specific inhibition of cyclin D/CDK4. Nature 1993;366:704–7.
171. Cairns P, Polascik TJ, Eby Y, et al. Frequency of homozygous deletion at p16/CDKN2 in primary human tumors. Nat Genet 1995;11:210–2.
172. Taylor SM. 5-Aza-2'-deoxycytidine: cell differentiation and DNA methylation. Leukemia 1993;7:3–8.
173. Jarrard DF, Bova GS, Ewing CM, et al. Deletional, mutational, and methylation analyses of CDKN2 (p16/MTS1) in primary metastatic prostate cancer. Genes Chromosomes Cancer 1997;19:90–6.
174. Gu K, Mes-Masson AM, Gauthier J, Saad F. Analysis of the p16 tumor suppressor gene in early-stage prostate cancer. Mol Carcinog 1998;21:164–70.
175. Lee WH, Morton RA, Epstein JI, et al. Cytidine methylation of regulatory sequences near the pi-class glutathione S-transferase gene accompanies human prostatic carcinogenesis. Proc Natl Acad Sci U S A 1994;91:11733–7.
176. Brooks JD, Weinstein M, Lin X, et al. CG island methylation changes near the GSTP1 gene in prostatic intraepithelial neoplasia. Cancer Epidemiol Biomarkers Prev 1998;7: 531–6.
177. Lee WH, Isaacs WB, Bova GS, Nelson WG. CG island methylation changes near the GSTP1 gene in prostatic carcinoma cells detected using the polymerase chain reaction: a new prostate cancer biomarker. Cancer Epidemiol Biomarkers Prev 1997;6:443–50.
178. Millar DS, Ow KK, Paul CL, et al. Detailed methylation analysis of the glutathione S-transferase pi (GSTP1) gene in prostate cancer. Oncogene 1999;18:1313–24.
179. Santourlidis S, Florl A, Ackermann R, et al. High frequency of alterations in DNA methylation in adenocarcinoma of the prostate. Prostate 1999;39:166–74.
180. Morton RA, Watkins JJ, Bova GS, et al. Hypermethylation of chromosome 17P locus D17S5 in human prostate tissue. J Urol 1996;156:512–6.
181. Lou W, Krill D, Dhir R, et al. Methylation of the CD44 metastasis suppressor gene in human prostate cancer. Cancer Res 1999;59:2329–31.
182. Nelson JB, Lee WH, Nguyen SH, et al. Methylation of the 5' CpG island of the endothelin B receptor gene is common in human prostate cancer. Cancer Res 1997;57:35–7.
183. LaSpada AR, Wilson EM, Lubahn DB, et al. Androgen receptor gene mutations in X-linked spinal and bulbar muscular atrophy. Nature 1991;352:77–9.
184. Giovannucci E, Stampfer MJ, Krithivas K, et al. The CAG repeat within the androgen receptor gene and its relationship to prostate cancer. Proc Natl Acad Sci U S A 1997; 94:3320–3.
185. Irvine RA, Yu MC, Ross RK, Coetzee GA. The CAG and GGC microsatellites of the androgen receptor gene are in linkage disequilibrium in men with prostate cancer. Cancer Res 1995;55:1937–40.
186. Stanford JL, Just JJ, Gibbs M, et al. Polymorphic repeats in the androgen receptor gene: molecular markers of prostate cancer risk. Cancer Res 1997;57:1194–8.
187. Hardy DO, Scher HI, Bogenreider T, et al. Androgen receptor CAG repeat lengths in prostate cancer: correlation with age of onset. J Clin Endocrinol Metab 1996;81:4400–5.
188. Edwards A, Hammond HA, Jin L, et al. Genetic variation at five trimeric and tetrameric tandem repeat loci in four human population groups. Genomics 1992;12:241–53.
189. Platz EA, Giovannucci E, Dahl DM, et al. The androgen receptor gene GGN microsatellite and prostate cancer risk. Cancer Epidemiol Biomarkers Prev 1998;7:379–84.
190. Visakorpi T, Hyytinen ER, Koivisto P, et al. In vivo amplification of the androgen receptor gene and progression of human prostate cancer. Nat Genet 1995;9:401–6.
191. Koivisto P, Kononen J, Palmberg C, et al. Androgen receptor gene amplification: a possible molecular mechanism for androgen deprivation therapy failure in prostate cancer. Cancer Res 1997;57:314–9.
192. Ruijter E, van de Kaa C, Miller G, et al. Molecular genetics and epidemiology of prostate cancer. Endocr Rev 1999; 20:22–45.
193. Taplin M-E, Bubley GJ, Shuster TD, et al. Mutation of the androgen-receptor gene in metastatic androgen-independent prostate cancer. N Engl J Med 1995;21:1393–8.
194. Gottlieb B, Lehvaslaiho H, Beitel LH, et al. The androgen receptor gene mutations database. Nucleic Acids Res 1998;26:234–8.
195. Castagnaro M, Yandell DW, Dockhorn-Dworniczak B, et al. Androgen receptor gene mutations and p53 gene analysis in advanced prostate cancer. Verh Dtsch Ges Pathol 1993; 77:119–23.
196. Takahashi H, Furusato M, Allsbrook WC Jr, et al. Prevalence of androgen receptor gene mutations in latent prostatic carcinomas from Japanese men. Cancer Res 1995;55: 1621–4.
197. Jenster G. The role of the androgen receptor in the development and progression of prostate cancer. Semin Oncol 1999;26:407–21.
198. Yeh S, Lin HK, Kang HY, et al. From HER2/neu signal cascade to androgen receptor and its coactivators: a novel pathway by induction of androgen target genes through MAP kinase in prostate cancer cells. Proc Natl Acad Sci U S A 1999;96:5458–63.
199. Devgan SA, Henderson BE, Yu MC, et al. Genetic variation of 3 beta-hydroxysteroid dehydrogenase type II in three racial/ethnic groups: implications for prostate cancer risk. Prostate 1997;33:9–12.
200. Davis DL, Russell DW. Unusual length polymorphism in human steroid 5 alpha-reductase type 2 gene (SRD5A2). Hum Mol Genet 1993;2:820.
201. Kantoff PW, Febbo PG, Giovannucci E, et al. A polymorphism of the 5 alpha-reductase gene and its association with prostate cancer: a case-control analysis. Cancer Epidemiol Biomarkers Prev 1997;6:189–92.
202. Reichardt JK, Makridakis N, Henderson BE, et al. Genetic variability of the human SRD5A2 gene: implications for prostate cancer risk. Cancer Res 1995;55:3973–5.
203. Makridakis NM, Ross RK, Pike MC, et al. Association of mis-sense substitution in *SRD5A2* gene with prostate cancer in African-American and Hispanic men in Los Angeles, USA. Lancet 1999;354:975–8.

4

Role of Stroma

GERALD R. CUNHA, PhD
ANNEMARIE A. DONJACOUR, PhD
SIMON W. HAYWARD, PhD
GARY D. GROSSFELD, MD, FACS
AXEL A. THOMSON, PhD
PAUL C. MARKER, PhD
RAJVIR DAHIYA, PhD

Greater than 95% of human prostatic cancers are adenocarcinomas, which arise from the epithelial cells that line the glands and ducts of the prostate. Consequently, most research on prostate cancer to date has examined changes occurring in the prostatic epithelial cell as it progresses from normal to malignant. There is, however, a growing body of evidence suggesting that as a carcinoma evolves, changes also occur in the stroma associated with the tumor. In many instances, these changes may serve to enhance or promote tumor progression. With this in mind, we have hypothesized that epigenetic influences originating from stromal cells in the immediate microenvironment of a prostatic tumor may be critical in determining whether a particular tumor assumes a slow-growing or an invasive phenotype.[1] It is possible that following genetic alteration to the prostatic epithelium, signaling from epithelium to the surrounding prostatic smooth muscle becomes aberrant. This may result in conversion of a predominantly smooth muscle stroma to a fibroblastic stroma. One of the consequences of such a transformation may be that the local microenvironment changes from promoting epithelial homeostasis to eliciting epithelial mitogenesis and dedifferentiation. These changes would be predicted to lead to increased epithelial proliferation and migration and ultimately could enhance the invasive potential of the emerging carcinoma cell.

This chapter (1) describes the role of prostatic mesenchyme and stroma in the normal development and homeostasis of the prostate, (2) presents evidence suggesting that stroma derived from nonmalignant sources may be able to alter the malignant phenotype of prostatic carcinoma cells, (3) summarizes the evidence in support of a "tumor stroma," and (4) summarizes data describing the role of tumor stroma in prostatic tumorigenesis.

STROMA OF THE NORMAL PROSTATE

The prostate is composed of two compartments: an epithelium, which includes the exocrine glands with their associated ductal structures, and a surrounding connective tissue stroma. The stroma of the human prostate consists of a number of different cell types. The most abundant cell type in the stromal compartment is smooth muscle, which is derived from the mesenchyme of the embryonic urogenital sinus (UGS). The prostate develops from the endoderm-derived urogenital sinus, the organogenesis of which is elicited by inductive signals from the urogenital sinus mesenchyme (UGM).[2] Regional differences in inductive activity of the UGM are responsible for the development of the well-defined lobar subdivisions of the rodent prostate. For example, the ventral mesenchymal pad lying ventral to the urethra has been shown experimentally to be able to induce the formation of the ventral prostate.[3] The outcome of epithelial-mesenchymal interactions is dependent not only on the source of the inducing mesenchyme but also the germ layer origin, responsiveness, and age of the epithelium. Although mesenchyme induces and specifies epithelial differentiation, developmental end points induced by mesenchyme are limited by the developmental repertoire unique to the germ layer origin of the epithelium. For example, prostatic development has been elicited only from endodermal epithelia derived from the urogenital sinus (vaginal, bladder, urethral, and prostatic epithelia). Attempts to induce prostatic differentiation from mesodermal epithelium derived from the wolffian duct or from foregut endoderm have been unsuccessful (GR Cunha, unpublished data, 1995).[4] Thus, the origin of the responding epithelium plays a critical role in determining the developmental outcome of experimental tissue recombinants.

Whereas the UGM induces urogenital sinus epithelial (UGE) differentiation, the UGE, in turn, induces the embryonic UGM to undergo smooth muscle differentiation. Indeed, differentiation and morphologic patterning of prostatic smooth muscle is regulated via cell-cell interactions with prostatic epithelium. When UGM was grafted and grown by itself in male hosts, little, if any, smooth muscle differentiated. However, when the UGM was grafted with rat or mouse urogenital sinus–derived epithelia, smooth muscle cells differentiated and became organized into thin sheaths characteristic for the rodent prostate.[5] Significantly, rat UGM differentiated into thick sheets of smooth muscle surrounding the epithelial ducts in tissue recombinants composed of rat UGM plus human prostatic epithelium.[6] Thick smooth muscle layers are characteristic of human prostate. Thus, the human prostatic epithelium not only induced the rat UGM to undergo smooth muscle differentiation, it also elicited the human smooth muscle pattern. These observations demonstrate that prostatic smooth muscle differentiation is induced and spatially patterned by epithelium.

The differentiation of prostatic smooth muscle occurs in an orderly manner with the sequential expression of a number of characteristic markers, including vimentin, α-actin, vinculin, myosin, and desmin.[5] The adult prostate, in which the stroma contains fully differentiated smooth muscle cells, is essentially growth quiescent and maintains very low and balanced levels of proliferation and cell death.[7] It should be emphasized that this growth-quiescent, homeostatic state exists in the presence of high levels of systemic androgens. In the adult rodent, androgens act directly on the prostatic smooth muscle cells to maintain this fully differentiated growth-quiescent state. We have postulated that androgens act in a similar fashion in the adult human prostate to maintain growth quiescence.[5] Given that growth quiescence of the prostate is a hallmark of smooth muscle-epithelium interactions, whereas fibroblast-epithelium interactions are associated with prostatic growth,[8] it is interesting that conversion of a prostatic smooth muscle stroma to a prostatic fibroblastic stroma is associated with a proliferative response to androgens. For example, after castration, there is an ordered loss of expression of the various smooth muscle differentiation markers in the prostate, which appears to reflect a change in the differentiation state of the smooth muscle cells. The loss of smooth muscle differentiation markers following castration occurs in the opposite order to which these markers were expressed during normal development.[5] The final result is a prostatic stroma in the long-term castrated animal that contains fibroblasts or mesenchymal cells that coexpress androgen receptor (AR) and vimentin and very few fully differentiated smooth muscle cells. If exogenous androgens are administered to such long-term castrates, prostatic tissue will respond in a highly coordinated manner with the massive proliferation followed subsequently by differentiation of both smooth muscle (again expressing its characteristic markers) and secretory epithelium.[9] Thus, in long-term castrates, the fibroblastic cells in prostatic stroma respond to androgens by inducing epithelial proliferation and columnar cytodifferentiation, and as these changes occur in the epithelium, the fibroblastic cells revert back to highly differentiated smooth muscle cells as proliferative activity subsides.

Prostatic development occurs as a result of androgenic stimulation of the AR-positive UGM. Analysis of tissue recombinants composed of AR-positive wild-type UGM plus AR-negative epithelium from testicular feminization mice indicates that androgens act through AR in the UGM to stimulate epithelial proliferation, ductal branching morphogenesis, and tall columnar epithelial cytodifferentiation.[2] In adulthood, AR-positive prostatic smooth muscle cells interact with epithelial cells and under androgenic conditions maintain the epithelium in a fully differentiated, growth-quiescent state.[10] These findings emphasize the paracrine nature of prostatic mesenchymal-epithelial interactions in the fetus and smooth muscle-epithelial interactions in adulthood. Human prostatic smooth muscle cells, which also express AR, are believed to play a similar role in maintaining prostatic homeostasis. In addition to smooth muscle cells, fibroblasts, which make up a large proportion of the stroma of the rodent prostate, are only found sporadically in the normal human prostate. In the rodent prostate, these fibroblastic cells have been suggested to be important in mediating epithelial proliferation in the prostate.[8]

In summary, low levels of circulating androgens act on the mesenchymal cells of the developing prostate to induce prostatic epithelial proliferation and differentiation.[11] In contrast, high circulating levels of androgen in the adult act through the prostatic smooth muscle to maintain a fully differentiated, growth-quiescent epithelium. Proliferative effects of mesenchyme or stroma on epithelium are mediated through stromal AR. The epithelial AR appears to be required only for synthesis of prostatic secretory proteins.[12] In long-term castrates, exogenous androgens initially promote prostatic epithelial proliferation and cytodifferentiation as well as the re-emergence of a smooth muscle stroma. Ultimately, androgen replacement leads to regeneration of a fully differentiated, growth-quiescent gland, in which both the epithelium and stroma are growth quiescent. These data suggest that the local control of prostatic epithelial proliferation and differentiation occurs through androgenic stimulation of the prostatic stroma and that the nature of the epithelial response to such stimulation is determined by the nature of the stromal cells. Androgen receptor–expressing prostatic smooth muscle cells appear to respond to androgenic stimulation by inhibiting epithelial proliferation and maintaining epithelial differentiation. In contrast, an AR-expressing fibroblastic stroma (either the UGM or the stroma from an androgen-deprived adult prostate) may respond to androgens by stimulating prostatic epithelial proliferation and eliciting columnar cytodifferentiation in rats and mice. The function of fibroblasts in human prostate remains unclear. Thus, it appears that the predominant cell type in the stroma plays a key role in determining if the effect of the stroma on the epithelium will be proliferative and morphogenetic, as is the case in development, or homeostatic, as is the case in adulthood.

EMBRYONIC PROSTATIC INDUCERS CAN ELICIT DIFFERENTIATION OF PROSTATIC CARCINOMA CELLS

We have hypothesized that undifferentiated phenotypically abnormal stroma associated with prostate cancer cells may promote epithelial proliferation and the loss of epithelial differentiation. A corollary to this idea described in detail below is that normal embryonic prostatic mesenchyme may be able to "normalize" a malignant prostatic epithelium. The idea that interactions between embryonic prostatic mesenchyme and malignant prostatic epithelium could possibly inhibit tumorigenic growth was examined by using the rat Dunning prostatic adenocarcinoma R3327 (DT). It is interesting that although the DT is considered an adenocarcinoma, through about 40 years of transplantation, a stroma of uncertain origin has been passaged along with the malignant epithelial cells. The stroma of the DT differs from that of the normal prostate, being composed of fibroblastic cells with a complete absence of smooth muscle. In addition, the basement membrane between the epithelium and the stroma is often discontinuous or excessively reduplicated.[13] Thus, the stromal and epithelial interactants in the DT clearly differ from those of the normal prostate. To test the hypothesis that the malignant DT epithelial cells might be modified by a more "normal" stromal environment, DT epithelial cells were grown for 1 month in male nude rodent hosts either alone or in combination with embryonic mesenchyme known to be able to induce prostatic development:

UGM or seminal vesicle mesenchyme (SVM).[14] Grafts of DT alone demonstrated a characteristic histology, forming tumors that contained small ducts, which were lined by one or more layers of epithelial cells. In contrast, DT epithelial cells grown in association with UGM or SVM differentiated into tall columnar epithelial cells arranged in large cystic ducts.[15] These changes in differentiation of the DT epithelium induced by UGM or SVM were associated with a markedly decreased tumorigenesis and a significantly lower proliferation rate than the parental Dunning tumor cells.[16] The ducts of primary SVM + DT recombinants were grafted directly into new male hosts or were combined with fresh SVM to form secondary SVM + DT recombinants. Both types of recombinants exhibited minimal growth during a 3-month period and maintained a highly differentiated state. Conversely, control grafts composed of DT alone formed large tumors, which weighed 5 to 7 g, during the same time period. The marked reduction in epithelial growth rate and the highly differentiated state of the SVM-induced DT epithelial cells were found to be associated with a dramatic decrease in cellular proliferation as determined by the ^{3}H-thymidine labeling index.[16] Significantly, smooth muscle cells, which were apparently derived from the SVM, were found in close apposition to the highly differentiated, relatively growth-quiescent DT epithelium in these tissue recombinants.[13]

TUMOR-ASSOCIATED STROMAL CELLS ARE PHENOTYPICALLY ABNORMAL

There is a growing body of evidence suggesting that in the course of carcinogenesis, changes occur in the surrounding connective tissue stroma that may serve to enhance the malignant potential of the associated carcinoma cells. The appearance of this so-called "tumor stroma" has been demonstrated in a number of epithelial malignancies. For example, the stroma associated with invasive breast carcinoma is composed of activated or abnormal myofibroblastic cells in close apposition to the tumor cells.[17] These myofibroblastic cells are unique to the tumor stroma and are not found in normal breast tissue. Myofibroblastic cells are certainly not specific to stroma of breast carcinomas. Myofibroblasts have also been identified in the stroma associated with cervical, colon, ovarian, and skin carcinomas.[17]

Carcinoma-associated fibroblasts (CAFs) have also been shown to produce elevated levels of growth-promoting agents or to overexpress enzymes that can potentially generate trophic agents. For example, cyclooxygenase (COX)-2, an enzyme involved in generating prostaglandins, is elevated in the myofibroblasts associated with colon carcinomas.[18] Carcinoma-associated fibroblasts have been shown to express a variety of growth factors, such as platelet-derived growth factor, insulin-like growth factors, transforming growth factor-ß1, hepatocyte growth factor/epithelial scatter factor, and keratinocyte growth factor. Other phenotypic changes have also been ascribed to CAF and include enhanced migratory behavior in vitro[19] and alterations in gene and protein expression. For example, CAFs isolated from breast, skin, and lower gastrointestinal tract malignancies overexpress metalloproteinases (MMPs).[20] Based on in situ hybridization studies, most MMPs are localized in tumor stroma and include stromelysin-3, gelatinase A, MT-MMP, interstitial collagenase, stromelysin-1 (SL-1), and cathepsin D. Other abnormalities in breast tumor stroma include expression and/or overexpression of (1) autocrine migration-stimulating factor and enhanced migratory behavior, (2) growth factors, (3) c-ets-1 transcription factor, (4) plasminogen activator inhibitor type 1, (5) urokinase-plasminogen activator, (6) plasminogen activator inhibitor type I, and (7) tissue inhibitor of MMP 1. The importance of one of the MMPs, SL-1, is emphasized by studies in transgenic mice that inappropriately express autoactivating SL-1. Mammary ducts of such SL-1 transgenic mice have supernumerary branches, show precocious alveolar development, inappropriately express casein, and exhibit unscheduled apoptosis during pregnancy. These changes are associated with progressive development of an altered stroma and development of mammary carcinoma.[21] In addition, proteins such as dipeptidyl-peptidase IV[22] and fibroblast activation protein-α[23] also appear to be selectively expressed by CAF. Because stromal cells contribute to the extracellular matrix, the appearance of a tumor stroma may also lead to changes in the extracellular matrix surrounding a carcinoma.[24] Tenascin is an extracellular matrix protein greatly elevated in the stroma associated with carcinoma cells.[25] Likewise, levels of hyaluronate are elevated in the stroma of certain carcinomas[17] and may enhance the invasive potential of malignant epithelial cells. Thus, it is evident that the behavior of carcinoma cells cannot be understood without considering the active and reciprocal dialogue with the surrounding stroma.

By altering the local microenvironment of a carcinoma cell, tumor stroma may be capable of modulating malignant phenotype and behavior. This hypothesis has been studied in experiments using MCF-7 breast carcinoma cells in coculture with various types of fibroblastic cells (embryonic or adult fibroblasts, normal or carcinoma-associated fibroblasts).[26] The phenotype of the MCF-7 cells, including their expression of estrogen receptor, progesterone receptor, pS2, and cathepsin D, was found to be dependent on the fibroblasts with which they were cocultured. Stromal modulation of epithelial cells appeared to take place through paracrine signaling mechanisms that were likely to be mediated by stroma-derived factors.

ABNORMAL STROMA AS A MEDIATOR OF TUMORIGENESIS IN THE PROSTATE

The idea that stromal cells may facilitate prostatic carcinogenesis has previously been investigated using an in vivo mouse prostatic reconstitution system. Thompson and colleagues infected either the urogenital sinus (prostatic anlagen) or its individual mesenchymal (UGM) or epithelial (UGE) components with a virus containing the MYC and RAS oncogenes.[27] In prostatic reconstitutions containing uninfected UGM + infected UGE, epithelial hyperplasias were observed. In prostatic reconstitutions composed of infected UGM + uninfected UGE, stromal desmoplasias were observed. Carcinomas were observed only when both UGM and UGE were infected.[27] These findings demonstrated that changes were required in both the epithelium and in the stromal microenvironment for prostatic carcinogenesis to occur.

Using highly anaplastic prostatic carcinoma cells, Chung and colleagues have examined the role of stromal cells in prostatic tumorigenesis. These investigators reported that coinoculation of tumorigenic (sarcomatous) NbF-1 fibroblasts with human PC-3 prostatic carcinoma cells accelerated tumor growth and shortened the tumor latency period.[28] The interaction between the sarcoma cells and the epithelial cells in this system was bidirectional in that PC-3 cells reciprocally enhanced the tumorigenesis of the sarcomatous NbF-1 fibroblasts. Similar studies were reported for the human LNCaP prostatic carcinoma cell line.[29] Coinoculation of LNCaP cells with various nontumorigenic fibroblasts demonstrated that fibroblasts differed in their ability to promote tumorigenesis.[29] Fibroblasts derived from rat UGM and human bone, but not NIH 3T3 cells, normal rat kidney fibroblasts, or normal human lung fibroblasts, enhanced tumorigenesis of the malignant highly anaplastic human LNCaP cells in vivo. Conditioned media from bone fibroblasts, rat UGM cells, or NbF-1 fibroblasts were effective in stimulating the growth of LNCaP cells in vitro, whereas conditioned media from 3T3 cells, normal rat kidney, and normal human lung were not nearly as effective. The effect was bidirectional since LNCaP conditioned medium-stimulated growth of rat UGM. These data support the concept that fibroblasts can enhance tumorigenesis of anaplastic human prostatic carcinoma cell lines and that the trophic effects of fibroblasts on prostatic carcinogenesis are not a property of fibroblasts in general but are enhanced in selected fibroblastic cells.

Given the volume and strength of cytogenetic data, it is likely that initiation of prostatic carcinogenesis involves genetic alteration of the prostatic epithelium. We hypothesize that following genetic alteration of the prostatic epithelium, there is a sequential disruption in the reciprocal homeostatic interactions between the prostatic smooth muscle and the epithelium.[1] This altered stromal-epithelial signaling leads to the dedifferentiation of both the emerging prostatic carcinoma cells and the surrounding smooth muscle. In this regard, we have shown that whereas the stroma associated with benign human prostatic ducts is composed almost exclusively of smooth muscle cells, the stroma associated with human prostatic carcinoma is mostly depleted of smooth muscle cells and instead consists of vimentin-positive fibroblastic cells. This phenotypic shift in the nature of human prostatic stroma is not associated with a major genetic change in the stromal cells.

Using an in vivo model system, we have examined the effects of CAFs on a nontumorigenic target epithelial cell. Our aim was to determine whether human prostatic CAFs have different effects on epithelial proliferation and differentiation than "normal" fibroblasts derived from benign human prostatic tissue. To test this hypothesis, we used a tissue recombination model in which benign or tumor-derived stromal cells isolated from human prostatic tissue were recombined with either phenotypically normal human prostatic ductal organoids (fragments of acini and ducts derived from benign prostate) or BPH-1 cells (a nontumorigenic, SV40T immortalized human prostatic epithelial cell line).[30] Transplants of BPH-1 cells survived and were identified in the graft site after many months, and tumors were not observed in any of the 226 transplants. The tissue recombinants were grown under the renal capsule of adult athymic rodent hosts. Control grafts were composed of either epithelial or stromal cells alone and were grown under conditions identical to the experimental tissue recombinants. The amount of tissue growth was determined by measuring wet weights. Histopathologic features of tissue recombinants were determined in tissue sections.

When grafted alone into intact male hosts, normal or tumor-derived stromal cells (CAFs), normal prostatic epithelial cells or the immortalized BPH-1 cells exhibited minimal growth during the experimental period. Tissue recombinants composed of normal human prostatic fibroblasts (NHPFs) plus BPH-1 cells (NHPF/BPH-1 tissue recombinants) exhibited minimal growth (Figure 4–1, A), forming solid cords of epithelial cells (Figure 4–1, E). In contrast, tissue recombinants composed of CAF plus BPH-1 cells (CAF/BPH-1 tissue recombinants) exhibited striking growth (see Figure 4–1, A). Some individual CAF/BPH-1 tissue recombinants achieved as much as 5-g wet weight after 41 days of in vivo growth (from an initial wet weight of approximately 10 mg).[31]

The CAF/BPH-1 tumors were composed of poorly differentiated, irregular epithelial cords (Figure 4–1, B to D).[31] Morphometric analysis demonstrated that these tumors were predominantly epithelial (80%), with a histologic appearance of poorly

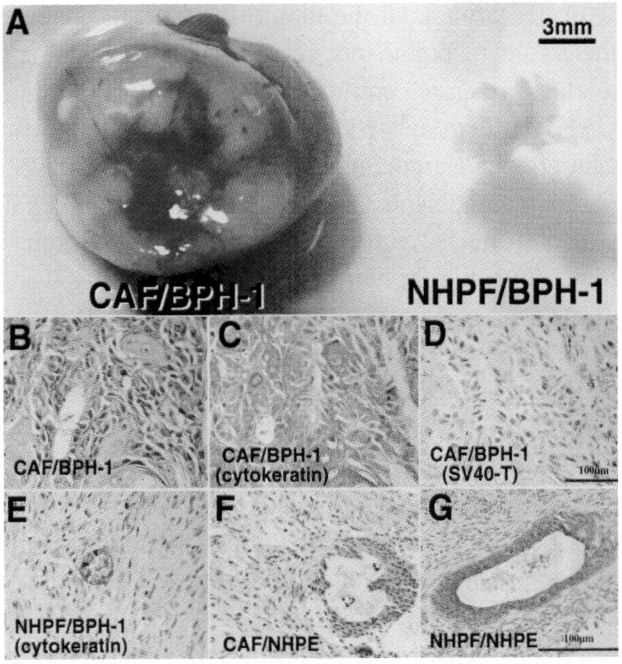

Figure 4–1. *A,* Gross appearance of tissue recombinants harvested after 85 days of growth in a male nude mouse host. Carcinoma-associated fibroblast (CAF)/BPH-1 tissue recombinant weighed 1,250 mg and normal human prostatic fibroblast (NHPF)/BPH-1 tissue recombinant weighed 10 mg (bar = 3 mm). *B* to *D,* Serial sections of a CAF/BPH-1 tissue recombinant. *B,* Hematoxylin and eosin–stained section demonstrates an appearance consistent with poorly differentiated adenocarcinoma. Note the presence of many loosely adherent, poorly differentiated epithelial cells as well as areas of squamous differentiation. *C,* Immunostaining with an antibody to cytokeratin confirms the epithelial nature of these poorly differentiated cells, whereas *D,* nuclear staining with an antibody to SV40-T in many of the epithelial cells confirms the derivation of the tumors from the BPH-1 cells that were immortalized with SV40 T antigen. *E,* Tissue recombinant composed of NHPF/BPH-1. This section was stained for cytokeratin. Note that the epithelial cells form discrete cordlike structures. *F,* Tissue recombinant composed of CAF/normal human prostatic epithelium (NHPE) (stained with hematoxylin and eosin). Note the epithelial ductal structure lined with an abnormal stratified squamous epithelium. *G,* Tissue recombinant composed of NHPF/NHPE stained to show prostate-specific antigen expression. Note the epithelial ductal structure lined with bilayered epithelium, apical cells of which are tall columnar epithelium and express human prostate-specific antigen. Scale bar for *B* to *G* = 100 μm.

differentiated prostatic adenocarcinoma. In some areas, epithelium formed small aberrant glands, whereas in other areas, epithelium appeared as single cells intermingled within a fibrous stroma. The epithelial nature of these cells was confirmed using a wide-spectrum anticytokeratin antibody (see Figure 4–1, C). Furthermore, epithelial cells within these tumors stained with an antibody to SV40T antigen (see Figure 4–1, D), confirming their BPH-1 origin. Stromal cells were intermingled between the epithelial cells throughout the tumor. In contrast, none of the tissue recombinants containing normal human ductal prostatic epithelium (NHPE), including CAF/NHPE tissue recombinants, exhibited significant growth. Carcinoma-associated fibroblast/NHPE tissue recombinants contained canalized epithelial structures lined with an abnormal stratified squamous epithelium (Figure 4–1, F). When NHPFs were grown in association with NHPE (NHPF/NHPE tissue recombinants), a bilayered epithelium developed, and the apical cells expressed prostate-specific antigen (Figure 4–1, G).

These studies demonstrated that stromal cells derived from benign and malignant sources differed significantly in their effects on nontumorigenic human prostatic epithelial cells in vivo. Carcinoma-associated fibroblasts, unlike normal fibroblasts, were capable of inducing an invasive phenotype in an immortalized but nontumorigenic human prostatic epithelial cell line. The same CAF cells were unable to induce this phenotype in genetically normal human prostatic epithelial cells even though effects on epithelial differentiation were observed. These data suggest (1) that both genetic and epigenetic changes may be important in human prostatic carcinogenesis; (2) that CAFs were able to stimulate progression of an initiated epithelium, whereas normal fibroblasts were incapable of stimulating progression; and (3) that CAFs were incapable of causing initiation in a genetically normal epithelium. Data obtained using an in vitro coculture system suggest that the CAFs may be capable of increasing proliferation and decreasing the death rates of the BPH-1 human prostatic epithelial cells.[31]

CONCLUSIONS

The data summarized above suggest that both genetic and epigenetic factors play important roles in the progression of prostate cancer. Our recent in vivo and in vitro studies have demonstrated that (1) CAFs do not form tumors when grown in the absence of epithelium, (2) CAFs stimulate progression of a genetically altered, nontumorigenic human prostatic epithelium toward a carcinomatous phenotype, (3) CAFs are unable to stimulate initiation of a genetically normal human prostatic epithelium, and (4) stromal cells from nonmalignant sources do not promote tumorigenesis in a genetically altered human prostatic epithelium under identical conditions. Our in vitro studies imply that interactions with the stromal microenvironment are important determinants in the progression from a normal prostatic epithelium to an invasive carcinoma.

Prostate cancer can exist in two forms: either as a clinically insignificant tumor or as an aggressive lesion that will progress without treatment. At the present time, we are unable to identify the specific factors that determine the behavior of any given tumor. The evidence presented above strongly suggests that the stromal microenvironment may be capable of modulating the biologic potential of a particular tumor. This may be accomplished through regulation of tumor neovascularity or through specific phenotypic changes in the surrounding stromal cells that result in altered expression of certain enzymes, cellular adhesion molecules, or growth factors, which affect epithelial behavior.

The implications of our studies regarding tumor growth are potentially very important from both a diagnostic and a therapeutic perspective. Traditional therapy for all epithelial malignancies, including prostate cancer, has been targeted at the malignant epithelial cell. Owing to its genetic instability, this cell represents a “moving therapeutic target.” Although CAFs are phenotypically abnormal, preliminary studies using karyotypic analysis and comparative genomic hybridization have demonstrated that these cells do not possess gross genetic alterations. Thus, CAFs may provide a more stationary target at which to direct treatment.

ACKNOWLEDGMENT

This work was supported by grants DK CA59831, DK47517, AG-16870, CA64872, DK52708, DK52721, CA89520, and CA76501 from the National Institutes of Health and grant PF-98-153-01 from the American Cancer Society.

REFERENCES

1. Hayward SW, Cunha GR, Dahiya R. Normal development and carcinogenesis of the prostate: a unifying hypothesis. Ann N Y Acad Sci 1996;784:50–62.

2. Cunha GR, Donjacour AA, Cooke PS, et al. The endocrinology and developmental biology of the prostate. Endocr Rev 1987;8:338–62.
3. Timms B, Lee C, Aumuller G, Seitz J. Instructive induction of prostate growth and differentiation by a defined urogenital sinus mesenchyme. Microsc Res Tech 1995;30:319–32.
4. Tsuji M, Shima H, Boutin G, et al. Effect of mesenchymal glandular inductors on the growth and cytodifferentiation of neonatal mouse seminal vesicle epithelium. J Androl 1994;15:565–74.
5. Hayward SW, Baskin LS, Haughney PC, et al. Stromal development in the ventral prostate, anterior prostate and seminal vesicle of the rat. Acta Anat (Basel) 1996;155:94–103.
6. Hayward SW, Haughney PC, Rosen MA, et al. Interactions between adult human prostatic epithelium and rat urogenital sinus mesenchyme in a tissue recombination model. Differentiation 1998;63:131–40.
7. Isaacs JT. Control of cell proliferation and death in the normal and neoplastic prostate: a stem cell model. In: Rogers CH, Coffey DS, Cunha GR, et al, editor. Benign prostatic hyperplasia. Vol. II. Bethesda (MD): National Institutes of Health; 1985. p. 85–94.
8. Nemeth JA, Lee C. Prostatic ductal system in rats: regional variation in stromal organization. Prostate 1996;28:124–8.
9. Bruchovsky N, Lesser B, van Doorn EV, Craven S. Hormonal effects on cell proliferation in rat prostate. Vitam Horm 1975;33:61–102.
10. Cunha GR, Hayward SW, Dahiya R, Foster BA. Smooth muscle-epithelial interactions in normal and neoplastic prostatic development. Acta Anat (Basel) 1996;155:63–72.
11. Donjacour AA, Cunha GR. The effect of androgen deprivation on branching morphogenesis in the mouse prostate. Dev Biol 1988;128:1–14.
12. Donjacour AA, Cunha GR. Assessment of prostatic protein secretion in tissue recombinants made of urogenital sinus mesenchyme and urothelium from normal or androgen-insensitive mice. Endocrinology 1993;131:2342–50.
13. Wong YC, Cunha GR, Hayashi N. Effects of mesenchyme of embryonic urogenital sinus and neonatal seminal vesicle on the cytodifferentiation of the Dunning tumor: ultrastructural study. Acta Anat (Basel) 1992;143:139–50.
14. Cunha GR. Epithelio–mesenchymal interactions in primordial gland structures which become responsive to androgenic stimulation. Anat Rec 1972;172:179–96.
15. Cunha GR, Hayashi N, Wong YC. Regulation of differentiation and growth of normal adult and neoplastic epithelial by inductive mesenchyme. In: Isaacs JT, editor. Prostate cancer: cell and molecular mechanisms in diagnosis and treatment. New York: Cold Spring Harbor Laboratory Press; 1991. p. 73–90.
16. Hayashi N, Cunha GR. Mesenchyme-induced changes in neoplastic characteristics of the Dunning prostatic adenocarcinoma. Cancer Res 1991;51:4924–30.
17. Ronnov-Jessen L, Petersen OW, Bissell MJ. Cellular changes involved in conversion of normal to malignant breast: importance of the stromal reaction. Physiol Rev 1996; 76:69–125.
18. Shattuck-Brandt RL, Varilek GW, Radhika A, et al. Cyclooxygenase 2 expression is increased in the stroma of colon carcinomas from IL-10(-/-) mice. Gastroenterology 2000;118:337–45.
19. Schor SL, Schor AM, Grey AM, Rushton G. Foetal and cancer patient fibroblasts produce an autocrine migration-stimulating factor not made by normal adult cells. J Cell Sci 1988;90:391–9.
20. Matrisian LM. Cancer biology: extracellular proteinases in malignancy. Curr Biol 1999;9:R776–8.
21. Werb Z, Ashkenas J, MacAuley A, Wiesen JF. Extracellular matrix remodeling as a regulator of stromal-epithelial interactions during mammary gland development, involution and carcinogenesis. Braz J Med Biol Res 1996;29:1087–97.
22. Atherton AJ, Monaghan P, Warburton MJ, et al. Dipeptidyl peptidase IV expression identifies a functional sub-population of breast fibroblasts. Int J Cancer 1992;50:15–9.
23. Scanlan MJ, Raj BK, Calvo B, et al. Molecular cloning of fibroblast activation protein alpha, a member of the serine protease family selectively expressed in stromal fibroblasts of epithelial cancers. Proc Natl Acad Sci U S A 1994;91:5657–61.
24. Bosman FT, de Bruine A, Flohil C, et al. Epithelial-stromal interactions in colon cancer. Int J Dev Biol 1993;37:203–11.
25. Chiquet-Ehrismann R, Mackie EJ, Pearson CA, Sakakura T. Tenascin: an extracellular matrix protein involved in tissue interactions during fetal development and oncogenesis. Cell 1986;47:131–9.
26. Adam L, Crepin M, Lelong JC, et al. Selective interactions between mammary epithelial cells and fibroblasts in co-culture. Int J Cancer 1994;59:262–8.
27. Thompson TC, Southgate J, Kitchener G, Land H. Multistage carcinogenesis induced by ras and myc oncogenes in a reconstituted organ. Cell 1989;56:917–30.
28. Camps JL, Chang S-M, Hsu TC, et al. Fibroblast-mediated acceleration of human epithelial tumor growth in vivo. Proc Natl Acad Sci U S A 1990;87:75–9.
29. Gleave M, Hsieh JT, Gao CA, et al. Acceleration of human prostate cancer growth in vivo by factors produced by prostate and bone fibroblasts. Cancer Res 1991;51: 3753–61.
30. Hayward SW, Dahiya R, Cunha GR, et al. Establishment and characterization of an immortalized but non-tumorigenic human prostate epithelial cell line: BPH-1. In Vitro 1995;31A:14–24.
31. Olumi AF, Grossfeld GD, Hayward SW, et al. Carcinoma-associated fibroblasts direct tumor progression of initiated human prostatic epithelium. Cancer Res 1999;59: 5002–11.

5

In Vitro and In Vivo Models

YUZHUO WANG, PHD
GERALD R. CUNHA, PHD
SIMON W. HAYWARD, PHD

Prostate carcinoma is one of the most common malignancies affecting males, resulting in a high rate of morbidity and mortality.[1] Human prostatic carcinogenesis has been viewed as a multistep process involving progression from prostatic intraepithelial neoplasia to carcinoma, even though the precise etiology and pathogenesis of human prostate cancer remain largely undefined. Features that have hampered our understanding of human prostate cancer are its extremely heterogeneous nature and the limited number of animal or human laboratory models. Some important concepts concerning human prostate cancer have been derived from studies using appropriate animal models,[2,3] which are of great value in the study of the biology of human prostate cancer. Integration of information from relevant in vivo and in vitro models of prostate cancer biology will enormously facilitate the rational design of prevention and treatment strategies to target prostate cancer progression.

At present, there is no single ideal model for all aspects of prostate cancer. We will attempt to identify attributes and drawbacks associated with specific models.

IN VITRO PROSTATE CANCER MODELS

Prostate cancer has been studied extensively in vitro. In common with many other disease and developmental paradigms, the appeal of in vitro study is the ability to perform clean and easily reproducible experiments. In vitro models, like all models, have positive and negative features. The price that is paid for their reproducibility is the loss of the normal biologic interactions between epithelial cells and their local microenvironment and with the overall milieu of the organism from which they were derived. This includes factors such as hormonal environment, growth factors, extracellular matrix, and interactions with the immune system. Thus, much care must be taken in extrapolating results obtained from in vitro models, such as cell lines, to whole organism biology.

In vitro culture techniques have their origins in the embryologic experiments of the late nineteenth century. In 1898, Ljunggren demonstrated that human skin could survive for several days in ascitic fluid. In 1903, Jolly maintained salamander leukocytes in hanging drops for up to a month, making detailed observations of cell division and death. By 1907, Harrison was able to reproducibly demonstrate the growth of nerve axons out of small pieces of spinal cord from embryonic frogs when aseptically cultivated in frog lymph clots.[4] Burrows introduced the use of the plasma clot to replace the lymph clot as a nutrient source. In 1917, he published the first in vitro prostate work.[5] This used the "hanging drop" method with various "culture media," including plasma and ascites fluid. One of the effects noted by these investigators was liquefaction of the growth substrates, which was probably caused by the production of proteases by the cultured cells. In 1949, Allgöwer described the culture of pieces of the benign prostatic hyperplasia (BPH) nodule from three patients. He used chicken plasma as a solid phase with a mixture of human serum, chicken embryonal extract, and Tyrode's solution as a liquid phase. Interestingly, he also used 20 mg/100 mL sulfathiazole as an antibiotic, noting that one of the main limitations to successful culture was infection. Again, liquefaction of the clot within 5 to 6 days was found to be a limiting factor in the culture of this tissue.[6]

In 1959, Röhl was able to report on the growth of cells from prostatic tissue samples derived from needle biopsies of prostatic carcinoma and tissue cut from the dorsal or dorsolateral margins of hyperplastic prostates removed by transvesical prostatectomy.[7] This work was performed by growing tiny pieces of tissue in a clot made from 50% fowl plasma, 45% Tyrode's solution, and 5% chicken embryo extract supplemented with penicillin and streptomycin. A total of 2,719 cultures were analyzed. Röhl described the growth of both fibroblasts and glandular epithelial cells from the tissue pieces. The only method available to distinguish between cell types was their morphology as determined by light microscopy. On this basis, he concluded that the stroma had a low growth potential in his system, whereas the epithelium was able to form extensive and apparently regular cell sheets. Röhl also used lysine ethyl ester to inhibit the fibrinolysin activity of the prostate cells and thus prevent the lysis of plasma clots. This method was reasonably successful and allowed him to investigate the effects of androgens on growth in his culture system. He found no statistically significant stimulation of growth when hyperplastic tissue was used as the starting material; however, in an investigation of stimulation of prostate cancer–derived tissue, he found significant stimulation of growth in one case of six investigated.

Thus, by the late 1950s, in vitro techniques had advanced to a stage at which growth of cells from some defined origins could be achieved and some of the mechanisms involved in growth could be investigated. At around this period, the mid to late 1950s, in vitro techniques started to diverge with the separation of tissue, organ, and cell culture techniques.

Cell and organ culture both rely on the use of small fragments of tissue, which are placed into medium and allowed to develop. The principal difference between organ culture and other forms of in vitro culture is that with this technique, efforts are made to maintain the architecture and differentiated functions of the tissue. Thus, the intimate relationships of the various components of the tissue are kept reasonably intact. Cell culture, on the other hand, is simply the growth of cells from a given piece of tissue, with no effort made to maintain structure.

The disadvantages of organ culture (some of which are common to in vivo systems) include the difficulty of separating effects owing to different cell types within the cultured material and, in the case of the prostate, the difficulty of effectively monitoring the exocrine function of the cultured tissue.

Much of the important historica organ culture work on the prostate was performed by Lasnitzki and various coworkers. She worked principally on mouse and human prostate and developed organ culture systems for these tissues. Early work described organ culture in watch glasses of prostate explants from young and adult mice and the influence of androgens on their structural integrity.[8] Atrophy was noted in glands from young animals in culture for up to 21 days but was absent in cultured adult glands. There was a loss in functional columnar epithelium with increasing culture periods in the young glands but not in those from adults. However, the addition of testosterone propionate to the culture medium led to the maintenance of structure in young glands in the short term and hyperplastic growth in the longer term. In prostate rudiments derived from adult mice, this treatment rapidly led to hyperplastic growth. This suggests that the mature epithelium was more sensitive to androgenic stimulus. It should be noted that workers at this time were using pharmacologic doses of steroids, and this may be a cause of the hyperplasia noted. In any case, significant differences were noted in the response of tissues derived from adult and immature sources.

The first report of organ culture of human BPH is that of Schrodt and Foreman.[9] These authors found that the tissue could be maintained in the short term but that longer-term culture led to changes in the secretory epithelium from tall columnar to cuboidal. A number of investigations of the effects of both androgens and estrogens have been performed using BPH organ culture systems.[10] Notable findings include the tolerance of this tissue to short-term androgen withdrawal without involution. Tissue deprived of androgen for a short period can be rescued from involutional change with testosterone or with dihydrotestosterone. At a histologic level, androgens maintained the secretory phenotype, whereas estrogens elicited loss of secretory cells. At a molecular level, androgen stimulation led to a rapid increase in total ribonucleic acid production, whereas estrogens had the opposite effect.[11]

Organ culture work on the rat prostate has shown that androgen withdrawal leads to a gradual involution with a relative increase in stroma (as occurs in vivo); this effect can be postponed, but not averted, by the addition of androgens to the culture medium.[12] Estrogens have the effect of rapidly producing squamous metaplasia of the prostatic epithelium in this organ culture system.

Many organ culture studies have demonstrated that androgens elicit epithelial proliferation and differentiation in the developing rat prostate (Figure 5–1).[13,14] Such studies have also demonstrated that growth factors, in particular members of the fibroblast growth factor family, can substitute for androgens in eliciting such epithelial development.[13,15]

In general, organ culture has been useful for the study of the developing prostate, which has many characteristics in common with prostate cancer. However, organ culture has not been a productive area for the direct study of prostatic carcinoma. This is attributable to many problems associated with defining areas of tumor before culture is initiated and with the generally slow-growing nature of prostate cancer.

Cell culture techniques have used immortalized cell lines and primary cell cultures derived directly from prostatic specimens. Cell lines have been derived from many sources and are representative of a number of different cell types. Their advantages include the fact that they are immortalized and cloned and thus should provide consistent and comparable results. They are generally fairly easy to maintain in culture. The disadvantages of cell lines are that they can diverge with increasing passage number from their source cell type. This is because cell culture exerts its own pressures, selecting for cells resistant to trypsin damage and able to grow rapidly in vitro. Other factors include the ability to grow on tissue culture plastic, lack of density dependence, and tolerance of pH fluctuations.

Immortalized cell lines tend to be less genetically stable than their normal in vivo counterparts. Many cell lines show considerable genetic drift with respect to characteristics such as steroid dependence and responsiveness. This means that even cloned lines grown in different conditions may produce subclones with entirely different characteristics from each other.[16]

A further potential problem in laboratories that grow a number of different cell types is cross-contamination between different lines. This problem is well illustrated by the finding that the first reported human prostate cell line (MA 160) and at least one subsequent prostate line (EB33), as well as a long list of other cell lines, carry HeLa marker chromo-

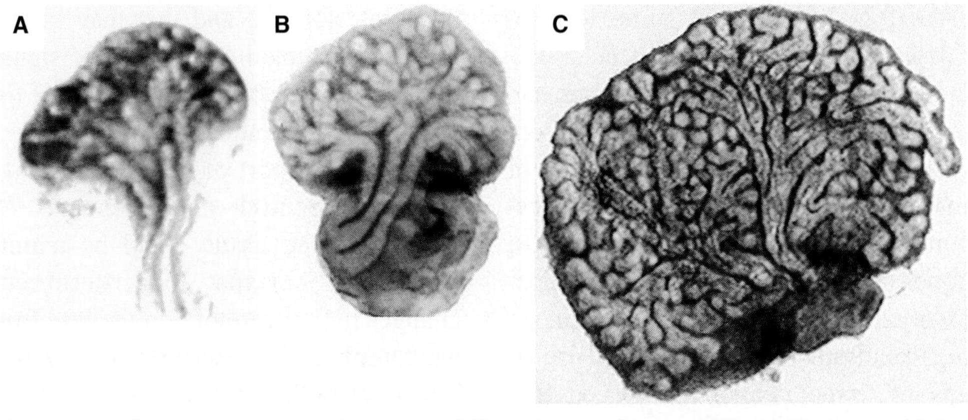

Figure 5–1. Organ culture of rat ventral prostate (VP) under serum-free conditions. *A,* Newborn rat VP has four main ducts and a small number of branches. *B,* When cultured for 6 days in the absence of testosterone the explant survives but undergoes a very limited amount of ductal branching morphogenesis. *C,* In contrast, culture in the presence of 10^{-8} M testosterone gives rise to extensive growth and branching.

somes.[17] This observation also reinforces the importance of obtaining cells from the originator or from a reputable facility rather than second or third hand through acquaintances.

Many human prostate epithelial cell lines have been developed. These were mostly derived from prostate cancer patients or from patients with BPH. All of these cells vary to a greater or lesser extent from prostate cells found in vivo. The most widely used human prostate cancer cell lines are DU145, PC-3, and LNCaP.

DU145 cells were derived in 1975 from a brain metastasis of a prostate adenocarcinoma in a 69-year-old white male. The original metastasis was identified as moderately differentiated with foci of poorly differentiated cells. DU145 cells grow very rapidly from low densities. They are neither hormone dependent nor hormone sensitive in terms of growth.[18]

The PC-3 line was isolated from a bone metastasis of a 62-year-old Caucasian diagnosed as having undifferentiated grade IV adenocarcinoma of the prostate. PC-3 will grow in soft agar, in suspension culture, and will form tumors in nude mice. It appears to be epithelial in nature but does not respond to androgens or various growth factors.[19]

LNCaP was derived in 1977 from a needle aspirate biopsy of a supraclavicular lymph node from a 50-year-old white male with stage D prostatic cancer. In culture, LNCaP cells produce human prostatic acid phosphatase, a trait that they maintain when transplanted into nude mice.[20] LNCaP cells are responsive to androgens in terms of growth (at least in the presence of serum); however, they exhibit aberrant responses to antiandrogens.[21]

Cell lines have great advantages in terms of ease of handling and reproducibility of results and can clearly be useful in answering well-defined questions that take their limitations into account. They have, however, lost many aspects of their original in vivo phenotype and therefore do not seem to provide a suitable model for the examination of many aspects of differentiated prostate biology or of tumor biology.

Beyond the three well-known cell lines, there are a number of other human and rodent prostate cancer cell lines. These include the human ND-1 line, which is unusual in that it was derived from a primary human prostate tumor.[22] Human prostate cancer cell lines were recently and thoroughly reviewed by Webber and colleagues in a three-part series.[23–25]

Another approach to prostatic cell culture is the use of artificially immortalized and transformed cell lines. A number of groups have used techniques such as the introduction of viral oncogenes to immortalize epithelial cells derived from nonmalignant human prostate.[26–30] In many of these cases, the resultant cells initially had a benign phenotype, not giving rise to tumors when grafted to athymic mice. However, these cell lines have proven capable of manipulation to give rise to a variety of malignant phenotypes. For example, the P69SV40T line, which has an extremely low tumorigenic potential, was cycled through nude mice to produce tumorigenic sublines with characteristic genetic defects.[31–33] Using a different route, Webber and colleagues took the SV40T-immortalized nontumorigenic RWPE-1 human prostatic cell line and stably introduced the VKIRAS oncogene, giving rise to a new cell line (RWPE-2) with malignant potential.[29,30]

Perhaps the most popular collection of prostate cancer cell lines is the series of cell lines derived from the Dunning tumor. These Dunning cell lines exhibit a wide variety of phenotypes from slow-growing to highly anaplastic lines with metastatic potential.[34] Another interesting pair of rat prostate epithelial cell lines is NRP 152 and NRP 154, derived from testosterone- and estradiol-treated Lobund-Wistar rats.[35] The NRP 152 line has basal cell–like characteristics in cell culture but can be made to form both basal and luminal cell phenotypes in culture and in tissue recombination models.[36,37] In contrast, the NRP 154 line is moderately tumorigenic.[34]

Most cell culture studies have concentrated on isolating epithelial cells of interest. It is clear, however, that one of the features of both a normal and a malignant prostate is the role of interactions between the epithelial and stromal populations, which are believed to play a role in the progression from genetically initiated epithelium to cancer.[38–40] For this reason, a few groups have now isolated and established human prostatic stromal cells in culture.[41–44]

Primary cell culture is a method of cultivating specific cell types from fresh tissue fragments. Such cells are not immortal and usually can be grown for a limited number of division cycles. The principal

extreme old age of these rats. Isaacs demonstrated that at the age of 24 months, 5% of the ACI/seg rats had prostatic carcinoma with metastatic capacity.[79]

In general, the low tumor incidence and very long latency periods limit the use of these spontaneous rat models. However, these models can be used to test putative enhancers of carcinogenesis (eg, carcinogens, high-fat diet, sex hormones). The transplantable tumors reportedly derived from spontaneous models would be valuable tools for studies on the biology of prostate cancer. However, in practice, the only commonly used transplantable rat prostate cancer model is the Dunning tumor.

Hormonal and Chemical Induction of Prostate Tumors

In general, as noted above, the incidence of spontaneous prostate cancer in animals is very low, with a very long latency. However, models of spontaneous prostate cancer have been used as a basis for tumor induction. Pollard reported that Lobund-Wistar rats developed a very low incidence of spontaneous metastatic prostatic cancer at 26 months.[75] Treating 3-month-old rats with testosterone increased the incidence of prostate cancer to 24% within 14 months. Surprisingly, dihydrotestosterone was not effective in inducing tumors.[80] In another study, Pollard and Luckert reported that 10% of Lobund-Wistar rats developed prostate cancer at 14 months after a single treatment of methylnitrosourea (MNU), and 14% developed prostate cancer within 14 months after subcutaneous administration of testosterone implants. A much higher incidence of carcinoma (77.5%) was found at an average age of 10.7 months after a single dose of MNU when combined with subcutaneous implants of testosterone.[81] Pollard and Luckert's description of their model suggested that the vast majority of the tumors originated within the anterior and dorsolateral prostate with rare seminal vesicle tumors.[82] However, it has since become clear that the vast majority (> 95%) of the grossly visible nodules/masses induced by combinations of a chemical carcinogen and testosterone originated in the seminal vesicles.[83,84] Therefore, the Lobund-Wistar model appears to be inappropriate to the study of prostatic carcinogenesis.

Other chemical carcinogens, for example, *N*-nitrosobis(oxopropyl)amine (BOP) have also been used to induce prostate cancer in rats. In Wistar-derived Medical Research Council rats, daily administration of BOP (either subcutaneously or intraperitoneally) for 3 days followed by testosterone given for life induced prostatic cancer in over 60% of rats.[85] Histologically, a large number of BOP-testosterone–induced prostatic tumors were adenocarcinomas of various histologic patterns that arose primarily in the dorsal lobe. In addition, squamous cell carcinomas were found in the ventral prostate.[85] These data suggest that testosterone plays an important role in the initiation of prostatic carcinogenesis, whereas tumor promotion is mediated by the interaction of testosterone with other factors.

Noble was the first to experimentally increase the low spontaneous incidence (0.48%) of prostate carcinoma to 20% in rats by prolonged treatment with pellets of testosterone propionate and estrone.[74,86] In another study, 73% of the rats subjected to testosterone plus estrogen (T + E2) treatment for 9 to 18 months (the same period as Noble) developed microscopic prostatic carcinoma. Of these, 10 to 15% developed grossly identifiable prostate tumors.[87] Wang and Wong developed a modified T + E2 induction protocol by increasing the testosterone level.[88] This protocol ensured a high incidence of prostate carcinogenesis and significantly shortened the induction period, producing a very useful model for prostate cancer research (Figure 5–2). Unfortunately, this rat model of prostatic cancer still has a long latency of 6 to 9 months.[88]

Transgenic Models

In recent years, transgenic mouse models have been instrumental in opening new avenues for exploring the mechanisms underlying cell growth and development. In terms of prostate carcinoma, a number of promoter sequences have been used to target various genes to the prostate. The promoters used include the rat C3(1) prostate steroid-binding protein promoter,[89–91] short and long versions of the rat probasin (PB) promoter,[92–95] the human PSA promoter,[96] the fetal globin (FG) promoter,[97] the mouse mammary tumor virus (MMTV) long terminal repeat (LTR),[98] and the mouse cryptdin-2 gene promotor.[99]

The PB promoters used in transgenic mice have been shown to be prostate epithelium specific with lobular variation in expression levels. Fetal globin and mouse cryptdin-2 promoters result in expression in prostatic neuroepithelial cells. C3(1), PSA, and MMTV regulatory sequences may also result in expression within nonprostatic epithelial cells. This was dramatically demonstrated in a transgenic line in which overexpression of the *FGF3/INT2* gene was achieved by placing it under the control of the MMTV LTR promoter.[100] Males of this line were reported to have greatly enlarged prostates and seminal vesicles, raising hopes that this may be a model of BPH.[98] However, careful dissection and critical examination of these mice revealed that the prostate was completely normal and did not even express the transgene, and the glandular enlargement was found to be an ampullary gland, a wolffian duct derivative. Expression of the transgene in these animals was found to be concentrated in wolffian duct derivatives.[101] The PSA promoter is also known to drive expression of transgenes in the salivary gland and gastrointestinal tract.[96]

The above targeting vectors have been used to express oncogenes, such as RAS, BCL2, SV40 large T antigen with or without small T, polyomavirus middle T (PYVMT), and keratinocyte growth factor (KGF) to the prostate epithelium of transgenic mice.

C3(1) and MMTV promoters have been used to target the expression of *BCL2* and KGF to the prostate. Male mice containing C3(1)/*BCL2* develop proliferative lesions in both epithelium and stroma.[89] Mice containing MMTV/KGF develop prostatic hyperplasia but not cancer[102]; it has yet to be independently confirmed that this hyperplasia is, in fact, in the prostate. These models may be useful for studying proliferative changes in the prostate but not for studying prostatic carcinogenesis.

The C3(1) promoter has also been used to target *PYVMT*. Male transgenic mice expressing *PYVMT* gene exhibited prostatic hyperplasia, dysplasia, and invasive carcinoma with lesions found in the ventral, dorsolateral, and anterior lobes of the prostate as well as in the vas deferens and epididymus.[103]

C3(1), PB, and FG have also been used to target SV40 early region (with large T and small T). When both large T and small T antigens were linked to the C3(1) promoter, tumors were induced in both the dorsolateral and ventral lobes.[91] In the so-called transgenic adenocarcinoma of the mouse prostate (TRAMP) model, the minimal PB promoter targets large and small T antigen expression to the prostate, giving rise to tumors predominantly within the dorsolateral lobes.[92] The FG promoter driving expression of the same viral oncogene gives rise to tumors in both the ventral and dorsolateral lobes.[97] In these models, the effective involvement of both large T and small T antigens makes the carcinogenesis very complicated as large T and small T antigens can easily disrupt many aspects of normal cell functions.

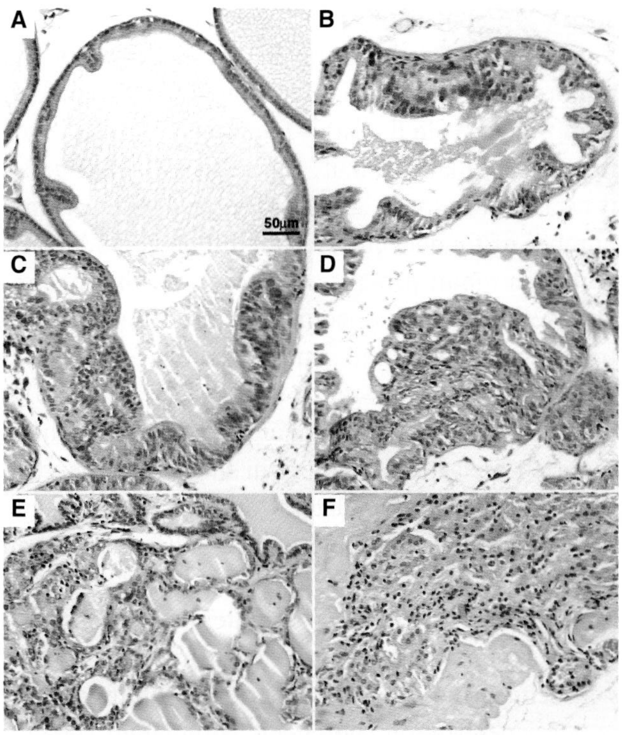

Figure 5–2. Response of the Noble rat dorsolateral prostate to testosterone and estradiol. *A,* The untreated prostate exhibits classic prostatic morphology with tall columnar luminal epithelial cells containing evenly shaped basally located nuclei. Exposure to testosterone and estradiol for 8 months gives rise to a range of histologic anomalies. *B* and *C,* These include low- and high-grade atypical hyperplasia, *D,* carcinoma in situ, and *E* and *F,* well- and poorly differentiated carcinoma. These conditions are characterized by progressive changes in the cell shape and nuclear-to-cytoplasmic ratio and by nuclear abnormalities. *F,* Cancer is characterized by invasion into the surrounding tissue exemplified by the coincidence of tumor and blood vessels. (Hematoxylin and eosin)

Kasper and colleagues reported on a series of transgenic mice carrying a large 12-kb fragment of the PB gene promoter (LPB) linked to SV40 large T deletion mutant (without small T).[94] This construct eliminates the role of small T antigen in tumorigenesis and results in more slow-growing tumors than those seen in the TRAMP model. Tumorigenesis in the LPB-Tag mice progressed in a manner similar to that observed in the human prostate. This study described mice derived from a number of founder lines that exhibited a wide variability in tumor progression and behavior, presumably related to the specific insertion point of the transgene. However, in general, there is a sequential development of high-grade dysplasia, carcinoma in situ, and locally invasive carcinoma without reported metastasis. Tumors in these mice develop primarily in the dorsolateral and anterior prostate and are responsive to androgen ablation, at least in the short term.

The mouse cryptdin-2 promoter has been used to direct expression of SV40T antigen to a subset of neuroendocrine cells.[99] Tumorigenesis in this model is not dependent on androgenic stimulation.

The targeting of viral oncogenes to the prostate results in a range of lesions. In the majority of cases, these are highly anaplastic and metastatic. Viral oncogenes (including *SV40T* and *PYVMT*) commonly work by disrupting the PRB and P53 pathways, making the cells susceptible to uncontrolled proliferation and genomic instability. Mutations in these pathways do occur in human prostate cancer but are generally considered to be late-stage events in the progression of the disease. Thus, these may not be ideal model systems with which to study the process of prostatic carcinogenesis. However, the ability of these tumors to metastasize and to mimic late-stage disease gives these transgenic models the potential to be useful in the study of late-stage disease. Another advantage of these models is that they exist in immunologically normal hosts, thus making them amenable to studies of the role of the immune system in cancer progression.

Transplantable Models

A small number of transplantable prostate tumors are available. Of these, the most widely used is the Dunning tumor. As noted above, the Dunning tumor was originally found at autopsy in a male Copenhagen rat.[73] This tumor has since been continuously passaged as subcutaneous grafts in Copenhagen, Fischer strain, and F1 hybrid rats. Over time, hosts have been chemically and hormonally manipulated, and tumors with various different characteristics have been isolated. A thorough review of the Dunning tumor is beyond the scope of this chapter; however, the history of the tumor and its various offshoots is provided by Isaacs.[3]

Serially transplantable human prostate tumors are problematic to grow and maintain. It has long been known that human prostate tumors are highly immunogenic in athymic mice.[104] In spite of this, a number of serially transplantable human tumors are available, of which the best known is probably PC-82.[105] This is a slow-growing tumor that produces human prostate-specific secretory proteins and is responsive to androgen ablation. The tumor does not metastasize. A number of other transplantable human prostate cancer xenograft models are also available.[106–111]

In addition to these serially transplantable tumors, a number of human prostatic cell lines can be grown in nude mice. These include the well-known LNCaP, DU145, and PC-3 lines. These lines have been used to study the phenomena of metastasis and progression from androgen dependence to independence. Extensive work performed by Chung and colleagues on LNCaP cells has led to the development and characterization of many sublines with different phenotypic and genotypic characteristics.[112,113] These models are being actively used to pursue the phenomena of bony metastasis and androgen independence.[113–115]

Transplantable models allow the examination of human or animal prostatic tumors in vivo. Their main disadvantages are that the human models require the use of immunocompromised hosts and that since these models are derived from preexisting tumors, they are not amenable to the study of early events in prostatic carcinogenesis.

Tissue Reconstitution Models

Prostate cancer research has historically focused on changes to epithelial cells. However, the role of prostatic stroma in the processes of carcinogenesis and tumor progression should not be overlooked.

The importance of the stromal microenvironment was demonstrated in a series of experiments by Thompson and colleagues. Using an in vivo mouse prostatic reconstitution system, these workers infected either the urogenital sinus or its individual mesenchymal (UGM) or epithelial (UGE) components using viruses carrying the *MYC* and the *RAS* oncogenes. Prostatic reconstitutions composed of uninfected UGM + infected UGE gave rise to epithelial hyperplasia. Stromal desmoplasia resulted from infection of UGM only. Carcinoma was induced only when both UGM and UGE were infected.[116–118] These findings demonstrated that stromal change may be a facilitator of the carcinogenic process.

We had long hypothesized that stromal changes play a role in the progression of human prostatic carcinoma.[38,39,68] Recently, we were able to demonstrate in another tissue recombination model that carcinoma-associated fibroblasts derived from human prostate tumors were able to induce genetically initiated but nontumorigenic human prostatic epithelial cells to form adenocarcinomas (Figure 5–3).[40]

Another application of tissue recombination models for prostate cancer research is the use of genetically modified tissue derived from gene knockout or transgenic animals. We have recently used prostatic epithelium derived from the retinoblastoma (*RB*) gene knockout mouse as the basis for a new model of prostatic carcinoma. Retinoblastoma knockout mice die in utero before the prostate rudiments form. Therefore, this model required the development of tissue rescue techniques to allow the generation of Rb–/– prostatic tissue. Rescued Rb–/– prostatic epithelium was recombined with rat UGM and grafted beneath the renal capsule of a nude mouse host. The host was then treated with T + E2 using Wang and Wong's modification of Noble's protocol.[88] In this model, the Rb–/– epithelium underwent a progressive stepwise progression toward prostatic carcinoma starting with dysplasia followed by carcinoma in situ and invasive cancer. Carcinomatous areas in T + E2–treated rUGM + Rb–/–prostatic epithelium tissue recombinants exhibited nuclear pleomorphism, elevated epithelial proliferation, increased mitoses and abnormal mitoses, loss of basal epithelial cells, complete loss of prostatic smooth muscle, loss of membrane staining for E-cadherin, and perturbation in ductal organization and epithelial polarity (Figure 5–4). In summary, prostatic carcinogenesis in the Rb–/– model parallels the early development of human prostatic carcinoma.[119]

Tissue recombination models are valuable in that they offer the ability to examine the effects of specific genetic insults to a known tissue layer and to examine the effects of such an insult in an in vivo environment while controlling for the complexities of the host environment. Thus, they can be used to address very specific genetic questions. One of their principal disadvantages is that, in most cases, they require the use of immunologically deficient host animals, making them unsuitable for examining phenomena and therapies based on the host immune system. There are also technical difficulties in that these models require extensive training and practice to be used successfully.

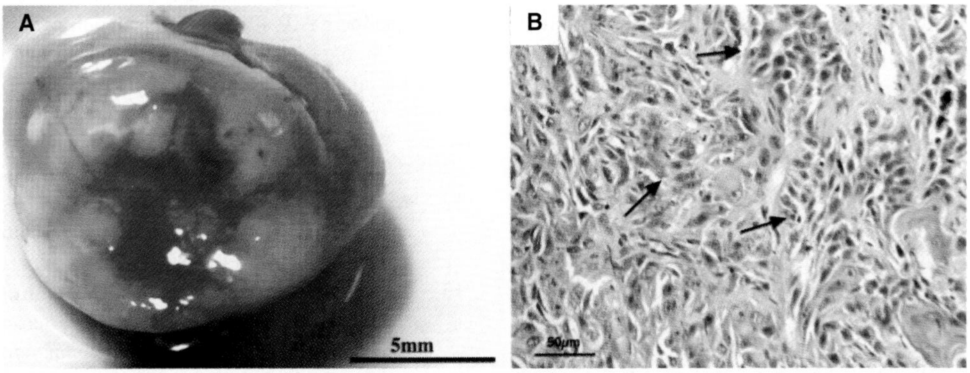

Figure 5–3. Tumor formed from a tissue recombinant composed of human prostatic carcinoma associated fibroblasts and BPH-1 human prostatic epithelial cells. As shown in *A*, the recombinant undergoes extensive growth to form a large bloody tumor. Histologically *B*, these tumors are characterized as adenocarcinoma based on the observation of abortive glandular structures (*arrows*). (Hematoxylin and eosin)

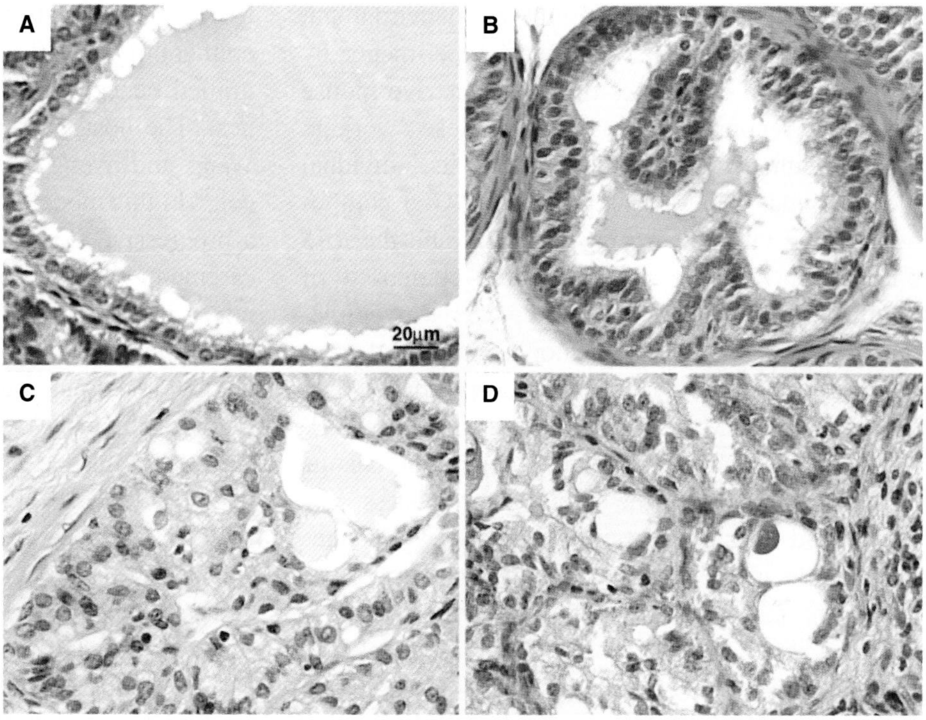

Figure 5–4. The response of a tissue recombinant composed of rat urogenital sinus mesenchyme and mouse retinoblastoma (*RB*) gene knockout prostatic epithelium to 8 weeks of treatment with testosterone and estradiol. A number of histologies are noted at this stage. *A,* There are large areas of normal-appearing prostatic tissue. *B,* Areas of hyperplastic histology are also seen; note the benign-appearing prostate histology with evenly shaped nuclei. *C,* Areas of atypical hyperplasia with disrupted glandular organization and irregularly shaped nuclei are seen. *D,* Areas of cancer with disrupted glandular organization and unevenly shaped nuclei are also found.

SUMMARY

There are many models of prostate cancer available to researchers today. One of the characteristics common to all of these models is that no single model is appropriate for investigation of all aspects of the progression of human prostatic carcinoma. Progress in prostate cancer research will require integration of the most informative model systems and, whenever possible, use of models that combine both in vitro and in vivo techniques.

ACKNOWLEDGMENT

The authors gratefully acknowledge research support from the National Institutes of Health through grants DK52721, DK 52708, CA 64872, DK 47517, CA 84294, and CA 59831.

REFERENCES

1. Chiarodo A. National Cancer Institute roundtable on prostate cancer: future research directions. Cancer Res 1991;51: 2498–505.
2. Coffey DS, Isaacs JT. Requirements for an idealized animal model of prostatic cancer. Prog Clin Biol Res 1980;37: 379–91.
3. Isaacs JT. Development and characteristics of the available animal model systems for the study of prostatic cancer. In: Coffey DS, Bruchovsky N, Gardner WW Jr, et al, editors. Current concepts and approaches to the study of prostate cancer. New York: AR Liss; 1987. p. 513–76.
4. Harrison RG. Observations on the living developing nerve fiber. Proc Soc Exp Biol N Y 1907;4:140–3.
5. Burrows MT, Burns JE, Suzuki Y. Studies on the growth of cells. The cultivation of bladder and prostatic tumors outside the body. J Urol 1917;1:3–15.
6. Allgöwer M. The cultivation of human prostatic adenomata *in vitro*. Exp Cell Res 1949;1 Suppl 1:456–9.
7. Röhl L. Prostatic hyperplasia and carcinoma studied with tissue culture technique. Acta Cirg Scand Suppl 1959;240.
8. Lasnitzki I. A hypervitaminosis on the effect of 20-methocholanthrene on mouse prostate glands grown in vitro. Br J Cancer 1955;9:434–41.
9. Schrodt GR, Foreman CD. *In vitro* maintenance of human hyperplastic prostate tissue. Invest Urol 1971;9:85–94.
10. Sandberg AA, Kadohama N. Regulation of prostatic growth in organ culture. Prog Clin Biol Res 1980;37:9–29.
11. Lasnitzki I. Human benign prostatic hyperplasia in cell and organ culture. In: Grayback JT, Wilson JD, Scherbenski MJ, editors. DHEW Publication no. (NIH) 76, 1113.1075. 1976. p. 235–48.
12. Martikainen PM, Makela SI, Santti RS, et al. Interaction of male and female sex hormones in cultured rat prostate. Prostate 1987;11:291–303.
13. Sugimura Y, Foster BA, Hom YK, et al. Keratinocyte growth factor (KGF) can replace testosterone in the ductal branching morphogenesis of the rat ventral prostate. Int J Dev Biol 1996;40:941–51.
14. Hayward SW, Baskin LS, Haughney PC, et al. Epithelial development in the rat ventral prostate, anterior prostate and seminal vesicle. Acta Anat (Basel) 1996;155:81–93.

15. Thomson AA, Cunha GR. Prostatic growth and development are regulated by FGF10. Development 1999;126:3693–701.
16. Darbre PD, King RJB. Progression to steroid insensitivity can occur irrespective of the presence of functional steroid receptors. Cell 1987;51:521–8.
17. Nelson-Rees WA, Flandermeyer RR. HeLa cultures defined. Science 1976;191:96–8.
18. Mickey DD, Stone KR, Wunderli H, et al. Characterization of a human prostate adenocarcinoma cell line (DU145) as a monolayer culture and as a solid tumour in athymic mice. Prog Clin Biol Res 1980;37:67–84.
19. Kaighn ME, Lechner JF, Babcock MS, et al. The Pasadena cell lines. Prog Clin Biol Res 1980;37:85–109.
20. Horoszewicz JS, Leong SS, Chu TM, et al. The LNCaP cell line—a new model for studies on human prostatic carcinoma. Prog Clin Biol Res 1980;37:115–32.
21. Wilding G, Chen M, Gelman EP. Aberrant response in vitro of hormone-responsive prostate cancer cells to antiandrogens. Prostate 1989;14:103–15.
22. Narayan P, Dahiya R. Establishment and characterization of a human primary prostatic adenocarcinoma cell line (ND-1). J Urol 1992;148:1600–4.
23. Webber MM, Bello D, Quader S. Immortalized and tumorigenic adult human prostatic epithelial cell lines: characteristics and applications. Part I. Cell markers and immortalized nontumorigenic cell lines. Prostate 1996;29:386–94.
24. Webber MM, Bello D, Quader S. Immortalized and tumorigenic adult human prostatic epithelial cell lines: characteristics and applications. Part 3. Oncogenes, suppressor genes, and applications. Prostate 1997;30:136–42.
25. Webber MM, Bello D, Quader S. Immortalized and tumorigenic adult human prostatic epithelial cell lines: characteristics and applications. Part 2. Tumorigenic cell lines. Prostate 1997;30:58–64.
26. Peehl DM, Wong ST, Sellers RG, et al. Loss of response to epidermal growth factor and retinoic acid accompanies the transformation of human prostatic epithelial cells to tumorigenicity with v-Ki-ras. Carcinogenesis 1997;18: 1643–50.
27. Kaighn ME, Reddel RR, Lechner JF, et al. Transformation of human neonatal prostate epithelial cells by strontium phosphate transfection with a plasmid containing SV40 early region genes. Cancer Res 1989;49:3050–6.
28. Hayward SW, Dahiya R, Cunha GR, et al. Establishment and characterization of an immortalized but non-tumorigenic human prostate epithelial cell line: BPH-1. In Vitro 1995;31A:14–24.
29. Bello D, Webber MM, Kleinman HK, et al. Androgen responsive adult human prostatic epithelial cell lines immortalized by human papillomavirus 18. Carcinogenesis 1997;18:1215–23.
30. Webber MM, Bello D, Kleinman HK, Hoffman MP. Acinar differentiation by nonmalignant immortalized human prostatic epithelial cells and its loss by malignant cells. Carcinogenesis 1997;18:1225–31.
31. Bae VL, Jackson-Cook CK, Maygarden SJ, et al. Metastatic sublines of an SV40 large T antigen immortalized human prostate epithelial cell line. Prostate 1998;34:275–82.
32. Bae VL, Jackson-Cook CK, Brothman AR, et al. Tumorigenicity of SV40 T antigen immortalized human prostate epithelial cells: association with decreased epidermal growth factor receptor (EGFR) expression. Int J Cancer 1994;58:721–9.
33. Jackson-Cook C, Bae V, Edelman W, et al. Cytogenetic characterization of the human prostate cancer cell line P69SV40T and its novel tumorigenic sublines M2182 and M15. Cancer Genet Cytogenet 1996;87:14–23.
34. Isaacs JT, Isaacs WB, Feitz WF, Scheres J. Establishment and characterization of seven Dunning rat prostatic cancer cell lines and their use in developing methods for predicting metastatic abilities of prostatic cancers. Prostate 1986; 9:261–81.
35. Danielpour D, Kadomatsu K, Anzano MA, et al. Development and characterization of nontumorigenic and tumorigenic epithelial cell lines from rat dorsal-lateral prostate. Cancer Res 1994;54:3413–21.
36. Hayward SW, Haughney PC, Lopes ES, et al. The rat prostatic epithelial cell line NRP-152 can differentiate in vivo in response to its stromal environment. Prostate 1999;39: 205–12.
37. Danielpour D. Transdifferentiation of NRP-152 rat prostatic basal epithelial cells toward luminal phenotype: regulation by glucocorticoid, insulin-like growth factor-I and transforming growth factor-beta. J Cell Sci 1999;112:169–79.
38. Hayward SW, Cunha GR, Dahiya R. Normal development and carcinogenesis of the prostate: a unifying hypothesis. Ann N Y Acad Sci 1996;784:50–62.
39. Cunha GR, Hayward SW, Dahiya R, Foster BA. Smooth muscle-epithelial interactions in normal and neoplastic prostatic development. Acta Anat (Basel) 1996;155:63–72.
40. Olumi AF, Grossfeld GD, Hayward SW, et al. Carcinoma-associated fibroblasts direct tumor progression of initiated human prostatic epithelium. Cancer Res 1999;59: 5002–11.
41. Webber MM, Trakul N, Thraves PS, et al. A human prostatic stromal myofibroblast cell line WPMY-1: a model for stromal-epithelial interactions in prostatic neoplasia. Carcinogenesis 1999;20:1185–92.
42. Peehl DM, Sellers RG. Basic FGF, EGF, and PDGF modify TGFbeta-induction of smooth muscle cell phenotype in human prostatic stromal cells. Prostate 1998;35:125–34.
43. Peehl DM, Sellers RG. Induction of smooth muscle cell phenotype in cultured human prostatic stromal cells. Exp Cell Res 1997;232:208–15.
44. Peehl DM, Sellers RG, Wong ST. Defined medium for normal adult human prostatic stromal cells. In Vitro Cell Dev Biol Anim 1998;34:555–60.
45. Webber M. Growth and maintenance of normal prostatic epithelium in vitro—a human cell model. Prog Clin Biol Res 1980;37:181–216.
46. Lasfargues EY. Cultivation and behaviour *in vitro* of the normal mammary epithelium of the adult mouse. Anat Rec 1957;127:117–29.
47. Webber MM. In vitro models for prostatic cancer: Summary. Prog Clin Biol Res 1980;37:133–47.
48. Hallowes RC, Cox S, Hayward S, et al. Effects of flutamide and hydroxy-flutamide on the growth of human benign prostatic hyperplasia cells in primary culture: a preliminary report. Anticancer Res 1991;11:1799–806.
49. Hayward S, Cox S, Mitchell I, et al. The effects of interferons on the activity of α-glycerolphosphate dehydrogenase in

benign prostatic hyperplasia cells in primary culture. J Urol 1987;138:648–53.
50. Merchant DJ. Terminally differentiating epithelial tissues in primary explant culture: a model of growth and development. In Vitro Cell Dev Biol Anim 1990;26:543–53.
51. Merchant DJ. Primary explant culture of human prostate tissue: a model for the study of prostate physiology and pathology. Prostate 1990;16:103–26.
52. Merchant DJ, Clarke SM, Ives K, Harris S. Primary explant culture: an in vitro model of the human prostate. Prostate 1988;4:523–42.
53. Peehl DM, Stamey TA. Serum-free growth of adult human prostatic epithelial cells. In Vitro Cell Dev Biol Anim 1986; 22:82–90.
54. Peehl DM, Stamey TA. Growth responses of normal, benign hyperplastic, and malignant human prostatic epithelial cells in vitro to cholera toxin, pituitary extract, and hydrocortisone. Prostate 1986;8:51–61.
55. Peehl DM, Wong ST, Stamey TA. Clonal growth characteristics of adult human prostatic epithelial cells. In Vitro Cell Dev Biol 1988;24:530–6.
56. Peehl DM, Wong ST, Terris MK, Stamey TA. Culture of prostatic epithelial cells from ultrasound-guided needle biopsies. Prostate 1991;19:141–7.
57. Kabalin JN, Peehl DM, Stamey TA. Clonal growth of human prostatic epithelial cells is stimulated by fibroblasts. Prostate 1989;14:251–63.
58. Mather JP, Sato GH. The use of hormone-supplemented serum-free media in primary cultures. Exp Cell Res 1979;124:215–21.
59. Hammond SL, Ham RG, Stampfer MR. Serum-free growth of human mammary epithelial cells: rapid clonal growth in defined medium and extended serial passage with pituitary extract. Proc Natl Acad Sci U S A 1984;81:5435–9.
60. Peehl DM, Stamey TA. Serial propagation of adult human prostatic epithelial cells with cholera toxin. In Vitro 1984;20:981–6.
61. Kan M, Shi E-G. Fibronectin, not laminin, mediates heparin-dependant heparin-binding growth factor type I binding to substrata and stimulation of endothelial cell growth. In Vitro 1990;26:1151–6.
62. Turner T, Bern HA. Growth responses of prostate epithelial cells from male mice neonatally exposed to diethylstilbestrol in serum-free collagen gel culture. Cancer Lett 1990;52:209–18.
63. Turner T, Bern HA, Young P, Cunha GR. Serum-free culture of enriched mouse anterior and ventral prostatic epithelial cells in collagen gel. In Vitro Cell Dev Biol 1990;26:722–30.
64. Taylor-Papadimitriou J, Purkis P, Fentiman IS. Cholera toxin and analogues of cyclic AMP stimulate the growth of cultured human mammary epithelial cells. J Cell Physiol 1980;102:317–21.
65. Green H. Cyclic AMP in relation to proliferation of the epidermal cell: a new view. Cell 1978;15:801–11.
66. McKeehan WL, Adams PS, Rosser MP. Direct mitogenic effects of insulin, epidermal growth factor, glucocorticoid, cholera toxin, unknown pituitary factors and possibly prolactin, but not androgen, on normal rat prostate epithelial cells in serum-free, primary cell culture. Cancer Res 1984;44:1998–2010.
67. Montpetit M, Abrahams P, Clark AF, Tenniswood M. Androgen-independent epithelial cells of the rat ventral prostate. Prostate 1988;12:13–28.
68. Hayward SW, Rosen MA, Cunha GR. Stromal-epithelial interactions in normal and neoplastic prostate. Br J Urol 1997;79 Suppl 2:18–26.
69. Pylkkanen L, Makela S, Santti R. Animal models for the preneoplastic lesions of the prostate. Eur Urol 1996;30:243–8.
70. Bell FW, Klausner JS, Hayden DW, et al. Clinical and pathologic features of prostatic adenocarcinoma in sexually intact and castrated dogs: 31 cases (1970–1987). J Am Vet Med Assoc 1991;199:1623–30.
71. Leav I, Ling GV. Adenocarcinoma of the canine prostate. Cancer 1968;22:1329–45.
72. Obradovich J, Walshaw R, Goullaud E. The influence of castration on the development of prostatic carcinoma in the dog. 43 cases (1978–1985). J Vet Intern Med 1987;1:183–7.
73. Dunning WF. Prostate cancer in the rat. Natl Cancer Inst Monogr 1963;12:351–70.
74. Noble RL. The development of prostatic adenocarcinoma in Nb rats following prolonged sex hormone administration. Cancer Res 1977;37:1929–33.
75. Pollard M. Spontaneous prostate adenocarcinomas in aged germfree Wistar rats. J Natl Cancer Inst 1973;51:1235–41.
76. Pollard M. The Lobund-Wistar rat model of prostate cancer. J Cell Biochem Suppl 1992:84–8.
77. Pollard M, Luckert PH. Patterns of spontaneous metastasis manifested by three rat prostate adenocarcinomas. J Surg Oncol 1979;12:371–7.
78. Ward JM, Reznik G, Stinson SF, et al. Histogenesis and morphology of naturally occurring prostatic carcinoma in the ACI/segHapBR rat. Lab Invest 1980;43:517–22.
79. Isaacs JT. The aging ACI/Seg versus Copenhagen male rat as a model system for the study of prostatic carcinogenesis. Cancer Res 1984;44:5785–96.
80. Pollard M, Snyder DL, Luckert PH. Dihydrotestosterone does not induce prostate adenocarcinoma in L-W rats. Prostate 1987;10:325–31.
81. Pollard M, Luckert PH. Autochthonous prostate adenocarcinomas in Lobund-Wistar rats: a model system. Prostate 1987;11:219–27.
82. Pollard M, Luckert PH. Early manifestations of induced prostate tumors in Lobund-Wistar rats. Cancer Lett 1992;67:113–6.
83. Lucia MS, Anzano MA, Slayter MV, et al. Chemopreventive activity of tamoxifen, N-(4-hydroxyphenyl)retinamide, and the vitamin D analogue Ro24-5531 for androgen-promoted carcinomas of the rat seminal vesicle and prostate. Cancer Res 1995;55:5621–7.
84. Tamano S, Rehm S, Waalkes MP, Ward JM. High incidence and histogenesis of seminal vesicle adenocarcinoma and lower incidence of prostate carcinomas in the Lobund-Wistar prostate cancer rat model using N-nitrosomethylurea and testosterone. Vet Pathol 1996;33:557–67.
85. Pour PM, Stepan K. Induction of prostatic carcinomas and lower urinary tract neoplasms by combined treatment of intact and castrated rats with testosterone propionate and N-nitrosobis(2-oxopropyl)amine. Cancer Res 1987;47: 5699–706.
86. Noble RL. Sex steroids as a cause of adenocarcinoma of the dorsal prostate in Nb rats, and their influence on the growth of transplants. Oncology 1977;34:138–41.

87. Drago JR. The induction of NB rat prostatic carcinomas. Anticancer Res 1984;4:255–6.
88. Wang YZ, Wong YC. Sex hormone-induced prostatic carcinogenesis in the noble rat: the role of insulin-like growth factor-I (IGF-I) and vascular endothelial growth factor (VEGF) in the development of prostate cancer. Prostate 1998;35:165–77.
89. Zhang X, Chen MW, Ng A, et al. Abnormal prostate development in C3(1)-bcl-2 transgenic mice. Prostate 1997; 32:16–26.
90. Maroulakou IG, Anver M, Garrett L, Green JE. Prostate and mammary adenocarcinoma in transgenic mice carrying a rat C3(1) simian virus 40 large tumor antigen fusion gene. Proc Natl Acad Sci U S A 1994;91:11236–40.
91. Shibata MA, Ward JM, Devor DE, et al. Progression of prostatic intraepithelial neoplasia to invasive carcinoma in C3(1)/SV40 large T antigen transgenic mice: histopathological and molecular biological alterations. Cancer Res 1996;56:4894–903.
92. Greenberg NM, DeMayo F, Finegold MJ, et al. Prostate cancer in a transgenic mouse. Proc Natl Acad Sci U S A 1995;92:3439–43.
93. Greenberg N, DeMayo F, Sheppard P, et al. The rat probasin gene promoter directs hormonally and developmentally regulated expression of a heterologous gene specifically to the prostate in transgenic mice. Mol Endocrinol 1994;8:230–9.
94. Kasper S, Sheppard PC, Yan Y, et al. Development, progression, and androgen-dependence of prostate tumors in probasin-large T antigen transgenic mice: a model for prostate cancer. Lab Invest 1998;78:319–33.
95. Yan Y, Sheppard PC, Kasper S, et al. Large fragment of the probasin promoter targets high levels of transgene expression to the prostate of transgenic mice. Prostate 1997; 32:129–39.
96. Schaffner DL, Barrios R, Shaker MR, et al. Transgenic mice carrying a PSArasT24 hybrid gene develop salivary gland and gastrointestinal tract neoplasms. Lab Invest 1995;72: 283–90.
97. Perez-Stable C, Altman NH, Mehta PP, et al. Prostate cancer progression, metastasis, and gene expression in transgenic mice. Cancer Res 1997;57:900–6.
98. Tutrone RF Jr, Ball RA, Ornitz DM, et al. Benign prostatic hyperplasia in a transgenic mouse: a new hormonally sensitive investigatory model. J Urol 1993;149:633–9.
99. Garabedian EM, Humphrey PA, Gordon JI. A transgenic mouse model of metastatic prostate cancer originating from neuroendocrine cells. Proc Natl Acad Sci U S A 1998;95:15382–7.
100. Muller JW, Lee FS, Dickson C, et al. The *int*-2 gene product acts as an epithelial growth factor in transgenic mice. EMBO J 1990;9:907–13.
101. Donjacour AA, Thomson AA, Cunha GR. Enlargement of the ampullary gland and seminal vesicle, but not the prostate in int-1/Fgf-3 transgenic mice. Differentiation 1998;62: 227–37.
102. Kitsberg DI, Leder P. Keratinocyte growth factor induces mammary and prostatic hyperplasia and mammary adenocarcinoma in transgenic mice. Oncogene 1996;13:2507–15.
103. Tehranian A, Morris DW, Min BH, et al. Neoplastic transformation of prostatic and urogenital epithelium by the polyoma virus middle T gene. Am J Pathol 1996;149:1177–91.
104. Reid LM, Minato N, Gresser I, et al. Influence of anti-mouse interferon serum on the growth and metastasis of tumor cells persistently infected with virus and of human prostatic tumors in athymic nude mice. Proc Natl Acad Sci U S A 1981;78:1171–5.
105. Hoehn W, Schroeder FH, Reimann JF, et al. Human prostatic adenocarcinoma: some characteristics of a serially transplantable line in nude mice (PC 82). Prostate 1980; 1:95–104.
106. Csapo Z, Brand K, Schrott KM, Schwindl B. Prostatic acid phosphatase in the serially transplantable human prostatic tumor lines PC-82 and PC-EW. Urol Res 1990;18:137–42.
107. Hoehn W, Wagner M, Riemann JF, et al. Prostatic adenocarcinoma PC EW, a new human tumor line transplantable in nude mice. Prostate 1984;5:445–52.
108. Ito YZ, Mashimo S, Nakazato Y, Takikawa H. Hormone dependency of a serially transplantable human prostatic cancer (HONDA) in nude mice. Cancer Res 1985;45: 5058–63.
109. Nagabhushan M, Miller CM, Pretlow TP, et al. CWR22: the first human prostate cancer xenograft with strongly androgen-dependent and relapsed strains both in vivo and in soft agar. Cancer Res 1996;56:3042–6.
110. Wainstein MA, He F, Robinson D, et al. CWR22: androgen-dependent xenograft model derived from a primary human prostatic carcinoma. Cancer Res 1994;54:6049–52.
111. Wright GL Jr, Haley CL, Csapo Z, van Steenbrugge GJ. Immunohistochemical evaluation of the expression of prostate tumor-association markers in the nude mouse human prostate carcinoma heterotransplant lines PC-82, PC-EW, and PC-EG. Prostate 1990;17:301–16.
112. Chung LW, Zhau HE, Wu TT. Development of human prostate cancer models for chemoprevention and experimental therapeutics studies. J Cell Biochem Suppl 1997;29:174–81.
113. Zhau HY, Chang SM, Chen BQ, et al. Androgen-repressed phenotype in human prostate cancer. Proc Natl Acad Sci U S A 1996;93:15152–7.
114. Nelson JB, Nguyen SH, Wu-Wong JR, et al. New bone formation in an osteoblastic tumor model is increased by endothelin-1 overexpression and decreased by endothelin A receptor blockade. Urology 1999;53:1063–9.
115. Wu TT, Sikes RA, Cui Q, et al. Establishing human prostate cancer cell xenografts in bone: induction of osteoblastic reaction by prostate-specific antigen-producing tumors in athymic and SCID/bg mice using LNCaP and lineage-derived metastatic sublines. Int J Cancer 1998;77:887–94.
116. Thompson TC. Growth factors and oncogenes in prostate cancer. Cancer Cells 1990;11:345–54.
117. Thompson TC, Southgate J, Kitchener G, Land H. Multistage carcinogenesis induced by ras and myc oncogenes in a reconstituted organ. Cell 1989;56:917–30.
118. Thompson TC, Timme TL, Kadmon D, et al. Genetic predisposition and mesenchymal-epithelial interactions in ras+myc-induced carcinogenesis in reconstituted mouse prostate. Mol Carcinog 1993;7:165–79.
119. Wang YZ, Hayward SW, Donjacour AA, et al. Sex hormone-induced prostatic carcinogenesis in Rb-deficient prostate tissue. Cancer Res 2000;60:6008–17.

6

Anatomy

RODMAN S. ROGERS, MD
PETER R. CARROLL, MD, FACS
EMIL TANAGHO, MD

GENERAL DESCRIPTION

The prostate is an ovoid structure with the appearance of an inverted bilobed cone, located between the urinary bladder superiorly and the pelvic floor inferiorly. The urethra traverses this gland, entering at the broad base of the cone just below the bladder neck and exiting near the narrowed apex of the cone at the level of the urogenital diaphragm. The rounded anterior surface is behind the pubis and the posterior surface is flattened with a midline depression (the median sulcus) that lies against the rectal ampulla (Figure 6–1). The lateral and inferior surfaces of the gland are in contact with the levator ani muscles. The ejaculatory ducts enter the posterior surface laterally and pass obliquely toward the midline, where they end at the verumontanum on the posterior surface of the prostatic urethra. Because of its location deep within the pelvis behind the pubic bone, surgical approaches to expose the prostate and protect surrounding structures can be challenging.

On surgical exposure of the retropubic space (of Retzius), with the bladder retracted superiorly, the anterior surface of the prostate and the adjacent lateral pelvic floor are covered with a glistening fascial layer. Covering the gland, this layer is formed by the prostatic and levator fasciae (together called the periprostatic fascia or prostatic sheath), which are closely applied to the prostatic capsule.[1] Lateral to the gland, this layer is called the endopelvic fascia and covers the pelvic floor with important underlying neurovascular structures. The prostatic venous plexus (of Santorini), a rich network of tributary veins that serve as the primary penile drainage, is seen within this fascial covering.[2] Erectile nerves to the corpora cavernosa travel outside the prostatic capsule in the lateral pelvic fascia between the prostate and the rectum.[3] Appreciating these anatomic relationships intraoperatively is essential to avoid unnecessary injury and bleeding.[4]

INTRINSIC ANATOMY

The internal structure of the prostate has been organized into two schemes described as lobes or zones. Lowsley's description of five lobes was based on the embryologic development of the prostate beginning as five groups of epithelial buds that branch off the urogenital sinus between the eleventh and sixteenth weeks of gestation. By successively branching and rebranching, a complex system of ducts is formed circumferentially around the urethra, forming five lobes: anterior, posterior, median, and two lateral lobes (Figure 6–2A). As these lobes grow, they meet side by side and abut their surrounding lobes. The tubules in each lobe do not intermingle with their neighboring lobe, and there are no fascial separations between these lobes.[5] By this description, the median lobe is bounded by the urethra anteriorly and the plane of the ejaculatory ducts posteriorly. The posterior lobe is located behind the plane of the ejaculatory ducts, in contact with that portion of the prostatic urethra lying below the level of the verumontanum (the inframontanal urethra). The lateral lobes are on each side of the urethra, and the anterior lobe joins the two lateral lobes anterior to the urethra. The

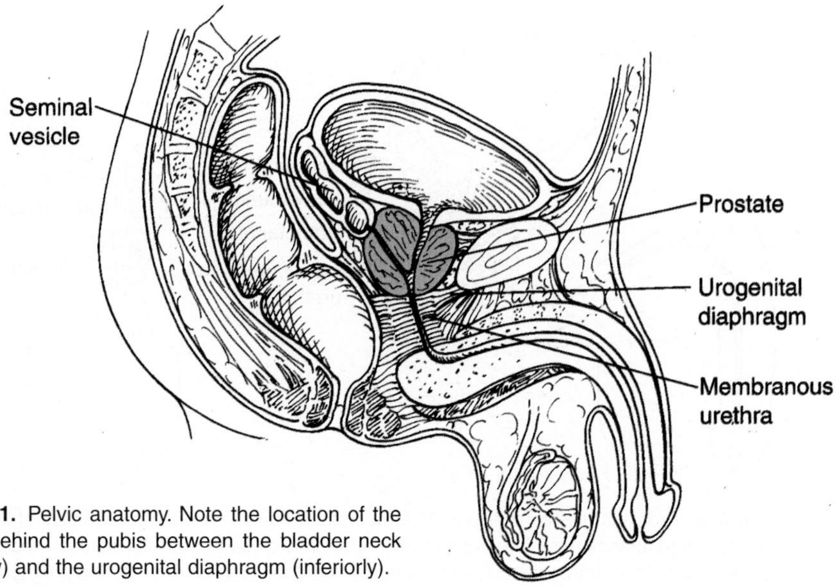

Figure 6–1. Pelvic anatomy. Note the location of the prostate behind the pubis between the bladder neck (superiorly) and the urogenital diaphragm (inferiorly).

zonal description of prostate structure[6] is based on more surgically oriented anatomy and therefore is more commonly used in clinical practice. According to this scheme (Figure 6–2B), the prostate consists of two primary areas: the peripheral zone and the central zone. In the absence of adenomatous hyperplasia, these two zones comprise up to 95 percent of the prostate mass.[7] The remaining gland consists of the transition zone, the anterior fibromuscular segment, and the periurethral glandular zone.

The peripheral zone is the largest portion of the prostate in young men, comprising 70 percent of the glandular mass.[8] It constitutes the bulk of the apical, posterior, and lateral prostatic tissue. Distal to the verumontanum, the peripheral zone may surround the urethra as it approaches the prostatic apex. At least

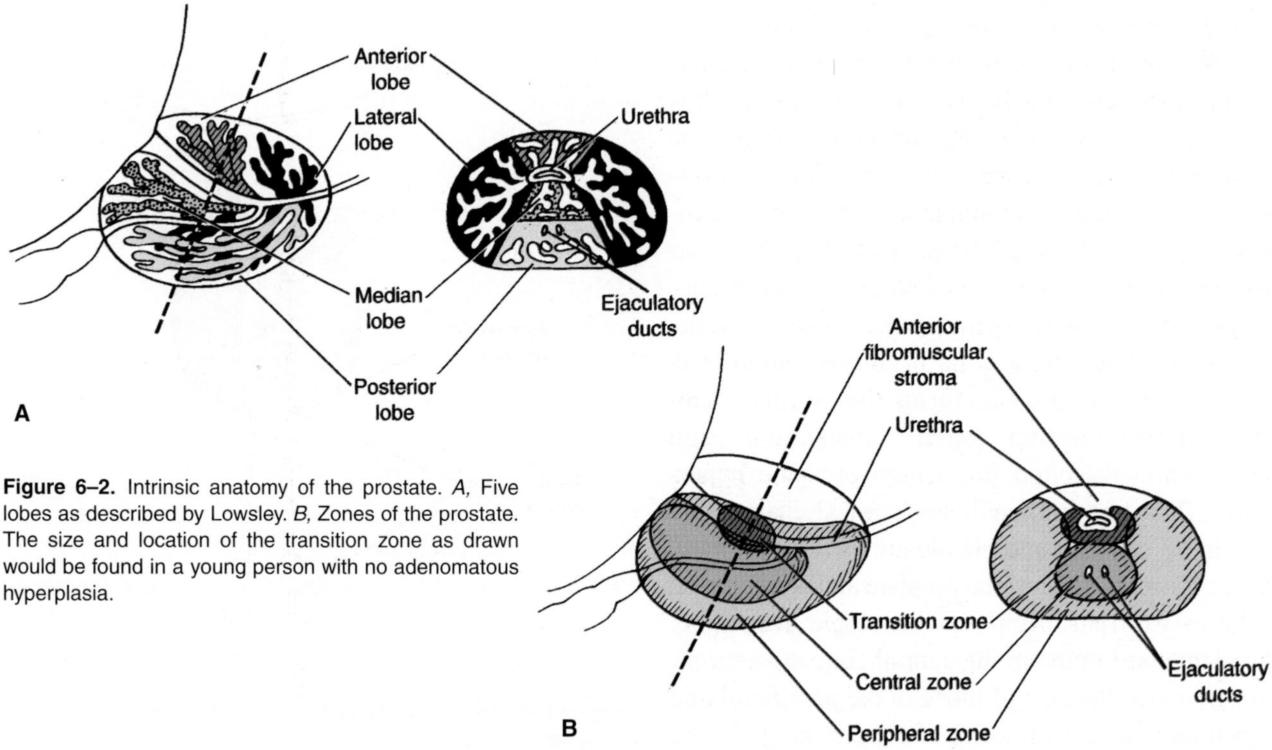

Figure 6–2. Intrinsic anatomy of the prostate. *A,* Five lobes as described by Lowsley. *B,* Zones of the prostate. The size and location of the transition zone as drawn would be found in a young person with no adenomatous hyperplasia.

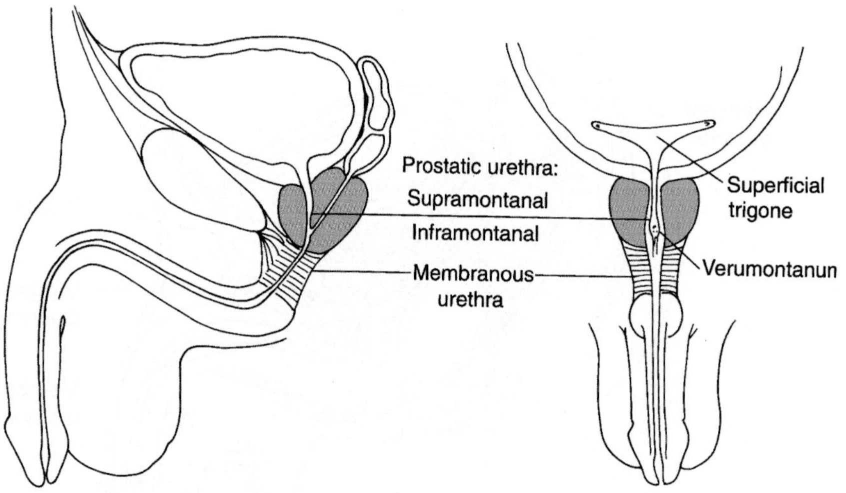

Figure 6–3. Prostatic urethra divisions. The prostatic urethra is divided functionally and structurally by the verumontanum. The supramontanal urethra extends from the bladder neck to the verumontanum. The inframontanal urethra extends from the verumontanum to the prostatic apex.

70 percent of prostate cancers occur in the peripheral zone.[9] Its location at the periphery of the gland, adjacent to the rectal ampulla over the prostate's broad posterior surface, explains the ability to detect pathology by digital rectal examination. In addition to hard nodules that may indicate cancer, a spongy consistency or prostatic tenderness and heat can herald prostatitis. The prostatic ducts drain into the prostatic sinus along the entire length of the inframontanal urethra,[6] which may explain why the peripheral zone is most commonly affected by chronic prostatitis.

The central zone surrounds the ejaculatory ducts and projects below the base of the bladder neck. It is almost cone shaped, with the flat surface of the cone at the base of the prostate and the pointed tip oriented toward the verumontanum. This zone comprises approximately 25 percent of total glandular tissue in the hyperplastic prostate.[10] As foci of adenomatous hyperplasia grow in the transition zone, the surrounding parenchyma becomes compressed, and this condensed tissue forms the "surgical capsule" noted during open enucleation and transurethral resection for benign prostatic hyperplasia. Based on immunohistochemical characteristics, these central zone glands are developmentally distinct from the rest of the prostate and are believed to be of wolffian origin. On histologic evaluation, the glandular lumina in the central zone are approximately twice the size of those in the peripheral and transition zones. A minority of cancers are believed to arise in this zone. McNeal and colleagues found that only 8 percent of cancers in their series of 104 radical prostatectomy specimens arose in this zone.[9]

The transition zone surrounds the urethra proximal to the ejaculatory ducts and comprises 5 to 10 percent of the glandular mass in the nonhyperplastic prostate. In patients with benign prostatic hyperplasia, however, this zone may constitute the bulk of the prostate and may be seen endoscopically as the "lat-

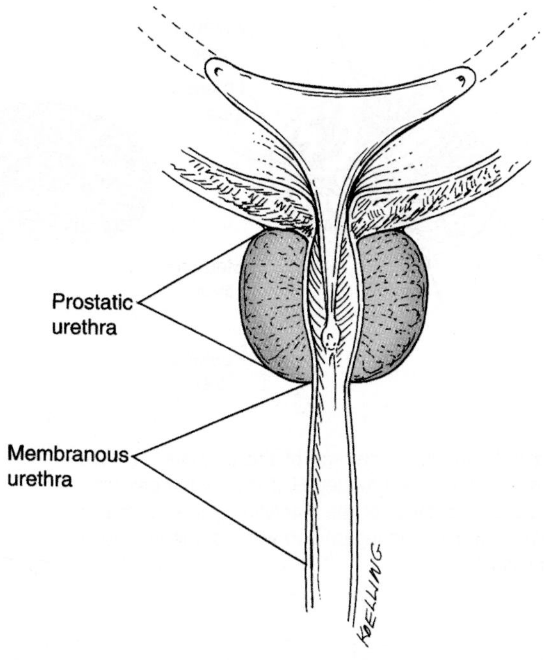

Figure 6–4. Prostatic and membranous urethra—the posterior urethral wall.

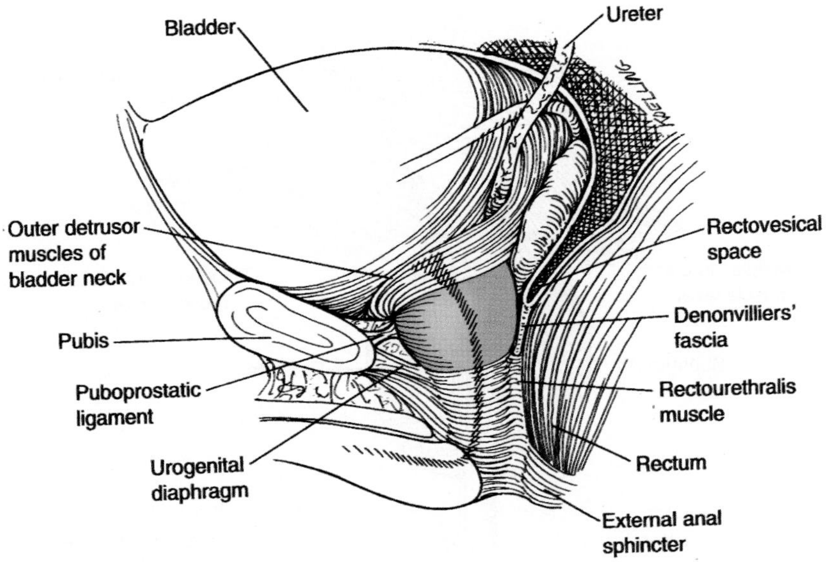

Figure 6–5. Prostatomembranous sphincter mechanisms — external view with urethral lumen shown (*hatched*).

eral lobes." Surrounding this zone is a dense fibromuscular band of tissue that may be easily appreciated by transrectal ultrasonography. According to McNeal and colleagues, 24 percent of evaluable cancers found after radical prostatectomy arose in the transition zone. Among cancers detected on pathologic examination of specimens from transurethral resection for benign prostatic hyperplasia (stage T1a or T1b), virtually all originated in the transition zone.[9]

The periurethral glandular zone describes a group of mucosal glands surrounding the prostatic urethra. Although this represents a small fraction of the glandular prostate, this zone is also prone to hyperplasia. The "median lobe" refers to benign prostatic hyperplasia within a subtrigonal group of these glands that may elevate and obstruct the bladder neck with increasing size.

THE PROSTATIC URETHRA

The normal prostatic urethra measures 3 to 4 cm in length and can be divided into two segments by the verumontanum. The proximal, supramontanal portion of the prostatic urethra extends from the bladder neck to the entrance of the ejaculatory ducts at the verumontanum. At this point, the urethra takes an approximate 35- to 45-degree turn anteriorly. The inframontanal portion extends over the distal prostate from the verumontanum to the membranous urethra (Figure 6–3). The supramontanal urethra is developmentally related to the bladder and lined with transitional epithelium. Muscular stroma in this portion of the gland is in continuity with the bladder detrusor muscle, as discussed below. The supramontanal urethra is lined with periurethral glands, which contribute minimally to seminal fluid, remain rudimentary structures, and are not connected to the vast network of prostatic acini. In contrast, the inframontanal urethra is lined with pseudostratified or stratified columnar epithelium, similar to the distal urethral lining. It is into this portion of the prostatic urethra that the bulk of secretions drains from prostatic acini to aid in sperm transport.[11]

The inner surface of the supramontanal prostatic urethra has a crest projecting into the lumen from the posterior midline, the crista urethralis, which represents a continuation of the superficial trigone (Figure 6–4).[12] The prostatic sinuses are the grooves to each side, between this crest and the lateral urethral wall. The bulk of glandular tubules from the deep network of prostatic acini drains into the supramontanal prostatic urethra with seminal emission. The verumontanum, also known as the seminal colliculus, contains the blind ending orifice of the prostatic utricle in the midline, a remnant of the müllerian duct system. Lateral to the utricle are the paired orifices of the ejaculatory ducts. During transurethral resection

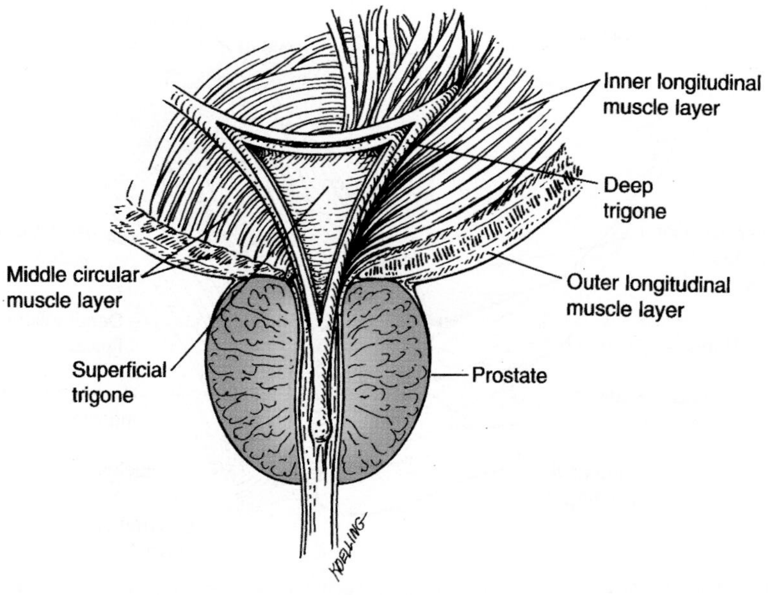

Figure 6–6. Muscle layers of the bladder neck and trigone in elation to the prostate.

of the prostate, the verumontanum is used as the landmark for the distal resection margin to avoid injury to the inframontanal prostatic musculature and sphincter mechanisms.[13]

SPHINCTER MECHANISMS

Understanding the normal sphincteric anatomy in the male may logically flow from basic information on the embryologic development of the prostatic urethra. As discussed previously, the glandular stroma of the prostate develops from glandular buds that begin as outpouchings from the epithelial lining of the proximal urethra.[14] As these buds grow through the muscular coat of the urethra, the primordial periurethral muscle becomes entangled between and around the glands as they develop and branch. Just as these periurethral muscle fibers provide tonus of the female urethra distal to the bladder neck, in the male these fibers are part of the developing prostate, become the muscular stroma, and contribute to closure of the prostatic urethra.[15] In the normal male, urinary continence occurs over the entire posterior urethra from the bladder neck through the distal membranous urethra. In addition to the prostatic stroma, there are two primary muscular zones that contribute to urethral pressure within this length that may be distinguished anatomically.[16] The proximal mechanism includes musculature of the bladder neck and continuation of the

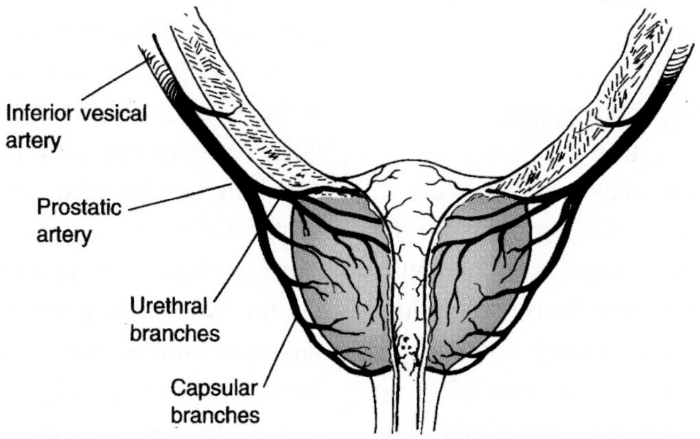

Figure 6–7. Prostatic arterial supply.

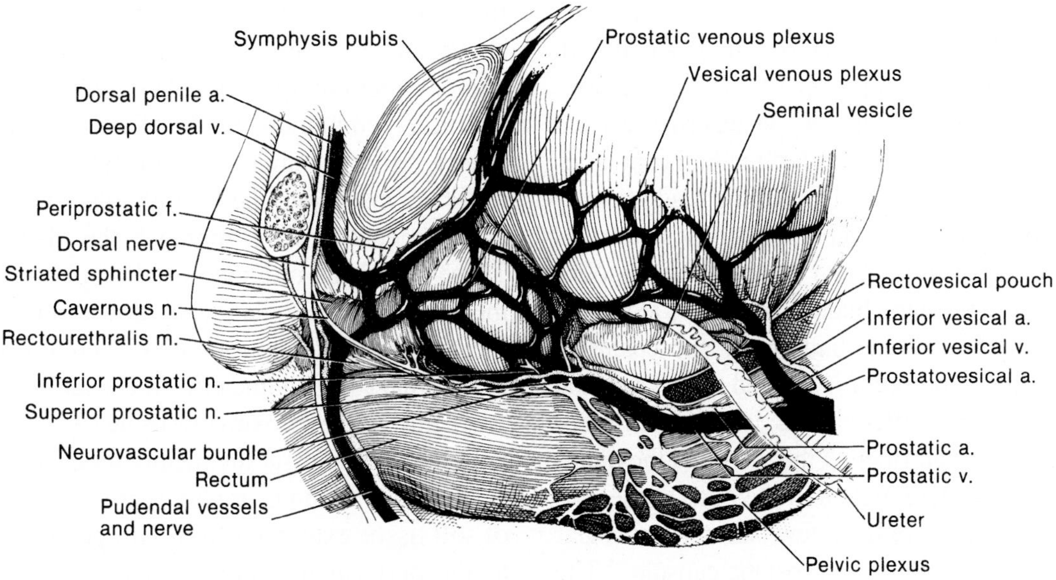

Figure 6–8. Prostatic venous drainage. Reproduced with permission from Human atlas.

detrusor fibers periurethrally to the level of the verumontanum. The distal mechanism involves both intrinsic and extrinsic components and extends from the verumontanum to the perineal membrane (Figure 6–5).

The prostate is in continuity with the bladder neck, and two layers of the detrusor fibers continue beyond the vesical neck to contribute to closure of the prostatic urethra (Figure 6–6). The middle circular detrusor fibers do not extend into the prostate but instead stop abruptly at the bladder neck.[17] The inner longitudinal layer of bladder muscle continues as the inner longitudinal smooth muscle layer throughout the prostatic urethra. The outer longitudinal muscle layer of the bladder encircles the proximal urethra for 1 to 1.5 cm (Figure 6–5) and connects distally with the prostatic musculature. These continuations of detrusor fibers have been described distinctly as the supramontanal (or preprostatic) sphincter or the smooth prostatic sphincter.[6] Within the loops of bladder neck musculature, fibers that originate in the superficial trigone of the bladder continue as the crista urethralis and insert in the musculature of the ejaculatory ducts, near the verumontanum.[12] These fibers are under sympathetic control and function to lift open the ejaculatory duct with contraction during ejaculation. Based on anatomic and physiologic studies, muscles originating in the deep trigone extend into and around the supramontanal prostatic urethra. These muscles are also under primarily sympathetic control and, with ejaculation, contract to provide resistance to retrograde flow of seminal fluid. This structure, therefore, functions as a genital sphincter and is separate functionally and structurally from the various urinary sphincter mechanisms.

The sphincteric mechanism distal to the verumontanum consists of both intrinsic and extrinsic components. Intrinsic components include the dense muscular stroma of the inframontanal prostate and the periurethral musculature. The periurethral musculature is composed of both smooth and striated muscle fibers that form a tube extending from the inframontanal prostate to the bulbar urethra. The periurethral striated muscle bundles are semicircular around the verumontanum and encircle the inframontanal urethra completely as they approach the membranous urethra, located between the inner longitudinal muscle layer and the external sphincter.[16] The so-called prostatomembranous or external sphincter is located where this tube of periurethral musculature traverses the pelvic floor. Therefore, urethral coaptation occurs owing to both of these intrinsic periurethral muscles and the striated muscle bundles of the adjacent pelvic floor.

The morphology of the intrinsic prostatic striated sphincter and prostatic apex has considerable anatomic variation between patients. The anatomic relationships, therefore, may be best understood with knowledge of the development of these structures. The sleeve-like primordium of the external striated sphincter extends from the level of the bulbospongiosus muscle primordia to the base of the bladder anteriorly but only to the mesonephric ducts posteriorly.[15] Its posterior surface is thin, and this cell layer encounters the growing prostatic buds as they arise along the developing urethra. As the buds grow and coalesce, the sphincteric primordium is pushed away from the urethral lumen and differentiates into circumferentially oriented striated fibers. Fibers around the membranous urethra differentiate into the bulk of the striated sphincter, with only a few striated muscular strands remaining around the prostatic capsule.[14] The lateral lobes of the prostate grow to surround the urethra and meet at an anterior commissure. The extent of distal fusion at this commissure and the thickness of prostatic parenchyma at this level determine the apical geometry and relationship between the sphincteric fibers and urethra at the prostatic apex. An anterior apical notch may be found in some glands such that glandular tissue does not cover the urethra to the apex of the prostate anteriorly, but, instead, sphincteric fibers remain in contact with the urethra within this gap.[16] In the adult, fibers of the striated sphincter are connected with the anterior capsule of the prostate and the vesicle neck. At the apex of the prostate, these fibers almost completely surround the gland, except for the variable posterior gap at the apex as mentioned above, and are continuous with muscles of the membranous urethral sphincter. The bulk of this muscle near the membranous urethra forms the shape of an omega. More proximally, the prostatic striated sphincter fibers insert into the laterally placed ischioprostatic ligaments as they approach the bladder neck.[16] These ligaments originate on the inferior surface of the ischia and pass diagonally down to meet the surface of the membranous urethra. Therefore, cross-sectional images of sphincteric fibers can vary in shape from tiny wings proximally to nearly encircling the urethra completely at the membranous urethra.

The membranous urethra represents that segment of soft tissue extending from the apex of the prostate to the perineal membrane. Coaptation of this segment is accomplished by contributions from multiple structures. From inside (luminal) to outside, these are (1) mucosal infolding, (2) fibroelastic tissue in the urethral wall including longitudinal and circular smooth muscle fibers, (3) intrinsic striated urethral sphincter, and (4) levator ani musculature. Fibers of the membranous striated sphincter encircle the urethra, originating at the anterior decussation of the prostatic sphincter and inserting at the perineal body at the level of the perineal membrane. These sphincteric fibers insert broadly over the surface of the prostatic fascia near the apex. Fibers of the membranous urethra distal to the apex play an important role in regaining continence following radical prostatectomy.[16]

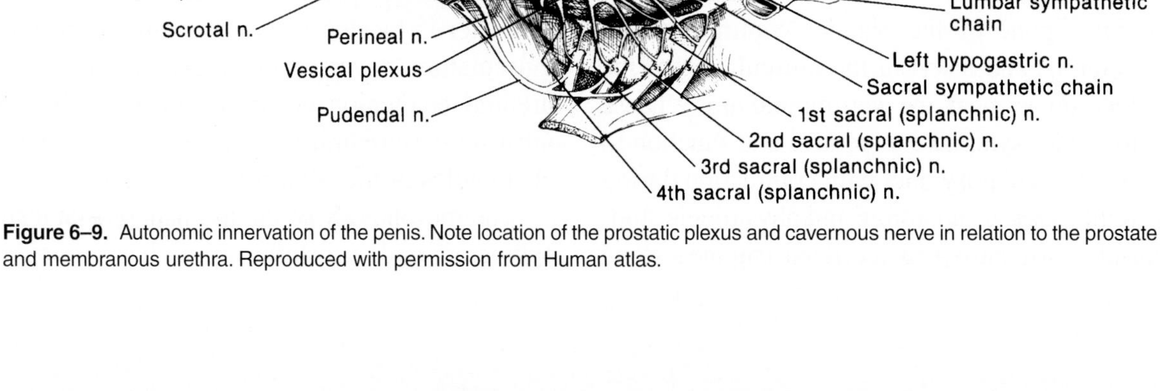

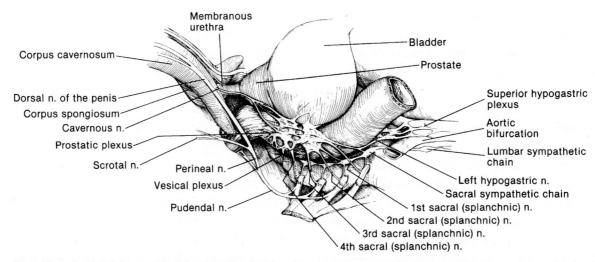

Figure 6–9. Autonomic innervation of the penis. Note location of the prostatic plexus and cavernous nerve in relation to the prostate and membranous urethra. Reproduced with permission from Human atlas.

HISTOLOGY

The prostatic parenchyma is composed of primarily glandular epithelium, yet 30 percent of its mass is composed of muscular elements.[10] The secretory epithelium of the prostate is contained within tubuloalveolar glands with a simple branching architecture. These glands are lined with simple cuboidal or columnar epithelium with flattened basal cells below. Fibers of the stromal smooth muscle and connective tissue weave throughout the gland, surrounding each acinus. Ducts draining each gland enter the urethra in several locations. Periurethral glands are not connected to the deep network of acini but extend within the longitudinal muscle fibers of the supramontanal sphincter. These open via short ducts into the supramontanal urethra. Ducts from transition zone glands pass beneath the supramontanal sphincter at the urethral angle and enter the posterior and lateral urethral wall. Central zone ducts enter the urethra circumferentially around the ejaculatory duct orifices. The peripheral zone comprises over 70 percent of the glandular tissue of the prostate, and its ducts enter the urethra at and below the level of the ejaculatory duct.[18]

Relationship of Prostate Gland to Surrounding Structures

Prostatic Sheath, Capsule, and Bone Fixation

Fascial layers of the retroperitoneum continue into the pelvis in three distinguishable layers: the outer, intermediate, and inner strata. The outer stratum is continuous with the transversalis faxcia of the anterior abdominal wall, lines the inner surface of the pelvic muscles, and is the superficial-most coat seen when the prostate is exposed retropubically. This layer continues to Cooper's ligament, the sacrospinous ligament, the ischial spine, and the tendinous arc of the levator ani. The intermediate stratum of the retroperitoneal fascia is a fatty layer that embeds the pelvic viscera, surrounding the prostate as the prostatic sheath or periprostatic fascia. This layer fuses with the outer stratum of retroperitoneal fascia as the endopelvic fascia anterolaterally. The periprostatic fascia is of great surgical importance as it encases the neurovascular bundle along the lateral margin of the gland.[1] Anteriorly, it continues to enclose the prostatic venous plexus (or dorsal vein complex) and extends posterolaterally to join the anterior lamella of Denonvilliers' fascia.

The prostatic capsule refers to a layer of condensed smooth muscle and connective tissue (collagen and elastin) of variable thickness. It blends with the prostatic sheath on the anterior and anterolateral surfaces of the gland and with the anterior lamella of Denonvilliers' fascia on the posterior surface of the gland. On the anterior surface and at the apex, this structure thins considerably such that on many surgical specimens, no capsule may be found in these areas.[19] The puboprostatic ligaments extend anterolaterally from the surface of the gland to fix the apex of the prostate to the pubis (see Figure 6–1). At both the apex and the base, no clear capsule separates the prostate from the striated urethral sphincter or bladder neck, respectively. Prostatic glands can be seen in the substance of the urethral sphincter, and smooth muscle fibers from the detrusor blend with the muscular coat of the prostate. For this reason, the prostate gland is not considered to have a true capsule.[18]

Levator Ani Muscles and "Urogenital Diaphragm"

Classically, the prostate has been depicted sitting atop a flat sheet of muscle that includes the urogenital diaphragm and striated urethral sphincter muscles sandwiched between the inferior and superior fasciae.[5] These descriptions were based on cadaver dissections, ex vivo pathologic examination, and intraoperative observation that likely suffered from distortion and destruction of the natural anatomic relationships and pelvic spatial orientation. Recent computer modeling of detailed in situ imaging using computed tomography, magnetic resonance imaging, and serial step sectioning has refined our understanding of the pelvic musculature and spatial relationships. Based on digitized reconstructions from the visible human data set,[20] the levator ani muscle has a near-vertical orientation with two superior wings posteriorly and funnels traveling inferiorly to surround the rectum. Viewed from below, this muscle forms the U-shaped urogenital hiatus bracketing the striated urethral sphincter. The prostate (covered by the prostatic sheath) and striated urethral sphincter are in contact with the levator ani along almost their entire lateral surface.

Denonvilliers' Fascia

Separating the prostate from the rectum is a layer of fusion-fascia derived from two layers of pelvic peritoneum in the retrovesical space. The anterior lamella of Denonvilliers' fascia (also called the rectoprostatic fascia) is adherent to the posterior surface of the prostate and merges laterally with the intermediate stratum of the retroperitoneal fascia (see Figure 6–5).[21] This layer is continuous with the lateral periprostatic fascia, prostatic sheath, and endopelvic fascia. The posterior lamella of Denonvilliers' fascia covers the anterior and anterolateral surfaces of the rectum.

Endopelvic Fascia

Fascial covering that overlies the pubococcygeal portion of the levator ani is called the endopelvic or lateral pelvic fascia. Overlying the prostate itself, the fascial layer is called the periprostatic fascia, which is continuous with the endopelvic fascia. Moving from lateral to medial toward the prostate, the endopelvic fascia separates from the prostatic capsule at a line called the arcus tendineus fasciae pelvis. Between the fascial covering and the prostate capsule are located fatty areolar tissue and the lateral portion of the dorsal vein complex. When incising the endopelvic fascia during a radical retropubic prostatectomy, it is important to cut lateral to this tendinous arch to avoid entering the dorsal vein complex.

Neurovascular Bundle

The cavernous nerves and branches of the prostatovesicular artery and veins run posterolateral to the prostate in the lateral prostatic fascia as the neurovascular bundle. The cavernous nerve arises from the pelvic plexus, contains both sympathetic and parasympathetic fibers, and passes beneath the arch of the pubis to supply the corpora cavernosa and the corpus spongiosum (Figure 6–9). These end in a network of nerve fibers around the cavernous vessels at the penile hilum. When performing a nerve-sparing prostatectomy, the endopelvic fascia must be incised anterior to the neurovascular bundle yet lateral to the prostatic venous complex to achieve an adequate surgical margin and also preserve erectile function.

ARTERIAL SUPPLY

Primary arterial supply to the prostate comes from the prostatovesical artery that descends inferiorly along the bladder base (Figure 6–7). The origin of this artery is variable, but it usually comes from the gluteopudendal trunk (also called the anterior division) of the internal iliac artery.[17] Variations include origins at the superior vesical, vesiculodeferential, internal pudendal, or obturator arteries. The prostatovesical artery divides into the inferior vesical and prostatic arteries. The prostatic artery divides at the base of the prostate to give the large posterolateral branch and the smaller anterior branch. The superolateral gland may receive arterial supply from the middle and superior rectal arteries.

Urethral branches from the prostatic artery enter the capsule posterolaterally below the bladder neck to supply the transition zone (see Figure 6–7). These traverse the gland perpendicular to the urethra and lie in the "lateral lobes" of the prostate (1 to 5 o'clock and 7 to 11 o'clock positions as viewed through the cystoscope). As these vessels approach the urethra, they turn caudally, parallel to the urethra, and are the primary arterial supply to benign adenoma located primarily in the transition zone and periurethral glands. Capsular branches enter the capsule more distally and laterally to supply the central and peripheral zones (see Figure 6–7).

VENOUS DRAINAGE

Prostate parenchymal veins, as well as veins draining all deep pelvic structures, intercommunicate with the prostatic venous plexus (Figure 6–8). This venous structure is thin-walled and lies within the periprostatic fascia on the anterior surface of the gland. The deep dorsal vein of the penis emerges beneath the symphysis pubis between the puboprostatic ligaments to join this plexus. Also in continuity are the inferior hypogastric venous system and the presacral prevertebral venous plexus. The majority of venous blood then drains directly into the prostatic and inferior vesical veins to the internal iliac veins. To a lesser extent, the prostatic venous plexus drains into the vesical venous plexus before reaching the inferior vesical veins.

INNERVATION

The two important physiologic processes occurring in the prostate, the secretion and emission of seminal fluid and contribution to urinary continence, follow directly from the nerve supply to this gland.[22] With sexual activity, parasympathetic nerve terminals stimulate the prostatic acini to produce secretions. Activity of sympathetic nerves closes the supramontanal sphincter, producing resistance to retrograde ejaculation, and increases smooth muscle tone in both the prostatic parenchyma and capsule to deposit secretions in the urethra (emission). Ejaculation occurs with contraction of the striated bulbospongiosus muscle.

Preganglionic sympathetic nerves to the supramontanal sphincter and smooth musculature of the prostate gland originate at spinal level L2–3 and pass through the sympathetic chain ganglia to the superior hypogastric plexus (see Figure 6–9). Here they synapse with postganglionic noradrenergic nerves, the cell bodies of which lie in the pelvic plexus lateral to the bladder and prostate. Parasympathetic innervation to the prostatic epithelium originates in the pelvic splanchnic nerves from spinal levels S2–4 (see Figure 6–9). These preganglionic neurons synapse in the prostatic plexus, located between the seminal vesicles and the prostate, and send short postganglionic fibers into the prostate stroma. Somatic motor output from the pudendal nerve arises from S1–3 and innervates the pubococcygeus muscle of the external striated sphincter. Some contribution to external sphincter tone may also come from the pelvic nerve.[22]

The prostatic nerve, which includes sympathetic, parasympathetic, and somatic fibers, travels with the neurovascular bundle and sends off main branches at the level of the prostate base. This nerve continues posterolaterally along the prostate and gives apical branches and a branch to the ejaculatory duct. The main branches pierce the prostatic capsule and then travel along the fibromuscular trabeculae as acinar branches before reaching their terminals at muscular and glandular cells. Afferent nerves from the prostate travel through the pelvic plexus to reach sensory tracts in the spinal cord.

LYMPHATIC DRAINAGE

Lymph capillaries emerge from the fibrous stroma and anastomose to form a perilobular network of channels. This pierces the capsule and then branches to form a periprostatic lymph network within the prostatic sheath. Lymphatic outflow thereafter travels along arterial pedicles: the prostatic artery laterally, the vesiculodeferential artery superiorly, the middle hemorrhoidal artery posteriorly, and the prostatovesical branch of the internal pudendal artery anteriorly (Figure 6–26). The major route of drainage is along the prostatic artery to the obturator and internal iliac nodes (Figure 6–27). Secondary lymphatic drainage occurs at the base of the prostate, where lymphatic trunks travel along the medial border of the seminal vesicles to drain into the external iliac nodes. Two lesser routes of drainage occur via capsular lymphatics on the posterior surface of the gland to the sacral nodes and via a separate trunk along the internal pudendal artery to the internal iliac nodes.

REFERENCES

1. Di Lollo S, Menchi I, Brizzi E, et al. The morphology of the prostatic capsule with particular regard to the posterosuperior region: an anatomical and clinical problem. Surg Radiol Anat 1997;19:143.
2. Aboseif SR, Breza J, Lue TF, et al. Penile venous drainage in erectile dysfunction. Anatomical, radiological and functional considerations. Br J Urol 1989;64:183.
3. Lepor H, Gregerman M, Crosby R, et al. Precise localization of the autonomic nerves from the pelvic plexus to the corpora cavernosa: a detailed anatomical study of the adult male pelvis. J Urol 1985;133:207.
4. Geary ES, Dendinger TE, Freiha FS, et al. Nerve sparing radical prostatectomy: a different view. J Urol 1995;154:145.
5. Hinman, F. Urosurgical atlas. 1993.
6. McNeal JE. The prostate and prostatic urethra: a morphologic synthesis. J Urol 1972;107:1008.
7. McNeal JE. Origin and evolution of benign prostatic enlargement. Invest Urol 1978;15:340.
8. Allen KS, Kressel HY, Arger PH, et al. Age-related changes of the prostate: evaluation by MR imaging. AJR Am J Roentgenol 1989;152:77.
9. McNeal JE, Redwine EA, Freiha FS, et al. Zonal distribution of prostatic adenocarcinoma. Correlation with histologic

pattern and direction of spread. Am J Surg Pathol 1988; 12:897.
10. McNeal JE. Regional morphology and pathology of the prostate. Am J Clin Pathol 1968;49:347.
11. McNeal JE. Normal histology of the prostate. Am J Surg Pathol 1988;12:619.
12. JB. In: Walsh PRA, Vaughan E, Wein A, editors.) Campbell's urology. Philadelphia: WB Saunders; 1998.
13. Mebust. In: Walsh PRA, Vaughan E, Wein A, editors. Campbell's urology. Philadelphia: WB Saunders; 1998.
14. Marshall FF. Embryology of the lower genitourinary tract. Urol Clin North Am 1978;5:3.
15. Oelrich TM. The urethral sphincter muscle in the male. Am J Anat 1980;158:229.
16. Myers RP. Male urethral sphincteric anatomy and radical prostatectomy. Urol Clin North Am 1991;18:211.
17. Bradley. In: Walsh PRA, Vaughan E, Wein A, editors. Campbell's urology. Philadelphia: WB Saunders; 1998.
18. Wheeler TM. Anatomic considerations in carcinoma of the prostate. Urol Clin North Am 1989;16:623.
19. Ayala AG, Ro JY, Babaian R, et al. The prostatic capsule: does it exist? Its importance in the staging and treatment of prostatic carcinoma. Am J Surg Pathol 1989;13:21.
20. Brooks JD, Chao WM, Kerr J. Male pelvic anatomy reconstructed from the visible human data set. J Urol 1998; 159:868.
21. Dietrich H. Giovanni Domenico Santorini (1681–1737) Charles-Pierre Denonvilliers (1808–1872). First description of urosurgically relevant structures in the small pelvis. Eur Urol 1997;32:124.
22. Vaalasti A, Hervonen A. Autonomic innervation of the human prostate. Invest Urol 1980;17:293.

7

Tumor Markers

MARC A. DALL'ERA, MD
CHRISTOPHER P. EVANS, MD, FACS

Tumor markers are biochemical indicators of cancer. When easily detectable in the serum, tumor markers become valuable in diagnosis and in monitoring treatment of several human cancers such as those of the ovary, testicle, colon, and prostate. The value of any tumor marker is measured by its ability to predict the presence of disease in an individual with cancer while correctly identifying patients without disease. From the early clinical applications of prostatic acid phosphatase (PAP) to the recent advances in prostate-specific antigen (PSA) analysis, tumor markers for prostate cancer have become the most important in all of oncology. Although PSA has essentially replaced PAP in diagnosis and in monitoring treatment of prostate cancer, novel markers for disease and innovative methods for analyzing PSA are under investigation to improve the sensitivity and specificity of tumor markers for prostate cancer. This chapter describes the historic use of PAP in managing prostate cancer before discussing the traditional and novel applications of PSA. Experimental tumor markers are also presented and discussed.

PROSTATIC ACID PHOSPHATASE

The acid phosphatases encompass a group of enzymes that hydrolyze esters of orthophosphoric acid in an acid medium to release phosphoric acid.[1] Acid phosphatases exist throughout the human body, and in 1936, Kutscher found high concentrations of acid phosphatases in semen and prostate tissue.[1a] Prostatic acid phosphatase was found to be under hormonal influence and was discovered to be markedly elevated in the serum of men with prostate cancer, especially with bone metastases.[1] Huggins and Hodges found that the growth of normal and malignant prostate tissue was dependent on the presence of androgens and that serum PAP decreased after androgen withdrawal.[2] This group also made the important observation that decreased serum PAP correlated with clinical regression of disease, thus paving the way for PAP as a tumor marker for prostate cancer.[2]

Prostatic acid phosphatase is neither prostate tissue nor tumor specific. Acid phosphatases are widely distributed throughout the body and can be increased in a variety of neoplasms including prostate, breast, stomach, and colon.[1] Despite the development of monoclonal immunologic assays and specific inhibitors aimed at detecting only acid phosphatases of prostatic origin, there remains significant interference with acid phosphatases from other sources. Compared with PSA, PAP experiences significant diurnal and random fluctuations over a 24-hour period, and serum concentrations are significantly affected by prostatic manipulation, resulting in more unreliable measurements. Prostatic acid phosphatase is less stable than PSA and requires very stringent handling precautions prior to analysis. These factors combine to give an overall poor specificity of PAP with fairly high false-positive rates. Elevated serum levels of PAP are related to the stage of disease, but the sensitivity of this enzyme for detecting prostate cancer increases with increasing stage. As most men with elevated PAP levels have metastasis, PAP is not very sensitive for identifying patients with early-stage disease who are most likely to benefit from early detection. Prostatic acid phosphatase has an overall positive predictive value of less than 5% and is not of use in screening men for prostate cancer.

As a tool for staging, an elevated serum PAP in the face of biopsy-proven prostate cancer almost inevitably suggests extensive disease. Oesterling and colleagues demonstrated in 275 patients with clinically localized prostate cancer who underwent radical prostatectomy and pelvic lymph node dissection that all patients with an elevated serum PAP had either capsular penetration or positive lymph nodes.[3] A normal serum PAP level, however, does not adequately predict localized disease. A study by Whitesel and colleagues found that in 318 patients with clinically localized disease and normal serum PAP, 22% had positive lymph nodes at the time of surgery.[4]

In 1987, Stamey and colleagues directly compared PSA and PAP in 127 men with prostate cancer and concluded that PSA was the more clinically useful tumor marker for this disease.[5] Serum PSA was elevated in 96% of the men with cancer, whereas PAP was abnormal in only 45% of cases. Prostate-specific antigen more strongly correlated with clinical stage and tumor volume than PAP and rapidly fell to undetectable levels after surgery, indicating superior tissue specificity over PAP. Moul and colleagues have reported that the preradical prostatectomy PAP is useful in predicting tumor recurrence.[6] The Kaplan-Meier disease-free survival rate at 4 years was 78% for PAP < 3 ng/mL and 39% for patients with PAP > 3 ng/mL. This applied to pretreatment PSA levels both < 10 ng/mL and > 10 ng/mL. However, PAP did not predict pathologic stage or margin status, and the clinical impact of this observation seems minimal. As data accumulated comparing PAP with PSA, the superiority of the latter for the screening, diagnosis, and monitoring of prostate cancer became indisputable, and the current role of PAP in clinical practice is limited.

PROSTATE-SPECIFIC ANTIGEN

Overview

Prostate-specific antigen is a 34-kDa glycoprotein composed of 237 amino acids that is primarily produced by the epithelial cells forming the acini and ducts of the prostate gland. The complete gene encoding PSA has been sequenced, localizes to chromosome 19, and is approximately 6-Kb pairs long. Prostate-specific antigen is a proteolytic enzyme that belongs to the kallikrein family of proteases and functions to liquify human semen. Prostate-specific antigen was first identified in seminal fluid by Hara and colleagues in 1969[6a]; however, it was not detected in adult male serum by Papsidero and colleagues until 1980.[6b] It was at this time that serum PSA measurement began to be recognized as clinically useful, and by the late 1980s, PSA emerged as the most important tumor marker for prostate cancer.

Once released from the prostate, PSA circulates in the serum as a free or complexed form. Prostate-specific antigen forms complexes by binding to two other circulating serum proteins, α_1-antichymotrypsin and α_2-macroglobulin. Most commercial PSA assays detect total PSA, free PSA, and PSA complexed with α_1-antichymotrypsin. When bound to α_2-macroglobulin, PSA is completely encapsulated and is not detected by immunologic assays. On average, the free PSA to α_1-antichymotrypsin bound PSA ratio is 1:4, but this ratio can vary with prostatic pathology.

A number of assays now exist for measuring PSA levels in the serum. The majority of data on the use of PSA in prostate cancer detection have been obtained using the Tandem-E and Tandem-R PSA assays (Hybritech Inc., San Diego, CA) and the PROS-CHECK PSA RIA kit (Yang Laboratories, Bellevue, WA). Different assays will have different reference ranges, and it is therefore important for clinicians to know which assay is being used to properly interpret the results.

In general, PSA is considered tissue, but not cancer, specific. Recent studies have shown that periurethral glands and some breast cancers also produce PSA, but for all intents and purposes, it can be considered a specific product of the prostate gland. Since PSA is produced by both malignant and benign prostate epithelium, conditions other than prostate cancer can cause increased serum PSA levels. Benign processes that disrupt normal prostate glandular structure such as benign prostatic hyperplasia (BPH) and acute and subclinical prostatitis may cause leakage of PSA and subsequent elevated serum levels. Several studies have examined the effect of ejaculation on serum PSA and suggest clinically significant elevations in older men within sev-

eral hours of ejaculation.[7,8] No studies have shown a significant elevation in serum PSA after routine digital rectal examination (DRE). Stamey and colleagues reported a fourfold increase in serum PSA after cystoscopy combined with prostatic massage, whereas several other studies have shown no effect.[5]

The widespread use of PSA in the clinical setting for prostate cancer screening has resulted in a dramatic shift in the proportion of prostate cancers that are organ confined at initial detection. Screening for prostate cancer with PSA measurement identifies patients with more organ-confined and therefore potentially curable disease over screening by DRE alone.[9] Today the most prevalent clinical stage of prostate cancer is T1c (nonpalpable, elevated PSA), and about 50% of tumors detected are pathologically organ confined.

Prostate-Specific Antigen: Use in Diagnosis

Total serum PSA measurement is useful for defining a patient's risk of having prostate cancer. The normal range for serum total PSA is generally regarded as 0 to 4 ng/mL. This range includes the 95% confidence interval of the average serum PSA concentration for a randomly selected population of American men over the age of 40 years with no clinical evidence of prostatic disease. It is generally agreed on that a PSA over 4 ng/mL warrants transrectal ultrasound (TRUS)-guided biopsy of the prostate. The American Urological Association and the American Cancer Society recommend PSA screening for all men 50 years or older and for all men 45 years or older with a family history of prostate cancer or of African descent (Table 7–1). Gann and colleagues found that a single PSA measurement > 4 ng/mL was 71% sensitive for detecting prostate cancer within 4 years of follow-up, with a total specificity of 91%.[10] A cross-sectional study by Catalona and colleagues reported an average sensitivity of 81% for PSA versus 56% for DRE for predicting the presence of prostate cancer in men aged 50 to 79 years.[9] In another study, they found that 63% of men diagnosed with prostate cancer with an elevated PSA on initial screening and an abnormal DRE had pathologically organ-confined disease, whereas 71% of men diagnosed with prostate cancer by serial-based PSA screening had organ-confined disease.[9] A large multicenter clinical trial directly comparing DRE and serum PSA in the early detection of prostate cancer found that a serum PSA > 4 ng/mL detected 82% of tumors versus 55% detection by DRE alone.[11] Seventy-five percent of the tumors detected by serum PSA alone were organ confined as opposed to 56% of the tumors detected by DRE. When used together, serum PSA and DRE increased the detection of organ-confined disease by 78%. These data suggest that PSA testing alone or in combination with DRE is superior to DRE alone in the diagnosis of localized prostate cancer.

Table 7–1. AMERICAN CANCER SOCIETY PROSTATE-SPECIFIC ANTIGEN SCREENING GUIDELINES

≥ Age 50 for men with greater than 10-year life expectancy
≥ Age 45 for men considered at higher risk
African American
Two or more affected first-degree relatives (father, brother)

The American Urological Association and the American Cancer Society recommend annual PSA screening for prostate cancer for all men over age 50. Prostate-specific antigen testing, however, should begin at age 45 for men of African descent and men with a family history of prostate cancer in a first-degree relative. Two recent studies have evaluated if the frequency of PSA testing can be reduced without compromising potentially curable cancer detection. Smith and colleagues reported only a 4% PSA conversion from 2.5 ng/mL or lower to > 4 ng/mL over 4 years of screening in white men over the age of 50 with normal DREs.[12] Forty-eight percent of men with initial PSA levels between 2.5 and 4 ng/mL converted to a level > 4 ng/mL over this 4-year period. Carter and colleagues concluded that curable prostate cancer is not likely to be missed with a 2-year PSA testing interval in men 55 years or older with a normal rectal examinaton and an initial PSA level less than 2 ng/mL.[13] More recently, Ross and colleagues compared prostate cancer mortality, PSA testing rates, and biopsy rates using various PSA screening strategies.[14] Initiating screening at age 45 followed by biennial testing prevented more prostate cancer deaths and used fewer PSA tests and prostate biopsies than the standard approach of annual tests beginning at age 50.

Prostate-specific antigen testing detects a significant number of tumors that would have been missed by DRE alone, and more cancers are now detected at an earlier stage.[15] Stage T1c cancer is the clinical stage that is increasing in incidence the most rapidly and represents a nonpalpable tumor in a patient with an elevated PSA. Although the advantage that serum PSA testing offers in the detection of early-stage, organ-confined prostate cancer is now clear, the impact on overall patient survival remains to be elucidated. A recent report by Ghavamian and colleagues compared disease-free survival in men with stage T1c versus stage T2 prostate cancer.[16] With respect to preoperative PSA, clinical stage T1c cancers resembled T2b and T2c disease. They found that clinical T1c tumors, however, were more likely to be organ confined and have a Gleason score less than 7 than stage T2b or T2c tumors. The authors concluded that stage T1c and T2a cancers differ significantly from T2b/c tumors in terms of disease-free survival and that there is a significant survival advantage at 5 and 7 years for both clinical T1c and T2a disease.

Efforts to improve the sensitivity and specificity of serum PSA measurements for the diagnosis of prostate cancer have resulted in the use of different contexts for analyzing the PSA level (Table 7–2). These include age-specific PSA reference ranges, free to total PSA ratio, PSA density (PSAD), and PSA velocity (PSAV). An algorithm for early detection of prostate cancer using serum PSA and its variations is summarized in Figure 7–1.

Age-Specific Prostate-Specific Antigen Reference Ranges

Several studies have analyzed the relationship between age, PSA production, and prostatic volume and have determined that a standard PSA reference range of 0 to 4 ng/mL does not adequately account for increases in serum PSA owing to age-related changes in prostate volume secondary to BPH. A direct and positive correlation exists between serum PSA and patient age.[17] In an effort to increase sensitivity, age-specific reference ranges for PSA have been determined to account for natural age-related differences in average PSA values with the goal of detecting early, potentially curable prostate cancers in younger men (Table 7–3). Prostate-specific antigen specificity would also increase by detecting fewer cancers in older men with life-limiting comorbidities and more likely indolent, clinically insignificant tumors. The proposed reference ranges for white patients are 0 to 2.5 ng/mL for ages 40 to 49 years, 0 to 3.5 ng/mL for ages 50 to 59 years, 0 to 4.5 ng/mL for ages 60 to 69 years, and 0 to 6.5 ng/mL for ages 70 to 79 years.[18] In an early prospective multi-institutional study by Catalona and colleagues, the effect that age-specific reference ranges had on biopsy rate and cancer detection in 6,600 asymptomatic men was evaluated.[11] In men older than age 60, they did not find a significant reduction in biopsy rate compared to the decrease in detection of organ-confined cancers. In younger men, they reported a 45% increase in the number of biopsies that would be performed, but the study was not designed to determine the number of cancers that would be detected had these biopsies been done. Using age-specific reference ranges, Partin and colleagues found 18% more tumors in men younger than 60 years old, while finding 22% fewer tumors in men 60 years or older than would have been detected using standard PSA cutoffs in a population of nearly 4,600 men with clinically localized prostate cancer.[19] Eighty-one percent of the additional tumors detected in younger men by using age-specific reference ranges had favorable pathologic findings, whereas 95% of the tumors missed in the older men were pathologically favorable. A study by Reissigl and colleagues found that

Table 7–2. PSA RELATED TESTS

Age-related PSA
Free/total PSA
PSA velocity
PSA density
Transition zone PSA

PSA = prostate-specific antigen.

Table 7–3. AGE-SPECIFIC PSA REFERENCE RANGES (ng/mL)

Age Range (yr)	White Pts.	Black Pts.	Asian Pts.
40–49	0.0–2.5	0.0–2.0	0.0–2.0
50–59	0.0–3.5	0.0–4.0	0.0–3.0
60–69	0.0–4.5	0.0–4.5	0.0–4.0
70–79	0.0–6.5	0.0–5.5	0.0–5.0

Reproduced with permission from Oesterling JE et al.[18]
Pts = patients; PSA = prostate-specific antigen.

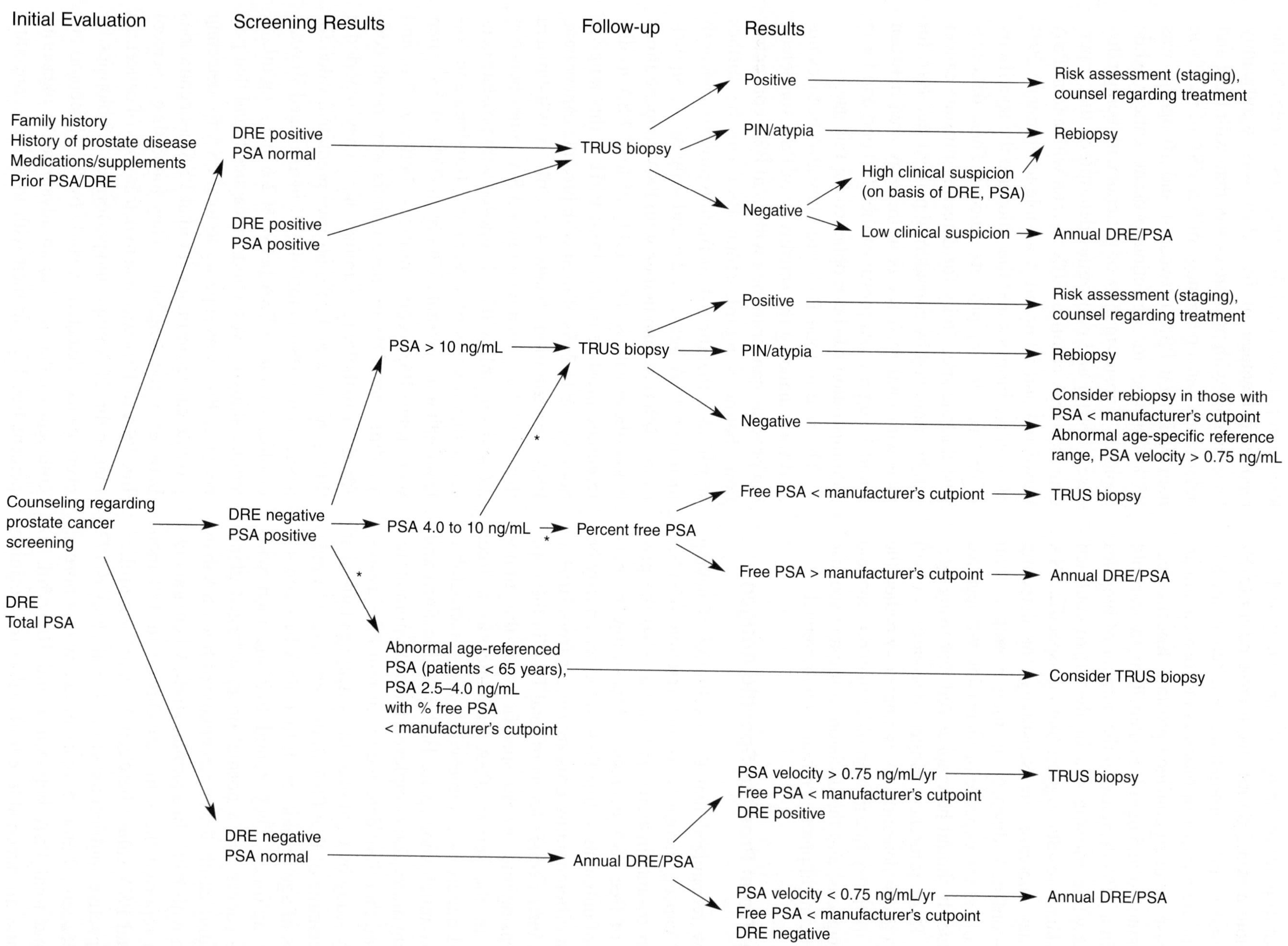

Figure 7–1. Algorithmn for the early detection of prostate cancer using total serum prostate-specific antigen (PSA) and its variations. DRE = digital rectal examination; PIN = prostatic intraepithelial neoplasia; TRUS = transrectal ultrasonography. Reproduced with permission from Carroll PR, Lee KL, Fuks ZY, Kantoff PW. Initial cancer staging and risk assessment. In: DeVita VT, Hellman S, Rosenberg SA, editors. Cancer: principles and practice of oncology. 6th ed. Philadelphia: Lippincott Williams and Wilkins; 2001. p. 1418–79.

using a cutoff point of 2.5 ng/mL for men aged 45 to 49 years old and 3.5 ng/mL for men aged 50 to 59 with normal rectal examinations resulted in an 8% increase in the number of biopsies performed and an 8% increase in organ-confined prostate cancer detection.[20] A cutoff of 6.5 ng/mL in men 70 to 75 years old resulted in a 21% decrease in the number of biopsies perfomed while missing 4% of the organ-confined cancers. These results suggest that age-specific PSA ranges may increase the sensitivity for detecting prostate-confined disease in men younger than 60 years old at the expense of increasing the negative biopsy rate. It should be emphasized that using age-specific PSA reference ranges decreases overall prostate cancer detection. It is unclear whether the decrease in biopsy rate in men older than 60 years old is advantageous, and the decision to use age-specific ranges in clinical practice remains controversial.

Free/Total Prostate-Specific Antigen

It is now recognized that the likelihood of having prostate cancer increases as the fraction of PSA bound to α_1-antichymotrypsin increases or the percentage of free PSA decreases. Measuring the percentage of unbound or free PSA in the serum may be useful in differentiating prostate cancer from BPH at low and intermediate levels of total PSA in the hope of increasing the overall specificity of this tumor marker. In the serum, PSA circulates as a free, unbound moiety or complexed with α_2-macroglobulin or α_1-antichymotrypsin. Both the free form and α_1-antichymotrypsin complexed form are immunoreactive and therefore detected by current PSA assays. An early study by Catalona and colleagues looked at the percentage of free PSA in the serum of 113 men 50 years of age or older with total PSA between 4.1 and 10 ng/mL.[21] They found that the men with prostate cancer and a normal or an enlarged gland had a significantly lower percentage of free PSA than the men with BPH. In a similar study, Chen and colleagues reported the same conclusion in 428 men with total PSA values between 2.5 and 10 ng/mL.[22] A prospective multicenter clinical trial studied 773 men between 50 and 75 years of age with a normal DRE and total PSA between 4 and 10 ng/mL to determine an acceptable cutoff value for defining abnormal percent free PSA. They confirmed that the median percentage of free PSA was significantly lower in men with prostate cancer than with BPH and determined that a percentage of free PSA of < 25% in men with total PSA between 4 and 10 ng/mL was 95% sensitive for detecting prostate cancer while avoiding biopsies in 20% of patients with benign disease.[23] Partin and colleagues determined that a percent free PSA cutoff of 20% in men with a total PSA between 4 and 10 ng/mL was able to eliminate 29% of negative biopsies and thus increase the specificity of PSA in detecting prostate cancer.[24] These data suggest that the specificity for detecting prostate cancer can be improved by considering percent free PSA for men with total PSA levels in the gray area between 4 and 10 ng/mL. Approval of the US Food and Drug Administration has been obtained for this use.

The free to total PSA ratio has also been evaluated for enhancing the sensitivity of PSA for detecting prostate cancer in men with total PSA concentrations below 4 ng/mL. Total PSA can be further stratified in that the risk of finding prostate cancer in men with PSA between 2.6 and 4 ng/mL is significantly different than in men with PSA concentrations below these values. The ability of total PSA to differentiate prostate cancer from BPH in this range is poor, yet up to 20% of men with prostate cancer have PSA concentrations below 4 ng/mL. It is estimated that 7 to 15% of men with initial PSA values between 2.6 and 4 ng/mL will be diagnosed with prostate cancer within 4 years of screening.[12] Catalona and colleagues found prostate cancer in 22% of 332 men with total PSA concentrations between 2.6 and 4 ng/mL, and 81% of these tumors were organ confined on pathologic examination.[25] They reported a 90% sensitivity and 24% positive predictive value for a percent free PSA cutoff of 27% in men aged 50 years or older with total PSA between 2.6 and 4 ng/mL. A similar study by Vashi and colleagues found that percent free PSA was superior to total PSA for detecting prostate cancer in men with total PSA concentrations between 3 and 4 ng/mL.[26] They found that a percent free PSA of 19% was able to detect 90% of cancers in men in this PSA range and performed 1.7 biopsies for every cancer detected. A study by Prestigiacomo and colleagues failed to find an advantage to measuring percent free PSA in men with total PSA concentra-

tions between 2 and 4 ng/mL; however, these data were based on only 17 patients and may have lacked sufficient power to detect a difference between total and percent free PSA.[27]

Recent studies have evaluated the ability of complexed PSA levels alone to provide the same clinical information as free to total PSA measurements. Brawer and colleagues proposed that measuring the amount of PSA bound to α_1-antichymotrypsin alone would aid in the diagnosis of prostate cancer, thus eliminating the need to measure two different values.[28] In men with total serum PSA values between 4 and 10 ng/mL, complexed PSA would have missed 1 cancer while eliminating 34 negative prostate biopsies. The authors concluded that measurement of complexed PSA has superior specificity over total PSA and free to total PSA calculations with only a slight reduction in sensitivity (81% versus 83% for total PSA).

Prostate-Specific Antigen Velocity

In 1992, Carter and colleagues reported on a case-control study evaluating the longitudinal changes in PSA levels in men with and without prostate cancer.[29] They found a significant difference in the rise of PSA with respect to time between men with and without prostate cancer 5 years prior to diagnosis. Prostate-specific antigen velocity takes into account the absolute value of PSA change over a certain period of time with the hypothesis that prostate cancer will show a greater rate of PSA change compared to BPH. Carter and colleagues found that a PSAV of 0.75 ng/mL/yr or greater was suggestive for prostate cancer with 72% sensitivity and 90% specificity.[29] Optimal calculation requires three consecutive PSA measurements (PSA1, PSA2, and PSA3) over a 1.5- to 2-year period.[30] Prostate-specific antigen velocity is then calculated as*[(PSA2–PSA1/time$_1$ years) + (PSA3–PSA2/time$_2$ years)]. These parameters are necessary as short-term intraindividual variability occurs with PSA measurements, and it has been shown that this variability does not differ significantly between men with and without prostate cancer.[30] A larger prospective study by Smith and Catalona confirmed these results and found that the predictive value of PSAV varied with patient age and initial PSA level.[31] For men age 70 and younger with an initial PSA level < 4.0 ng/mL, a PSAV of > 0.75 ng/mL/yr detected 47% of cancers and was 79% specific and 66% sensitive for detecting prostate cancer. Only 11% of men with PSAV < 0.75 ng/mL/yr were subsequently diagnosed with prostate cancer. The study also found that the sensitivity of PSAV decreased for men older than 70 years. In men whose initial PSA measurements were above 4.0 ng/mL, a lower PSAV of 0.4 ng/mL/yr maximized the sensitivity and specificity for detecting prostate cancer at 63% and 62%, respectively. In this group of men, cancer was diagnosed in 33% of patients with PSAV greater than 0.4 ng/mL/yr compared with 15% of men with PSAV less than this value. Overall, Carter and Pearson estimate that three consecutive PSA measurements taken over a period of 1.5 to 2 years will reveal that < 5% of men without prostate cancer will have a PSAV of 0.75 ng/mL/yr or greater, whereas about 70% of men with prostate cancer will have such a PSAV.[30] Measuring and calculating PSAV is probably most useful for assessing the risk of prostate cancer in an individual with a normal yet rising total PSA. It may also be useful in determining the need for repeat prostate biopsy in men with total PSA > 4 ng/mL and normal previous biopsies.

Prostate-Specific Antigen Density

In an effort to better differentiate BPH from clinically significant prostate cancer in men with elevated PSA, the concept of PSAD was introduced. Prostate-specific antigen density accounts for the differences in PSA secretion per unit volume of prostate gland between prostate cancer and benign processes.[32] Prostate-specific antigen density is defined as the total serum PSA (ng/mL) divided by prostatic volume in cubic centimeters as estimated by TRUS. In an early case-control study by Benson and colleagues, PSAD was calculated for 41 patients with prostate cancer and 20 patients with BPH.[32] The mean PSAD for the men with prostate cancer was 0.581 compared with 0.044 for the men with BPH, which was statistically significant. In a second study including 127 men with intermediate PSA levels (between 4.0 and 10.0 ng/mL), the mean PSADs for men with and without prostate cancer were 0.279 and

0.204, respectively (p = .012).[32] Seaman and colleagues determined that a PSAD cutoff of 0.15 enhanced prostate cancer detection in men with intermediate serum PSA levels between 4.1 and 10 ng/mL.[33] Other studies have failed to find enhanced cancer detection by using PSAD over total PSA alone.[34,35] A large prospective multicenter study by Catalona and colleagues compared PSAD to serum PSA alone in the early detection of prostate cancer. A PSAD of 0.15 was only 52% sensitive in predicting cancer in men with total serum PSA between 4.1 and 9.9 ng/mL, normal DRE, and normal TRUS, thus missing nearly half of the tumors in this group.[35] Brawer and colleagues were similarly unable to find a diagnostic advantage to using PSAD alone to predict prostate cancer in 218 men with intermediate serum PSA levels.[34] Recent efforts have looked at transition zone PSAD (PSAT) to improve overall specificity based on the almost exclusive development of hyperplasia in the transition zone of the prostate. Benign hyperplasia of glands in the peripheral and central zones is believed to be a less common event and therefore a less significant and constant source of PSA.[36] In 939 men with total serum PSA < 10 ng/mL, Djavan and colleagues determined that a cutoff PSAT, calculated as serum PSA (ng/mL)/transition zone volume (cc), of 0.35 ng/mL/cc yielded a positive predictive value of 74% for prostate cancer detection.[37] Further studies are required to better define the clinical usefulness of this parameter in the diagnosis of prostate cancer. Major limitations of PSAD and PSAT include operator-dependent TRUS estimation of total prostate or transition zone volume with a 10% error margin and the lack of accurate correlation between BPH volume and PSA production attributable to variations in stromal and epithelial content.

Prostate-Specific Antigen: Use in Staging

Accurate clinical staging at the time of diagnosis is critical when counseling patients on appropriate treatment options for prostate cancer. Several methods of analyzing PSA have been evaluated for use in prostate cancer staging (Table 7–4). Large studies have shown that total serum PSA correlates with increasing clinical stage, final pathologic stage, and tumor volume.[5,38] Ercole and colleagues found that 93% of patients with a preoperative serum PSA > 10 ng/mL had extracapsular disease on final pathologic examination but concluded that values between 4 and 10 ng/mL were not useful for predicting stage.[39] Lange and colleagues similarly found that 83% of patients with a minimum preoperative PSA of 10 ng/mL had evidence of extracapsular disease.[40] The positive predictive value of serum PSA > 10 ng/mL for extracapsular disease, however, was 78%, which was considered too low for clinical utility. Oesterling and colleagues found a 65% false-positive rate when using a PSA cutoff of 10 ng/mL for predicting the presence of extracapsular disease.[41] These early studies determined that total serum PSA lacks the sensitivity and specificity to be used alone in the prediction of most pathologic stages of prostate cancer.

Table 7–4. PSA TESTING FOR CLINICAL STAGING
PSA < 20
< 0.5% likelihood of skeletal metastasis[1]
PSA < 10, Gleason score ≤ 6
< 1% likelihood of lymph node metastasis[2]
PSA < 25, Gleason score ≤ 6, and clinical stage T1c
< 3% likelihood of lymph node metastasis[3]

PSA = prostate-specific antigen (ng/mL).

Total serum PSA is sensitive enough, however, to be used alone for predicting the presence of bone metastasis or stage D2 disease. A study by Chybowski and colleagues found that in 306 men with newly diagnosed, untreated prostate cancer and a total PSA of < 20 ng/mL, only 1 patient had bone metastasis, independent of clinical stage or tumor grade.[42] They concluded that a serum PSA concentration of less than 20 ng/mL had a negative predictive value of 99.7% for bone metastasis and that costly staging radionuclide bone scans could be safely eliminated in this population of patients. Bone scans are no longer routinely obtained for staging prostate cancer in a patient with no skeletal symptoms and with a total serum PSA < 10 ng/mL.

Other studies have looked at the utility of serum PSA in combination with other factors in predicting pelvic lymph node tumor involvement preoperatively. Narayan and colleagues evaluated the ability of serum PSA and Gleason score to predict the presence of pelvic lymph node metastasis in 932 men with newly diagnosed prostate cancer.[43] They determined that a biopsy Gleason score of 6 or less and serum PSA < 10 ng/mL predicted lymph node involvement adequately enough to eliminate the need for staging pelvic lymph node dissections prior to radical prostatectomy. Rees and colleagues identified a subset of patients with a less than 3% chance of having pelvic lymph node metastasis on final pathologic examination.[44] These patients with newly diagnosed prostate cancer had either a serum PSA < 5 ng/mL, a Gleason score < 5 or a combination of a PSA < 25 ng/mL, a Gleason score < 7, and a negative DRE. Eliminating routine staging pelvic lymph node dissections on patients preoperatively determined to have a low probability of metastatic disease leads to decreased morbidity and overall cost savings.

Using multivariate analysis, serum PSA has been combined with clinical stage and Gleason score to increase the use of each factor in predicting pathologic stage. In a multi-institutional analysis including 4,133 patients with untreated prostate cancer, Partin and colleagues constructed nomograms to better predict the percent probability of having organ-confined disease based on serum PSA, clinical stage, and Gleason score (Table 7–5).[45] They found that these three variables in combination could better predict pathologic stage than any variable alone and performed a validation study to determine that the nomograms correctly predicted a given pathologic stage 72.4% of the time. These data are useful when counseling patients on treatment options for prostate cancer based on predicted extent of disease. Meng and Carroll used formal decision analysis and reported that pelvic lymph node dissection is unnecessary in patients with a risk of lymph node metastasis < 18%, as determined by nomograms such as Partin and colleagues'.[46] This 18% cutoff corresponds to Gleason score ≤ 6 and PSA ≤ 10 ng/mL and thereby supports the observations of others.

Percentage-free PSA has also been evaluated for use in staging prostate cancer. Initial studies reported conflicting results on the ability of percent free PSA to accurately predict pathologic stage even when analyzed in combination with clinical stage and Gleason score.[47–49] These early studies, however, differed in study designs, PSA assays, and definitions of pathologic outcomes, making direct comparisons difficult. A later retrospective study by Pannek and colleagues using frozen sera reported a significant difference in percent free PSA between men with organ confined and non–organ-confined disease in 263 men with clinically localized prostate cancer.[50] A 15% free PSA cutoff resulted in a 76% positive predictive value for extracapsular disease in these patients. A large prospective multicenter clinical trial by Southwick and colleagues also concluded that percent free PSA in combination with Gleason score was useful for predicting final pathologic stage in 379 men with clinical stage T1c prostate cancer and total serum PSA in the diagnostic gray zone of 4 to 10 ng/mL.[51] Logistic regression analysis revealed that in these patients, percent free PSA was the most significant predictor of an unfavorable pathologic outcome followed by Gleason score. Patients with > 15% free PSA and Gleason score < 7 had the greatest probability of a favorable pathologic outcome. As the usefulness of percent free PSA measurement for predicting disease stage becomes elucidated, it is possible that this marker may gain increased use in clinical practice.

Prostate-Specific Antigen: Use in Follow-up After Localized Surgical Therapy

Serial PSA measurements after radical prostatectomy offer the most effective means for diagnosing disease recurrence. An early study by Oesterling and colleagues demonstrated that the percentage of patients with elevated follow-up PSA after radical prostatectomy increased with increasing pathologic stage and that all patients with clinical recurrence over a 2-year period had concomitant elevated serum PSA levels.[41] As prostatic epithelium is the most important source of PSA in the adult male, total serum PSA, with a half-life of 3 days, rapidly declines after radical prostatectomy unless extraglandular disease exists. Following radical prostatectomy, 25 to 45% of patients will eventually have a serum PSA elevation, and the persistence of a measurable serum PSA immediately after surgery suggests the presence of metastatic disease regardless of residual local disease.[52] PSA recurrence precedes clinical recurrence by 3 to 5 years.[53]

In 1997, Pound and colleagues reported on the patterns of PSA and disease recurrence in 1,623 men

Table 7–5. NOMOGRAM FOR PREDICTION OF FINAL PATHOLOGIC STAGE BASED ON PRETREATMENT SERUM PSA, CLINICAL STAGE, AND GLEASON GRADE

	PSA (0.0–4.0 ng/mL)							PSA (4.1–10.0 ng/mL)						
	Clinical Stage							Clinical Stage						
Gleason Score	T1a	T1b	T1c	T2a	T2b	T2c	T3a	T1a	T1b	T1c	T2a	T2b	T2c	T3a
Organ-confined disease														
2–4	90 (84–95)	80 (72–86)	89 (86–92)	81 (75–86)	72 (65–79)	77 (69–83)	—	84 (75–92)	70 (60–79)	83 (78–88)	71 (64–78)	61 (52–69)	66 (57–74)	43 (27–58)
5	82 (73–90)	66 (57–73)	81 (76–84)	68 (63–72)	57 (50–62)	62 (55–69)	40 (26–53)	72 (60–85)	53 (44–63)	71 (67–75)	55 (51–60)	43 (38–49)	49 (42–55)	27 (17–39)
6	78 (68–88)	61 (52–69)	78 (74-81)	64 (59–68)	52 (46–57)	57 (51–64)	35 (22–48)	67 (55–82)	47 (38–57)	67 (64–70)	51 (47–54)	38 (34–43)	43 (38–49)	23 (14–34)
7	—	43 (34–53)	63 (68–68)	47 (41–52)	34 (29–39)	38 (32–45)	19 (11–29)	49 (34–68)	29 (21–38)	49 (45–54)	33 (29–38)	22 (18–26)	25 (20–30)	11 (6–17)
8–10	—	31 (20–43)	52 (41–62)	36 (27–45)	24 (17–32)	27 (18–36)	—	35 (18–62)	18 (11–28)	37 (28–46)	23 (16–31)	14 (9–19)	15 (10–22)	6 (3–10)
Established capsular penetration														
2–4	9 (4–15)	19 (13–26)	10 (7–14)	18 (13–23)	25 (19–32)	21 (14–28)	—	14 (7–23)	27 (18–37)	15 (11–20)	26 (19–33)	35 (26–43)	29 (21–37)	44 (30–59)
5	17 (9–26)	32 (24–40)	18 (15–22)	30 (26–35)	40 (34–46)	34 (27–40)	51 (38–65)	25 (14–36)	42 (32–51)	27 (23–30)	41 (36–46)	50 (45–55)	43 (37–50)	57 (46–68)
6	19 (11–29)	35 (27–43)	21 (18–25)	34 (30–38)	43 (38–48)	37 (31–43)	53 (41–65)	27 (15–39)	44 (35–53)	30 (27–33)	44 (41–48)	52 (48–56)	46 (40–51)	57 (47–67)
7	—	44 (35–54)	31 (26–36)	45 (40–50)	51 (46–57)	45 (38-52)	52 (40–63)	36 (20–51)	48 (38–60)	40 (35–44)	52 (48–57)	54 (49–59)	48 (42–54)	48 (37–58)
8–10	—	43 (32–56)	34 (27–44)	47 (38–56)	48 (40–57)	42 (33–52)	—	34 (17–58)	42 (28–57)	40 (33–49)	49 (42–57)	46 (39–53)	40 (31–48)	34 (24–46)
Seminal vesicle involvement														
2–4	0 (0–2)	1 (0–3)	1 (0–1)	1 (0–2)	2 (1–5)	2 (1–5)	—	1 (0–4)	2 (0–6)	1 (0–3)	2 (1–5)	4 (1–9)	5 (1–10)	10 (3–23)
5	1 (0–3)	2 (0–4)	1 (1–2)	2 (1–3)	3 (2–4)	3 (2–6)	7 (3–14)	2 (0–5)	3 (1–7)	2 (1–3)	3 (2–5)	5 (3–8)	6 (4–10)	12 (6–20)
6	1 (0–3)	2 (0–4)	1 (1–2)	2 (1–3)	3 (2–4)	4 (2–5)	7 (4–13)	2 (0–6)	3 (1–6)	2 (2–3)	3 (2–4)	5 (4–7)	6 (4–9)	11 (6–18)
7	—	6 (1–13)	4 (2–7)	6 (4–9)	10 (6–14)	12 (7–17)	19 (10–31)	6 (1–19)	9 (2–18)	8 (5–11)	10 (8–13)	5 (11–19)	18 (13–24)	26 (17–36)
8–10	—	11 (2–23)	9 (5–16)	12 (7–19)	17 (11–25)	21 (12–31)	—	10 (0–34)	15 (4–29)	15 (10–22)	19 (13–26)	24 (17–31)	28 (20–37)	35 (23–48)
Lymph node involvement														
2–4	0 (0–1)	0 (0–1)	0 (0–0)	0 (0–0)	0 (0–1)	0 (0–1)	—	0 (0–2)	1 (0–3)	0 (0–1)	0 (0–1)	1 (0–2)	1 (0–2)	1 (0–5)
5	0 (0–2)	1 (0–2)	0 (0–0)	0 (0–1)	1 (0–2)	1 (0–2)	2 (0–4)	1 (0–5)	2 (1–5)	0 (0–1)	1 (0–1)	2 (1–3)	2 (1–3)	3 (1–7)
6	1 (0–7)	2 (1–5)	0 (0–1)	1 (0–1)	2 (1–3)	2 (1–4)	5 (2–9)	3 (0–15)	5 (2–11)	1 (1–2)	2 (1–3)	4 (3–6)	4 (3–6)	9 (5–15)
7	—	6 (2–13)	1 (1–3)	2 (1–4)	5 (2–8)	5 (2–9)	9 (4–17)	8 (0–32)	12 (5–23)	3 (2.–5)	4 (3–6)	9 (6–12)	9 (6–13)	15 (8–23)
8–10	—	14 (5–27)	4 (2–7)	5 (2–9)	10 (5–17)	10 (4–18)	—	18 (0–55)	23 (10–43)	8 (4–12)	9 (5–13)	16 (11–24)	17 (10–26)	24 (13–38)

Reproduced with permission from Partin AW et al.[45]

Table 7–5. CONTINUED

Gleason Score	PSA (10.1–20.0 ng/mL) Clinical Stage							PSA (> 20.0 ng/mL) Clinical Stage						
	T1a	T1b	T1c	T2a	T2b	T2c	T3a	T1a	T1b	T1c	T2a	T2b	T2c	T3a
Organ-confined disease														
2–4	76 (65–88)	58 (46–69)	75 (68–82)	60 (52–70)	48 (39–58)	53 (42–64)	—	—	38 (26–52)	58 (46–68)	41 (31–52)	29 (20–40)	—	—
5	61 (47–78)	40 (31–50)	60 (54–65)	43 (38–49)	32 (26–37)	36 (29–43)	18 (10–27)	—	23 (15–32)	40 (32–49)	26 (19–33)	17 (12–22)	19 (14–26)	8 (4–14)
6	—	33 (25–42)	55 (51–59)	38 (34–43)	26 (23–31)	31 (25–37)	14 (8–22)	—	17 (11–25)	35 (27–42)	22 (16–27)	13 (10–17)	15 (11–20)	6 (3–10)
7	33 (19–57)	17 (11–24)	35 (31–40)	22 (18–26)	13 (11–16)	15 (11–19)	6 (3–10)	—	—	18 (13–23)	10 (7–14)	5 (4–8)	6 (4–9)	2 (1–4)
8–10	—	9 (5–16)	23 (16–32)	14 (9–19)	7 (5–11)	8 (5–12)	3 (1–5)	—	3 (2–7)	10 (6–16)	5 (3–9)	3 (2–4)	3 (2–5)	1 (0–2)
Established capsular penetration														
2–4	20 (10–32)	36 (26–46)	22 (16–29)	35 (26–43)	43 (34–53)	37 (27–47)	—	—	47 (33–61)	34 (24–44)	48 (36–58)	52 (39–65)	—	—
5	33 (18–47)	50 (39–59)	35 (30–40)	50 (45–56)	57 (51–63)	51 (43–57)	59 (47–69)	—	57 (44–68)	48 (40–56)	60 (52–68)	61 (53–69)	55 (46–64)	54 (40–67)
6	—	49 (38–59)	38 (34–42)	52 (48–57)	57 (51–62)	50 (44–57)	54 (44–64)	—	51 (37–64)	49 (43–56)	60 (53–66)	57 (50–64)	51 (43–59)	46 (34–58)
7	38 (18–61)	46 (34–60)	45 (40–50)	55 (50–60)	51 (45–57)	45 (39–52)	40 (30–50)	—	—	46 (39–54)	51 (44–58)	43 (35–50)	37 (29–45)	29 (19–40)
8–10	—	33 (21–51)	40 (33–49)	46 (38–55)	38 (30–47)	33 (24–42)	26 (17–37)	—	24 (13–42)	34 (27–45)	37 (28–48)	28 (20–37)	23 (16–31)	17 (11–26)
Seminal vesicle involvement														
2–4	2 (0–7)	4 (1–10)	2 (1–5)	4 (1–8)	7 (2–14)	8 (2–16)	—	—	9 (1–22)	7 (2–15)	10 (3–20)	14 (4–29)	—	—
5	3 (0–9)	5 (1–10)	3 (2–5)	5 (3–8)	8 (5–11)	9 (6–15)	15 (8–25)	—	10 (2–21)	9 (5–14)	11 (6–17)	15 (9–23)	19 (11–28)	26 (14–41)
6	—	4 (1–9)	4 (3–5)	5 (3–7)	7 (5–10)	9 (6–13)	14 (8–21)	—	8 (2–17)	8 (6–12)	10 (7–15)	13 (9–19)	17 (11–24)	21 (13–33)
7	8 (0–28)	11 (3–22)	12 (8–16)	14 (10–19)	18 (13–24)	22 (16–29)	28 (18–39)	—	—	22 (15–28)	24 (17–32)	27 (20–34)	32 (24–42)	36 (25–49)
8–10	—	15 (4–32)	20 (13–28)	22 (15–31)	25 (18–34)	30 (21–40)	34 (21–47)	—	20 (6–43)	31 (21–42)	33 (22–45)	33 (24–45)	38 (26–51)	40 (25–55)
Lymph node involvement														
2–4	0 (0–7)	2 (0–8)	0 (0–2)	1 (0–2)	1 (0–5)	1 (0–6)	—	—	4 (0–17)	1 (0–4)	1 (0–5)	3 (0–11)	—	—
5	3 (0–14)	5 (2–11)	1 (0–2)	2 (1–3)	4 (1–7)	4 (1–7)	7 (3–15)	—	10 (3–21)	3 (1–6)	3 (1–7)	7 (3–13)	7 (3–13)	11 (4–22)
6	—	13 (6–24)	3 (2–5)	4 (3–6)	10 (7–13)	10 (6–14)	18 (10–27)	—	23 (10–40)	7 (4–11)	8 (5–13)	16 (11–23)	17 (11–25)	26 (16–38)
7	18 (0–57)	24 (10-41)	8 (5–11)	9 (6–13)	17 (12–23)	18 (12–25)	26 (16–38)	—	—	14 (9–21)	14 (9–22)	25 (18–33)	25 (16–34)	32 (20–45)
8–10	—	40 (19–60)	16 (10–24)	17 (11–25)	29 (21–38)	29 (19–40)	37 (24–52)	—	51 (25–72)	24 (15–36)	24 (15–35)	36 (25–48)	35 (23–48)	42 (27–58)

Reproduced with permission from Partin AW et al.[45]

Number represent predictive probability (95% confidence interval). Dashes indicate lack of sufficient data to calculate probability.

PSA = prostate-specific antigen.

having undergone radical retropubic prostatectomy for clinically localized prostate cancer.[54] Overall actuarial 5- and 10-year recurrence-free likelihood was 80% and 68%, respectively, in this series. They reported a significant difference in the likelihood of recurrence between men with preoperative PSA values between 4 and 10 ng/mL and between 10 and 20 ng/mL and those with a level greater than 20 ng/mL. The 10-year actuarial recurrence-free rates in these groups were 75%, 30%, and 28%, respectively. The authors also found that in 129 men with clinical failure, the timing of PSA recurrence was the most predictive variable for distinguishing local recurrence from distant metastasis. Within 1 year of surgery, only 7% of patients with a local recurrence had a PSA recurrence as compared with 93% of men with distant metastasis. Patel and colleagues found that once PSA became detectable after radical prostatectomy, PSA doubling time became the best predictor of risk and time to clinical recurrence over preoperative PSA, Gleason score, and pathologic stage.[55] Two years after PSA recurrence, for example, a PSA doubling time between 4.6 and 6.9 months estimated a 33% rate of clinical recurrence, and the risk of clinical recurrence doubled with each 9-month decrease in PSA doubling time. Short PSA doubling times (< 6 months) were associated with distant metastasis, whereas longer doubling times were associated with local recurrence. Over a mean 3-year follow-up, 33% of patients with PSA doubling times less than 6 months had distant clinical recurrence, whereas only 2% of patients with doubling times greater than 6 months did. Local clinical recurrence occurred in 18% of 44 patients with PSA doubling times greater than 6 months but occurred in only 3% of patients with doubling times less than 6 months.

Prostate-specific antigen velocity, Gleason score, and pathologic stage were combined in a multivariate analysis by Partin and colleagues to predict distant from local disease recurrence in men with elevated serum PSA levels within 1 year of radical prostatectomy (Table 7–6).[56] Ninety-four percent of men with local recurrence had a PSAV of less than 0.75 ng/mL/yr, whereas 50% of men with distant recurrence had a PSAV greater than this value. Patients with eventual distant metastasis were more likely to experience PSA recurrence within 2 years of surgery and have adverse pathologic conditions such as Gleason score > 7, seminal vesicle involvement, or pelvic lymph node involvement. A low PSAV with a long interval between treatment and PSA recurrence suggests local disease progression as opposed to a rapidly increasing serum PSA soon after surgery, which suggests distant metastasis.

Serum PSA measurement is the most important tool for following patients after radical prostatectomy. A recent study of 1,916 men followed after radical prostatectomy reported that no men with an undetectable serum PSA had local recurrence or distant metastasis for an average of 5 years after surgery.[57] The authors concluded that screening radiographic imaging and DRE for disease recurrence are unnecessary for follow-up after radical prostatectomy in asymptomatic men with an undetectable total serum PSA.

Total serum PSA has also been evaluated for predicting bone scan positivity in men with increasing serum PSA after radical prostatectomy. In a retrospective analysis of 122 bone scans performed in 93 men with rising PSA after surgery, Cher and colleagues found that positive bone scans were significantly associated with higher mean serum PSA levels postoperatively.[58] Through logistic regression, the authors showed that total serum PSA was the only significant predictor of a positive bone scan over pretreatment PSA, Gleason score, pathologic stage, or time to PSA recurrence. They concluded that the probability of a positive bone scan in a patient with PSA recurrence after radical prostatectomy with no adjuvant hormonal therapy is less than 5% until serum PSA exceeds 30 to 40 ng/mL.

Prostate-Specific Antigen: Use after Antiandrogen Therapy

Men with advanced prostate cancer commonly receive androgen withdrawal therapy with one or more modalities for therapy and palliation. Although PSA gene expression is androgen sensitive and therefore dependent on the hormonal status of the individual, serum PSA has been evaluated for follow-up use in hormonally treated patients with prostate cancer to predict the rate of disease progression and overall survival. It is generally believed that three consecutive

Table 7–6. RISK FACTORS FOR RECURRENCE OF CARCINOMA OF THE PROSTATE: PSA ELEVATIONS AFTER RADICAL PROSTATECTOMY

Local recurrence
PSA velocity < 0.75 ng/mL/yr
Metastatic recurrence
PSA velocity > 0.75 ng/mL/yr
Gleason score > 7
Seminal vesicle involvement (PT3cNxMx)

increases in serum PSA after treatment signify a true biochemical recurrence. In 1989, Stamey and colleagues reported on 45 men receiving antiandrogen therapy for previously untreated stage D2 prostate cancer. They found that the patients who tended to survive longer than 2 years had normal or undetectable total serum PSA levels 6 months after initiation of therapy.[59] Arai and colleagues found that the rate of decrease in PSA after endocrine therapy predicted survival as patients who had an 80% decrease in total serum PSA within 1 month of beginning therapy survived significantly longer than patients without such a rapid decline.[60] Patients whose serum PSA levels reached a nadir within 1 month of therapy had the best prognosis, whereas patients with elevated PSA 3 months after the initiation of therapy had the highest risk of disease progression. In 49 patients undergoing orchiectomy for metastatic prostate cancer, Evans and colleagues reported that the 6-month proportional decrease in PSA from preoperative levels was the best predictor of patient survival after hormonal therapy (Table 7–7).[61]

Although the best clinical application of PSA monitoring after hormonal therapy for prostate cancer remains to be determined, a few generalizations can be made. Patients with the best prognosis tend to have a rapid decline in total serum PSA that persists for greater than 6 months after the initiation of therapy. As hormonally treated patients progress from androgen-sensitive to androgen-insensitive disease, PSA recurrence acts as a sentinel for poor prognosis.

Prostate-Specific Antigen: Use After Radiation Therapy

Serum PSA provides a valuable tool for monitoring the response of prostate cancer patients to radiation therapy and predicting disease progression after treatment. As seen with antiandrogen therapy, PSA decline after radiation therapy is widely variable in rate and magnitude and may not become completely undetectable. In an early study, Zietman and colleagues reported that pretreatment PSA was a more significant factor predicting outcome after radiation therapy than even clinical stage.[62] They found that patients with stage T1-T2 prostate cancer and a pretreatment serum PSA > 15 ng/mL had a similarly poor outcome after radiation therapy as men with T3 disease and a PSA > 15 ng/mL. Other studies suggested that a pretreatment PSA < 4 ng/mL was required for optimal outcomes after radiation therapy.[63,64] A recent study by Preston and colleagues of men treated with external beam radiation therapy for prostate cancer assessed the ability of pre- and posttreatment PSA to predict overall response to therapy.[65] As shown in previous studies, they found that pretreatment PSA was a strong predictor of treatment outcome. In their series of 371 men, a pretreatment PSA of < 20 ng/mL predicted the best response with a 5-year disease-free survival of 60%. In multivariate analysis, however, PSA nadir was the strongest predictor of long-term outcome, with patients achieving a PSA nadir < 0.5 ng/mL having the best prognosis. Critz and colleagues evaluated PSA patterns in 489 men with T1-T2 prostate cancer who received iodine 125 seed implantation followed by external beam radiation.[66] Ninety-two percent of men who had a PSA nadir of 0.2 ng/mL or less had no evidence of biochemical recurrence after 10 years compared with 41% of men with a PSA nadir between 0.3 and 1 ng/mL. Biochemical recurrence was defined as three consecutive increases in PSA after the nadir value was achieved. This is the definition of postirradiation failure as defined by the American Society

Table 7–7. SIGNIFICANCE OF ALTERNATIVE MODELS EVALUATING EFFECTS OF PSA IN PREDICTING SURVIVAL AFTER HORMONAL ABLATION

As Function of Initial Bone Scan, Patient Age, and	*p*
Preorchiectomy PSA level	.61
Absolute 6-month PSA level	.08
6-month decrease in PSA*	.49
6-month proportional decrease in PSA*	.006

Reproduced with permission from Evans CP et al.[61]
*From preorchiectomy level
PSA = prostate-specific antigen.

for Therapeutic Radiation and Oncology, although it awaits clinical validation. The authors concluded that a PSA nadir of 0.2 ng/mL or less should be the definition of freedom from disease in men with prostate cancer treated with radiotherapy.

Reverse Transcriptase Polymerase Chain Reaction for Prostate-Specific Antigen

Although PSA screening has resulted in an increased number of men with less advanced disease at the time of diagnosis, one-third to one half of men undergoing radical prostatectomy for clinically localized prostate cancer will fail on the basis of rising serum PSA.[53] Several series have also shown that up to 40% of patients will have tumor extension into the surgical margin at the time of surgery, prompting the need for improved staging of prostate cancer. A number of investigators have evaluated the "molecular staging" of prostate cancer using the reverse transcriptase polymerase chain reaction (RT-PCR) assay for PSA in the hope of more accurately predicting clinical stage.

The RT-PCR assay provides a rapid and sensitive method for detecting metastatic dissemination of prostate cancer by the ability to identify a single PSA-producing cell among a large, heterogeneous population of cells in a clinical sample. Investigators report the ability to detect a single PSA-producing cell among 1×10^7 to 1×10^8 leukocytes.[67] This assay uses the retroviral enzyme reverse transcriptase to produce a DNA copy of all messenger RNA transcripts in the sample followed by PCR amplification of the tissue-specific PSA gene. As all cells contain the genomic DNA for PSA, by only amplifying the complementary DNA of messenger ribonucleic acid (mRNA) transcripts, RT-PCR successfully identifies only the cells actively expressing PSA.

Several independent studies have revealed that RT-PCR for PSA in serum is appropriately negative in patients with benign disease while being able to correctly identify patients with known metastasis.[68] The use of RT-PCR for detecting PSA-expressing cells in lymph nodes and bone marrow aspirates from patients with metastatic prostate cancer was first reported in 1992.[69] Since then, a number of investigators have applied PSA RT-PCR to detect PSA-producing cells in a variety of clinical specimens including serum, lymph nodes, and bone marrow aspirates. A large study by Katz and colleagues in 1994 found a positive correlation between RT-PCR PSA positivity in serum and the presence of capsular penetration and positive surgical margins in 65 men undergoing radical prostatectomy for clinically localized prostate cancer.[70] This study also detected PSA mRNA in the systemic circulation of 78% of patients with known metastatic disease. Olsson and colleagues performed RT-PCR for PSA on the serum of 100 men and found a significant correlation of RT-PCR positivity and pathologic stage with a sensitivity and specificity of 73% and 90%, respectively, for detecting extracapsular disease.[68] Other studies, however, have reported conflicting results. A recent study by Gao and colleagues found that PSA RT-PCR performed on serum samples from 85 men prior to radical prostatectomy for clinically localized disease was not able to predict pathologic stage or early serum PSA recurrence.[71] Compared with patients with negative results, patients with RT-PCR positivity for PSA were less likely to have positive surgical margins or PSA recurrence at a mean follow-up of 26 months. The authors suggested that difference in sample handling, processing, and assay parameters may account for the conflicting experiences reported for RT-PCR. Ignatoff and colleagues similarly found no advantage in preoperative staging using PSA RT-PCR on serum samples.[72] Gao and colleagues also evaluated RT-PCR positivity in bone marrow aspirates from 116 men undergoing radical prostatectomy and found no significant correlation with pathologic stage, grade, or margin positivity.[73]

The significance of finding PSA-expressing cells in the circulation by RT-PCR remains to be determined. There is no evidence that a single circulating prostate cell harbors the genetic changes necessary for it to become invasive and form a distant metastatic focus. Finding a prostate cell in the bone marrow or a lymph node may also represent normal physiologic filtration and elimination of cells in these compartments. Great disparity exists between laboratories in terms of patient selection, sample handling, sample preparation, and RT-PCR technique. Although some early reports were encouraging, many subsequent studies produced conflicting results, and the ability of PSA RT-PCR to act as a staging tool for prostate cancer and to predict patterns of disease recurrence after localized therapy remains to be determined.

Haese and colleagues described an ultrasensitive method for detecting PSA by concentrating serum samples prior to standard immunologic analysis.[74] They prospectively obtained sera from 442 men undergoing radical prostatectomy for clinically localized prostate cancer and measured PSA in unconcentrated samples and in fourfold concentrated samples prepared by lyophilization. With a mean follow-up of 449 days, 20.8% of patients experienced biochemical recurrence, 31% of whom demonstrated failure by the concentrated assay before becoming positive on the standard assay. The concentrated assay detected PSA relapse a mean of 267 days before the standard assay, and the authors concluded that this method provides a significant reduction in time to diagnosis of recurrent disease after radical prostatectomy with the same accuracy as conventional PSA assays. The relationship between earlier detection of disease recurrence and patient outcome is yet to be determined.

PROSTATE-SPECIFIC MEMBRANE ANTIGEN

Horoszewicz and colleagues described prostate-specific membrane antigen (PSMA) in 1987 after isolating monoclonal antibody 7E11-C5.3 from mice immunized with purified fractions of cell membrane from a human prostate cancer cell line.[75] Prostate-specific membrane antigen is a 100,000 kDa transmembrane glycoprotein with intracellular and extracellular domains, the function of which is not entirely clear. Prostate-specific membrane antigen has been evaluated as a new diagnostic and prognostic marker for prostate cancer as well as a target for antibody-directed imaging studies.

By immunohistochemistry, PSMA appears to show differential staining between benign and malignant prostate tissue. In their original paper, Horoszewicz and colleagues describe more intense staining for PSMA in malignant prostate epithelial cells than in normal or hyperplastic tissue.[75] Sweat and colleagues also found that primary prostate cancers and lymph node metastasis stained more heavily for PSMA than benign prostatic tissue, with the lymph node metastasis staining less heavily than the primary tumor.[76] Other investigators reported immunohistochemical staining for PSMA in primary prostate tumors, prostate cancer lymph node metastasis, and prostate cancer bone metastasis.[77,78] Prostate-specific membrane antigen is not prostate tissue specific, however, and a variety of other tissues including colon, brain, salivary glands, muscle, and renal tubules will stain positive for PSMA. Liu and colleagues recently reported positive PSMA staining in vascular endothelial cells from a variety of tumors.[79]

The value of serum PSMA measurements in the staging and prognosis of prostate cancer has also been investigated. In a population of 226 asymptomatic men, serum PSMA was not significantly elevated in men with biopsy-proven prostate cancer; however, it correlated with the stage of disease ($r = .85$).[80] Beckett and colleagues used Western blot to study PSMA levels in serum samples from 236 men and women with and without cancer.[81] Prostate-specific membrane antigen was detected in the serum of normal men and women as well as in serum from men with BPH or prostate cancer and women with breast cancer. Although they found increasing serum PSMA levels with patient age, there was no correlation between PSMA levels and cancer stage or overall prognosis. Prostate-specific membrane antigen appears to be under hormonal regulation as androgen withdrawal therapy results in increased expression of PSMA by prostatic epithelial cells.[82]

Reverse transcriptase polymerase chain reaction technology has also been applied to detect PSMA-producing cells in the circulation and bone marrow of men with prostate cancer in an effort to improve clinical staging. Current studies have not shown a significant correlation between serum PSMA RT-PCR positivity and pathologic stage or Gleason score in men with prostate cancer.[83,84]

A clinical application for PSMA is the ProstaScint scan, which uses immunoscintigraphy to identify PSMA expression anywhere in the body for staging prostate cancer. Prostate-specific membrane antigen serves as a target for an antibody-based scan as its expression is increased in metastatic, poorly differentiated, and hormonally treated prostate cancer. The ProstaScint scan is about 75% sensitive and 66% specific, suggesting clinical use for detecting metastatic disease to regional lymph nodes.[85] Kahn and colleagues found that the ProstaScint scan enhanced PSA response prediction after salvage radiotherapy in men with prostate cancer who failed radical prostatectomy.[86] The ProstaScint scan is not frequently employed clinically as PSA kinetics and other clinicopathologic correlates may indicate whether disease recurrence is localized or metastatic. In addition, the decision for immediate versus delayed hormonal ablation in the context of prostate cancer disease progression remains unproved and controversial.

Prostate-specific membrane antigen does not appear to be prostate tissue or prostate cancer specific. As new antibodies to PSMA and improved assays are developed, the value and efficacy of this tumor marker in the diagnosis and treatment of prostate cancer will be determined.

NEW MARKERS

Despite significant advances in the diagnosis and treatment of prostate cancer, up to 31% of patients treated with radical prostatectomy and up to 53% of men undergoing radiotherapy for prostate cancer will experience a recurrence of their disease.[52] A number of novel molecular markers are under investigation for their potential use in the more accurate prediction of tumor aggressiveness and response to therapy.

The Ki-67 labeling index (LI) is a marker for cellular proliferation, which is expressed in all stages of the cell cycle except during G_0. Several investigators have reported that Ki-67 LI correlates with Gleason grade and that a high proliferative index is significantly associated with disease recurrence and a poorer prognosis.[87–91] The *P53* tumor suppressor gene plays an important role in cell cycle control during times of cell stress and DNA damage. *P53* mutations are the most common known genetic lesions in human cancers and lead to high levels of nonfunctional, intracellular levels of P53 protein.[92] Increased P53 staining by immunohistochemistry is associated with high Gleason grade and with decreased survival in men with prostate cancer.[90,93–96] Bubendorf and colleagues studied P53 staining in core needle biopsies of men with prostate cancer and concluded that the prognostic significance of P53 staining may provide valuable information for predicting tumor aggressiveness and prognosis.[88] Increased staining for P53 and the *BCL2* oncogene are associated with treatment failure after external beam radiation therapy for clinically localized prostate cancer.[97] Determination of P53 and *BCL2* staining in 54 core needle biopsy specimens showed a statistically significant correlation between increased staining for these two molecular markers and failure to reach a PSA nadir of less than 1 ng/mL after radiotherapy. Although not ready for widespread use in clinical practice, these molecular markers offer potential for improving the prediction of prostate cancer progression and patterns of recurrence for the application of more tailored therapeutic strategies.

Recent developments in understanding the role of angiogenesis in prostate cancer metastasis have led to studies evaluating the use of prostatic microvessel density (MVD) as a prognostic sign in patients with prostate cancer. Several studies of MVD in radical prostatectomy specimens have found a positive correlation between MVD and pathologic stage.[98,99] Other studies reported that MVD can predict biochemical recurrence in patients with prostate cancer treated with surgery or external beam radiation.[100–102] A recent study by Rubin and colleagues looked at MVD in 100 radical prostatectomy specimens by endothelium-specific antibody CD31 staining.[103] The authors failed to find a correlation between MVD and pathologic stage or biochemical recurrence and concluded that MVD is not a useful prognostic indicator for men with clinically localized prostate cancer.

Recent studies have evaluated the ability of serum levels of human glandular kallikrein 2 (hK2) to differentiate men with BPH from men with prostate cancer. Similar to PSA, hK2 is a serine protease with high levels of expression in the prostate.[104,105] In 1997, Darson and colleagues reported higher hK2 expression in prostate adenocarcinoma than in normal prostate tissue.[106] Becker and colleagues compared serum hK2 levels to total and free PSA levels in men with prostate disease. All healthy male controls had hK2 levels below the level of detection for the immunoassay used in this study.[107] Concentrations of hK2 were significantly higher in men with clinically localized prostate cancer compared with men with BPH and in men with advanced prostate cancer versus men with clinically localized disease. The authors reported the greatest discrimination of men with BPH from those with prostate cancer when serum hK2 levels were analyzed in combination with total PSA and free PSA and concluded that further studies are required to confirm these findings and better define the clinical use of this assay. Partin and colleagues reported that the total hK2 to percentage of free PSA ratio in patients with PSA levels between 2 and 4 ng/mL would identify up to 40% of prostate cancers and require biopsy in only 17% of men in this PSA range.[108] The total hK2 to percentage of free PSA ratio provided additional specificity for cancer detection and may have a clinical role once validated.

REFERENCES

1. Romas NA, Kwan DJ. Prostatic acid phosphatase. Urol Clin North Am 1993;20:581–8.

1a. Kutscher W, Worner A. Prostatophosphatase. Physiol Chem 1936;239:109–12.

2. Huggins C, Hodges C. Studies on prostatic cancer: the effect of castration, of estrogen, and of androgen injection on serum phosphatases in metastatic carcinoma of the prostate. Cancer Res 1941;1:293–7.

3. Oesterling JE, Brendler CB, Epstein JI, et al. Correlation of clinical stage, serum prostatic acid phosphatase, and preoperative Gleason grade with final pathological stage in 275 patients with clinically localized adenocarcinoma of the prostate. J Urol 1987;138:92–8.

4. Whitesel JA, Donohue RE, Mani JH, et al. Acid phosphatase: its influence on the management of carcinoma of the prostate. J Urol 1984;131:70–2.

5. Stamey TA, Yang N, Hay AR, et al. Prostate-specific antigen as a serum marker for adenocarcinoma of the prostate. N Engl J Med 1987;317:909–16.

6. Moul JW, Connelly RR, Perahia B, McLeod DG. The contemporary value of pretreatment prostatic acid phosphatase to predict pathological stage and recurrence in radical prostatectomy cases. J Urol 1998;159:935–40.

6a. Hara M, Inoue T, Koyanagi Y, et al. [Immunoelectrophoretic studies of the protein components in human seminal plasma (especially its specific component). (Forensic immunological study of body fluids and secretions. VI)]. Nippon Hoigaku Zasshi 1972;26:78–80.

6b. Papsidero CD, Wang MC, Valenzuela LA, et al. A prostate antigen in sera of prostatic cancer patients. Cancer Res 1980;40:2428–32.

7. Herschman JD, Smith DS, Catalona WJ. Effect of ejaculation on serum total and free prostate specific antigen concentrations. Urology 1997;50:239–43.

8. Tchetgen MB, Song JT, Strawderman M, et al. Ejaculation increases the serum prostate-specific antigen concentration. Urology 1996;47:511–6.

9. Catalona WJ, Smith DS, Ratliff TL, Basler JW. Detection of organ confined prostate cancer is increased through prostate specific antigen-based screening. JAMA 1993;270:948–54.

10. Gann PH, Hennekens CH, Stampfer MJ. A prospective evaluation of plasma prostate-specific antigen for detection of prostatic cancer. JAMA 1995;273:289–94.

11. Catalona WJ, Richie JP, Ahmann FR, et al. Comparison of digital rectal examination and serum prostate specific antigen in the early detection of prostate cancer: results of a multicenter clinical trial of 6,630 men. J Urol 1994;151:1283–90.

12. Smith DS, Catalona WJ, Herschman JD. Longitudinal screening for prostate cancer with prostate-specific antigen. JAMA 1996;276:1309–15.

13. Carter HB, Epstein JI, Chan DW, et al. Recommended prostate-specific antigen testing intervals for the detection of curable prostate cancer. JAMA 1997;277:1456–60.

14. Ross KS, Carter HB, Pearson JD, Guess HA. Comparative efficiency of prostate-specific antigen screening strategies for prostate cancer detection. JAMA 2000;284:1399–405.

15. Cooner WH, Mosley BR, Rutherford CLJ, et al. Prostate cancer detection in a clinical urological practice by ultrasonography, digital rectal examination, and prostate specific antigen. J Urol 1990;143:1146–52.

16. Ghavamian R, Blute ML, Bergstralh EJ, et al. Comparison of clinically nonpalpable prostate-specific antigen-detected (cT1c) versus palpable (cT2) prostate cancers in patients undergoing radical retropubic prostatectomy. Urology 1999;54:105–10.

17. Oesterling JE. Prostate specific antigen: a critical assessment of the most useful tumor marker for adenocarcinoma of the prostate. J Urol 1991;145:907–23.

18. Oesterling JE, Jacobsen SJ, Chute CG, et al. Serum prostate-specific antigen in a community-based population of healthy men. JAMA 1993;270:860–4.

19. Partin AW, Criley SR, Subong ENP, et al. Standard versus age-specific prostate specific antigen reference ranges among men with clinically localized prostate cancer: a pathological analysis. J Urol 1996;155:1336–9.

20. Reissigl A, Pointner J, Horninger W, et al. Comparison of different prostate-specific antigen cutpoints for early detection of prostate cancer: results of a large screening study. Urology 1995;46:662–5.

21. Catalona WJ, Smith DS, Wolfert RL, et al. Evaluation of percentage of free serum prostate-specific antigen to improve specificity of prostate cancer screening. JAMA 1995;274:1214–20.

22. Chen YT, Luderer AA, Thiel RP, et al. Using proportions of free to total prostate-specific antigen, age, and total prostate-specific antigen to predict the probability of prostate cancer. Urology 1996;47:518–24.

23. Catalona WJ, Partin AW, Slawin KM, et al. Use of the percentage of free prostate-specific antigen to enhance differentiation of prostate cancer from benign prostatic disease. JAMA 1998;279:1542–7.

24. Partin AW, Catalona WJ, Southwick PC, et al. Analysis of percent free prostate specific antigen (PSA) for prostate cancer detection: influence of total PSA, prostate volume, and age. Urology 1996;Suppl 48:55–61.

25. Catalona WJ, Smith DS, Ornstein DK. Prostate cancer detection in men with serum PSA concentrations of 2.6 to

4.0 ng/mL and benign prostate examination. JAMA 1997; 277:1452–5.
26. Vashi AR, Wojno KJ, Henricks W, et al. Determination of the "reflex range" and appropriate cutpoints for percent free prostate-specific antigen in 413 men referred for prostatic evaluation using the AxSYM system. Urology 1997; 49:19–27.
27. Prestigiacomo AF, Lilja H, Pettersson K, et al. A comparison of the free fraction of serum prostate specific antigen in men with benign and cancerous prostates: the best case scenario. J Urol 1996;156:350–4.
28. Brawer MK, Meyer GE, Letran JL, et al. Measurement of complexed PSA improves specificity for early detection of prostate cancer. Urology 1998;52:372–8.
29. Carter HB, Pearson JD, Metter J, et al. Longitudinal evaluation of prostate-specific antigen levels in men with and without prostate disease. JAMA 1992;267:2215–20.
30. Carter HB, Pearson JD. PSA velocity for the diagnosis of early prostate cancer: a new concept. Urol Clin North Am 1993;20:665.
31. Smith DS, Catalona WJ. Rate of change in serum prostate specific antigen levels as a method for prostate cancer detection. J Urol 1994;152:1163–7.
32. Benson MC, Whang IS, Pontuk A, et al. Prostate specific antigen density: a means of distinguishing benign prostatic hypertrophy and prostate cancer. J Urol 1992;147:815–6.
33. Seaman E, Whang M, Olsson CA, et al. PSA density (PSAD): role in patient evaluation and management. Urol Clin North Am 1993;20:653–63.
34. Brawer MK, Aramburu EAG, Chen GL, et al. The inability of prostate specific antigen index to enhance the predictive value of prostate specific antigen in the diagnosis of prostatic carcinoma. J Urol 1993;150:369–73.
35. Catalona WJ, Richie JP, deKernion JB, et al. Comparison of prostate specific antigen concentration versus prostate specific antigen density in the early detection of prostate cancer: receiver operating characteristic curves. J Urol 1994;152:2031–6.
36. Kalish J, Cooner WH, Graham SD. Serum PSA adjusted for volume of transition zone (PSAT) is more accurate than PSA adjusted for total gland volume (PSAD) in detecting adenocarcinoma of the prostate. Urology 1994;43:601–6.
37. Djavan B, Marberger M, Zlotta A, Schulman CC. PSA, f/t-PSA, PSAD, PSA-TZ, and PSA-velocity for prostate cancer prediction: a multivariate analysis [abstract]. J Urol 1998;159(Pt 2):235.
38. Myrtle JF, Klinley PG, Ivor LP, et al. Clinical utility of prostate specific antigen in the management of prostate cancer. XVth Annual meeting ISOBM, Quebec, 1987. Tumor Biol 1987;8:353.
39. Ercole CJ, Lange PH, Mathisen M, et al. Prostate specific antigen and prostatic acid phosphatase in the monitoring and staging of patients with prostatic cancer. J Urol 1987; 138:1181–4.
40. Lange PH, Ercole CJ, Lightner DJ, et al. The value of serum prostate specific antigen determinations before and after radical retropubic prostatectomy. J Urol 1989;141:873–9.
41. Oesterling JE, Chan DW, Epstein JI, et al. Prostate specific antigen in the preoperative and postoperative evaluation of localized prostatic cancer treated with radical prostatectomy. J Urol 1988;139:766–72.
42. Chybowski FM, Keller JJL, Bergstralh EJ, Oesterling JE. Predicting radionuclide bone scan findings in patients with newly diagnosed, untreated prostate cancer: prostate specific antigen is superior to all other clinical parameters. J Urol 1991;145:313–8.
43. Narayan P, Fournier G, Gajendran V, et al. Utility of preoperative serum prostate-specific antigen concentration and biopsy Gleason score in predicting risk of pelvic lymph node metastases in prostate cancer. Urology 1994;44: 519–24.
44. Rees MA, McHugh TA, Dorr RP, et al. Assessment of the utility of bone scan, CT scan and lymph node dissection in staging of patients with newly diagnosed prostate cancer [abstract]. J Urol 1995;153:352A.
45. Partin AW, Kattan MW, Subong ENP, et al. Combination of prostate-specific antigen, clinical stage, and Gleason score to predict pathological stage of localized prostate cancer. JAMA 1997;277:1445–51.
46. Meng MV, Carroll PR. When is pelvic lymph node dissection necessary before radical prostatectomy? A decision analysis. J Urol 2000;164:1235–40.
47. Pannek J, Subong EN, Jones KA, et al. The role of free/total prostate-specific antigen ratio in the prediction of final pathologic stage for men with clinically localized prostate cancer. Urology 1996;48:51.
48. Graefen M, Hammerer P, Henke P, et al. Percentage of free-PSA does not correlate with pathological outcome [abstract]. J Urol 1996;155(Pt 2):370A.
49. Arcangeli CG, Shepherd DL, Smith DS, et al. Correlation of percent free PSA with pathologic features of prostatic carcinomas [abstact]. J Urol 1996;155(Pt 2):415A.
50. Pannek J, Rittenhouse HG, Chan DW, et al. The use of percent free prostate specific antigen for staging clinically localized prostate cancer. J Urol 1998;159:1238–42.
51. Southwick PC, Catalona WJ, Partin AW, et al. Prediction of post-radical prostatectomy pathological outcome for stage T1c prostate cancer with percent free prostate specific antigen: a prospective multicenter clinical trial. J Urol 1999;162:1346–51.
52. Lange PH. Tumor markers in prostate cancer. In: Raghavan D, Scher HI, Leibel SA, Lange PH, editors. Principles and practice of genitourinary oncology. Philadelphia: Lippincott-Raven; 1997. p. 417–25.
53. Paulson DF. Impact of radical prostatectomy in the management of clinically localized disease. J Urol 1994;152: 1826–30.
54. Pound CR, Partin AW, Epstein JI, Walsh PC. Prostate-specific antigen after anatomic radical retropubic prostatectomy. Urol Clin North Am 1997;24:395–406.
55. Patel A, Dorey F, Franklin J, deKernion JB. Recurrence patterns after radical retropubic prostatectomy: clinical usefulness of prostate specific antigen doubling times and log slope prostate specific antigen. J Urol 1997;158:1441–5.
56. Partin AW, Pearson JD, Landis PK, et al. Evaluation of serum prostate-specific antigen velocity after radical prostatectomy to distinguish local recurrence from distant metastases. Urology 1994;43:649.

57. Pound CR, Christens-Barry OW, Gurganus RT, et al. Digital rectal examination and imaging studies are unnecessary in men with undetectable prostate specific antigen following radical prostatectomy. J Urol 1999;162:1337–40.
58. Cher ML, Bianco FJ Jr, Lam JS, et al. Limited role of radionuclide bone scintigraphy in patients with prostate specific antigen elevations after radical prostatectomy. J Urol 1998;160:1387–91.
59. Stamey TA, Kabalin JN, Ferrari M, Yang N. Prostate specific antigen in the diagnosis and treatment of adenocarcinoma of the prostate. IV. Anti-androgen treated patients. J Urol 1989;141:1088–90.
60. Arai Y, Yoshiki T, Yoshida O. Prognostic significance of prostate specific antigen in endocrine treatment for prostatic cancer. J Urol 1990;144:1415–9.
61. Evans CP, Gajendran V, Tewari A, et al. The proportional decrease in prostate specific antigen level best predicts the duration of survival after hormonal therapy in patients with metastatic carcinoma of the prostate. Br J Urol 1996;78:426–31.
62. Zietman AL, Coen JJ, Shipley WU, et al. Radical radiation therapy in the management of prostatic adenocarcinoma: the initial prostate-specific antigen value as a predictor of treatment outcome. J Urol 1994;151:640–5.
63. Kuban D, El-mahdi A, Schellhammer P. Prostate-specific antigen for pretreatment prediction and posttreatment evaluation of outcome after definitive irradiation for prostate cancer. Int J Radiat Oncol Biol Phys 1995;32:307–16.
64. Zagars GK. Serum PSA as a tumor marker for patients undergoing definitive radiation therapy. Urol Clin North Am 1993;20:737–48.
65. Preston DM, Bauer JJ, Connelly RR, et al. Prostate-specific antigen to predict outcome of external beam radiation for prostate cancer: Walter Reed Army Medical Center experience 1988–1995. Urology 1999;53:131–8.
66. Critz FA, Williams WH, Holladay CT, et al. Post-treatment PSA $\leq$ 0.2 ng/mL defines disease freedom after radiotherapy for prostate cancer using modern techniques. Urology 1999;54:968–71.
67. Gomella LG, Raj GV, Moreno JG. Reverse transcriptase polymerase chain reaction for prostate specific antigen in the management of prostate cancer. J Urol 1997;158:326–37.
68. Olsson CA, de Vries GM, Buttyan R, Katz AE. Reverse transcriptase-polymerase chain reaction assays for prostate cancer. Urol Clin North Am 1997;24:367–78.
69. Vessella RL, Blouke KA, Stray JE, et al. The use of the polymerase chain reaction to detect metastatic prostate cancer in lymph nodes and bone marrow. Proceedings of 83rd annual meeting of the Am Assoc Cancer Res, May 20–23, 1992, San Diego, California [abstract No. 2367]. Proc Am Assoc Cancer Res 1992;33:396.
70. Katz AE, Olsson CA, Raffo AJ, et al. Molecular staging of prostate cancer with the use of an enhanced reverse transcriptase-PCR assay. Urology 1994;43:765–75.
71. Gao CL, Maheshwar S, Dean RC, et al. Blinded evaluation of reverse transcriptase-polymerase chain reaction prostate-specific antigen peripheral blood assay for molecular staging of prostate cancer. Urology 1999;53:714–21.
72. Ignatoff JM, Oefelein MG, Watkin W, et al. Prostate specific antigen reverse transcriptase-polymerase chain reaction assay in preoperative staging of prostate cancer. J Urol 1997;158:1870–5.
73. Gao CL, Dean RC, Pinto A, et al. Detection of circulating prostate specific antigen expressing prostatic cells in the bone marrow of radical prostatectomy patients by sensitive reverse transcriptase polymerase chain reaction. J Urol 1999;161:1070–6.
74. Haese A, Huland E, Graefen M, et al. Ultrasensitive detection of prostate specific antigen in the followup of 422 patients after radical prostatectomy. J Urol 1999;161:1206–11.
75. Horoszewicz JS, Kawinski E, Murphy GP. Monoclonal antibodies to a new antigenic marker in epithelial prostatic cells and serum of prostatic cancer patients. Anticancer Res 1987;7:927–36.
76. Sweat SD, Pacelli A, Murphy GP, Bostwick DG. Prostate-specific membrane antigen expression is greatest in prostate adenocarcinoma and lymph node metastases. Urology 1998;52:637–40.
77. Silver DA, Pellicer I, Fair WR, et al. Prostate-specific membrane antigen expression in normal and malignant human tissue. Clin Cancer Res 1997;3:81–5.
78. Troyer JK, Becket ML, Wright GLJ. Detection and characterization of prostate-specific membrane antigen (PSMA) in tissue extract and body fluids. Int J Cancer 1995;62:552–8.
79. Liu H, Moy P, Kim S, et al. Monoclonal antibodies to the extracellular domain of prostate-specific membrane antigen also react with tumor vascular endothelium. Cancer Res 1997;57:3629–34.
80. Murphy GP, Barren RJ, Erickson SJ, et al. Evaluation and comparison of two new prostate carcinoma markers. Cancer 1996;78:809–18.
81. Beckett ML, Cazares LH, Vlahou A, et al. Prostate-specific membrane antigen levels in sera from healthy men and patients with benign prostate hyperplasia or prostate cancer. Clin Cancer Res 1999;5:4034–40.
82. Wright GL, Grob BM, Haley C, et al. Up-regulation of prostate-specific membrane antigen after androgen deprivation therapy. Urology 1996;48:326–34.
83. Israili RS, Miller WH, Su SL, et al. Sensitive nested reverse transcription polymerase chain reaction detection of circulating prostatic tumor cells: comparison of prostate-specific membrane antigen and prostate-specific antigen-based assays. Cancer Res 1994;54:6303–10.
84. Sokoloff MH, Tso CL, Kaboo R, et al. Quantitative polymerase chain reaction does not improve preoperative prostate cancer staging: a clinicopathological molecular analysis of 121 patients. J Urol 1996;156:1560–6.
85. Elgamal AA, Holmes EH, Su SL, et al. Prostate-specific membrane antigen (PSMA): current benefits and future value. Semin Surg Oncol 2000;18:10–6.
86. Kahn D, Williams RD, Haseman MK, et al. Radioimmunoscintigraphy with In-111-labeled capromab pendetide predicts prostate cancer response to salvage radiotherapy after failed radical prostatectomy. J Clin Oncol 1998;16:284–9.
87. Bubendorf L, Sauter G, Moch H, et al. Ki67 labeling index: an independent predictor of progression in prostate cancer treated by radical prostatectomy. J Pathol 1996;178:437–41.

88. Bubendorf L, Tapia C, Gasser TC, et al. Ki67 labeling index in core needle biopsies independently predicts tumor-specific survival in prostate cancer. Hum Pathol 1998;29:949–54.
89. Bettencourt MC, Bauer JJ, Sesterhenn IA, et al. Ki-67 expression is a prognostic marker of prostate cancer recurrence after radical prostatectomy. J Urol 1996;156:1064–8.
90. Grossfeld GD, Olumi AF, Connolly JA, et al. Locally recurrent prostate tumors following either radiation therapy or radical prostatectomy have changes in KI-67 labeling index, P53 and BCL-2 immunoreactivity. J Urol 1998; 159:1437–43.
91. Stattin P, Damber JE, Karlberg L, et al. Cell proliferation assessed by Ki-67 immunoreactivity on formalin fixed tissues is a predictive factor for survival in prostate cancer. J Urol 1997;157:219–22.
92. Alberts B, Bray D, Lewis J, et al. Molecular biology of the cell. New York: Garland; 1994.
93. Bauer JJ, Sesterhenn IA, Mostofi FK. Elevated levels of apoptosis regulator proteins p53 and bcl-2 are independent prognostic biomarkers in surgically treated clinically localized prostate cancer. J Urol 1996;156:1511–6.
94. Grignon DJ, Caplan R, Sarkar FH, et al. p53 status and prognosis of locally advanced prostatic carcinoma: a study based on RTOG 8610. J Natl Cancer Inst 1997;89:158–65.
95. Shurbaji MS, Kalbfleisch KH, Thurmond TS. Immunohistochemical detection of p53 protein as a prognostic indicator in prostate cancer. Hum Pathol 1995;26:106–9.
96. Stricker HJ, Kay JK, Linden MD, et al. Determining prognosis of clinically localized prostate cancer by immunohistochemical detection of mutant p53. Urology 1996;47: 366–9.
97. Scherr DS, Vaughan EDJ, Wei J, et al. BCL-2 and p53 expression in clinically localized prostate cancer predicts response to external beam radiotherapy. J Urol 1999;162:12–6.
98. Rogatsch H, Hittmair A, Reissigl A, et al. Microvessel density in core biopsies of prostatic adenocarcinoma: a stage predictor? J Pathol 1997;182:205–10.
99. Wakui S, Furusato M, Itoh T, et al. Tumor angiogenesis in prostate carcinoma with and without bone marrow metastasis: a morphometric study. J Pathol 1992;168:257–62.
100. Fregene T, Khanuja P, Noto AC, et al. Tumor associated angiogenesis in prostate cancer. Anticancer Res 1993;13: 2377–82.
101. Hall MC, Troncoso P, Pollack A, et al. Significance of tumor angiogenesis in clinically localized prostate carcinoma treated with external beam radiotherapy. Urology 1994; 44:869–75.
102. Silbermann MA, Partin AW, Veltri RW, et al. Tumor angiogenesis correlates with progression after radical prostatectomy but not with pathological stage in Gleason sum 5 to 7 adenocarcinoma of the prostate. Cancer 1996;79: 772–9.
103. Rubin MA, Buyyounouski M, Bagiella E, et al. Microvessel density in prostate cancer: lack of correlation with tumor grade, pathologic stage, and clinical outcome. Urology 1999;53:542–7.
104. Chapdelaine P, Paradis G, Tremblay RR, Dube JY. High level of expression in the prostate of a human glandular kallikrein mRNA related to prostate specific antigen. FEBS Lett 1988;236:205–8.
105. Lilja H. A kallikrein-like serine protease in prostatic fluid cleaves the predominant seminal vesicle protein. J Clin Invest 1985;76:1899–903.
106. Darson MF, Pacelli A, Roche P, et al. Human glandular kallikrein 2 (hK2) expression in prostatic intraepithelial neoplasia and adenocarcinoma: a novel prostate cancer marker. Urology 1997;49:857–62.
107. Becker C, Piironen T, Pettersson K, et al. Discrimination of men with prostate cancer from those with benign disease by measurements of human glandular kallikrein 2 (hK2) in serum. J Urol 2000;163:311–6.
108. Partin AW, Catalona WJ, Finlay JA, et al. Use of human glandular kallikrein 2 for the detection of prostate cancer; preliminary analysis. Urology 1999;54:839–45.

8

Detection: Evolving Role of Systematic Biopsy

JOSEPH C. PRESTI JR, MD

Systematic sextant biopsy of the prostate under transrectal ultrasound (TRUS) guidance was introduced just over 10 years ago and revolutionized our ability to detect carcinoma of the prostate (CaP). Prior to systematic sampling, prostate biopsies were usually performed under digital guidance and were directed at palpable nodules. With the introduction of prostate-specific antigen (PSA), detection rates of CaP increased, and many patients with normal digital rectal examinations (DREs), yet elevated PSA levels, were found to have cancer. Such cancers are detected by systematic biopsies and represent the largest growing clinical stage of CaP today (T1c).

As originally described, systematic sextant biopsies are usually performed in the parasagittal line halfway between the lateral border and midline of the prostate on both right and left sides from the base, midgland, and apex (Figure 8–1).[1] This scheme samples the peripheral zone (PZ) of the prostate in which approximately 80% of prostate cancers are felt to originate.[2] The superiority of this biopsy scheme over conventional lesion-directed biopsies is well established. Later, Stamey recommended shifting the biopsies laterally to better sample the anterior horn of the PZ.[3] This important contribution recognized that the needle trajectory of the originally described systematic scheme, while sampling the PZ, also sampled the transition zone (TZ). Lateral direction of these same sextant biopsies would result in a more extensive sampling of the PZ (Figure 8–2).

Several investigators have demonstrated that prostate cancer detection rates are inversely proportional to prostate size. In a referral population undergoing systematic sextant biopsies, one study demonstrated a 23% cancer detection rate in men with prostates ≥ 50 cc in size compared with 38% in men with prostates < 50 cc.[4] In a large prospective study of 1,974 men with a normal DRE and TRUS and an elevated PSA who underwent systematic sextant biopsy, cancer detection rates incrementally decreased with incremental increases in prostate size.[5] These observations prompted many investigators to explore extended systematic biopsy schemes of the prostate. Approaches to investigate biopsy schemes have used one of two approaches: computer modeling of biopsy schemes, or prospective evaluations of different biopsy schemes on referral-based populations.

COMPUTER MODELING SCHEMES

Several investigators have used computer simulations and modeling to better refine systematic biopsy schemes of the prostate. One approach uses step-sectioned radical prostatectomy specimens. Data are obtained from well-mapped specimens,

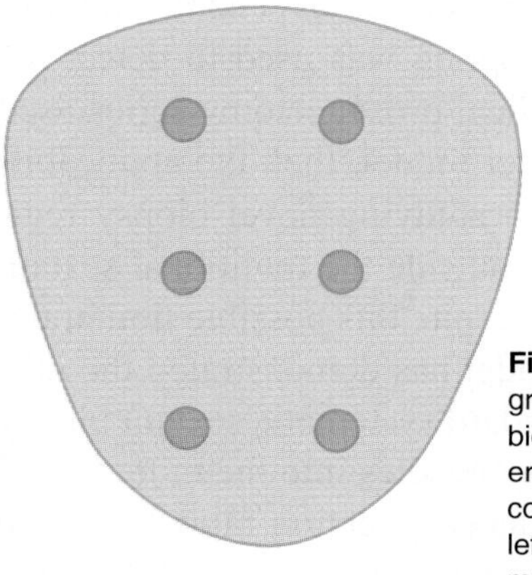

Figure 8–1. Schematic diagram of the standard sextant biopsy scheme of the peripheral zone of the prostate in the coronal plane on the right and left sides at the base (*top*), midgland, and apex (*bottom*).

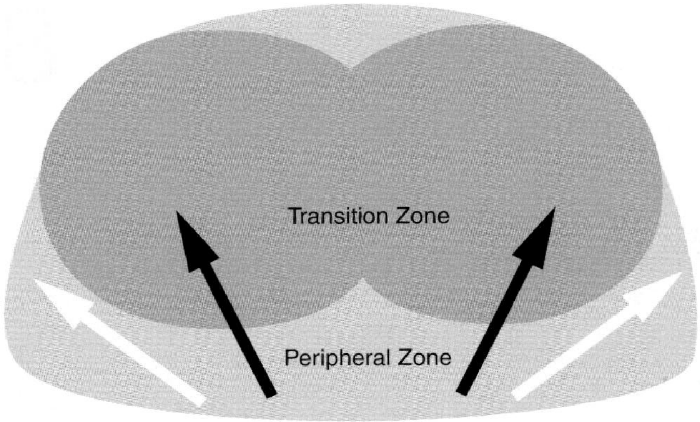

Figure 8–2. Schematic diagram of the prostate in the transverse plane demonstrating the needle trajectory in the standard midlobar plane and in the laterally directed plane. Notice that the laterally directed biopsy (*lighter arrows*) actually samples more of the peripheral zone than the midlobar biopsy (*darker arrows*), which also samples some of the transition zone.

including total prostate volume measurements as well as total tumor volume measurements. Computer-generated prostate models with varying tumor sizes are then created, and systematic sampling is then simulated. Different biopsy schemes can be tested to determine their efficiency for cancer detection. One study demonstrated that systematic sextant biopsies could miss cancers as large as 6 cc.[6] Limitations of simulated models, as described here, include the fact that tumors must typically be simulated as spheres within the prostate, and the differential zonal incidence of carcinoma is often neglected. Additionally, as most data for these models are derived from radical prostatectomy specimens, the means of cancer detection that resulted in a patient undergoing surgery must be acknowledged. In the study mentioned above, cancers were detected by a lesion-directed approach alone. Such models may not be useful in refining cancer detection schemes for T1c lesions. If sextant sampling was used to detect the cancers in a given radical prostatectomy series used to construct a computer model, then the applicability of these models in studying novel biopsy regimens employing sites outside the traditional sextant regions is unknown. Despite this possible limitation, a recent computer model has demonstrated the utility of altering the standard systematic sextant biopsy by directing the biopsy needles into the more lateral aspect of the PZ.[7] Cancer detection rates increased by 23% with this simple manipulation. Additional biopsies resulted in only a modest increase in cancer detection rates (Table 8–1). Another computer model has also demonstrated increasing cancer detection rates by increasing the number of systematic biopsies; however, reported detection rates demonstrate significant variations between series (see Table 8–1).[8]

Another computer-assisted approach involved the retrospective review of 156 consecutive patients diagnosed with T1c prostate cancer.[9] In this model, a computer randomly deleted one of the biopsies from both the right and left lobes and then evaluated the number of cancers that would have been missed if only four biopsies had been obtained. This model demonstrated that between 4 and 19% of the cancers would have been missed if only four rather than six biopsies were performed. One confounding issue that the authors point out is that if a four-biopsy regimen was used, the four sites would most likely not correspond to four of the six sites from the sextant regimen. However, this model also seems to support the concept that the clinically positive biopsy rate may depend in part on the extent of gland sampling.

Recently, one group has attempted to define the number of biopsies required for a given prostate size

Table 8–1. DETECTION RATES IN SEVERAL BIOPSY SERIES

Series	Number of Biopsies	Cancers Detected (%)
Computer modeling schemes		
Bauer et al[7] (N = 201)	6	73
	6 (lateral)	95
	10	99
	14	99
	16	100
Chen et al[8] (N = 180)	4	59
	6	63
	8	65
	13	74
	18	77
Prospectively evaluated schemes		
Eskew et al[10] (N = 48)	6	65
	13	100
Norberg et al[11] (N = 276)	6	85
	8	96
Chang et al[12] (N = 121)	6	82
	10	96
Presti et al[13] (N = 202)	6	80
	8	95
	10	96

N = number of cancers in each series.

and patient age to detect a clinically significant cancer.[4] This complex computer model gives consideration to both tumor and host factors, including an estimate of tumor doubling time of 4 years, and assumes that a tumor volume of 20 cc results in the death of the host. Other assumptions of this model include a spherical tumor size and a random distribution of the tumor throughout the entire volume of the prostate. This model demonstrated that for a given age of patient, the number of biopsies required increases with increasing prostate size. A 55-year-old man with a 20-, 30-, or 40-cc prostate was recommended to undergo 10, 15, and 20 biopsies, respectively. A 60-year-old man with comparable prostate size was recommended to undergo 7, 10, and 13 biopsies, respectively. As described above, this model makes several assumptions; however, the introduction of host factors (age relates to life expectancy) is novel.

PROSPECTIVELY EVALUATED SCHEMES

Over the past 5 years, several investigators have prospectively evaluated new systematic biopsy regimens in referral-based populations. One group studied a five-region technique of systematic biopsy in a series of 119 patients.[10] The five regions included the standard sextant biopsy regimen obtained halfway between the lateral border and midline of the prostate on both the right and left sides (regions 2 and 4) but also obtained two biopsies from each lateral aspect of the prostate (regions 1 and 5) and three biopsies from the midline at the apex, midgland, and base (region 3). Of the 119 patients, 48 (40%) had cancer on the biopsy, of which 17 (35% of cancers detected) were detected only in regions 1, 3, and 5. Of note, only 2 cancers were detected by the three centrally placed biopsies of region 3. With respect to complications, these investigators reported an 80% incidence of gross hematuria, which they attributed to the region 3 biopsies, which probably penetrated the urethra (see Table 8–1).

Another group prospectively evaluated an 8- or 10-biopsy regimen depending on gland size in 512 patients.[11] In this protocol, all patients underwent 8 biopsies of the PZ, 4 from each lobe at the apex, midgland, base, and lateral midgland. When prostate length exceeded 4 cm, 2 additional biopsies were obtained from the TZ. When comparing the standard sextant biopsy regimen with the extended biopsy regimen, overall cancer detection rates increased from 85 to 97%. If lesion-directed biopsies had been added to the standard sextant biopsy regimen, then cancer detection rates would have increased to 93% (see Table 8–1).

Another approach taken by one group has been to investigate the utility of performing two consecutive sets of sextant biopsies of the prostate in a single office visit in 137 consecutive patients in a referral-based population.[15] A total of 43 cancers were detected in the entire study population (31% cancer detection rate). Using the first sextant biopsy set as the reference set, 30 cancers were detected (70% of all cancers), so the second biopsy set increased the detection rate by 30%. However, if the second biopsy set had been used as the reference, 40 cancers were detected (93% of all cancers), whereas the first biopsy set would have increased the detection rate only by 7%. The benefit of this type of approach needs further study with a larger patient cohort as two sextant samplings, presumably from similar locations, resulted in a large disparity in detection rates (70% versus 93%).

Since the majority of carcinomas arise in the PZ, it seemed logical that systematic biopsies should focus on better sampling of this zone. Stamey had suggested moving the standard sextant biopsies more laterally to better sample the anterior extension of the PZ.[3] The work of Eskew and colleagues[10] and Norberg and colleagues,[15] as well as the report by Stamey, prompted us to prospectively evaluate the utility of adding four lateral biopsies of the PZ to the routine sextant biopsy regimen (Figure 8–3). A total of 273 consecutive patients referred for an abnormal DRE and/or PSA ≥ 4.0 ng/mL underwent TRUS and systematic biopsies along with lesion-directed biopsies.[12] Sextant biopsies were obtained in the midlobar parasagittal plane, halfway between the lateral edge and midline of the prostate gland, at the base, midgland, and apex. The lateral PZ biopsies were performed by positioning the probe just medial to the lateral edge of the prostate. The lateral PZ biopsies were obtained at the midgland and base only as apical biopsies are, in fact, lateral as the prostate narrows in this area. Forty-four percent of the patients had cancer on biopsy (121/273). Whereas the routine sextant biopsies detected 82% of the cancers, the lateral PZ biopsies detected 77% (17/22) of the missed cancers. Lateral PZ biopsies increased cancer detection rates by 14% (see Table 8–1). In the subset of the 147 patients with lesions on TRUS imaging, cancer was found in 50% (74/147); routine sextant biopsies detected 76% of the cancers (56/74), whereas the lateral PZ biopsies detected 80% (59/74). This finding is striking when considering that this comparison is between a 4-biopsy (lateral biopsy) and a 6-biopsy regimen (sextant biopsy). Fifteen of these 74 patients (20%) had positive lateral PZ biopsies with negative sextant biopsies. Lesion-directed biopsies uniquely identified only 1 cancer. Our conclusion from this study was that the performance of 10 biopsies of the PZ increased cancer detection rates by 14% and nearly eliminated the need for lesion-directed biopsies, thus minimizing the operator dependence of the TRUS examination.

We recently completed a prospective evaluation of 483 consecutive patients in an attempt to define the optimal systematic biopsy regimen.[13] Prior to biopsy, a thorough TRUS examination was performed. Then, using a spinal needle, approximately 5 cc of 1% lidocaine were infiltrated into each of the periprostatic neurovascular bundles at the right and left base of the gland under TRUS guidance. All identified hypoechoic lesions were first biopsied prior to obtaining systematic biopsies. Sextant biopsies were obtained in the midlobar parasagittal plane,

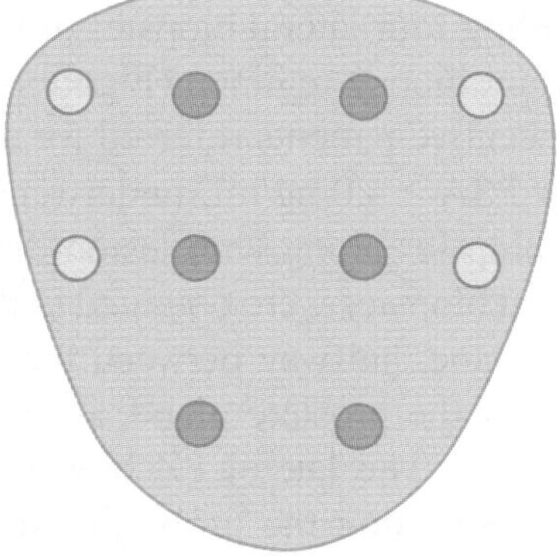

Figure 8–3. Schematic diagram of the 10-biopsy scheme of the peripheral zone of the prostate in the coronal plane using the standard sextant scheme (*dark circles*) and additional biopsies obtained from the lateral aspect of the peripheral zone at the base and mid gland (*open circles*).

halfway between the lateral edge and midline of the prostate gland, at the base, midgland, and apex. The lateral biopsies were performed by positioning the probe just medial to the lateral edge of the prostate at the mid and base portions of the gland. Patients with prostate sizes exceeding 50 cc also underwent systematic sextant TZ biopsies in the midlobar parasagittal plane. The needle was advanced to within 1.5 cm of the anterior prostate capsule prior to firing the biopsy gun. Procedures were well tolerated without the need for intravenous sedation. Forty-two percent of the patients had cancer on biopsy (202/483). Routine sextant biopsies detected 161 cancers (80% of all cancers detected), whereas the combination of sextant and lateral biopsies, for a total of 10 PZ biopsies, detected 194 cancers (96% of all cancers detected). The 8 missed cancers were detected by the lesion-directed (n = 5) or the TZ biopsies (n = 3). We noted several important results from this study: (1) traditional sextant biopsies may miss over 20% of cancers; (2) a lateral sextant regimen (apex, lateral mid, lateral base) outperforms the traditional midlobar sextant regimen (88.6% versus 79.7%, respectively; $p = .027$); (3) regardless of the number of systematic biopsies performed (6 versus 8 versus 10), variations in cancer detection rates were most pronounced in patients with PSA levels < 10 ng/mL or in patients with prostate sizes ≥ 50 cc, reflecting the importance of sampling as patients with lower PSA levels or larger prostates more commonly may have smaller cancer volumes per unit of prostate tissue; and (4) when comparing the detection rates of the five systematic PZ regions in the 10-biopsy scheme, the midlobar base region demonstrated the lowest detection rate and the lowest unique cancer detection rate. From the latter observation, we felt that the midlobar base biopsy could be omitted from the systematic biopsy scheme. The low yield from this site might be because this biopsy site may, in part, be sampling the central zone, where the incidence of cancer is low (Figure 8–4). In this study, we only crudely addressed prostate size (< 50 cc versus ≥ 50 cc), and future work is needed to more carefully address variations in prostate configuration.

Approximately 25 to 30% of prostate cancers originate in the TZ of the prostate.[16] Appropriate indications for TZ biopsies remain an area of debate.

One retrospective series demonstrated a low unique cancer detection rate in TZ biopsies when performed in all patients (TZ biopsy was the only site of positive biopsy in 2% of patients with cancer).[17] A prospective evaluation of the performance of two TZ biopsies in all patients was performed by one group and also demonstrated a low unique cancer detection rate for the TZ biopsies. For all patients, TZ biopsies were the only positive site in 8 of 279 cancers (2.9%), and if considering only patients with a normal DRE, TZ biopsies were the unique site of cancer in 6 of 145 (4.1%) cancers.[18] As the prostate enlarges, preferential zonal growth tends to occur in the TZ. We thus felt it important to control for prostate size in determining the need for TZ biopsies. Recently, we prospectively evaluated 213 consecutive patients from a referral-based population who had calculated prostate sizes greater than 50 cc.[19] All patients underwent the conventional sextant biopsies of the PZ as well as additional sextant biopsies of the TZ, for a total of 12 biopsies. The PZ biopsy specimens were obtained in the parasagittal plane midway between the lateral border and the midline of the gland. Three specimens were obtained from each lobe at the apex, midportion, and base of the gland. The TZ biopsies were obtained just lateral to midline, and the needles were advanced into the gland to approximately 1.5 cm from the anterior capsule prior to firing the gun to minimize sampling of the PZ. Three cores were obtained from each side at the apex, midportion, and base of the prostate. Fifty-five cases of carcinoma were found, for a 26% detection rate. The TZ biopsies detected cancer in 30 of the 55 patients (55%) compared with the 47 patients in whom cancer was detected by the PZ biopsies (85%). Seven cancers (13% of cancers) were detected only by the additional TZ biopsies. Subsequently, an additional prospective evaluation of TZ biopsies has been reported.[20] This study obtained two biopsies of the TZ and did not control for prostate size. Seven of 151 (5%) of the cancers were detected only by the TZ biopsies. The results were stratified for race; however, no racial differences were observed in the yield of TZ biopsies.

Most investigators agree that TZ biopsies are indicated in patients with a high suspicion of prostate cancer who have had negative prior systematic biopsies. One retrospective series demonstrated that in this scenario, 9 of 47 patients with cancer (19%) demonstrated cancer only in the TZ biopsies.[21] Other investigators have retrospectively demonstrated similar detection rates in this population, specifically 8 of 58 patients with cancer (14%) in one series and 2 of 19 patients with cancer (10%) in another series.[22,23]

As the number of biopsy cores in a systematic biopsy scheme has increased, the question of patient tolerance in the clinic setting has needed to be addressed. Two major types of local anesthesia have been described: a periprostatic block using a lidocaine injection or intrarectal lidocaine jelly. In the former, a spinal needle is placed under transrectal ultrasound guidance adjacent to the vascular pedicles at the base of the prostate and a 1% lidocaine solution is injected. In the latter, a 2% lidocaine jelly is instilled into the rectum prior to the ultrasound probe. Several investigators have reported on these methods in randomized, placebo-controlled trials. With respect to lidocaine jelly, no statistical differ-

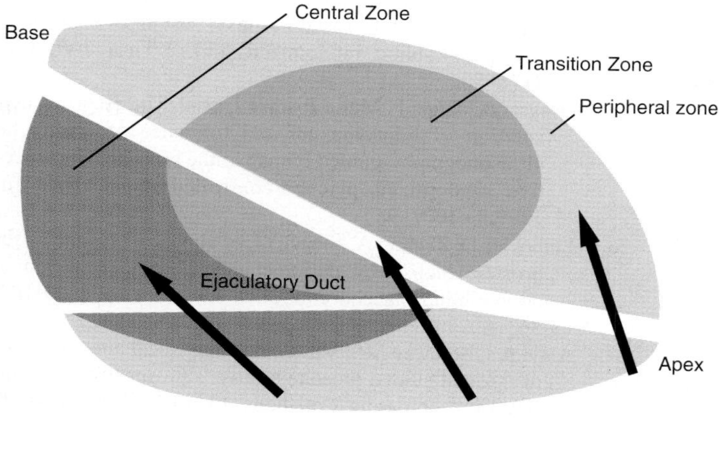

Figure 8–4. Schematic diagram of the prostate in the sagittal plane demonstrating the needle trajectory in the standard midlobar plane. Notice that the standard midlobar base biopsy also samples the central zone, perhaps contributing to its lower cancer detection rate.

ence was observed in pain relief between the placebo groups and the lidocaine groups in two studies.[24,25] A randomized, placebo-controlled study using a lidocaine block demonstrated a significant reduction in pain in the patients receiving lidocaine.[26] A randomized trial between these methods has been completed, and superior pain relief was reported in the patients receiving the lidocaine block compared to the group receiving lidocaine jelly.[27]

CONCLUSIONS

Systematic biopsy of the prostate has been part of urologic practice for just over 10 years. However, recent work suggests that 6 biopsies are probably not adequate for all prostates. An 8- or 10-biopsy regimen appears superior to a 6-biopsy regimen and should replace the standard sextant biopsy scheme. It is quite likely that the number of systematic biopsies should be directly related to prostate size. Laterally directed PZ biopsies appear to increase the efficiency of prostate sampling. Additional work is needed to better determine the optimal location and number of such biopsy schemes for a given prostate size and PSA level.

REFERENCES

1. Hodge KK, McNeal JE, Terris MK, Stamey TA. Random systematic versus directed ultrasound guided transrectal core biopsies of the prostate. J Urol 1989;142:71–5.
2. McNeal JE, Redwine EA, Freiha FS, Stamey TA. Zonal distribution of prostatic adenocarcinoma: correlation with histologic pattern and direction of spread. Am J Surg Pathol 1988;12:897–906.
3. Stamey TA. Making the most out of six systematic sextant biopsies. Urology 1995;45:2–12.
4. Uzzo RG, Wei JT, Waldbaum RS, et al. The influence of prostate size on cancer detection. Urology 1995;46:831–6.
5. Karakiewicz PI, Bazinet M, Aprikian AG, et al. Outcome of sextant biopsy according to gland volume. Urology 1997;49:55–9.
6. Daneshgari F, Taylor GD, Miller GJ, Crawford D. Computer simulation of the probability of detecting low volume carcinoma of the prostate with six random systematic core biopsies. Urology 1995;45:604–9.
7. Bauer JJ, Zeng J, Weir J, et al. Three-dimensional computer-simulated prostate models: lateral prostate biopsies increase the detection rate of prostate cancer. Urology 1999;53:961–7.
8. Chen ME, Troncoso P, Tang K, et al. Comparison of prostate biopsy schemes by computer simulation. Urology 1999; 53:951–60.
9. Karakiewicz PI, Aprikian AG, Meshref AW, Bazinet M. Computer-assisted comparative analysis of four-sector and six-sector biopsies of the prostate. Urology 1996;48:747–50.
10. Eskew LA, Bare RL, McCullough DL. Systematic 5 region prostate biopsy is superior to sextant method for diagnosing carcinoma of the prostate. J Urol 1997;157:199–203.
11. Norberg M, Egevad L, Holmberg L, et al. The sextant protocol for ultrasound-guided core biopsies of the prostate underestimates the presence of cancer. Urology 1997;50:562–6.
12. Chang JJ, Shinohara K, Bhargava V, Presti JC Jr. Prospective evaluation of lateral biopsies of the peripheral zone for prostate cancer detection. J Urol 1998;160:2111–4.
13. Presti JC Jr, Chang JJ, Bhargava V, Shinohara K. The optimal systematic prostate biopsy scheme should include eight rather than six biopsies—results of a prospective clinical trial. J Urol 2000;163:163–6.
14. Vashi AR, Wojno KJ, Gillespie B, Oesterling JE. A model for the number of cores per prostate biopsy based on patient age and prostate gland volume. J Urol 1998;159:920–4.
15. Levine MA, Ittman M, Melamed J, Lepor H. Two consecutive sets of transrectal ultrasound guided sextant biopsies of the prostate for the detection of prostate cancer. J Urol 1998;159:471–6.
16. McNeal JE, Villers AA, Redwine EA, et al. Capsular penetration in prostate cancer: significance for natural history and treatment. Am J Surg Pathol 1990;14:240–7.
17. Terris MK, Pham TQ, Issa MM, Kabalin JN. Routine transition zone and seminal vesicle biopsies in all patients undergoing transrectal ultrasound guided prostate biopsies are not indicated. J Urol 1997;157:204–6.
18. Bazinet M, Karakiewicz PI, Aprikian AG, et al. Value of systematic transition zone biopsies in the early detection of prostate cancer. J Urol 1996;155:605–6.
19. Chang JJ, Shinohara K, Hovey RM, et al. Prospective evaluation of systematic sextant transition zone biopsies in large prostates for cancer detection Urology 1998;52:89–93.
20. Fowler JE Jr, Bigler SA, Kilambi NK, Land SA. Results of transition zone biopsy in Black and White men with suspected prostate cancer. Urology 1999;53:346–50.
21. Lui PD, Terris MK, McNeal JE, Stamey TA. Indications for ultrasound guided transition zone biopsies in the detection of prostate cancer. J Urol 1995;153:1000–3.
22. Keetch DW, Catalona WJ. Prostatic transition zone biopsies in men with previous negative biopsies and persistently elevated serum prostate specific antigen values. J Urol 1995;154:1795–7.
23. Fleshner NE, Fair WR. Indications for transition zone biopsy in the detection of prostatic carcinoma. J Urol 1997;157: 556–8.
24. Chang SS, Alberts G, Wells N, et al. Intrarectal lidocaine during transrectal prostate biopsy: results of a prospective double-blind randomized trial. J Urol 2001;166: 2178–80.
25. Desgrandchamps F, Meria P, Irani J, et al. The rectal administration of lidocaine gel and tolerance of transrectal ultrasonography-guided biopsy of the prostate: a prospective randomized placebo-controlled study. BJU Int 1999;83:1007–9.
26. Leibovici D, Zisman A, Siegel YI, et al. Local anesthesia for prostate biopsy by periprostatic lidocaine injection: a double-blind placebo controlled study. J Urol 2002;167: 563–5.
27. Alavi AS, Soloway MS, Vaidya A, et al. Local anesthesia for ultrasound guided prostate biopsy: a prospective randomized trial comparing 2 methods. J Urol 2001;166:1343–5.

9

Imaging

MAYA D. MEUX, MD
MICHAEL B. GOTWAY, MD
FERGUS V. COAKLEY, MD

Prostate cancer (adenocarcinoma) is the most common noncutaneous malignancy in American men.[1,2] For the year 2000, the number of new cases of prostate cancer in the United States is estimated to be 180,400, with 31,900 expected deaths.[3] The rapid rise in the number of prostate cancer diagnoses in the 1990s may be attributed to the increasing age of the population and early diagnosis with the measurement of serum prostate-specific antigen (PSA).[4]

The clinical management of prostate cancer continues to be controversial, with no consensus on the need for cancer screening, choice of diagnostic tests for pretreatment evaluation, and the need for and appropriateness of treatment for any stage of disease. Controversies in management can be attributed to several unique biologic features of the disease. Some prostate cancers may not lead to serious morbidity or death. Autopsy studies have shown that 30 to 40% of men older than age 50 have microscopic prostate cancer, yet less than 20% of men develop clinical prostate cancer in their lifetime. Unlike many other cancers such as lung, breast, colon, or ovarian, which behave aggressively and are more rapidly and uniformly fatal if untreated, prostate cancer behaves in a less predictable fashion. Some cancers are small, well differentiated, and unlikely to cause clinically significant disease, whereas others are large, poorly differentiated, and likely metastasize, causing death. Although a number of tumor prognostic factors, including serum PSA, tumor grade, and tumor stage, can generally predict disease at either end of the spectrum, most cancers fall into an intermediate range, where it is difficult to distinguish those cancers likely to progress from those that can be observed.[5]

The diagnosis and evaluation of prostate cancer have great potential impact on patient care and economics in the United States, underscoring the importance of a critical assessment of the currently employed staging modalities.[6] The successful treatment of patients with newly diagnosed prostate cancer is dependent on the early diagnosis and the ability to monitor the progression and regression of malignancy. The presence of cancer outside the confines of the prostate either by extracapsular extension (ECE) or seminal vesicle invasion (SVI) often results in treatment failure following radical prostatectomy or radiation therapy. Extracapsular extension is known to occur in 27 to 60% of patients undergoing radical prostatectomy when careful step-sectioning techniques are used to examine the surgical specimen. Such patients may still benefit from radical prostatectomy if the ECE is focal, the tumor is of low to moderate grade, and negative surgical margins are achieved. For example, if ECE can accurately be identified preoperatively, surgeons may elect to widely excise the ipsilateral neurovascular bundle to increase the likelihood of attaining negative surgical margins.[7]

Prostate cancer is usually suspected because of an abnormal digital rectal examination (DRE) or elevated serum PSA. American Cancer Society recommendations for annual prostate cancer screening include DRE and serum PSA testing for men 50 years of age or older or for younger men with risk factors for the disease, including black race or family history. To date, imaging has not proven useful in screening for prostate cancer. Transrectal ultrasound (TRUS)-guided sextant or extended pattern core biopsies of the prostate are recommended to maximize the diagnostic yield of biopsy and to allow estimation of tumor grade and volume.[5,8] Biopsy results may provide a great deal of information for risk assessment before radical prostatectomy or radiation therapy.

However, imaging does play an important role in the diagnosis of the disease. For example, TRUS assists in the diagnosis by guiding biopsies of the prostate gland in patients with an abnormal DRE or serum PSA level. Imaging may also play a role in prostate cancer staging. Magnetic resonance imaging (MRI) may help to assess more accurately the local extent of disease, and computed tomography (CT) and bone scintigraphy (bone scan) are valuable techniques for assessing distant spread of disease.[5] Since optimal decision making regarding treatment depends on accurate tumor staging prior to treatment,[9] the accurate localization of cancer within the prostate gland is becoming increasingly important. Such a determinate, if accurate, may influence the choice of treatment, surgical and radiation treatment planning, and possibly the extent and localization of focal therapy.[10] The purpose of this chapter is to describe the role of imaging in the detection and staging of prostate carcinoma.

TRANSRECTAL ULTRASONOGRAPHY

Clinical staging of prostate cancer has traditionally relied on DRE, bone scan, and CT of the abdomen and pelvis. The advent of TRUS of the prostate in the mid-1980s added an office-based imaging modality to the evaluation of patients at risk for cancer.[11] Transrectal ultrasonography produces high-resolution images of the prostate by placing a high-frequency (5 to 7.5 MHz) endorectal transducer in close proximity to the prostate. The imaging protocol for TRUS should include assessment of the prostate gland (Figure 9–1) and seminal vesicles in both the sagittal and axial planes. This allows for accurate estimation of gland volume using the prolate ellipse formula ($0.5 \times D1 \times D2 \times D3$), with dimensions obtained in the axial, anteroposterior, and sagittal planes. The weight of the prostate in grams is essentially equal to prostate volume as the specific gravity of prostate tissue is approximately 1.0.[5]

The normal prostate of the young adult male is composed of homogeneous, low-level echoes on ultrasonographic examination. The central and peripheral zones (both in the peripheral gland) comprise the bulk of the normal prostate in such patients. Both are uniformly hyperechoic, with no distinct boundaries that allow for differentiation between these zones on TRUS. The transition zone lies in the midline of the normal prostate (central gland) and is less echogenic than the surrounding tissue. In younger patients without benign prostatic hyperplasia (BPH), the transition zone is small and inconspicuous. Bright linear echoes that appear to represent a fibrous capsule define the margin of the normal prostate. This margin is distinct from the periprostatic fascia, which surrounds the gland. Young adults do not demonstrate well-defined central glandular anatomy until the end of the fourth decade, after which BPH begins to develop in the transition zone in the majority of men. With aging, the transition zone (central gland) enlarges and becomes the dominant part of the gland. In men with BPH, the central gland typically appears as hypoechoic when compared with the peripheral portions of the gland and may be identified as a clearly defined,

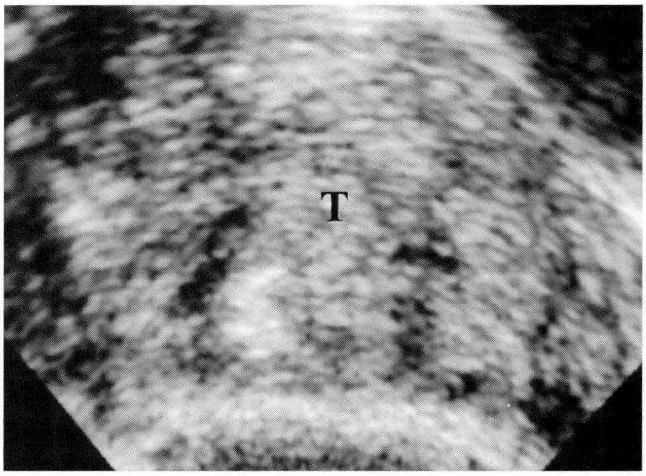

Figure 9–1. Normal prostate gland on transrectal ultrasonography. Transaxial ultrasonographic image obtained through the prostate gland at the level of the midgland. The transition zone (*T*) is heterogeneous in echotexture and contains an echogenic focus compatible with calcification.

well-demarcated area on TRUS. Benign prostatic hypertrophy has a variable ultrasonographic appearance, which can make differentiation from other processes including cancer or prostatitis difficult.[12]

The appearance of prostate cancer on ultrasonography may vary depending on lesion size, location, and transducer specifications. To differentiate benign from malignant tissue, the comparison of symmetry, echotexture, and echogenicity may be useful. The most common ultrasonographic appearance of prostate cancer is a hypoechoic peripheral zone lesion (60 to 70%) (Figure 9–2). Hypoechoic areas have a 17 to 57% chance of being malignant.[13] The normal echogenic pattern of the prostate is generated by the interface between the prostatic stroma and fluid-filled acini. The hypoechoic appearance of cancer is attributed to the relative decrease in the number of acinar stromal interfaces. Tiguret and colleagues and Shinohara and colleagues found that high-grade tumors were more hypoechoic, presumably owing to the progressive loss of glandular elements and acoustic interfaces.[11,14] This finding was supported by Lee and colleagues,[15] who reported that a hypoechoic lesion carries a high risk for cancer and that biopsy is indicated even for the smallest lesions. This group also found that the size of the hypoechoic lesions was related to risk for cancer, with a large lesion more likely to be malignant than a small one. The positive predictive value for hypoechoic lesions was found to increase in the face of a positive DRE and an elevated PSA (> 2.6 ng/mL). The finding of a hypoechoic lesion on TRUS is not specific for cancer, however, as benign processes, such as prostatitis, frequently appear hypoechoic. Up to 40% of lesions are isoechoic and are therefore not detected on ultrasonography. Hyperechoic lesions are rare, representing 1 to 5% of lesions.[5]

Transrectal ultrasonography has its limitations since the interpretation of images is dependent on the expertise of the user and restricted by the limitations of visual perception.[13] A relative lack of sensitivity and specificity and the low positive predictive value of gray-scale ultrasonography of 18 to 52% have limited the role of TRUS in screening for prostate cancer.[5,16,17]

The reported staging accuracy of TRUS varies widely in published reports, ranging from 46 to 66%,

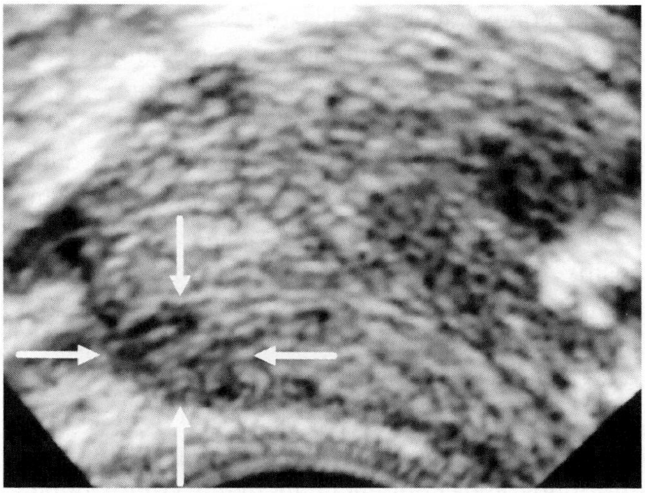

Figure 9–2. Prostate carcinoma on transrectal ultrasonography. Transaxial ultrasonographic image obtained at the level of the right midgand demostrates a hypoechoic focus in the peripheral zone (*arrows*). No capsular bulge is identified.

and a recent study funded by the National Institutes of Health compared TRUS with DRE for the determination of the local extent of prostate cancer in 386 patients and found no significant difference. Factors that influence the staging accuracy of TRUS include its operator-dependent nature,[6,11] tumor characteristics, and criteria for pathologic correlation. The importance of tumor characteristics is highlighted by the findings of a study involving 343 men who underwent TRUS before radical prostatectomy.[3] In that study, nearly 40% of cancers detected pathologically were not identified by TRUS. Lack of identification makes staging of these lesions using TRUS impossible. That less than 60% of lesions will have a classic hypoechoic pattern (see Figure 9–2) adds to a decreased sensitivity in lesions detected by TRUS.

Rorvik and colleagues found that using a 7-mHz transducer, understaging and overstaging were 32% and 37%, respectively.[16] These authors concluded that TRUS was an unreliable tool in the staging protocol prior to radical prostatectomy. The overall sensitivity, specificity, and positive and negative predictive values for detection of ECE were found to be 0.68, 0.63, 0.85, and 0.38, respectively, in the same study. A relative lack of sensitivity and specificity has limited the role of TRUS in screening for prostate cancer.[16,17]

For recognized hypoechoic lesions, recent investigators have described a new ultrasound staging criterion, contact length. This refers to the extent of contact between the tumor and the fibromuscular capsule of the prostate. Receiver operating characteristic curves based on data from 95 men with hypoechoic lesions determined that the best cutoff value for contact length was 23.0 mm, resulting in a sensitivity for ECE of 65%, a specificity of 88%, a positive predictive value of 83%, and an overall accuracy of 77% compared with 30%, 88%, 70%, and 60%, respectively, for conventional extraprostatic extension criteria.[6]

Since the introduction of TRUS in clinical practice, there have been progressive improvements in ultrasonography equipment, including color Doppler, which has enhanced the ability to identify prostatic lesions.[11,18] However, recent evidence has suggested that systematic sextant biopsies plus two lateral biopsies of the prostate have the same cancer yield as lesion-directed biopsies using state-of-the-art equipment.[11] Therefore, many urologists use TRUS to guide systematic biopsy rather than to guide biopsy of suspicious lesions selectively. However, Tiguert and colleagues, in a retrospective study, found that patients who had the pure definition of clinical T1c cancer, that is, a normal DRE and TRUS with abnormal PSA, had a significantly better pathologic stage and improved disease-free survival compared with those with abnormal DRE or abnormal TRUS, possibly supporting the use of ultrasonographic findings in risk assessment of prostate cancer.[11]

One potential way to improve the diagnosis of prostate cancer using ultrasonography is by addition of Doppler technology. In addition to traditional grayscale imaging, ultrasonography may be used to estimate the velocity of moving particles in the ultrasound beam using the Doppler principle, a technique of measuring frequency shifts caused by movement, named after the physicist Christian Johann Doppler. This technique was first reported in 1959, and it has developed into a well-accepted clinical tool.[13] Blood flow can be detected either by pulsed-wave Doppler (which displays the frequency shift or velocity as spectral waves) or color Doppler imaging, also known as color-flow imaging. Color-flow imaging provides a two-dimensional, cross-sectional, real-time, color-coded Doppler shift that is superimposed on the real-time, gray-scale, anatomic display. It displays the range of the mean frequency shift or velocities of red blood cells within flowing blood as colors of the spectrum.[3] This technique enables the user to examine local changes in tissue blood supply and vascularization. Because tumor growth appears to depend on neovascularization, it is assumed that malignant tissue in the prostate, or any other organ, has increased blood perfusion compared with nonmalignant tissue. Evaluating blood flow measurements in areas suspicious for prostatic malignancy may increase the sensitivity of TRUS of the prostate.[13]

Normally, the prostate gland should demonstrate symmetric, low-to-absent color-flow signal intensity, with the periurethral area exhibiting some flow and the outer gland showing minimal to no flow.[3,19] Several studies have demonstrated that malignant prostate tissue can sometimes be associated with abnormal vascular patterns.[20–22] Detection of these abnormal blood flow patterns within prostatic tumors is the main application of Doppler ultrasonography in prostate cancer imaging. To date, clinical results have varied. Louvar and colleagues confirmed significantly higher mean Gleason scores for cancers with increased color Doppler flow, compared with lesions demonstrating normal blood flow.[18] Kelly and colleagues reported a sensitivity of 96% for TRUS alone and 87% for color Doppler imaging. The addition of color Doppler imaging increased the positive predictive value from 0.53 to 0.77, but at a cost of reduced sensitivity. Color Doppler imaging suggested the diagnosis of malignancy independently of TRUS in only 1 of 158 cases. The authors concluded that color Doppler imaging improves the positive predictive value but has no demonstrable value over TRUS alone in the diagnosis of prostate cancer.[3] Rifkin and colleagues demonstrated abnormal Doppler flow in 9 of 132 cancers (7%) that had no identifiable gray-scale abnormality.[19] Newman and colleagues correlated color Doppler imaging results with the histologic findings from site-specific transrectal core biopsies and demonstrated that color Doppler imaging had a sensitivity of 49%, a specificity of 93%, and a positive predictive value of 62%.[23] Additionally, at least one focus of carcinoma was found in seven patients with no gray-scale abnormality.

The prognostic significance of detecting increased flow within a tumor has also been investigated. Tumor-associated angiogenesis, measured as vascular density, has been shown to give prognostic information in a variety of solid tumors, including prostate cancer.[20] Several studies have suggested that the degree of tumor vascularization may correlate with its potential for rapid growth and distant metastases, although, overall, the results have been mixed.[21,22] Ismail and colleagues have demonstrated that color Doppler flow within prostate cancer correlates with both tumor grade and stage and that increased flow is associated with a higher Gleason score, higher incidence of SVI, and increased risk of relapse.[24]

Early results when comparing gray-scale ultrasonography to color Doppler imaging have been disappointing. Unfortunately, one drawback to Doppler ultrasonography is the difficulty in demonstrating slow blood flow in small vessels owing to limited spatial resolution.[13,25] There are also problems in detection of low volume flow because slow movement results in frequency shifts below the noise level that are not detected.[3,13] Thus, one reason behind the difficulty in identifying prostatic tumor sites by color Doppler ultrasonography may be the relationship between vascularity and tumor size, with no vascularity noted in small lesions (< 2 mm) or large lesions, secondary to central necrosis. To combat the problem of slow flow, "power" Doppler imaging has been investigated as a modality with which to detect cancer in the prostate gland with greater sensitivity. The main advantage of power Doppler is the ability to detect slower flow with less reliance on Doppler angle. To date, it remains to be seen whether this type of imaging will significantly improve sensitivity in the detection of prostate cancer.

A relatively new method of Doppler imaging includes the use of a contrast agent, in the form of microbubbles. The amplitude of the detected Doppler signal is directly related to the number of moving particles. Because air bubbles in ultrasound contrast agents are restricted to the blood vessels, only the vessel is imaged.[13,26] This may provide important additional dynamic information to quantify vascular blood flow, although the spread of microbubbles throughout the body leads to an unknown concentration at the site of interest.[13] Unfortunately, the microbubble agents will not necessarily provide improved tissue specificity.[27] Further investigation in this technique with regard to prostate cancer is needed.

Conventional TRUS uses two-dimensional imaging to visualize three-dimensional anatomy and disease processes. Any technique that could overcome this spatial limitation would likely result in improved staging of disease.[28] Garg and colleagues and Seghal and colleagues used digitized TRUS information and computer postprocessing to determine the volume of the prostate gland and noted that the technique was more accurate and faster than planimetric methods.[28,29] Garg and colleagues found that visualization of a lesion in three planes allowed improved assessment of capsular disruption. For detection of extracapsular tumor extension, sensitivity with this method was 80%, specificity 96%, positive predictive value 90%, and negative predictive value 96%. Overall staging accuracy was 94%.[28] An important caveat in the interpretation of three-dimensional images is that vascular areas that lie just outside the prostate can imperceptibly merge with visible areas of cancer, which can lead to an erroneous impression of ECE. The static nature of three-dimensional ultrasonography makes this distinction more difficult. Careful study of real-time two-dimensional Doppler ultrasonographic images should prevent this error by identifying features such as blood flow and pulsation.[28]

Transrectal ultrasonography is a useful test to identify local disease recurrence following radical prostatectomy (RP). Detection of recurrent disease rises significantly with serum PSA levels.[30,31] The normal anatomy after RP as demonstrated by TRUS has been defined.[30,32] Tissue at the bladder neck can often be seen as a hyperechoic, homogeneous, well-marginated ring as a result of the vesicuourethral anastomosis. In 50% of patients, a hyperechoic tissue mass can also be visualized anterior to the bladder neck, representing pulled-down bladder tissue at the time of the anastomosis. Recurrent disease after RP is usually visualized as a hypoechoic mass in the region of the anastomosis.[32,33] Up to 30% of tumor recurrences, however, may be isoechoic and therefore more difficult to detect by TRUS.

Identifying tumor recurrence by TRUS after primary radiation therapy and cryosurgery has been more problematic. The fibrosis caused by radiation therapy distorts normal tissue planes and creates a small, more hyperechoic gland on ultrasonography. The sensitivity of TRUS following radiation therapy to detect persistent or recurrent disease is only around 50%.[30,32,33] Transrectal ultrasonography does, however, remain useful for guiding biopsies following radiation therapy. Following cryosurgery, the prostate appears more ill-defined owing to cell death from the freezing process. Areas suspicious for recurrence can be visualized as hypoechoic lesions.[32]

MAGNETIC RESONANCE IMAGING

Like TRUS, MRI currently has no established role as a screening modality in prostate cancer detection.[5] Magnetic resonance imaging has been available for use as a staging modality for prostate cancer since 1984. Although the role of MRI for preoperative staging in the radiology literature is still debated, many radiologists consider MRI the best local staging modality currently available.[4,34] However, the use of MRI to select patients with prostate cancer for curative therapy is justified only if implementation of MRI will improve patient outcome and if there is a real justification on the basis of cost, risk, and benefit.[4] Currently, urologists do not routinely use MRI in staging, with only 10% of US urologists reporting its use.[4,35,36]

The advantage of MRI over other imaging modalities is the capability of visualizing zonal anatomy of the prostate gland (Figure 9–3). Magnetic resonance imaging has a potential for further improvements in image quality using equipment with higher field strengths, different coil designs, and new pulse sequences.[14] Owing to its high spatial and contrast resolution, MRI does have potential as a local staging modality. The development of endorectal surface coils has enabled performance of high-resolution MRI[37,38] and has allowed application of localized three-dimensional proton MR spectroscopic imaging to the evaluation of the prostate gland,[39] in a clinically reasonable period of time.

Recent improvements in MRI include the use of combined endorectal and phased array coils for signal reception, analytic image correction, faster imaging sequences, a better understanding of morphologic criteria used to diagnose extraprostatic disease, and increased reader experience.[34,40,41] The use of the body coil for excitation and a combined endorectal coil and pelvic phased array coil for reception allows the acquisition of MRI and MR spectroscopic imaging data from the prostate with a higher spatial resolution than is otherwise possible using a body coil alone. Postprocessing correction, by eliminating near-field high signal intensity artifacts, has resulted in a dramatic improvement in the ability to interpret endorectal coil images.[40] The use of fast spin echo (FSE) imaging with improved gradient and radiofrequency technology has significantly reduced the imaging time from over an hour to less than 30 minutes using conventional T2-weighted MRI.

The MRI protocol should include axial T2-weighted images (FSE if available) through the prostate gland (Figure 9–4) and seminal vesicles to allow assessment of zonal anatomy.[42,43] Additional coronal or sagittal T2-weighted images are useful for assessing the anatomy (Figure 9–5) and pathology of the seminal vesicles as well as disease at the prostatic base and apex (Figure 9–6). Axial T1-weighted images, to the level of the aortic bifurcation (Figure 9–7), should be obtained for tissue characterization and detection of pelvic lymph node metastases. Thin slices (3 to 4 mm) and a small field

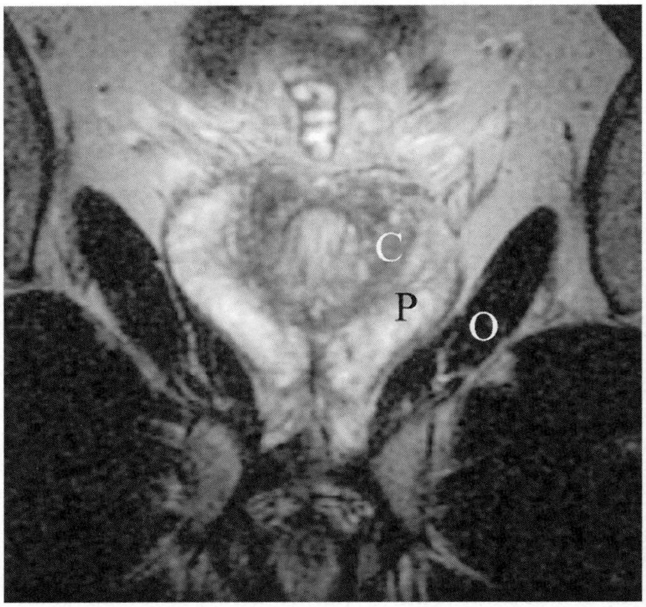

Figure 9–3. Normal zonal anatomy on magnetic resonance imaging. Coronal T2-weighted image demonstrates a clear distinction between the central zone (*C*) and the relatively hyperintense peripheral zone (*P*). O = obterator internus muscle.

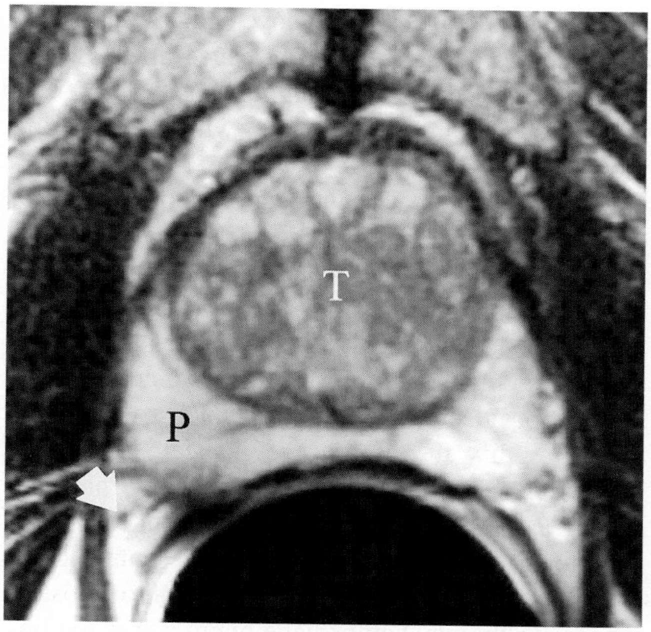

Figure 9–4. Benign prostatic hypertrophy on magnetic resonance imaging. Transaxial T2-weighted image demonstrates an enlarged and heterogeneous transition zone (*T*) and a normal hyperintense peripheral zone (*P*). Arrow = right neurovascular bundle.

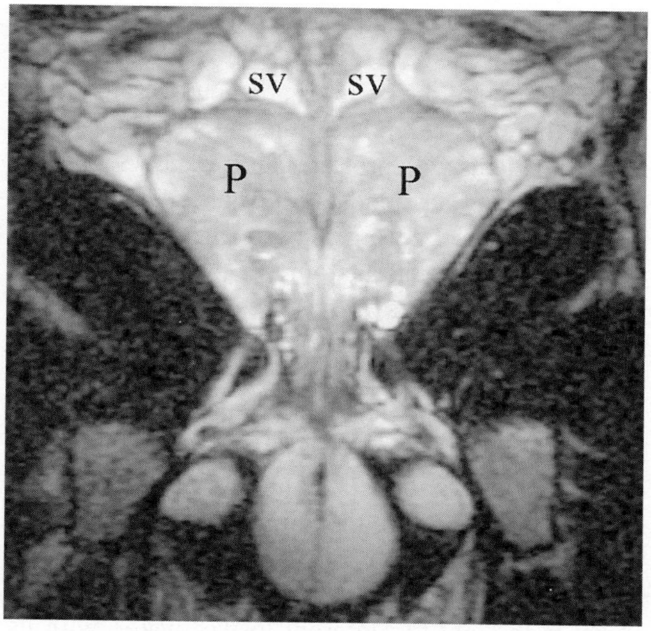

Figure 9–5. Normal zonal anatomy on magnetic resonance imaging. Coronal T2-weighted image. The seminal vesicles (SV) demonstrate low signal intensity walls and contain high signal fluid. P = prostate gland.

of view (14 cm) should be used to maximize image resolution in all three dimensions.[5]

On T1-weighted images,[44] the prostate, seminal vesicles, and periprostatic veins all demonstrate a low signal and appear uniform (Figure 9–8). The internal architecture of the prostate is not visible. In contrast to the low signal of these structures, the periprostatic fat is of a very high signal and sharply outlines the pelvic soft tissues, including the prostate, nerves, muscles, vessels, and lymphatics. The neurovascular bundles are usually visible on these images (see Figure 9–8) and run in the triangle of fat in the left and

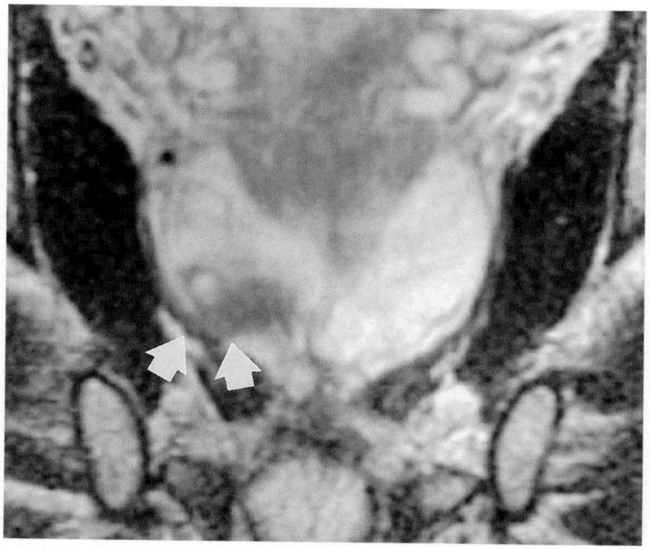

Figure 9–6. Prostate carcinoma on magnetic resonance imaging. Coronal T2-weighted image demonstrates a focus of low signal intensity (*arrows*) in the right prostatic apex. No capsular bulge is seen.

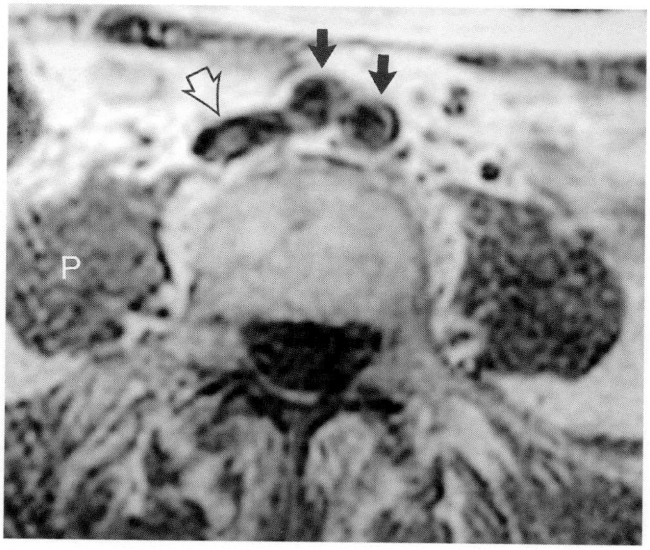

Figure 9–7. Normal retroperitoneal anatomy. Axial T1-weighted image. P = right psoas muscle; open white arrow = inferior vena cava; solid black arrows = aortic bifurcation.

right rectoprostatic angles and contain the cavernosal nerves, believed to be responsible for potency. The demonstration of the periprostatic neurovascular bundles is therefore essential in the preoperative assessment of patients with prostate cancer. The various fascial layers that surround the prostate gland are also well seen on the T1-weighted sequences.

The normal zonal anatomy of the prostate gland and seminal vesicles is best seen on T2-weighted images.[5,12,42,44] The peripheral zone is hyperintense, as are the seminal vesicles, on the T2-weighted sequences, whereas the central and transition zones are hypointense[45] (see Figures 9–3 and 9–5). Prostate cancer usually manifests as abnormal areas of low signal intensity within the homogeneous high signal intensity background of the normal peripheral zone[5,44] (Figures 9–9 and 9–10). (The decrease in T2 signal is thought to represent loss of water, with its long T2, in luminal ducts.[38])

Technical considerations[46] include proper placement of the endorectal coil, use of glucagon (to diminish artifact related to peristalsing bowel), and the use of faster sequences. The endorectal coil must be appropriately positioned. Harris and colleagues found a tendency for the coil to migrate in a cephalad direction when the balloon is being inflated.[46] This tendency should be counteracted by gentle traction on the coil as the balloon is being filled. Malposition of the balloon can result in suboptimal visualization of the prostatic apex. Glucagon is recommended to decrease movement of the colon and rectum and hence motion-related artifacts. The FSE technique decreases imaging time, and thereby increases patient compliance, while decreasing motion artifact.

A normal-appearing prostate gland does not exclude the presence of cancer. Cancer may not be detected if it does not demonstrate low signal on the T2-weighted sequences, if it is located primarily within the central gland, or if the peripheral zone does not demonstrate uniform high signal intensity. In addition, decreased T2 signal intensity does not always signify the presence of cancer. Postbiopsy hemorrhage, prostatitis, and prior therapy may also appear as a low T2 signal in the peripheral zone. Postbiopsy hemorrhage, in fact, represents a common impedance to the accurate detection of prostate cancer. Postbiopsy hemorrhage manifests as regions of increased signal intensity on the T1-weighted sequences; however, it can manifest as either high or low signal intensity on T2-weighted sequences, more commonly the latter (Figure 9–11). Additionally, it is possible for areas of postbiopsy hemorrhage to obscure underlying cancer. It has been demonstrated that there is a statistically significant overestimation of tumor and ECE in patients who undergo MRI less than 21 days after biopsy,[47] therefore, staging accuracy has significantly improved when MRI was deferred for 21 days following biopsy.[40,47] For example, White and colleagues

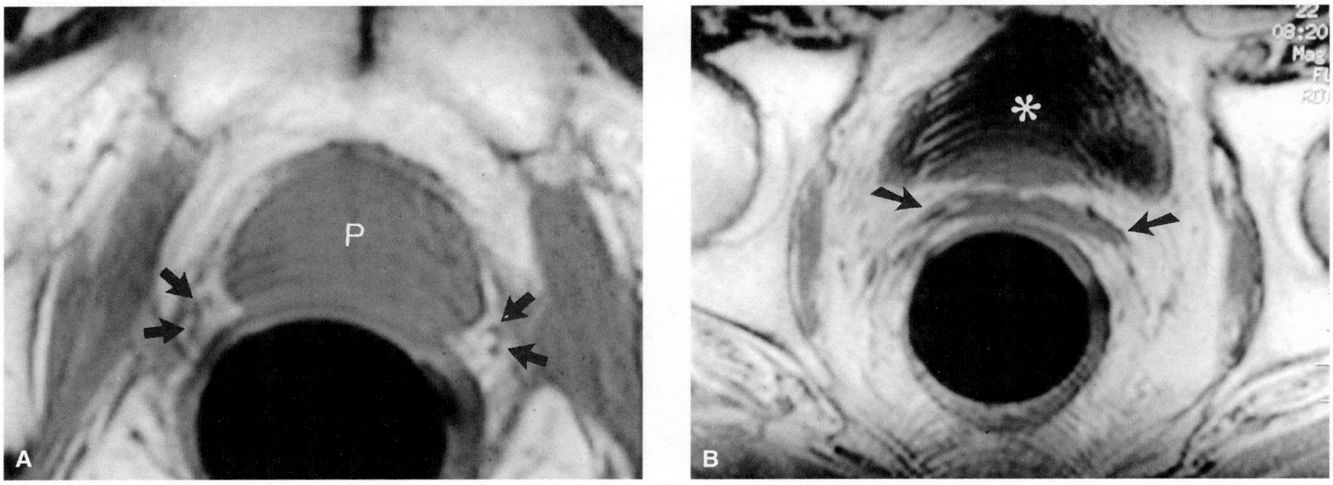

Figure 9–8. Normal anatomy on magnetic resonance imaging. Axial T1-weighted images. *A*, The prostate gland (*P*) demonstrates homogeneous intermediate signal intensity. Neurovascular bundles (*arrows*) are surrounded by high signal intensity fat. *B*, Seminal vesicles (*arrows*) are also of homogeneous intermediate signal intensity. Asterisk = urinary bladder.

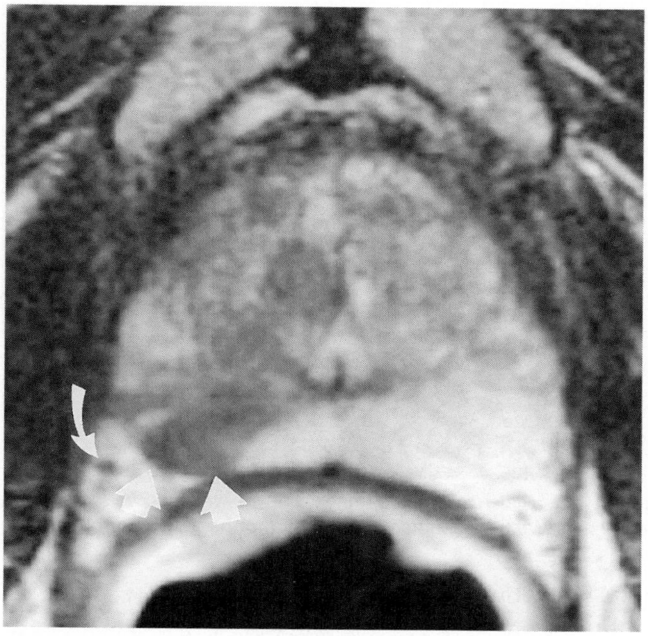

Figure 9–9. Prostate carcinoma on magnetic resonance imaging. Transaxial T2-weighted image demonstrates focal low signal intensity in the right peripheral zone (*arrows*). The prostatic capsule is intact. The right neurovascular bundle is distinctly seen (*curved arrow*) and surrounded by high signal intensity fat.

found that staging accuracy improved from 46 to 83% after 21 days.[47] Low or high signal intensity postbiopsy artifacts, however, may persist for an indeterminate amount of time and have been described as being detected up to 4.5 months after biopsy.[47] Hence, the metabolic information provided by MR spectroscopy can help in the determination of whether tissues underlying a region of postbiopsy hemorrhage contain cancer[40] (Figure 9–12).

In a study comparing MRI results and histopathologic results from radical prostatectomy specimens, Ikonen and colleagues demonstrated a 62% accuracy in tumor detection by MRI, as well as a sensitivity of 56% and a specificity of 70%.[48] They also found a linear relationship between sensitivity in tumor detection and the size of the prostate gland, with sensitivity falling as the prostatectomy specimen increased in weight. Explanations include flattening of the peripheral zone, where cancers are most often located, by the central gland hyperplasia, technical problems with the endorectal coil, and the presence of heterogeneous nodules in the central gland of a hyperplastic prostate (see Figure 9–4). As the prostate increases in size, correct positioning of the endorectal coil can become problematic, leading to inadequate contact between the coil and the prostate, leading to images of lower quality.

Enthusiasm for prostate cancer detection by MRI has been limited owing to significant interobserver variability, as evidenced by the wide range of diagnostic accuracies reported in the literature. Problems that have been found to contribute to the high variability in diagnostic accuracy include a steep learning curve for the interpretation of endorectal MRI and the lack of standardized diagnostic criteria.[39,41,46,49]

Variable results have been reported for local staging of prostate cancer by endorectal MRI, with accuracy as low as 54% in a large multicenter trial to as high as 82 to 88% in two recently published studies. The corresponding sensitivities and specificities range from 51 to 89% and 67 to 87%, respectively.[5,39,41] Yu and colleagues proposed that the diagnosis of ECE should be standardized and based on MRI features found to be the most predictive for ECE, specifically the presence of an irregular capsular bulge (Figures 9–13 and 9–14), obliteration of the rectoprostatic angle, and asymmetry of the neurovascular bundles.[39,41,49] Application of these criteria allowed reproducible high specificity of 94 to

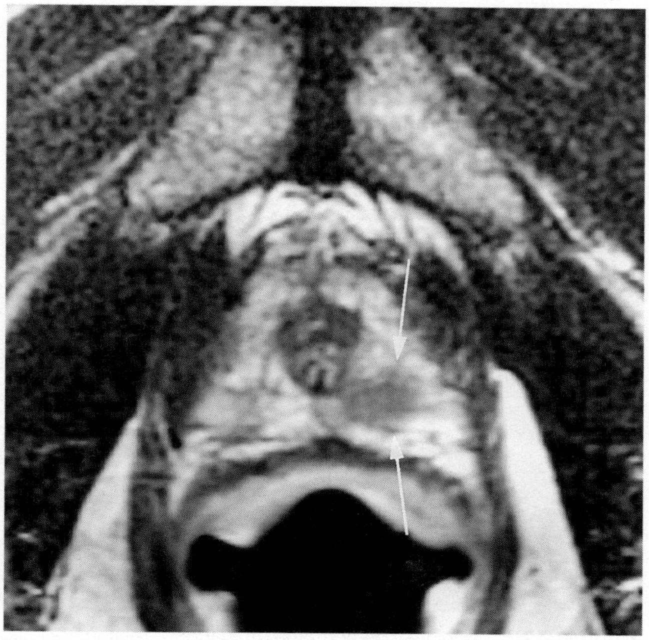

Figure 9–10. Prostate carcinoma on magnetic resonance imaging. Transaxial T2-weighted image demonstrates focal low signal in the left prostatic apex (*arrows*). There is no evidence of extracapsular extension.

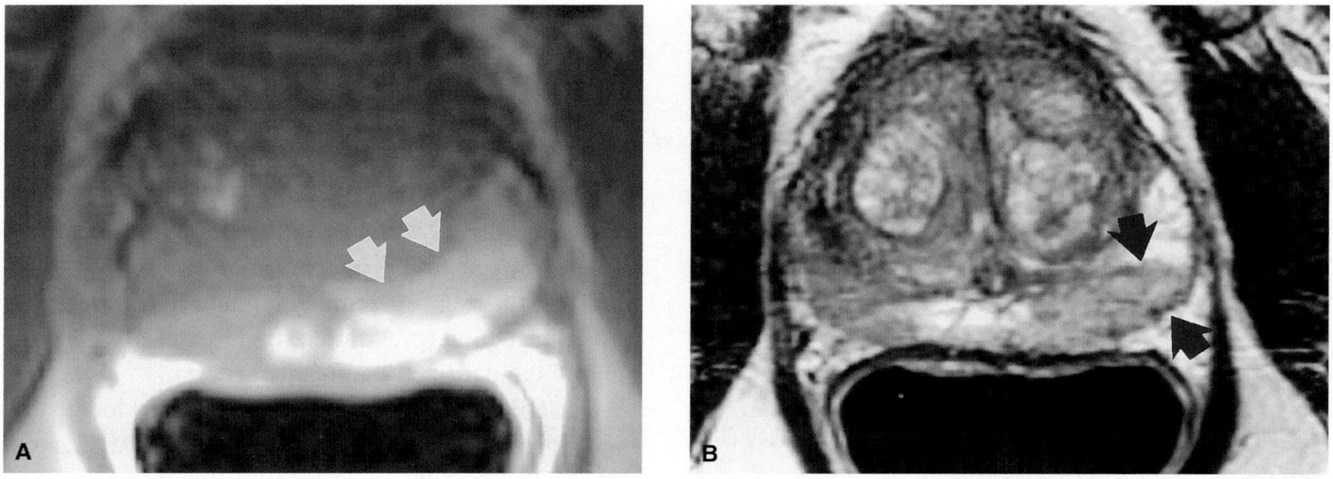

Figure 9–11. Postbiopsy hemorrhage. *A,* Transaxial T1-weighted image. *B,* Transaxial T2-weighted image. The T1-weighted image demonstrates focal increased high signal involving predominantly the left peripheral zone (*arrows*), compatible with hemorrhage. Hemorrhage manifests as low signal intensity on the T2-weighted image (*arrows*).

95% but low sensitivities of 17% and 54%. Lower sensitivity may have reflected a shift toward lower-stage disease in the patient population in this study, with a lower prevalence of ECE. However, because high diagnostic specificity minimizes false-positive results and helps ensure that few patients will be deprived of potentially curative surgery, it is a test characteristic desirable in treatment selection.[40]

Endorectal MRI may be more useful when applied to specific groups of patients based on disease characteristics. D'Amico and colleagues performed a retrospective review of the pathologic findings of 347 patients with prostate cancer treated with radical retropubic prostatectomy.[50] Preoperative clinical indicators including PSA, clinical stage, Gleason score, and endorectal MRI data were employed in a multivariate analysis to identify patients who were at high risk for ECE or SVI. In the patient subgroup with a PSA > 10 to 20 ng/mL and a Gleason score of 5 to 7, the addition of the endorectal coil MRI results allowed for identification of an additional 71% and 27% of patients with SVI (Figure 9–15) and ECE, respectively. Rorvik and colleagues demonstrated sensitivity and specificity for SVI of 71% and 83%, respectively, but sensitivity and specificity of 71% and 47% for ECE.[51]

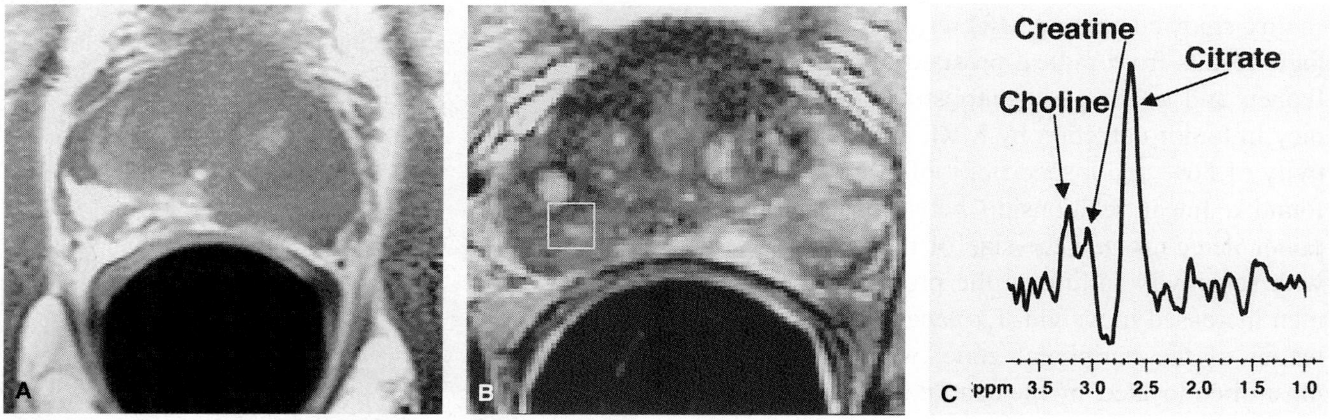

Figure 9–12. Postbiopsy hemorrhage on magnetic resonance imaging (MRI) and magnetic resonance spectroscopy. *A,* T1-weighted MRI indicates focal high signal intensity in the right peripheral zone compatible with postbiopsy hemorrhage. *B,* The corresponding T2-weighted images demonstrate low signal intensity in the same location. *C,* The presence of cancer could not be definitely determined. The magnetic resonance spectroscopic spectrum from the same region demonstrates choline and citrate levels indicative of normal peripheral zone tissue, compatible with postbiopsy change. Images courtesy of John Kurhanewicz, MD, University of California at San Francisco.

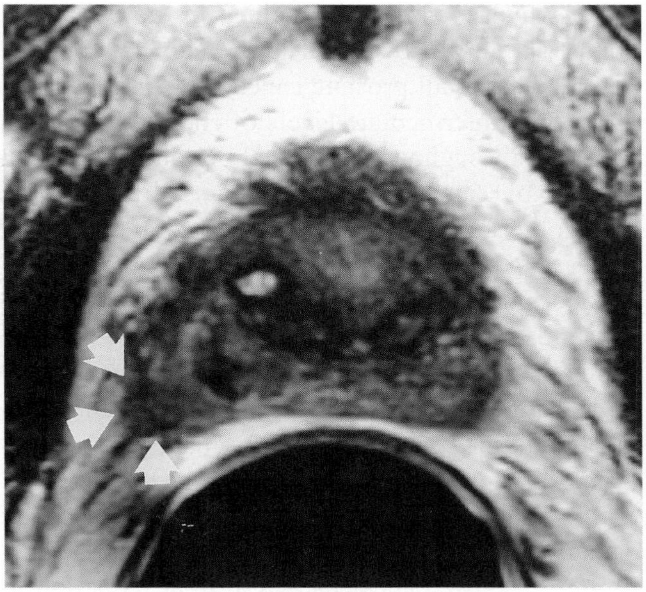

Figure 9–13. Prostate carcinoma with extracapsular extension on magnetic resonance imaging. Transaxial T2-weighted image at the level of the base demonstrates low signal intensity throughout the peripheral zone, with a contour bulge of the prostatic capsule (*arrows*). The right neurovascular bundle is not discretely seen, which is suspicious for tumor involvement.

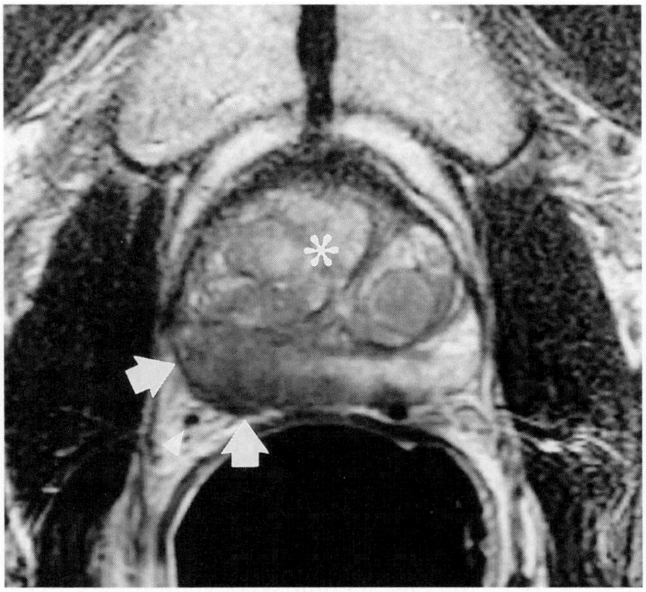

Figure 9–14. Prostate carcinoma with possible extracapsular extension. Transaxial T2-weighted image demonstrates focal low signal intensity (*arrows*) in the right peripheral zone compatible with prostatic carcinoma. There is a subtle bulge of the capsule suggestive of extracapsular extension. The right neurovascular bundle (*arrowhead*) is discretely seen, surrounded by high signal intensity fat. The transition zone is enlarged and heterogeneous in signal intensity compatible with benign prostatic hyperplasia (*asterisk*).

Some studies concerning MRI of prostate cancer have emphasized detection of tumors differing in Gleason scores, with results varying considerably. Ikonen and colleagues retrospectively reviewed and compared the MRI findings and histopathologic results of RP specimens from 63 patients and found a highly significant difference in the detection of cancer lesions based on their differentiation grade.[48] In the entire series, there were no tumors of Gleason score 2 or 3. Percentage rate of MRI detection of tumor ranged from 41% in patients with a Gleason score of 4, to 70% with a Gleason score of 7, to 94% with a Gleason score of 10. Overall accuracy in detecting cancer lesions was consistent with that of previous studies and found to be 62%. In contrast, other studies, including those of Carrol and colleagues and Carter and colleagues,[48] found that the likelihood of tumor identification did not appear to correlate with total Gleason score.

Manzone and colleagues found that patients whose staging endorectal MR studies show definite extracapsular disease (see Figure 9–13) are significantly more likely to demonstrate biochemical failure after radical prostatectomy than are patients whose MR studies show definitely localized or only questionable ECE. An MR finding of definite ECE was highly specific (93.9%) for the prediction of tumor recurrence, although sensitivity was limited (23.5%). A patient with definitely advanced disease, if treated surgically, was found to be two to three

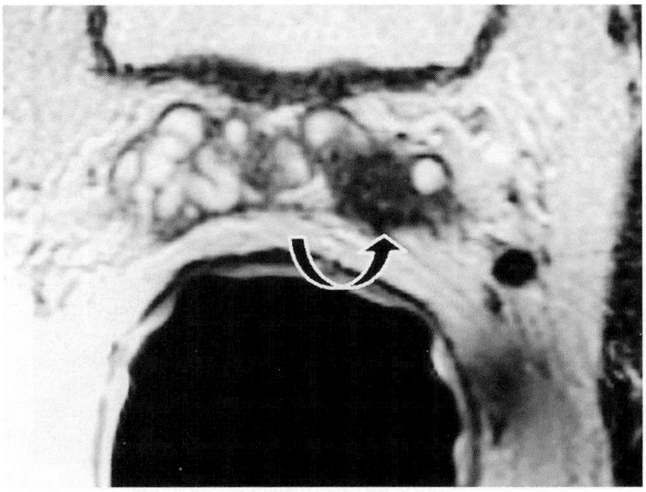

Figure 9–15. Seminal vesicle invasion on magnetic resonance imaging. Transaxial T2-weighted image through the seminal vesicles demonstrates focal low signal in the left seminal vesicle (*curved arrow*), surrounding normal high signal intensity fluid.

times more likely to have a tumor recurrence than a patient with a clearly negative or equivocal MR study. Patients in the same study cohort, with definitely localized disease at MRI, even if they had disease recurrence, enjoyed about twice as long a disease-free interval after surgery as those patients with questionable advanced disease.[9]

MAGNETIC RESONANCE SPECTROSCOPY

The addition of metabolic information from three-dimensional MR spectroscopic imaging to morphologic data from MRI may allow more specific diagnosis and localization of prostate cancer.[40] Magnetic resonance spectroscopy has been used to obtain metabolic data from tumors in situ[10] (Figures 9–15 and 9–16). Recent technical developments have allowed the application of localized three-dimensional proton MR spectroscopic imaging to the in vivo evaluation of the human prostate.[10,38]

The prostate is a secretory gland that provides a signficant proportion of the human male ejaculate. However, the normal prostate is not a homogeneous organ but is composed of several anatomic zones that differ in morphology, function, and pathologic significance. Human prostatic secretions contain high concentrations of citrate that are 240 to 1,300 times greater than blood plasma concentrations. Citrate production, secretion, and storage are associated only with prostatic glandular tissues, the majority of which (75%) are contained in the peripheral zone[40] (Figure 9–18). This is the site for approximately 68% of all prostate cancers.[40] High levels of citrate and intermediate levels of choline have been observed throughout the normal peripheral zone. In regions of cancer, two significant differences in metabolite levels have been observed: a significant increase in prostate choline levels relative to the normal peripheral zone and a significant reduction in prostate citrate levels (see Figure 9–15). The decrease in citrate in prostate cancer is caused by both changes in cellular function[40,52] and in the organization of the tissue that loses its characteristic ductal morphology.[40,53,54] In prostate cancer, malignant epithelial cells have demonstrated diminished capacity for net citrate production and secretion.[40,38,52] Also, cancer causes a great reduction in the volume of glandular ducts, which normally contain high levels of citrate.[40,53,54]

With the use of three-dimensional MR spectroscopic imaging, significantly higher choline levels and significantly lower citrate levels were observed in regions of cancer compared with areas of BPH and normal prostatic tissue (see Figures 9–15 and 9–17). The ratio of these metabolites (choline to citrate) in regions of cancer appears not to overlap with ratios in the normal peripheral zone, which suggests that three-dimensional MR spectroscopic imaging combined with MRI may improve tumor detection and localization compared to MRI alone.[10,38] Scheidler and col-

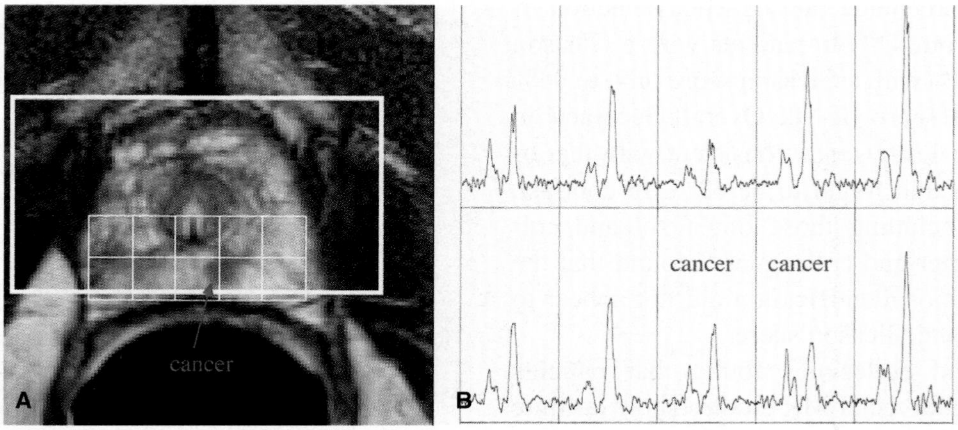

Figure 9–16. Prostate carcinoma on magnetic resonance spectroscopy. A 56-year-old man with a prostate-specific antigen level of 5.5 ng/mL and biopsy-positive cancer at the left apex. *A,* T2-weighted magnetic resonance imaging indicates a focal low signal intensity lesion. *B,* The corresponding spectra demonstrate elevated choline and reduced citrate relative to surrounding healthy tissue compatible with prostate cancer. Images courtesy of John Kurhanewicz, MD, University of California at San Francisco.

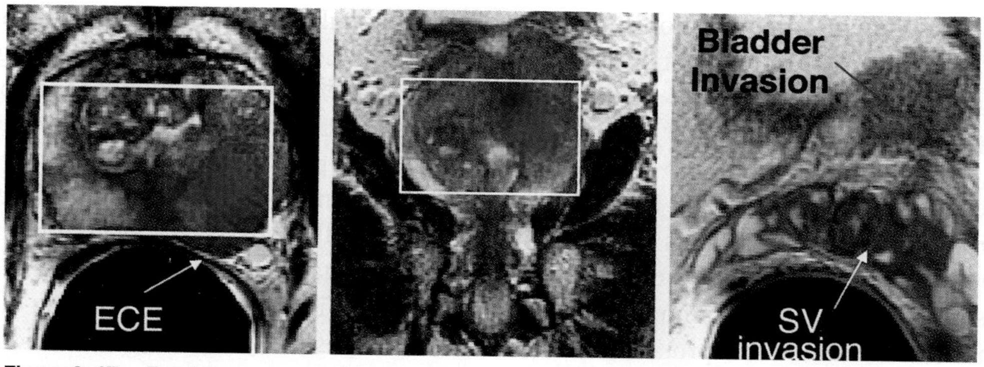

Figure 9–17. Prostate carcinoma with extracapsular extension (*ECE*) and adjacent organ involvement on magnetic resonance spectroscopy: 67-year-old patient with a prostate-specific antigen level of 13 ng/mL, Gleason score of 7 (4 + 3), and a clinical stage T2b tumor, who wanted brachytherapy. Magnetic resonance imaging/magnetic resonance spectroscopy demonstrates a large volume tumor with ECE on the left side, bilateral seminal vesicle (*SV*) invasion, and invasion of the bladder neck. These findings are compatible with stage T3c. Images courtesy of John Kurhanewicz, MD, University of California at San Francisco.

leagues found that a positive result with combined MRI and three-dimensional MR spectroscopic imaging indicated the presence of tumor with high probability (positive predictive value of 89% to 92%).[10] The combination that was most useful for excluding the presence of cancer in a sextant (negative predictive value of 74 to 82%) was the absence of cancer with either aforementioned modality.[40] Magnetic resonance spectroscopy has been effective in discriminating residual cancer from necrosis and other residual tissues after cryosurgery.[55–57]

Magnetic resonance spectroscopic imaging information may also provide insight into tumor aggressiveness, which may lead to improved risk assessment in patients with prostate cancer. Early biochemical studies have indicated that citrate levels in prostatic cancer are grade dependent, with citrate levels being low in well-differentiated prostate cancers and effectively absent in poorly differentiated prostate cancer.[40]

More recent developments to improve MRI include contrast-enhanced fast dynamic MRI. On contrast-enhanced images, prostate cancer shows a typical early and rapidly accelerating enhancement compared with normal tissues.[46] A current problem with this technique is the large variation in enhancement patterns among patients with prostate cancer and the overlapping enhancement pattern of BPH.[5] To date,

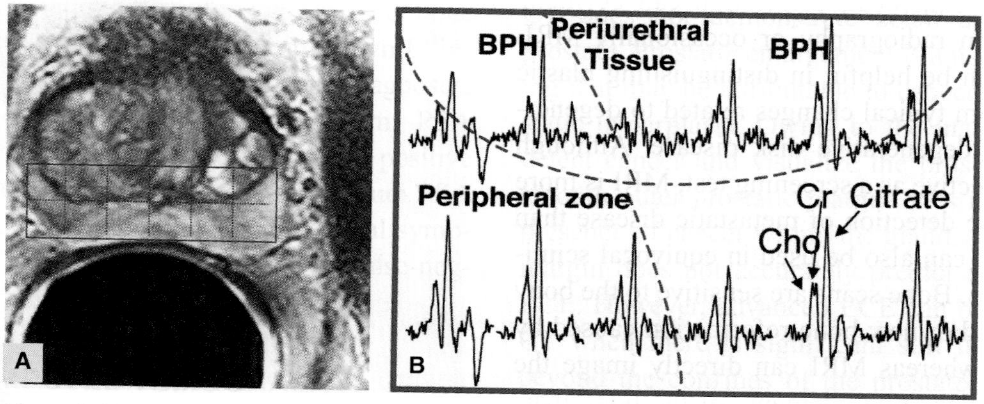

Figure 9–18. Normal magnetic resonance spectroscopy: a man with an elevated prostate-specific antigen level of 8.5 ng/mL who was biopsy negative for cancer. *A*, T2-weighted magnetic resonance image indicates high signal intensity throughout the peripheral zone indicative of healthy peripheral zone tissue. *B*, Magnetic resonance spectroscopy demonstrates high levels of citrate and indeterminate levels of choline (*Cho*) and creatine (*Cr*), also indicative of healthy peripheral zone tissue. BPH = benign prostatic hyperplasia. Images courtesy of John Kurhanewicz, MD, University of California at San Francisco.

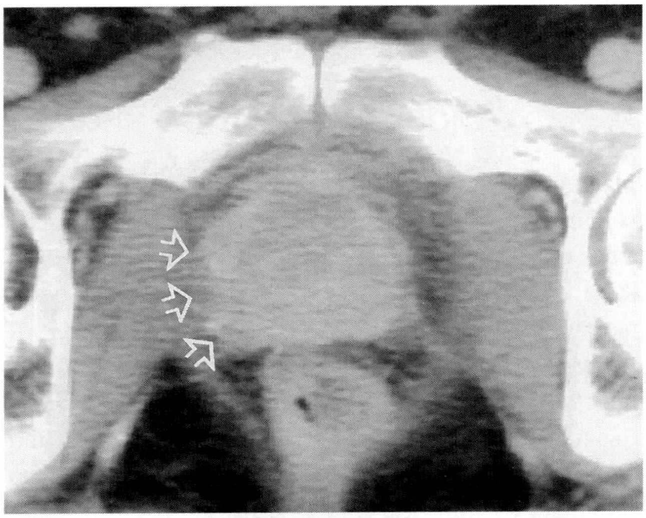

Figure 9–21. Extracapsular extension on computed tomography (CT). Contrast-enhanced helical CT image through the pelvis at the level of the symphysis pubis. Capsular irregularity and contour bulge on the right (*open arrows*), with obliteration of the fat plane between the prostate gland and the obturator internus muscle, is compatible with extracapsular extension.

icant advance in CT technology, it is unlikely that the inherent limitation of low soft tissue contrast can be sufficiently overcome to improve staging accuracy.

One potential role for CT is in the evaluation of patients suspected of having advanced disease with spread of tumor into adjacent organs (Figures 9–22 to 9–24) or in patients at risk for local or distant lymph node metastases (Figures 9–25 to 9–28). The presence of locally advanced disease and/or nodal metastases in contemporary series of patients newly diagnosed with prostate cancer is low. Therefore, it has been suggested that CT can be eliminated from routine staging in patients with PSA less than 20 or a Gleason score of 7 or less.[63]

Computed tomography has virtually supplanted bipedal lymphography in the detection of lymphadenopathy.[32] Sensitivity in the detection of lymph node metastases has varied. Van Poppel and colleagues, in a study of 285 patients (using a nonhelical scanner), noted 78% sensitivity and 97% specificity in the detection of pelvic lymph node metastases prior to RP.[44] Oyen and colleagues performed fine-needle aspiration biopsy on 43 patients with positive CT (asymmetric lymph node greater than 6 mm) and demonstrated sensitivity, specificity, and accuracy of 77.8, 100, and 96.5%, respectively.[64] Wolf and colleagues performed a thorough review of the literature to determine the sensitivity and specificity of CT in predicting lymph node metastases.[65] Eighteen series were reviewed in which pathologic confirmation of lymph node metastases was required. Based on review of the literature, CT was found to have a sensitivity of 36% and a specificity of 97% for detecting lymph node metastases. These same authors performed a decision analysis and reported that for imaging to be beneficial, the probability of lymph node metastases in an individual patient must be at least 32%. Such patients include those with a serum PSA > 20 ng/mL, Gleason score of 8 to 10, palpably advanced local disease, or a positive seminal vesicle biopsy. An important limitation of CT imaging in the evaluation of nodal metastases continues to be dependence on enlargement of lymph nodes as a criterion for metastatic involvement, when metastases may also be present in normal-sized nodes.[51] Computed tomography offers advantages over MRI in the detection of lymphadenopathy, including lower cost, decreased scan time and motion artifact, relatively easy availability, and the ability to perform concomitant CT-guided fine-needle aspiration, as needed.

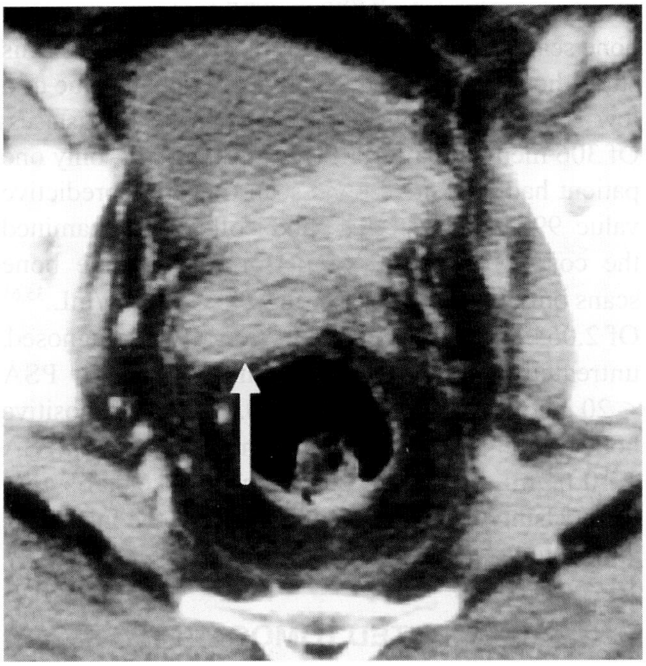

Figure 9–22. Seminal vesicle invasion on computed tomography (CT). Contrast enhanced helical CT image at the level of the seminal vesicles demonstrates asymmetric enlargement of the right seminal vesicle (*arrow*) compatible with seminal vesicle invasion. Thickening along the posterior wall of the bladder suggests metastatic involvement also.

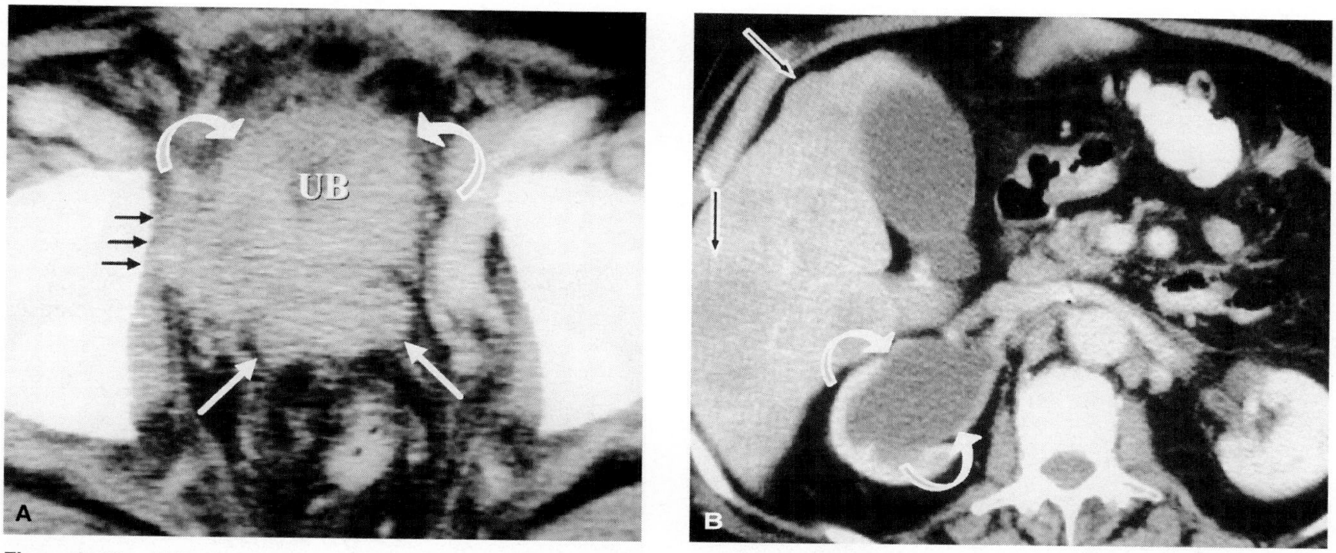

Figure 9–23. Extensive metastatic disease on computed tomography (CT). Contrast-enhanced CT at the level of the renal hila and lower pelvis. *A,* Marked thickening of the bladder wall (*curved arrows*) is compatible with metastatic involvement and accounts for the hydronephrosis in *B.* Enlargement of the seminal vesicles (*long white arrows*) and soft tissue (*black arrows*) interposed between the urinary bladder (*UB*) and the right obturator internus muscle are also findings of metastatic disease. *B,* Multiple hypoattenuating lesions in the liver (*black arrows*) are compatible with visceral metastases. Marked right hydronephrosis (*curved white arrows*) and associated thinning of the renal parenchyma are findings of an ureteral obstruction.

Computed tomography is able to detect visceral and osseous metastatic disease[32] (Figures 9–29 and 9–30) and in this regard may be used to evaluate patients with rising PSA after definitive local therapy and without a documented site of recurrence.

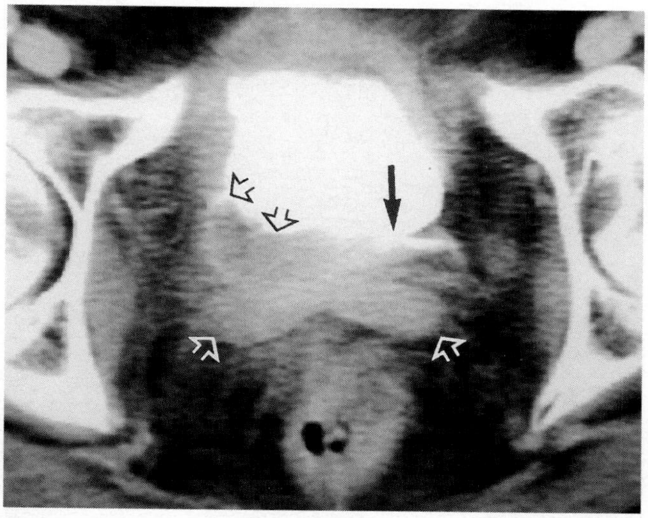

Figure 9–24. Invasion of the bladder wall on computed tomography (CT). Contrast-enhanced delayed helical CT image at the level of the seminal vesicles (*open arrows*) demonstrates nodular thickening of most of the bladder wall, most prominent along the posterior wall (*open black arrows*), with obliteration of the right ureterovesicle junction, compatible with bladder invasion. The left ureterovesicle junction is well visualized (*black arrow*).

Because CT is limited to the transaxial plane of section, tumor invasion of the bladder base cannot always be detected reliably; however, the presence of hydronephrosis is a useful imaging finding in that it suggests bladder invasion, with involvement of the ipsilateral ureterovesical junction.[5] Focal eccentric bladder wall thickening in the proper context would be considered suspicious for bladder invasion (see Figure 9–23).

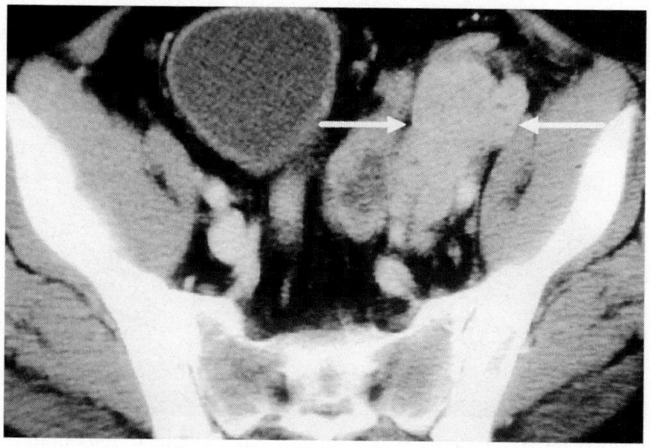

Figure 9–25. Metastatic adenopathy on computed tomography (CT). Contrast-enhanced helical CT image through the lower abdomen demonstrates a large nodal mass in the left external iliac nodal chain (*arrows*).

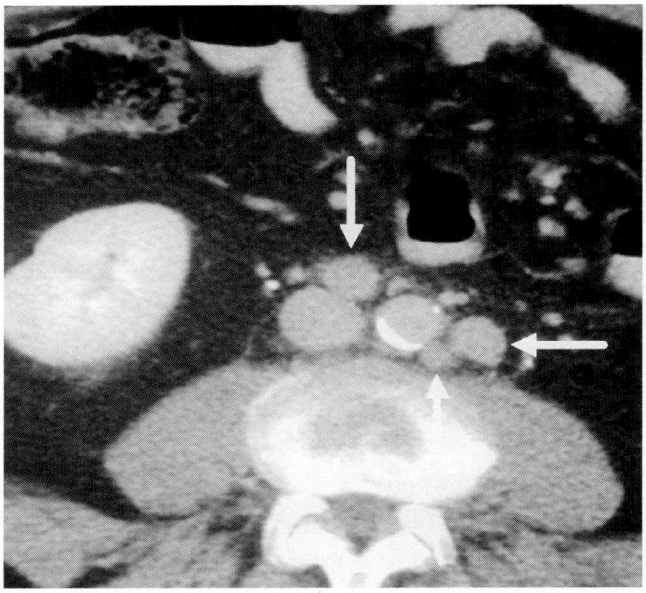

Figure 9–26. Metastatic adenopathy on computed tomography (CT). Contrast-enhanced helical CT image through the abdomen demonstrates several nodal masses (*arrows*) in the retroperitoneum and in the interaortocaval and left para-aortic spaces.

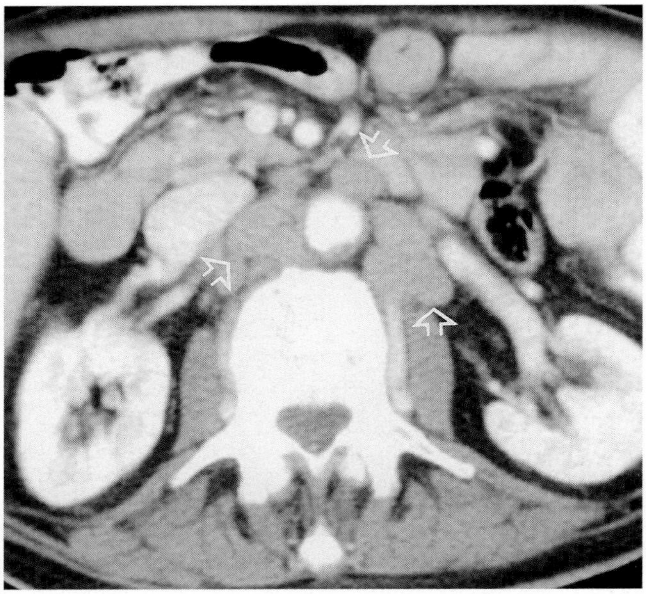

Figure 9–27. Metastatic adenopathy on computed tomography (CT). Contrast-enhanced helical CT image through the abdomen demonstrates retroperitoneal adenopathy (*open arrows*) (retrocaval, interaortocaval, and left para-aortic) at the level of the renal hila.

SCINTIGRAPHY

Indium 111 capromab pendetide is a conjugate of a monoclonal antibody (7E11-C5.3), a linker-chelator, and a gamma-emitting radioisotope (In 111). The antibody is directed toward a membrane-associated antigen (prostate specific membrane antigen) of prostate cells that is more highly expressed in malignant than nonmalignant cells and in metastatic than primary prostate carcinoma.[32,66] The compound is administered intravenously and single-photon emission computed tomography of the abdomen and

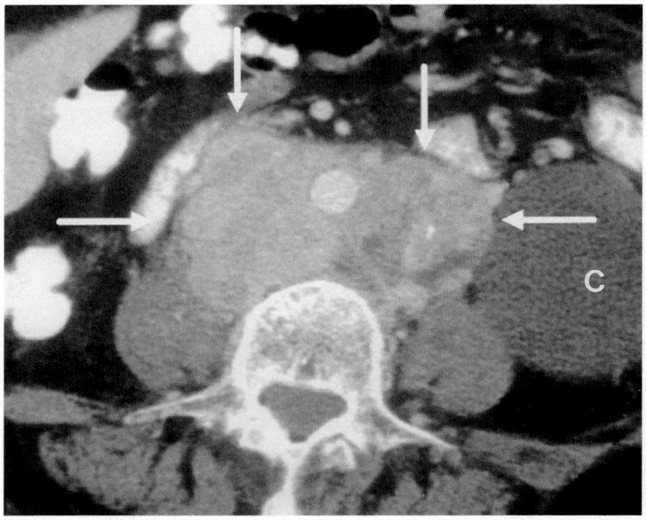

Figure 9–28. Extensive adenopathy on computed tomography (CT). Contrast-enhanced helical CT image through the abdomen demonstrates massive retroperitoneal adenopathy (*arrows*), which surrounds the aorta, obscures the inferior vena cava, and deviates loops of small bowel anteriorly. C = exophytic left renal cyst.

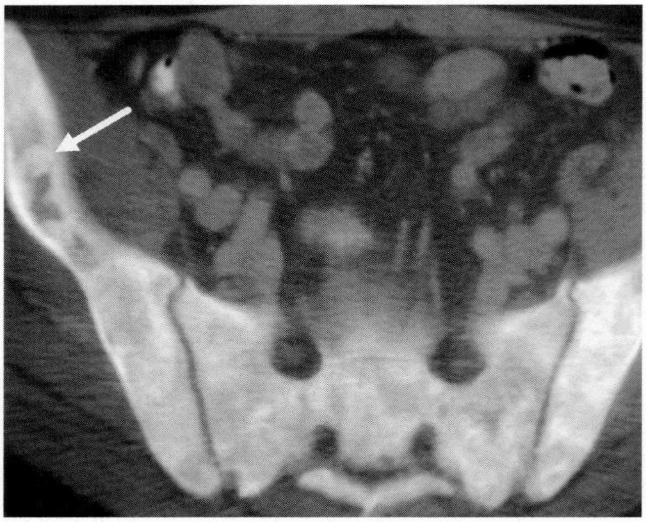

Figure 9–29. Osseous metastatic disease on computed tomography (CT). Contrast-enhanced helical CT image through the lower abdomen (bone window) demonstrates extensive blastic osseous metastatic disease involving the sacrum and iliac wings diffusely. Arrow = discrete blastic metastasis in right iliac wing.

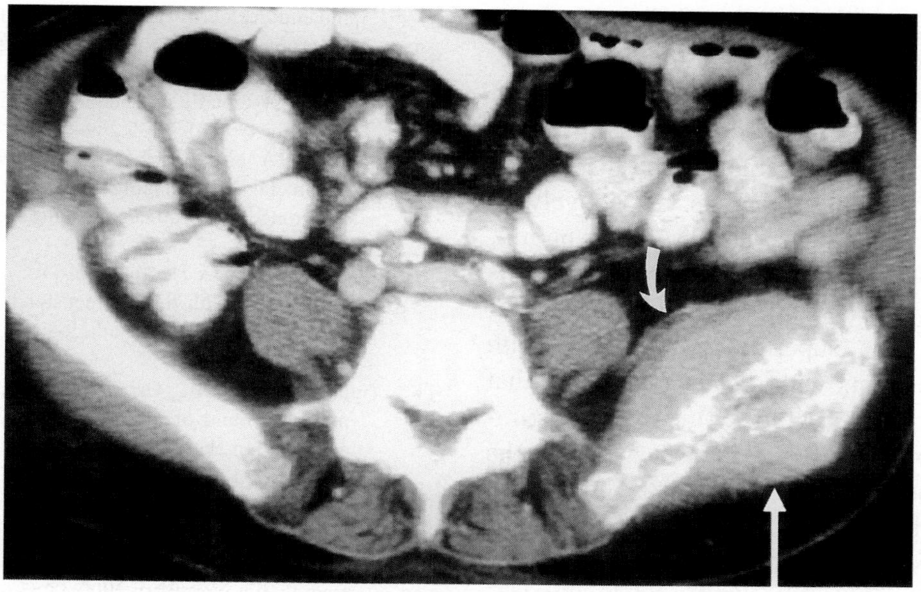

Figure 9–30. Osseous metastatic disease on computed tomography (CT). Contrast-enhanced helical CT image through the lower abdomen demonstrates an expansile lytic lesion in the left iliac wing, associated with expansion of the left iliacus (*curved arrow*) and gluteus (*long arrow*) muscles.

pelvis are performed at 30 minutes (blood pool) and again 96 to 120 hours later (delayed images). Additional views may consist of whole-body or spot planar images.[32] In 1996, the US Food and Drug Administration approved the In 111–labeled monoclonal antibody also known as ProstaScint for the detection of soft tissue metastases in patients with prostate cancer who are at high risk for metastatic disease. This approval was based on clinical trials that showed increased sensitivity for detecting soft tissue metastases often found in pelvic and extrapelvic nodes.[33] Performance characteristics in an initial clinical trial, in newly diagnosed patients, demonstrated a sensitivity of 62%, a specificity of 72%, a positive predictive value of 62%, a negative predictive value of 72%, and an overall accuracy of 68%.

ProstaScint may be used to predict occult lymph node metastases in patients newly diagnosed with prostate cancer who are contemplating definitive local therapy and for the detection and localization of recurrent disease following failed local therapy. Its high cost and difficult interpretation have limited the role of ProstaScint in the initial evaluation of patients with prostate cancer. Instead, most clinicians currently use this modality to evaluate a patient with an increasing serum PSA following treatment. In this setting, conventional imaging studies, such as CT, MRI, and bone scan, have limited sensitivity, and the use of immunoscintigraphy with a monoclonal antibody directed against a PSMA offers the theoretic advantage of specific tissue binding and high sensitivity, requiring small doses of antibody. However, the results to date using monoclonal antibody imaging for such patients have been confusing as most studies have not included tissue sampling to confirm the results of the ProstaScint scan. In a study of 158 patients with PSA recurrence following RP who underwent biopsy of the prostatic fossa, the sensitivity, specificity, positive predictive value and negative predictive value of the ProstaScint scan to detect residual or recurrent cancer in the prostatic fossa was 49%, 71%, 50%, and 70%, respectively.[33,67] Similarly, ProstaScint has a sensitivity for detecting lymph node metastases of 44 to 63% with a specificity, positive predictive value, and negative predictive value of 72 to 86%, 50 to 62%, and 72 to 83%, respectively.[68,69] In a recent study of 45 patients with an elevated serum PSA following definitive local therapy, Seltzer and colleagues compared the detection of metastatic disease by spiral CT, positron emission tomography (PET), and ProstaScint.[70] The median PSA in this group of patients was 3.8 ng/mL. These authors demonstrated that both CT and PET were superior to ProstaScint in the detection of metastatic disease in this setting and that such detection was dependent on the serum PSA at the time of evaluation. In patients with a serum PSA < 4.0 ng/mL, PET and CT demonstrated distant disease in only 4 and 17% of patients, respectively. In contrast, for patients with a serum PSA > 4.0 ng/mL, distant disease was identified in 50% of patients using either imaging modality. The detection rate for both modalities was superior to that seen with ProstaScint. In patients with distant metastases that were confirmed with CT-guided fine-needle aspiration, the sensitivity of PET was 67% whereas the sensitivity of ProstaScint was only 17%. Given these results, most clinicians currently recommend a ProstaScint study only when there is a persistently detectable or rising PSA following radical prostatectomy or radiation therapy with no identifiable site of recurrence by the standard imaging modalities or by local biopsies.[32]

Technologic advances in imaging hardware and software are expected to continue at a rapid rate, and further improvements in modalities used to image the prostate can be anticipated, with the potential for even greater diagnostic capabilities. Development of new contrast media for ultrasonography and MRI, monoclonal antibodies specific for prostatic tissue, and metabolic imaging by MR spectroscopy and PET hold the promise of greater diagnostic accuracy in the evaluation of prostate cancer.[5]

REFERENCES

1. Costello LC, Franklin RB, Narayan P. Citrate in the diagnosis of prostate cancer. Prostate 1999;38:237–45.
2. Fleshner N, Rakovitch E, Klotz L. Differences between urologists in the United States and Canada in the approach to prostate cancer. J Urol 2000;163:1461–6.
3. El-Gabry EA, Halpern EJ, Strup SE, Gomella LG. Imaging prostate cancer: current and future applications. Oncology 2001;15:325–36.
4. Jager GJ, et al. Prostate cancer staging: should MR imaging be used? A decision analytic approach. Radiology 2000; 215:445–51.
5. Yu KK, Hricak H. Imaging prostate cancer. Radiol Clin North Am 2000;38:59–85.
6. Perrotti M, Pantuck A, Rabbani F, et al. Review of staging modalities in clinically localized prostate cancer. Urology 1999;54:208–14.
7. Presti JC, Hricak H, Narayan PA, et al. Local staging of prostatic carcinoma: comparison of transrectal sonography and endorectal MR imaging. AJR Am J Roentgenol 1996; 166:103–8.
8. Salomon L, Colombel M, Patard J, et al. Value of ultrasound-guided systematic sextant biopsies in prostate tumor mapping. Eur Urol 1999;35:289–93.
9. Manzone TA, Malkowicz SB, Tomaszewski JE, et al. Use of endorectal MR imaging to predict prostate carcinoma recurrence after radical prostatectomy. Radiology 1998; 209:537–42.
10. Scheidler J, Hricak H, Vigneron DB, et al. Prostate cancer: localization with three-dimensional proton MR spectroscopic imaging-clinicopathologic study. Radiology 1999; 213:473–80.
11. Tiguret R, Gheiler EL, Grignon DJ, et al. Patients with abnormal ultrasound of the prostate but normal digital rectal examination should be classified as having clinical stage T_2 tumors. J Urol 2000;163:1486–90.
12. Grossfeld GD, Coakley FV. Benign prostatic hyperplasia: clinical overview and value of diagnostic imaging, the prostate gland: a clinically relevant approach to imaging. Radiol Clin North Am 2000;38:31–47.
13. Aarnink RG, Beerlage HP, De La Rosette JJ, et al. Transrectal ultrasound of the prostate: innovations and future applications. J Urol 1998;159:1568–79.
14. Shinohara K, Wheeler TM, Scardino PT. The appearance of prostate cancer on transrectal ultrasonography: correlation of imaging and pathological examinations. J Urol 1989;142:76–82.
15. Lee F, Torp-Pedersen S, Littrup PJ, et al. Hypoechoic lesions of the prostate: clinical relevance of tumor size, digital rectal examination, and prostate-specific antigen. Radiology 1989;170:29–32.
16. Rorvik J, Halvorsen OJ, Servoll E, Haukaas S. Transrectal ultrasonography to assess local extent of prostatic cancer before radical prostatectomy. 1994;73:65–9.
17. Smith JA, Scardino PT, Resnik MI, et al. Transrectal ultrasound versus digital rectal examination for the staging of carcinoma of the prostate: results of a prospective, multi-institutional trial. J Urol 1997;157:902–6.
18. Louvar E, Littrup PJ, Goldstein A, et al. Correlation of color Doppler flow in the prostate with tissue microvascularity. Cancer 1998;83:135–9.
19. Rifkin MD, Sudakoff GS, Alexander AA. Prostate: techniques, results, and potential applications of color Doppler US scanning. Radiology 1993;186:509–13.
20. Lissbrant IF, Stattin P, Damber JE, Bergh A. Vascular density is a predictor of cancer-specific survival in prostatic carcinoma. Prostate 1997;33:38–45.
21. Brawer MK, Deering RE, Brown M, et al. Predictors of pathologic stage in prostate carcinoma. Cancer 1994;73:678–87.
22. Bostwick DG, Wheeler TM, Blute M, et al. Optimized microvessel density analysis improves prediction of cancer stage from prostate needle biopsies. Urology 1996;48: 47–57.
23. Newman JS, Bree RL, Rubin JM. Prostate cancer: diagnosis with color Doppler sonography with histologic correlation of each biopsy site. Radiology 1995;195:86–90.
24. Ismail M, Peterson RO, Alexander AA, et al. Color Doppler imaging in predicting the biologic behavior of prostate

cancer: correlation with disease-free survival. Urology 1997;50:906–12.
25. Rogers HA, Sedelaar JM, Beerlage HP, et al. Contrast-enhanced three-dimensional power Doppler angiography of the human prostate: correlation with biopsy outcome. Urology 1999;54:97–104.
26. Albrech T, Urbank A, Mahlr M, et al. Prolongation and optimization of Doppler enhancement with a microbubble US contrast agent by using continuous infusion: preliminary experience. Radiology 1998;207:339–47.
27. Thornbury JR, Ornstein DK, Choyke PL, et al. Prostate cancer: what is the future role for imaging? AJR Am J Roentgenol 2001;176:17–22.
28. Garg S, Fortling B, Chadwick D, et al. Staging of prostate cancer using 3-dimensional transrectal ultrasound images: a pilot study. J Urol 1999;162:1318–21.
29. Sehgal CM, Broderick GA, Whittington R, et al. Three-dimensional US and volumetric assessment of the prostate. Radiology 1994;192:274–8.
30. Goldenberg SL, Carter M, Dashefsky S, Cooperberg PL. Sonographic characteristics of the urethrovesical anastomosis in the early post-radical prostatectomy patient. J Urol 1992;147:1307–9.
31. Catalona WJ, Smith DS. Cancer recurrence and survival rates after anatomic radical retropubic prostatectomy for prostate cancer: intermediate-term results. J Urol 1998; 160:2428.
32. Nudell DM, Wefer AE, Hricak H, Carroll PR. Imaging for recurrent prostate cancer. Radiol Clin North Am 2000; 38:213–29.
33. Quintana JC, Blend MJ. The dual-isotope ProstaScint imaging procedure clinical experience and staging results in 145 patients. Clin Nucl Med 1999;25:33–40.
34. Seltzer SE, Getty DJ, Tempany CM, et al. Staging prostate cancer with MR imaging: a combined radiologist-computer system. Radiology 1997;202:219–26.
35. O'Dowd GJ, Veltri RW, Orozco R, et al. Update on the appropriate staging evaluation for newly diagnosed prostate cancer. J Urol 1997;158:687–98.
36. Plawker MW, Fleisher JM, Vapnek EM, Macchia RJ. Current trends in prostate cancer diagnosis and staging among United States urologists. J Urol 1997;158:1853–8.
37. Rorvik J, Halvorsen OJ, Albrektsen G, et al. Use of pelvic surface coil MR imaging for assessment of clinically localized prostate cancer with histopathogical correlation. Clin Radiol 1999;54:164–9.
38. Kurhanewicz J, Vigneron DB, Hricak H, et al. Three-dimensional H-1 MR spectroscopic imaging of the in situ human prostate with high (0.24-0.7 cm^3) spatial resolution. Radiology 1996;198:795–805.
39. Yu KK, Scheidler J, Hricak H, et al. Prostate cancer: prediction of extracapsular extension with endorectal MR imaging and three-dimensional proton MR spectroscopic imaging. Radiology 1999;213:481–8.
40. Kurhanewicz J, Vigneron DB, Males RG, et al. The prostate: MR imaging and spectroscopy. Radiol Clin North Am 2000;38:115–38.
41. Yu KK, Hricak H, Alagappan R, et al. Detection of extracapsular extension of prostate carcinoma with endorectal and phased-array coil MR imaging: multivariate analysis. Radiology 1997;202:697–702.
42. Parra RO, Wolf RM, Huben RP. Use of transrectal ultrasound in the detection and evaluation of local pelvic recurrences after a radical urological pelvic operation. J Urol 1990; 144:707–9.
43. Kier R, Wain S. Fast spin-echo MR images of the pelvis obtained with a phased-array coil: value in localizing and staging prostate carcinoma AJR Am J Roentgenol 1993; 161:601.
44. Schnall MD, Pollack HM. Magnetic resonance imaging of the prostate gland. Urol Radiol 1990;12:109–14.
45. Kubik-Huch RA, Hailemariam S, Hamm B. CT and MRI of the male genital tract: radiologic-pathologic correlation. Eur Radiol 1999;9:16–28.
46. Harris RD, Schned AR, Heaney JA. Staging of prostate cancer with endorectal imaging: lessons from a learning curve. Radiographics 1995;15:813–29.
47. White S, Hricak H, Forstner R, et al. Prostate cancer: effect of postbiopsy hemorrhage on interpretation of MR images. Radiology 1995;195:385–90.
48. Ikonen S, Karkkainen P, Kivisaari L, et al. Magnetic resonance imaging of prostate cancer: does detection vary between high and low Gleason score tumors? Prostate 2000;43:43–8.
49. Outwater EK, Petersen RO, Siegelman ES, et al. Prostate carcinoma assessment of diagnostic criteria for capsular penetration on endorectal coil MR images. Radiology 1994; 193:333–9.
50. D'Amico AV, Whittington R, Schnall M, et al. The impact of the inclusion of endorectal coil magnetic resonance imaging in a multivariate analysis to predict clincally unsuspected extraprostatic cancer. Cancer 1995;75: 2368–72.
51. Rorvik J, Halvorsen OJ, Albrektsen G, et al. MRI with an endorectal coil for staging of clinically localized prostate cancer prior to radical prostatectomy. Eur Radiol 1999; 9:29–34.
52. Costello LC, Franklin RB. Concepts of citrate production and secretion by prostate 1. Metabolic relationships. Prostate 1991;18:25–46.
53. Kahn T, Burrig K, Schmitz-Drager B, et al. Prostatic carcinoma and benign prostatic hyperplasia: MR imaging with histopathologic correlation. Radiology 1989;173:847–51.
54. Scheibler ML, Tomaszewski JE, Bezzi M, et al. Prostatic carcinoma and benign prostatic hyperplasia: correlation of high-resolution MR and histopathologic findings. Radiology 1989;172:131–7.
55. Kaji Y, Kurhanewicz J, Hricak H, et al. Localizing prostate cancer in the presence of postbiopsy changes on MR images: role of proton MR spectroscopic imaging. Radiology 1998;206:785–90.
56. Kurhanewicz J, Vigneron DB, Hricak H, et al. Prostate cancer: metabolic response to cryosurgery as detected with 3D H-1 MR spectroscopic imaging. Radiology 1996;200:489–96.
57. Parivar F, Hricak H, Shinohara K, et al. Detection of locally recurrent prostate cancer after cryosurgery: evaluation by transrectal ultrasound, magnetic resonance imaging, and three-dimensional proton magnetic spectroscopy. Urology 1996;48:594–9.

58. Lin K, Szabo Z, Chin BB, Civelek C. The value of a baseline bone scan in patients with newly diagnosed prostate cancer. Clin Nucl Med 1998;24:579–82.
59. Freedman GM, Negendank WG, Hudes GR, et al. Preliminary results of a bone marrow magnetic resonance imaging protocol for patients with high-risk prostate cancer. Urology 1999;54:118–23.
60. Chybowski FM, Keller JJ, Bergstralh EJ, Oesterling JE. Predicting radionuclide bone scan findings in patients with newly diagnosed, untreated prostate cancer: prostate specific antigen is superior to all other clinical parameters. J Urol 1991;145:313.
61. Oesterling JE, Martin SK, Bergstralh MS, Lowe FC. The use of prostate-specific antigen in staging patients with newly diagnosed prostate cancer. JAMA 1993;269:57–60.
62. Salo JO, Kivisaari L, Rannikko S, Lehtonen T. Computerized tomography and transrectal ultrasound in the assessment of local extension of prostatic cancer before radical retropubic prostatectomy. J Urol 1987;137:435–8.
63. Lee N, Newhouse JH, Olsson CA, et al. Which patients with newly diagnosed prostate cancer need a computed tomography scan of the abdomen and pelvis? An analysis based on 588 patients. Urology 1999;54:490–4.
64. Oyen RH, Van Poppel HP, Ameye FE, et al. Lymph node staging of localized prostatic carcinoma with CT and CT-guided fine-needle aspiration biopsy: prospective study of 285 patients. Radiology 1994;190:315–22.
65. Wolf JS, Cher M, Dall'era M, et al. The use and accuracy of cross-sectional imaging and fine needle aspiration cytology for detection of pelvic lymph node metastases before radical prostatectomy. J Urol 1995;153(3 Pt 2):993–9.
66. Kahn D, Williams RD, Manyak MJ, et al. 111-Indium-capromab pendetide in the evaluation of patients with residual or recurrent prostate cancer after radical prostatectomy. J Urol 1998;159:2041–7.
67. Kahn D, Williams RD, Seldin DW, et al., Radioimmunoscintigraphy with In-111 labeled CYT-356 for the detection of occult prostate cancer recurrence. J Urol 1994;152:1952.
68. Texter JH, Neal CE. The role of monoclonal antibody in the management of prostate adenocarcinoma. J Urol 1998; 160:2393.
69. Babaian RJ, Sayer J, Podoloff DA, et al. Radioimmunoscintigraphy of pelvic lymph nodes with 111 indium-labeled monoclonal antibody CYT-356. J Urol 1994;152:1952.
70. Seltzer MA, Barbaric Z, Belldegrun A, et al. Comparison of helical computerized tomography, positron emission tomography and monoclonal antibody scans for evaluation of lymph node metastases in patients with prostate specific antigen relapse after treatment for localized prostate cancer. J Urol 1999;162:1322.

10

Staging: Initial Risk Assessment

JOSEPH C. PRESTI JR, MD

Accurate clinical staging is critical to the management of patients with prostate cancer. Treatment selection and treatment planning are influenced by local staging assessment. Most importantly, clinicians must distinguish between pathologically organ-confined disease (pT1–2) and non–organ-confined disease (pT3–4).

Physicians must use clinical parameters including digital rectal examination (DRE), tumor grade, serum prostate-specific antigen (PSA), transrectal ultrasonography (TRUS), endorectal magnetic resonance imaging (MRI), and needle biopsy information as they contribute to the prediction of pathologic stage and risk of relapse. The focus of this chapter is on studies that have correlated preoperative clinical information with the ability to predict pathologic stage and/or clinical outcome following radical prostatectomy. We recognize that this may introduce a verification bias as this information may not be generally applicable to the entire population of patients with prostate cancer since patients with locally advanced disease (gross pT3 or pT4) are usually not considered surgical candidates. However, with respect to local staging, radical prostatectomy specimens must be considered the gold standard.

TUMOR VOLUME AND STAGE

The progression of most, if not all, cancers is linked to cell division and tumor growth.[1] This observation has led to the hypothesis that the biologic behavior of a given prostate cancer will be directly related to the tumor volume. Careful step-sectioned histopathologic analyses of radical prostatectomy specimens have demonstrated a direct correlation between measured tumor volume and probability of extracapsular extension (ECE), seminal vesicle invasion, and lymph node metastases.[2,3] Extracapsular extension is rare in tumors less than 4 cc in size and is almost uniformly present in tumors larger than 12 cc in size. Risk of seminal vesicle invasion and lymph node metastases, although also related to tumor volume, is difficult to ascertain as a result of verification bias (patients with these features identified preoperatively are not taken to surgery). The importance of preoperative identification of tumor volume is clear from the above discussion; however, estimates of tumor volume must be based on clinically available information. Such preoperative information includes the results of the DRE, tumor grade, serum PSA, needle biopsy, and imaging.

A model to predict prostate cancer volume on the basis of preoperative clinical parameters has been proposed.[4] The model estimates the volume of prostate cancer (V_{ca}) and is defined as:

$$V_{ca} = \frac{\text{cancer-specific PSA/PSA leak into}}{\text{/PSA leak into serum per cc of cancer}}$$

Prostate-specific antigen leak is a constant as a function of Gleason sum, as defined in Table 10–1. Cancer-specific PSA is the preoperative serum PSA level (PSA_{preop}) corrected for the amount of PSA contributed from benign prostatic hyperplasia tissue and is defined as:

$$PSA_{preop} - [0.2 \times 0.33 \times \text{prostate volume}]$$

The prostate volume can be estimated by the TRUS measurement, whereas the coefficients are

Table 10–1. PSA LEAK AS A FUNCTION OF GLEASON GRADE

Gleason Sum	PSA Leak
2	20
3	15
4	10
5	7
6	4
7	3
8	2
9	1.5
10	1

PSA = prostate-specific antigen.

derived from an estimation of the fraction of total gland volume comprised of epithelium (0.2) and the estimated leakage of PSA into the serum per cc of benign epithelial tissue (0.33). Further validation of this model is needed by other centers to determine its widespread applicability.

DIGITAL RECTAL EXAMINATION

When palpable, prostate cancer is usually appreciated as induration of the prostate on DRE. Whitmore first described palpation of the prostate for staging in 1956, and the first staging system using the DRE result was reported by Jewett in 1975.[5,6] The subjectivity of DRE is well described, and significant understaging and, to a lesser extent, overstaging are seen when correlated with step-sectioned radical prostatectomy specimens. The frequency of pathologic understaging is partly related to clinical stage, ranging from 30% in clinical stage T1b to 60% in clinical stage T2 disease.[7,8] The utility of DRE in the staging of nonpalpable (T1c) prostate cancer is limited. This stage of disease is the most commonly diagnosed stage of disease at presentation today because of the widespread use of PSA. Parameters other than DRE are critical in staging these patients.

TUMOR GRADE

The Gleason grading system is the most commonly employed grading system for prostate cancer in the United States.[9] It is truly a system that relies on the "low-power" appearance of the glandular architecture under the microscope. In assigning a grade to a given tumor, pathologists assign a primary grade to the pattern of cancer that is most commonly observed and a secondary grade to the pattern of cancer that is the second most commonly observed grade in the specimen. Grades range from 1 to 5. If the entire specimen has only one pattern present, then both the primary and the secondary grade are reported as the same grade. The Gleason score or sum is obtained by adding the primary and secondary grades together. As Gleason grades range from 1 to 5, Gleason scores or sums will thus range from 2 to 10. Well-differentiated tumors have a Gleason sum of 2 to 4, moderately differentiated tumors have a Gleason sum of 5 to 6, and poorly differentiated tumors have a Gleason sum of 8 to 10. Historically, tumors with a Gleason sum of 7 have sometimes been grouped with the moderately differentiated tumors and at other times with the poorly differentiated tumors. One point that needs to be clarified is that it is perhaps the primary Gleason grade that is the most important with respect to placing patients into prognostic groups.[10] This is most important in assessing patients with a Gleason sum of 7. Patients who have a primary Gleason grade of 4 (4 + 3), tend to have a worse prognosis than patients with a primary Gleason grade of 3 (3+4). Many clinical series have failed to distinguish between these two populations, and in reviewing these series, caution must be exercised.

In general, the likelihood of having organ-confined disease decreases with increasing tumor grade. One report demonstrated organ-confined rates of 77%, 69%, 57%, 30%, and 13% for Gleason scores of 2 to 4, 5, 6, 7, and 8 to 10, respectively.[11] The reported rates of ECE, seminal vesicle invasion, and lymph node metastases increase with increasing tumor grade.

PROSTATE-SPECIFIC ANTIGEN

Prostate-specific antigen levels have been shown to correlate with both intraprostatic and extraprostatic tumor volume (correlation coefficient = .70).[12] Early reports demonstrated that the PSA level rises at a rate of approximately 3.5 ng/mL per cc of cancer and by 0.3 ng/mL per cc of benign prostatic hyperplasia by the Stamey and colleagues assay.[13] However, tumor grade may impact on the amount of PSA production in an individual patient, with higher-grade tumors producing less PSA than lower-grade tumors.[14] In addition, the amount and type of benign prostatic hyperplasia tissue (epithelial versus stromal) in a given patient is an extra variable that can alter an individual's PSA level. Although PSA may be helpful in studying large groups of patients, the accuracy in a single patient may be limited. In general, men with PSA levels < 4 ng/mL have organ-confined disease, whereas approximately 50% of patients with PSA levels > 10 ng/mL have ECE. Much overlap exists in men with PSA levels between 4 and 10 ng/mL.

NOMOGRAMS USING PROSTATE-SPECIFIC ANTIGEN, TUMOR GRADE, AND DIGITAL RECTAL EXAMINATION STAGE

As described above, individual use of DRE result, tumor grade, or PSA provides some information regarding the local stage of prostate cancer. However, combining these three preoperative parameters in a multinomial log-linear regression model has resulted in a more powerful predictor of pathologic tumor stage than any single parameter alone. One of the earliest and most widely used nomograms to predict pathologic tumor stage, the Partin nomogram (see Chapter 8), has been updated by combining data from three institutions.[15] Several other nomograms have been described that may be equally useful in providing physicians and patients with important information with respect to risk assessment and local staging.

Using information from these nomograms, patients may be assigned into one of three broadly defined risk groups for disease recurrence following local therapy based on PSA at diagnosis, tumor stage, and tumor grade. In general, low-risk patients are defined by low clinical stage (T1c–T2a), serum PSA at diagnosis < 10 ng/mL, and biopsy Gleason score of 6 or less, with no Gleason 4 or 5 pattern. Such patients appear to fare well after receiving local therapy alone, with a risk of disease recurrence ranging from 6 to 20%.[16] Indeed, some low-risk patients may not require local therapy owing to advanced age or comorbid conditions. Intermediate-risk patients are those with a serum PSA at diagnosis of 10 to 20 ng/mL, Gleason score of 7, or clinical stage T2b–T3a disease. For such patients, the risk of disease recurrence following local therapy is approximately 40 to 65%. High-risk patients have a serum PSA at diagnosis > 20 ng/mL or a Gleason score of 8 to 10. The risk of disease recurrence following local therapy alone in these patients may reach as high as 50 to 100%.[16]

PROSTATE-SPECIFIC ANTIGEN DENSITY

Prostate-specific antigen density (PSAD) is defined as the total serum PSA level (in ng/mL) divided by the volume of the prostate gland (in cc). Typically, the prostate volume is estimated using TRUS and a prolate ellipse formula; the volume equals $\pi/6 \times$ length $\times$ width $\times$ height, where length is obtained in the longitudinal plane and height and width are obtained in the axial plane. Conflicting results have been reported studying the utility of PSAD in comparison to PSA for cancer detection.[17–20]

Conflicting data on the utility of PSAD in predicting local stage and treatment failure following radical prostatectomy have been reported. One study of 107 patients demonstrated that using a PSAD cutoff of 0.35 stratified patients into two distinct groups: those with a PSAD > 0.35 had a failure rate of 66%, whereas those with a PSAD < 0.35 had a failure rate of 10%.[21] Another series failed to demonstrate a difference between PSA and PSAD in predicting local stage or risk of recurrence.[22] More recently, one group performed a multivariate analysis in a series of 198 radical prostatectomy patients with a PSA level < 10 ng/mL.[23] The model included Gleason score, serum PSA, percent free PSA, PSAD of the entire prostate, and PSAD of the transition zone. Prostate-specific antigen density of the transition zone and Gleason score were the most powerful predictors of extracapsular disease (relative risk of 60.5 and 1.4, respectively).

PERCENT FREE PROSTATE-SPECIFIC ANTIGEN

Recently, it has been recognized that there are different molecular forms of PSA in the serum, free PSA and protein-bound PSA. Approximately 90% of the serum PSA is bound to α_1-antichymotrypsin, whereas lesser amounts are free or bound to α_2-macroglobulins. In the latter form, no epitopes are available to the antibodies used in the current assays, whereas PSA bound to α_1-antichymotrypsin may have three of its five epitopes masked. The measurement of the ratio between unbound or free PSA to total PSA levels (percent free PSA or F/T PSA) has demonstrated utility in distinguishing between patients with PSA elevations resulting from benign prostatic hyperplasia from those with prostate cancer.[24]

Several studies have attempted to determine whether F/T PSA can aid in distinguishing between organ-confined and non–organ-confined prostate cancer. The two largest series have led to opposite results; however, it should be noted that these two studies used different F/T PSA assays. One study using the Dianon assay demonstrated no utility in predicting local staging in 301 radical prostatectomy patients.[25] A second study using the Hybritech assay demonstrated some utility in predicting local staging in 263 radical prostatectomy patients.[26] In the latter study, a F/T PSA cutoff of 15% resulted in a positive and negative predictive value for organ confinement of 76% and 53%, respectively. Further studies are ongoing to better define the utility of the F/T PSA assay in staging and risk of relapse.

SYSTEMATIC NEEDLE BIOPSY

Systematic sextant biopsy of the prostate has been shown to be superior to the use of lesion-directed biopsies in detecting prostate cancer.[27] Currently, most detection strategies include a systematic sextant technique that samples the prostate in the apex, mid, and base of the gland on the right and left sides (see Figure 8–1 in Chapter 8). However, the information from systematic prostate biopsy has been underused by clinicians. Typically, needle biopsy information is used to identify the presence or absence of cancer and assess the grade of the tumor. Needle biopsy information can also contribute to the estimation of tumor volume. Potential information from this systematic sampling regarding staging and/or risk of treatment failure has been neglected until recently.

SYSTEMATIC NEEDLE BIOPSY AND TUMOR VOLUME

Some investigators have demonstrated the utility of measuring the length of core involved with cancer as contributing to the prediction of tumor volume. This correlation appears to be highest for large cancers. A large degree of involvement of the core biopsies with cancer is strongly suggestive of high-stage disease.[28,29] A threshold of 3 mm of core length involvement on one core biopsy reliably predicts cancer volumes of 0.5 cc or larger.[30] However, the converse is not always true; focal cancer on the needle biopsy is not always associated with an insignificant cancer volume at radical prostatectomy. In a series of 33 consecutive radical prostatectomy patients who were identified as having focal prostate cancer on needle biopsy (single focus less than 3 mm in length on only one biopsy without any Gleason pattern 4 or 5), only 2 patients had a measured tumor volume of less than 0.5 mL in the radical prostatectomy specimen.[31] Such attempts at quantifying the length of needle core involvement are labor intensive and subject to interpretative variability. One study demonstrated no advantage of quantifying the total length of cancer involvement on all needle biopsies over the percentage of core biopsies involved (correlation coefficients of .47 and .49, respectively).[32] Another study demonstrated that PSAD, in conjunction with the maximum length of cancer involvement in any one core, was the most valuable means of predicting insignificant cancer at radical prostatectomy.[33]

A recent study has suggested that the performance of additional systematic biopsies may more accurately assess tumor volume. A scheme using 10 biopsies (conventional sextant biopsies in the peripheral zone bilaterally from the apex, mid, and base of the gland and adding bilateral biopsies of the transition zone and laterally directed biopsies of the peripheral zone in the midgland) more accurately predicted tumor volume than sextant biopsies alone (correlation coefficients of .56 and .39, respectively).[34] Further work is needed to define the optimal biopsy strategies for a given prostate size. The number and position of systematic biopsies would most likely vary with prostate size as differential zonal growth of the prostate occurs with enlargement (transition zone preferentially enlarges with benign growth), whereas propensity for malignancy preferentially resides within the peripheral zone.

SYSTEMATIC NEEDLE BIOPSY AND RISK OF EXTRACAPSULAR EXTENSION OR RECURRENCE

Analysis of the number of positive biopsies has been suggested by several investigators to contribute to the prediction of ECE at radical prostatectomy. This type of information might, in fact, differ from the quantitation of core length involvement as it represents a "mapping" of the prostate. This regional sampling of the prostate may be a surrogate to tumor volume and thus may contribute to the prediction of ECE and/or risk of treatment failure.

In one series, 100 radical prostatectomy patients were analyzed and several preoperative clinical parameters were studied in their ability to predict ECE and recurrence. Several parameters correlated with ECE, including a palpable nodule greater than one half of one lobe, a PSA > 25 ng/mL, a PSAD ≥ 0.6, perineural invasion on the needle core, and the involvement of ≥ 67% of the core biopsies obtained. The same parameters also correlated with serologic recurrence, but, in addition, the presence of bilaterally positive biopsies and the presence of Gleason score ≥ 7 on the biopsy also contributed to predicting recurrence.[35]

Peller and colleagues also demonstrated that the number of positive systematic sextant biopsies could be useful in predicting ECE at radical prostatectomy. These authors examined tumor extent in 102 radical prostatectomy specimens. ECE was discovered in 20% of specimens from patients with 3 or fewer positive prostate biopsies versus 76% of specimens from patients with 4 or more positive biopsies. Tumor grade also appeared to be important in this regards, as patients with 4 or more positive biopsies and a total Gleason score ≥ 7 had an increased risk of ECE when compared to patients with fewer positive biopsies and lower grade tumors.[36]

Huland and colleagues examined radical prostatectomy specimens from 257 consecutive patients to determine whether digital rectal examination, preoperative serum PSA level, tumor grade and systematic sextant biopsy results could be used to predict final pathologic tumor stage and the likelihood of tumor recurrence following surgery. With respect to tumor stage, preoperative serum PSA level, the number of positive prostate biopsies and biopsy tumor grade were significant predictors of capsular penetration and positive surgical margins. The number of positive prostate biopsies and biopsy Gleason score were the best predictors of tumor recurrence. Only 13% of patients with fewer than 3 positive biopsies and a total Gleason score ≤ 7 demonstrated biochemical diseasea recurrence within 2 years of surgery.[37]

Another series of 480 patients demonstrated that the probability of having organ-confined prostate cancer at radical prostatectomy decreased with the increasing percentage of positive sextant biopsies. Patients with < 33%, between 33 and 50%, and ≥ 50% of positive biopsies had an 84%, 62%, and 38% probability of being organ confined, respectively. Patients with < 50% of systematic biopsies positive demonstrated a disease-free survival of over 80% at 2 years.[38] These authors updated their results by examining the impact of percent positive biopsies on disease recurrence in 960 patients undergoing radical prostatectomy at two academic institutions.[39] Patients were placed into one of three risk groups (low, intermediate, or high) based on PSA at diagnosis, tumor grade, and tumor stage, as previously described. These investigators reported that the percentage of positive biopsies added significant information to other clinical measures when predicting outcome for intermediate-risk patients undergoing radical prostatectomy. Such information was clinically useful for 80% of intermediate-risk patients who could be classified as having either an 11% or an 86% risk of disease recurrence.[39]

Borirakchanyavat and colleagues reported on 104 patients who had undergone systematic sextant biopsy prior to radical prostatectomy. In the study, they performed a side-for-side analysis and demonstrated that the risk of ECE was 8% and 14% on sides containing none or one of three positive biopsies, whereas it was 37% and 43% in sides containing two or three positive biopsies, respectively.[40]

Presti and colleagues reported on a different patient population consisting of 109 patients who had undergone systematic sextant biopsy prior to radical prostatectomy.[41] No patients in this series received neoadjuvant or adjuvant therapy. This study correlated preoperative clinical parameters with the risk of serologic recurrence. Presti and colleagues demonstrated that patients who had four or more positive sextant biopsies were at a significantly higher risk of failure following radical prostatectomy than patients with three or less positive biopsies (relative risk = 2.4). In a multivariate Cox regression model, systematic biopsy results and tumor grade were the most powerful predictors of serologic relapse (relative risk = 2.3 and 1.9, respectively). It was interesting to note that in the multivariate analysis, PSA dropped out of the model. This may be because systematic biopsies are a better surrogate of tumor volume than PSA.

Information from the systematic set of prostate biopsies has also been shown to be an important predictor of extraprostatic disease extension and outcome following radical prostatectomy using data from CaPSURE, a large national disease registry of patients with prostate cancer treated predominantly in community-based practice settings. In a group of 1,313 patients undergoing radical prostatectomy, univariate and multivariate analyses demonstrated that PSA at diagnosis, biopsy Gleason score, and the percentage of positive biopsies were all important predictors of extraprostatic disease extension, whereas the percentage of positive biopsies was the strongest predictor of understaging on multivariate analysis.[42] This effect was most evident for patients with intermediate- or high-risk disease based on serum PSA at diagnosis and biopsy Gleason score. In a follow-up study, serum PSA at diagnosis, biopsy Gleason score, and percent positive biopsies were also found to be significant independent predictors of disease recurrence in 1,265 CaPSURE patients undergoing radical prostatectomy.[43] When assigning patients into risk groups, as described above, the percentage of positive prostate biopsies was found to be a significant predictor of disease recurrence for patients in the low-, intermediate-, and high-risk groups. For patients with high-risk disease, the likelihood of disease recurrence 5 years following surgery was 24%, 34%, and 59% for patients with 0 to 33%, 34 to 66%, and > 66% positive biopsies, respectively ($p < .0001$).

Several investigators have recently reported that increasing the number of systematic biopsies results in an increase in cancer detection rate. One group reported the results of a five-region biopsy technique that included laterally directed biopsies of the peripheral zone and a central region of biopsy in addition to the usual sextant biopsy samples.[44] A 35% improvement in detection rate compared to sextant biopsy alone was achieved, with nearly all of the improvement found in the far lateral biopsies. We recently reported on our prospective study comparing routine sextant biopsies with sextant plus additional lateral peripheral zone biopsies (lateral midgland and lateral base; see Figure 8–3 in Chapter 8) and demonstrated a 14% increase in cancer detection with the addition of the lateral peripheral zone biopsies.[45] We have previously demonstrated an increased cancer detection rate in large prostates (> 50 cc) by performing six systematic biopsies of the transition zone in addition to the sextant biopsies of the peripheral zone.[46] These studies demonstrate that six biopsies are probably not adequate systematic sampling for all prostates with respect to cancer detection. Additional studies are needed to assess the possible role of these extended systematic biopsy schemes in cancer volume estimates, local staging, and risk of relapse.

IMAGING

Transrectal ultrasonography has consistently been proven to be more accurate for local staging than DRE.[47–49] Magnetic resonance imaging using a body coil has also been used in the local staging of prostate cancer and has provided better information than DRE alone.[50,51] However, a comparative trial of TRUS with body coil MRI in the staging of prostate cancer did not demonstrate a statistical difference between the two modalities.[52] Since that study, numerous technical advances have been made for MRI most notably the development of an endorectal surface coil.[53] One report demonstrated that endorectal MRI has a 58% sensitivity and a 78% specificity in detecting ECE and an overall staging accuracy of 68%.[54] A second study reported an overall staging accuracy of 51% for endorectal MRI.[55] One prospective comparative trial assessing the relative merit of TRUS and endorectal MRI in assessing the local stage of carcinoma of the prostate failed to demonstrate any significant difference in the imaging modalities.[56] The costs associated with endorectal MRI are high, and until this methodology is demonstrated to provide superior clinical information that alters patient management, its use should be limited. Attempts at defining patients who could potentially benefit from this imaging are ongoing.

CONCLUSIONS

Refinement in the local staging and risk assessment for patients with prostate cancer using clinical parameters is ongoing. Digital rectal examination, tumor grade, and PSA provide some useful information for risk assessment in individual patients. More recent studies employing percent free PSA levels and systematic biopsy results have added additional staging information and may play a more significant role in the future in risk assessment. This information should supplement additional imaging tests in the management of these patients.

REFERENCES

1. Cohen SM, Ellwein LB. Cell proliferation in carcinogenesis. Science 1990;249:1007–11.
2. McNeal JE, Villers AA, Redwine EA, et al. Histologic differentiation, cancer volume and pelvic lymph node metastasis in adenocarcinoma of the prostate. Cancer 1990;66:1225–33.
3. McNeal JE. Cancer volume and site of origin of adenocarcinoma in the prostate: relationship to local and distant spread. Hum Pathol 1992;23:258–66.
4. D'Amico AV, Whittington R, Schultz D, et al. Outcome based staging for clinically localized adenocarcinoma of the prostate. J Urol 1997;158:1422–6.
5. Whitmore WF Jr. Hormone therapy in prostate cancer. Am J Med 1956;21:697–713.
6. Jewett HJ. The present status of radical prostatectomy for stages A and B prostatic cancer. Urol Clin North Am 1975;2:105–24.
7. Zincke H, Oesterling JE, Blute ML, et al. Long term (15 year) results after radical prostatectomy for clinically localized (stage T2c or lower) prostate cancer. J Urol 1994;152:1850–7.
8. Paulson DF. The impact of radical prostatectomy in the management of clinically localized disease. J Urol 1994;152:1826–30.
9. Gleason DF, Mellinger GT, and the Veterans Administration Cooperative Urological Research Group. Prediction of prognosis for prostatic adenocarcinoma by combined histological grading and clinical staging. J Urol 1974;111:58–64.
10. Epstein JI, Partin AW, Sauvageot J, Walsh PC. Prediction of progression following radical prostatectomy: a multivariate analysis of 721 men with long-term follow-up. Am J Surg Pathol 1996;20:286–92.
11. Partin AW, Yoo JK, Carter HB, et al. The use of prostate-specific antigen, clinical stage and Gleason score to predict pathological stage in men with localized prostate cancer. J Urol 1993;150:110–4.
12. Stamey TA, Kabalin JN, McNeal JE, et al. Prostate specific antigen in the diagnosis and treatment of adenocarcinoma of the prostate. II. Radical prostatectomy treated patients. J Urol 1989;141:1076–83.
13. Stamey TA, Yang N, Hay AR, et al. Prostate-specific antigen as a serum marker for adenocarcinoma of the prostate. N Engl J Med 1987;317:909–16.
14. Partin AW, Carter B, Chan DW, et al. Prostate specific antigen in the staging of localized prostate cancer: influence of tumor differentiation, tumor volume and benign hyperplasia. J Urol 1990;143:747–52.
15. Partin AW, Kattan MW, Subong EN, et al. Combination of prostate-specific antigen, clinical stage, and Gleason score to predict pathological stage of localized prostate cancer. JAMA 1997;277:1445–51.
16. Carroll PR, Lee KL, Fuks ZY, Kantoff PW. Cancer of the prostate. In: DeVita VT, Hellman S, Rosenberg SA, editors. Cancer: principles and practice of oncology. 6th ed. Philadelphia: Lippincott Williams and Wilkins; 2001. p. 1418–79.
17. Benson MC, Whang IS, Pantuck A, et al. Prostate-specific antigen density: a means of distinguishing benign prostatic hypertrophy and prostate cancer. J Urol 1992;147:815–6.
18. Brawer MK, Aramburu EAG, Chen GL, et al. The inability of prostate specific antigen index to enhance the predictive value of prostate specific antigen in the diagnosis of prostatic carcinoma. J Urol 1993;150:369–73.
19. Catalona WJ, Richie JP, deKernion JB, et al. Comparison of prostate specific antigen concentration versus prostate specific antigen density in the early detection of prostate cancer: receiver operating characteristic curves. J Urol 1994;152:2031–6.
20. Presti JC Jr, Hovey R, Bhargava V, et al. Prospective evaluation of prostate specific antigen and prostate specific antigen density in the detection of carcinoma of the prostate: ethnic variations. J Urol 1997;157:907–12.
21. Seaman E, Whang M, Olsson CA, et al. PSA density (PSAD): role in patient evaluation and management. Urol Clin North Am 1993;20:653–63.
22. Shinohara K, Wolf JS Jr, Narayan P, Carroll PR. Comparison of prostate specific antigen with prostate specific antigen density for 3 clinical applications. J Urol 1994;152:120–3.
23. Zlotta AR, Petein DM, Susani M, et al. Prostate specific antigen density of the transition zone for predicting pathological stage of localized prostate cancer in patients with serum prostate specific antigen less than 10 ng/ml. J Urol 1998;160:2089–95.
24. Catalona WJ, Partin AW, Slawin KM, et al. Use of the percentage of free prostate-specific antigen to enhance differentiation of prostate cancer from benign prostatic disease: a prospective multicenter clinical trial. JAMA 1998;279:1542–7.
25. Pannek J, Subong ENP, Jones K, et al. The role of free/total prostate-specific antigen ratio in the prediction of final pathological stage for men with clinically localized prostate cancer. Urology 1996;48:51–4.
26. Pannek J, Rittenhouse HG, Chan DW, et al. The use of per-

cent free prostate specific antigen for staging clinically localized prostate cancer. J Urol 1988;159:1238–42.
27. Hodge KK, McNeal JE, Terris MK, Stamey TA. Random systematic versus directed ultrasound guided transrectal core biopsies of the prostate. J Urol 1989;142:71–5.
28. Terris MK, McNeal JE, Stamey TA. Detection of clinically significant prostate cancer by transrectal ultrasound-guided systematic biopsies. J Urol 1992;148:829–32.
29. Hammerer P, Huland H, Sparenberg A. Digital rectal examination, imaging, and systematic sextant biopsy in identifying operable lymph node-negative prostatic carcinoma. Eur Urol 1992;22:281–7.
30. Dietrick DD, McNeal JE, Stamey TA. Core cancer length in ultrasound-guided systematic sextant biopsies: a preoperative evaluation of prostate cancer volume. Urology 1995; 45:987–92.
31. Weldon VE, Tavel FR, Neuwirth H, Cohen R. Failure of focal prostate cancer on biopsy to predict focal prostate cancer: the importance of prevalence. J Urol 1995;154:1074–7.
32. Cupp MR, Bostwick DG, Myers RP, Oesterling JE. The volume of prostate cancer in the biopsy specimen cannot reliably predict the quantity of cancer in the radical prostatectomy specimen on an individual basis. J Urol 1995;153:1543–8.
33. Goto Y, Ohori M, Arakawa A, et al. Distinguishing clinically important from unimportant prostate cancers before treatment: value of systematic biopsies. J Urol 1996;156: 1059–63.
34. Egevad L, Norberg M, Mattson S, et al. Estimation of prostate cancer volume by multiple core biopsies before radical prostatectomy. Urology 1998;52:653–8.
35. Ravery V, Boccon-Gibod LA, Dauge-Geffroy MC, et al. Systematic biopsies accurately predict extracapsular extension of prostate cancer and persistent/recurrent detectable PSA after radical prostatectomy. Urology 1994;44:371–6.
36. Peller PA, Young DC, Marmaduke DP, et al. Sextant prostate biopsies. A histopathologic correlation with radical prostatectomy specimens. Cancer 1995;75:530–8.
37. Huland H, Hammerer P, Henke RP, Huland E. Preoperative prediction of tumor heterogeneity and recurrence after radical prostatectomy for localized prostatic carcinoma with digital rectal examination, prostate specific antigen and the results of 6 systematic biopsies. J Urol 1996;155:1344–7.
38. D'Amico AV, Whittington R, Malkowicz SB, et al. Combined modality staging of prostate carcinoma and its utility in predicting pathologic stage and postoperative prostate specific antigen failure. Urology 1997;49:23–30.
39. D'Amico AV, Whittington R, Malkowicz SB, et al. Clinical utility of the percentage of positive prostate biopsies in defining biochemical outcome after radical prostatectomy for patients with clinically localized prostate cancer. J Clin Oncol 2000;18:1164–72.
40. Borirakchanyavat S, Bhargava V, Shinohara K, et al. Systematic sextant biopsies in the prediction of extracapsular extension at radical prostatectomy. Urology 1997;50:373–8.
41. Presti JC Jr, Shinohara K, Bacchetti P, et al. The positive fraction of systematic biopsies predicts risk of relapse following radical prostatectomy. Urology 1998;52:1079–84.
42. Grossfeld GD, Chang JJ, Broering JM, et al. Under staging and under grading in a contemporary series of patients undergoing radical prostatectomy: results from the Cancer of the Prostate Strategic Urologic Research Endeavor database. J Urol 2001;165:851–6.
43. Grossfeld GD, Latini DM, Lubech DP, et al. Predicting disease recurrence in intermediate and high-risk patients undergoing medical prostatectomy using percent positive biopsies: results from CAPSURE. Urology 2002;59:560–5.
44. Eskew LA, Bare RL, McCullough DL. Systematic 5 region prostate biopsy is superior to sextant method for diagnosing carcinoma of the prostate. J Urol 1997;157:199–203.
45. Chang JJ, Shinohara K, Bhargava V, Presti JC Jr. Prospective evaluation of lateral biopsies of the peripheral zone for prostate cancer detection. J Urol 1998;160:2111–4.
46. Chang JJ, Shinohara K, Hovey RM, et al. Prospective evaluation of systematic sextant transition zone biopsies in large prostates for cancer detection. Urology 1998;52::89–93.
47. Perrapato SD, Carothers GG, Maatman TJ, Soechtig CE. Comparing clinical staging plus transrectal ultrasound with surgical-pathological staging of prostate cancer. Urology 1989;33:103–5.
48. Scardino PT, Shinohara K, Wheeler TM, St. C. Carter S. Staging of prostate cancer: value of ultrasonography. Urol Clin North Am 1989;16:713–34.
49. Andriole GL, Coplen DE, Mikkelsen DJ, Catalona WJ. Sonographic and pathological staging of patients with clinically localized prostate cancer. J Urol 1989;142:1259–61.
50. Hricak H, Dooms GC, Jeffrey RB, et al. Prostatic carcinoma: staging by clinical assessment, CT and MR imaging. Radiology 1987;162:331–6.
51. Bezzi M, Kressel HY, Allen KS, et al. Prostatic carcinoma: staging with MR imaging at 1.5 T. Radiology 1988;169: 339–46.
52. Rifkin MD, Zerhouni EA, Gatsonis CA, et al. Comparison of magnetic resonance imaging and ultrasonography in staging early prostate cancer: results of a multi-institutional cooperative trial. N Engl J Med 1990;323:621–6.
53. Pollack HM, Schnall MD. Magnetic resonance imaging in carcinoma of the prostate. Prostate 1992;4:17–31.
54. Chelsky MJ, Schnall MD, Seidmon EJ, Pollack HM. Use of endorectal surface coil magnetic resonance imaging for local staging of prostate cancer. J Urol 1993;150:391–5.
55. Quinn SF, Franzini DA, Demlow TA, et al. MR imaging of prostate cancer with an endorectal surface coil technique: correlation with whole-mount specimens. Radiology 1994;190:323–7.
56. Presti JC Jr, Hricak H, Narayan PA, et al. Local staging of prostatic carcinoma: comparison of transrectal sonography and endorectal MR imaging. AJR Am J Roentgenol 1996;166:103–8.

11

Natural History

GARY D. GROSSFELD, MD, FACS
PETER R. CARROLL, MD, FACS

Neoplastic disease is a proliferative disorder that is characterized by uncontrolled cellular growth.[1] Such unregulated proliferation of genetically altered cells often has a predictable natural history, beginning with a marked increase in the local tumor burden. This exponential increase in cell number may predispose the malignant cells to acquire additional genetic alterations, some of which may enable a population of cells to break off from the primary tumor mass and travel to distant metastatic sites. Metastatic tumor growth often results in the compromise and eventual demise of the host.

Whereas the natural history of many solid malignancies may follow such a predictable course that eventually leads to the death of the patient, the natural history of prostate cancer is not as well defined. Prostate cancer is the most commonly diagnosed solid tumor in American men and the second leading cause of cancer-related death in this population. Indeed, it was estimated that 179,300 new cases of prostate cancer would be diagnosed in 1999, leading to 37,000 deaths caused by this disease.[2] Although the risk of developing prostate cancer from birth in men living in the United States is approximately 9 to 11%, the risk of dying of prostate cancer in the same men is only 2.6 to 4.3%.[3] Thus, only 25 to 33% of men who develop prostate cancer will eventually die of the disease.[3,4]

Despite the frequency with which it is detected, prostate cancer initiation is likely a more common event than is clinically identified. It has been estimated that one in every three men over the age of 45 will demonstrate histologic evidence of prostate cancer during his lifetime.[5] This frequency increases with age; histologic evidence of prostate cancer may be present in up to 80% of men by age 80.[6] Even though a significant proportion of men will harbor histologic evidence of prostate cancer, the disease does not become clinically evident in all cases. This had led some to use the term "latent prostate cancer" to describe tumors that are histologically detectable but clinically unrecognized during the patient's lifetime. In still other men, the disease may follow a protracted course, and because the incidence of prostate cancer increases with age, death from competing causes may render such clinically recognized prostate cancers insignificant with respect to the patient's overall survival. Thus, when the natural history of prostate cancer is considered, one must consider not only the malignant potential of the tumor but also the natural history of the host.[7] Despite the protracted natural history of prostate cancer in some patients, it is clear that the disease pursues a more aggressive course in others. Unfortunately, the mechanism by which prostate cancer becomes a clinically detectable, life-threatening disease remains unknown.

This variable natural history has led some authors to advocate conservative treatment, or "watchful waiting," as management for patients newly diagnosed with prostate cancer. Reports of conservative treatment date back many years, and provide some insight into the natural history of prostate cancer. In 1926, Bumpus described disease-specific outcomes for untreated patients diagnosed with prostate cancer.[8] This report included patients with and without evidence of metastatic disease. For patients without metastases, the average time from diagnosis until death was approximately 1 year, with 58% of patients dying of disease during that time interval. In contrast, nearly two-thirds of patients with distant metastases died within 9 months of diagnosis. In 1946, Nesbit and Plumb examined 477 men with prostate cancer and no evidence of metastases and compared them with 260 patients with prostate cancer who presented with metastatic disease at diagnosis.[9] For patients with no evidence of metastases, the mean interval from diagnosis until death was 23.6 months (median = 12.8 months, range = 1 to 180 months). In contrast, the mean interval from diagnosis until death was only 16.9 months (median = 9.6 months, range = 1 to 176 months) for patients with metastatic disease. Similarly, in 1950, Nesbitt and Baum reported the 1-, 3-, and 5-year survivals for patients with prostate cancer with and without metastases at diagnosis.[10] Survival was 54%, 22%, and 10% at 1, 3, and 5 years after diagnosis, respectively, for patients without metastases, and 47%, 11%, and 6% for patients with documented metastatic disease at presentation.

Whitmore has defined the natural history of prostate cancer as "the evolution of clinical and pathologic manifestations" from the inception of the tumor until the death of the untreated host.[7] Although there are many series in the literature that document disease-specific outcomes in patients with prostate cancer treated "conservatively," contemporary reports documenting the true natural history of the disease are difficult to find. This is because most contemporary series include patients who receive some type of anticancer treatment, usually androgen deprivation, at some point during the course of their disease. Nevertheless, these "watchful waiting" series do provide the best available information regarding the natural history of prostate cancer in large groups of patients who are followed for many years after diagnosis without receiving curative treatment.

The purpose of this chapter is to summarize the most current information available regarding the natural history of untreated prostate cancer and prostate cancer in patients treated with noncurative intent. To accomplish this goal, the following topics will be addressed: (1) the natural history of incidentally discovered low-volume prostate cancer, (2) local and metastatic tumor progression in patients treated with noncurative intent, (3) disease-specific survival in patients treated with noncurative intent, (4) the need for additional cancer-specific treatment in these patients, and (5) predictors of tumor progression.

NATURAL HISTORY OF INCIDENTALLY DISCOVERED LOW-VOLUME PROSTATE CANCER

Although watchful waiting is a treatment option for patients with all stages of prostate cancer, conservative management has traditionally been the preferred treatment option for patients with incidentally discovered stage T1a prostate cancer. A patient becomes aware that he has stage T1 prostate cancer following pathologic examination of tissue removed by transurethral resection of the prostate (TURP) or open enucleation for presumed benign prostatic hyperplasia (BPH). Approximately 10% of men undergoing such procedures will be diagnosed with incidental prostate cancer.[11–16] In 1975, Jewett proposed that stage A (T1) tumors be subdivided into those of low biologic potential that pursue an indolent course and rarely progress (low stage and low grade) and those with a more aggressive biologic potential and a high likelihood of progression if left untreated (high grade and/or high volume).[17] The most recent American Joint Committee on Cancer staging system for prostate cancer categorizes incidentally discovered tumors into stages T1a and T1b disease based on tumor volume in the resected specimen.[18] Stage T1a disease is defined by tumor in less than 5% of the resected specimen, whereas stage T1b is defined by 5% or more of the specimen containing prostate cancer. Tumor grade is not considered in this staging system.

Given that stage T1a tumors cause no symptoms and that these tumors are presumed indolent based on low stage and grade at diagnosis, conservative management is the recommended treatment course for many of these patients. This makes such patients appropriate subjects in whom to investigate the natural history of low-stage prostate cancer. Prior to discussing the natural history of these tumors, however, it is important to determine whether stage T1a prostate cancers represent incidental, low-volume, unifocal tumors or whether they actually represent the "tip of the iceberg" for a larger, peripherally based malignancy. To address this issue, several studies have examined radical prostatectomy specimens from patients with clinical stage T1a disease and described the incidence and characteristics of any residual prostatic cancers. On average, these series report that 20% of patients with stage T1a prostate cancer have no evidence of residual tumor in the prostatectomy specimen (range = 0 to 53%), 40% of patients have minimal residual disease (range, 14 to 74%), and 40% have substantial residual disease that justifies a higher pathologic tumor stage (range = 13 to 86%).[19–24] Included with the patients who are upstaged are 8 to 17% who either have evidence of extracapsular disease extension, positive surgical margins, seminal vesicle invasion, or lymph node metastases.

McNeal and colleagues described the morphologic features of radical prostatectomy specimens obtained from 11 patients with clinical stage T1 prostate cancer and compared these tumors with specimens obtained from 73 patients with clinical stage T2 disease.[25] This study demonstrated that all stage T1 cancers were located anteromedially (commonly invading the anterior fibromuscular stroma), whereas most stage T2 cancers were located posteriorly. Other than location, the stage T1 and T2 cancers were similar with respect to range of tumor volume and degree of differentiation. Both stages of tumor demonstrated progressive dedifferentiation with increasing tumor volume. These results strongly suggested that although different in their sites of origin, stage T1 and T2 tumors were similar with respect to their biologic potentials. In a related study from Voges and colleagues, morphometric analysis was performed on 44 radical prostatectomy specimens removed from patients with clinical stage T1 tumors (22 patients with stage T1a and 22 patients with stage T1b cancer).[24] Six of the 22 specimens (27%) removed for clinical stage T1a disease demonstrated extracapsular disease extension on final pathologic analysis, whereas 5 of the 22 specimens (23%) demonstrated positive surgical margins. Furthermore, 90% of the specimens from patients with clinical stage T1a disease demonstrated unsuspected cancers that were apparently unrelated to the index tumor identified at the time of transurethral resection. Eighty-three percent of these unsuspected tumors were located outside of the transition zone and 26% measured greater than 0.2 cm^3 in volume.

It is evident from these radical prostatectomy studies that a significant percentage of patients with clinical stage T1a prostate cancer will have substantial residual tumor present after the initial transurethral resection. In some instances, these tumors may be multifocal and exhibit adverse pathologic characteristics (including extracapsular disease extension and positive surgical margins). Thus, examining the clinical outcomes of such patients who are managed expectantly may provide important insight into the natural history of the disease.

Most early studies suggested that stage T1a prostate cancer had little impact on either overall or prostate cancer–specific survival. Generally, a 10-year disease-specific mortality rate of less than 5% was associated with expectant management of such patients, likely attributable to a high prevalence of comorbid conditions in this patient population leading to death from intercurrent illness.[16] In a study of 847 consecutive patients undergoing suprapubic prostatectomy for BPH, Bauer and colleagues found that 28 patients had well-differentiated prostate cancer at the time of surgery.[26] Overall survival rates for these patients at 5 and 10 years following diagnosis were 75% and 47%, respectively. Consequently, these authors suggested that small, well differentiated, incidentally discovered prostate cancers may require no further treatment. Hanash and colleagues reported disease-specific outcomes for 21 patients with incidentally discovered, low-grade prostate cancers who were managed expectantly.[27] Overall survival 5 years after diagnosis was reported to be 100% for these patients, and survival in this group of patients continued to be superior to expected survival (based on life table analysis) for up to 15 years after diagnosis.

Because of the high rate of intercurrent illness in this patient population, disease progression has replaced overall survival as the end point for measuring the biologic potential of stage T1a prostate cancer. In 1981, Cantrell and colleagues examined the rate of disease progression in 49 patients with stage T1a disease and at least 4 years of follow-up after diagnosis.[28] Disease progression was reported in only 1 patient (2%) during this period (Table 11–1), confirming the low biologic potential of this stage of disease. However, because of increasing life expectancy, patients with stage T1a prostate cancer who are managed expectantly will now spend more time alive with their prostate cancer. Consequently, the policy of expectant management for these patients has recently been challenged. Several studies have demonstrated the potential not only for disease progression but also for death owing to disease in these patients.[15,29,30] More recent studies, with long-term follow-up, suggest that disease progression can occur in 10 to 27% of patients with stage T1a prostate cancer who are managed expectantly for 7 to 10 years after diagnosis (see Table 11–1). Epstein and colleagues reported the results of 50 men with stage T1a prostate cancer who were managed expectantly and followed for at least 8 years after diagnosis.[30] In this study, 8 patients (16%) experienced disease progression, and 6 of these 8 patients died of prostate cancer within an average of 2 years after progression. Neither tumor volume in the TURP specimen nor tumor grade predicted which patients would ultimately progress. Thompson and Zeidman followed 60 patients with stage T1a prostate cancer for an average of 7.5 years after diagnosis.[15] Although the overall rate of disease progression was low in this group of patients (5%), 8% of patients at risk for at least 7 years demonstrated progressive disease, and all 3 patients who progressed died of disease within 1 year of progression. Similar to the findings of Epstein and colleagues, these authors reported no correlation between tumor volume at TURP and disease progression. Blute and colleagues reported progressive disease in 27% of men with stage T1a prostate cancer managed expectantly, with the median time to progression being 10.2 years.[31] Three of the 4 patients who progressed in this study were found to have systemic disease. Finally, Ingerman and colleagues reported disease progression in 13% of patients with stage T1a prostate cancer presumed to be at low risk owing to a negative staging TURP.[32] Of the 3 patients who progressed, 1 did so with metastatic disease.

Table 11–1. NATURAL HISTORY OF UNTREATED STAGE T1a PROSTATE CANCER

Lead Author	Year	N	Number with Progression (%)	Follow-up (yr)
Heaney[65]	1977	50*	3 (6)	NS
Correa[66]	1974	39*	3 (8)	NS
Cantrell[28]	1981	49	1 (2)	At least 4
Blute[31]	1986	15	4 (27)	10.2†
Epstein[30]	1986	50	8 (16)	At least 8
Thompson[15]	1989	60	3 (5)	7.5
Lowe[67]	1990	80	12 (15)	8.4
Roy[29]	1990	19	3 (16)	NS
Zhang[68]	1991	132	13 (10)	8.2
Ingerman[32]	1993	24‡	3 (13)	7

NS = not specified.
*Some patients in these series were treated with radical prostatectomy or hormonal therapy.
†Median time to progression.
‡All patients without residual carcinoma on repeat transurethral resection of the prostate.

Additional evidence in support of the observation that stage T1a prostate cancer may progress over time comes from a study performed by Brawn.[33] In this study, Brawn examined TURP specimens from 54 patients with prostate cancer who required two separate transurethral resections. The second procedure was performed from 3 to 11 years after the initial TURP. Of 26 patients with grade 1 prostate cancer at the time of initial TURP, 19 (73%) had higher-grade tumors at repeat resection. In addition, 75% of grade 2 lesions and 88% of grade 3 lesions dedifferentiated into a higher grade at repeat TURP. All 8 poorly differentiated tumors (grade 4) remained poorly differentiated on both resections. Grade was unchanged in only 10 (19%) patients, and only 1 lesion demonstrated a lower grade at repeat resection (from grade 2 to grade 1). Moreover, the presence of metastases was associated with tumor grade. Whereas no grade 1 tumors demonstrated metastases, 19% of the grade 2 lesions, 55% of the grade 3 lesions, and 80% of the grade 4 lesions were associated with metastatic disease. These data suggest that low-grade prostate cancers may have the ability to dedifferentiate over time and that progression of disease may be a consequence of such dedifferentiation.

Therefore, studies that have examined the natural history of untreated stage T1a prostate cancer suggest that a significant percentage of these tumors have the potential for progression with long-term follow-up. Not only can these tumors progress locally, but there is also evidence to suggest that systemic progression, leading to death from disease, may be possible. It does not appear that the likelihood of progression can be reliably predicted from the findings at TURP, but the major risk factor for progression appears to be extended follow-up.

NATURAL HISTORY OF PROSTATE CANCER: DISEASE PROGRESSION

In most instances, solid malignancies that remain untreated will continue to grow locally and eventually progress to metastatic disease. Although this progression is likely to occur in many patients with prostate cancer, factors such as patient age at diagnosis and tumor grade and stage at presentation may significantly impact which patients with prostate cancer will ultimately demonstrate progressive disease. Prostate cancer is often a disease of older men. Thus, some patients will succumb to comorbid conditions prior to experiencing tumor progression, especially older patients with low-grade, low-stage disease at diagnosis. The determination of local disease progression is also complicated by imprecise measures of local tumor extent. Local disease progression is often based on digital rectal examination, which is a crude measure of tumor volume. Despite these issues, several studies have determined the likelihood of local tumor progression and progression to metastatic disease in patients with prostate cancer who remain untreated or those who are treated with noncurative intent. These studies differ from those summarized in Table 11–1 as they not only include patients with incidentally diagnosed low-grade, low-stage disease, they also include patients diagnosed with prostate cancer by digital rectal examination and patients with more extensive disease at the time of TURP.

Table 11–2 summarizes the risk of local and distant tumor progression in patients with prostate cancer who remain untreated and those who are treated conservatively with immediate or deferred androgen deprivation. The risk of local progression in these series ranges from 8 to 84%, whereas the risk of progression to metastatic disease ranges from 6 to 74% (see Table 11–2). It is important to emphasize several points when interpreting these results. Although the age at diagnosis differs among patients in these studies, the average age at prostate cancer diagnosis is greater than 70 years in many of these series. Thus, these figures may underestimate the risk of disease progression for younger patients with prostate cancer who are likely to live longer with their disease. In addition, follow-up in these studies ranges from 4 to 14 years after diagnosis, and such differences likely account for the wide range of local and distant progression reported. Many studies

Table 11–2. ESTIMATES OF LOCAL AND METASTATIC TUMOR PROGRESSION IN PROSTATE CANCER PATIENTS WHO REMAIN UNTREATED AND THOSE WHO ARE TREATED WITH NONCURATIVE INTENT

Lead Author	Year	N	Mean Follow-up (yr)	Local Tumor Progression	Metastatic Tumor Progression
Egawa[34]	1993	107	6.2	8% of patients	23% of patients
George[39]	1988	120	7	84% of patients	11% of patients
Warner[41]	1994	75	11.2–13.5	77.3% of patients; median time to progression 78 mo	Median time to progression 186 mo
Byar[48]	1981	50	6.8–7.7	NS	6% of patients
Adolfsson[36] (clinical T3)	1999	50	7.75	66% of patients	22% at 5 yr, 34% at 10 yr
Adolfsson[37] (clinically localized)	1997	122	9.1	NS	18% at 10 yr, 52% at 15 yr
Adolfsson[38] (age < 70)	1991	61	8.0	49% at 5 yr, 72% at 10 yr	8% at 5 yr, 23% at 10 yr
Rana[35]	1994	199	4.2	26% of patients	46% of patients
Johansson[40]	1997	223	14	33% of untreated patients with localized disease	13% of untreated patients with localized disease
Chodak[49]	1994	828	6.6	NS	19% of grade 1, 42% of grade 2, 74% of grade 3 at 10 yr

NS = not specified.

include a preponderance of patients with low-grade and/or low-stage disease who were selected for watchful waiting or conservative treatment from a larger group of patients presenting with prostate cancer. This selection bias certainly will lead to underestimation of disease progression in the general population of patients with untreated prostate cancer. As stated above, the definition of local progression in the majority of these series was based on changes in digital rectal examination that were suggestive of local tumor growth or disease spread outside of the prostatic capsule. This is an imprecise measure that may influence the reporting of local tumor progression. It is interesting to note that Egawa and colleagues and Rana and colleagues defined local progression by the development of bladder outlet obstruction, necessitating surgical intervention.[34,35] These were the only studies in Table 11–2 in which distant progression exceeded local progression. Finally, it must be emphasized that the proportion of patients receiving endocrine therapy, as well as the timing and indications for such treatment, differed among the different studies. In some studies, patients were treated at the time of tumor progression only,[36–41] whereas in others, a proportion of patients received immediate androgen deprivation at the time of diagnosis.[34,35]

Recognizing these limitations, the estimates in Table 11–2 still represent the best and most contemporary data available regarding local and metastatic tumor progression in patients with prostate cancer who are treated conservatively with either observation or immediate or deferred androgen deprivation. Thus, these data provide some insight into the natural history of prostate cancer progression. Differences between the studies with respect to patient age at diagnosis, clinical tumor stage and histologic tumor grade, and their impact on disease progression and cancer-specific survival are discussed below.

NATURAL HISTORY OF PROSTATE CANCER: DISEASE-SPECIFIC SURVIVAL

The most important measure of the natural history of any malignancy is its ability to cause the death of the patient. Previous studies have attempted to quantify the lethality of untreated prostate cancer by determining how often it is the underlying cause leading to the death of the patient. Similar to the studies cited above regarding disease progression, it is difficult to compare these series given the different age and risk characteristics of the population under consideration, different periods of follow-up after diagnosis, inconsistent use of endocrine therapy, and the different methods used to report disease-specific mortality. Nevertheless, some insight into the natural history of prostate cancer can be gained from analyzing these studies as they estimate disease-specific mortality in patients with prostate cancer who remain untreated or who are treated with noncurative intent.

One method that has been used to quantify disease-specific mortality in conservatively treated patients with prostate cancer has been determination of the proportion of such patients in whom prostate cancer ultimately caused or contributed to death. Such a measure has been reported in several studies, and, overall, prostate cancer caused or contributed to death in 34 to 62% of the patients who died in these series.[42–47] In a study of 514 patients with prostate cancer, all of whom died between 1988 and 1991 and received immediate or deferred androgen deprivation therapy only, Aus and colleagues reported that prostate cancer caused or contributed to death in 62% of the study population.[43] When analyzing only those patients with clinically localized disease at diagnosis (M0), 50% still died as a result of this disease. Gronberg and colleagues analyzed 6,514 similar patients all diagnosed with prostate cancer in northern Sweden between 1971 and 1987.[44] Follow-up in this series ranged from 7 to 23 years after diagnosis. Of the patients who died during this time period, 55% died as a result of prostate cancer. Finally, in a series of 451 patients with prostate cancer from the Connecticut Tumor Registry, Albertsen and colleagues reported that prostate cancer was the cause of death in 34% of the patients who died, with a mean follow-up of 15.5 years.[42]

Other authors have attempted to quantify the excess mortality and/or decrease in life expectancy caused by prostate cancer in patients who remained untreated or who were treated with immediate or deferred androgen deprivation. Brasso and colleagues reported that prostate cancer caused a significant excess mortality in such patients, with the number of actual deaths being approximately 1.6 times greater than the expected number of deaths in the general population.[45] Similarly, Rana and colleagues reported that actuarial survival was 17% less at 5 years following diagnosis and 15% less at 10 years following diagnosis for a group of 199 patients with prostate cancer who were managed conservatively when compared with age-matched controls.[35] Both Albertsen and colleagues and Stattin and colleagues determined the number of lost years of life expectancy attributable to prostate cancer in patients who were treated with noncurative intent.[42,47] Stattin and colleagues reported a life expectancy of 6.3 years in 186 consecutive patients with prostate cancer who were managed with delayed androgen deprivation after TURP for obstructive voiding symptoms.[47] This was in contrast to a 10.2-year life expectancy for age-matched controls. Albertsen and colleagues performed a similar analysis in 451 patients with an average of 15.5 years of follow-up after prostate cancer diagnosis.[42] These authors found that loss of life expectancy was dependent on histologic tumor grade at diagnosis. For patients with well-differentiated tumors with a Gleason score of 2 to 4, no loss of life expectancy was found. In contrast, for patients with moderately (Gleason 5 to 7) or poorly differentiated (Gleason 8 to 10) tumors, maximum estimated lost life expectancy was 4 to 5 years and 6 to 9 years, respectively.

Finally, several studies have reported estimates of disease-specific survival for patients with prostate cancer who remained untreated or those who were treated with noncurative intent. Table 11–3 summarizes disease-specific survival and follow-up for the most contemporary series in the literature. Disease-specific survival ranged from 60 to 98% at 5 years, 34 to 92% at 10 years, and 62 to 81% at 15 years following diagnosis.[34–41,48,49] Average follow-up in these series ranged from 4.2 to 14 years.

NATURAL HISTORY OF PROSTATE CANCER: DISEASE-SPECIFIC SURVIVAL IN PATIENTS WHO SURVIVE AT LEAST 10 YEARS FOLLOWING DIAGNOSIS

A few studies have examined disease-specific survival in conservatively treated patients with prostate cancer who survived at least 10 years following diagnosis. Such patients represent an interesting population to study for a number of reasons. First, since they exhibit prolonged survival without receiving curative treatment, these patients are presumed to have low-grade, low-stage, nonmetastatic disease at presentation. Such disease is likely to be organ confined. In addition, these patients obviously have an extended life expectancy, exceeding 10 years. Thus, these patients are the most likely to benefit from definitive local therapy if it is offered, and by virtue of their favorable disease characteristics, they are also the most likely to harbor "latent" prostate cancer at diagnosis, if such an entity exists. These studies appear to demonstrate that the natural history of prostate cancer, even in patients who survive

Table 11–3. ESTIMATES OF DISEASE-SPECIFIC SURVIVAL IN PROSTATE CANCER PATIENTS WHO REMAIN UNTREATED AND THOSE WHO ARE TREATED WITH NONCURATIVE INTENT

Lead Author	Year	N	Follow-up (yr)	Disease-Specific Survival
George[39]	1988	120	7.0	80% at 5 yr, 75% at 7 yr following diagnosis
Byar[48]	1981	50	6.8–7.7	60–84% at 5 yr (overall survival)
Johansson[40]	1997	223	14	86% at 10 yr, 81% at 15 yr following diagnosis
Chodak[49]	1994	828	6.6	87% well or moderately differentiated, 34% poorly differentiated at 10 yr following diagnosis
Rana[35]	1994	199	4.2	70% at 5 yr, 50% at 10 yr following diagnosis
Warner[41]	1994	75	11.2–13.5	Median survival 156 mo following diagnosis
Egawa[34]	1993	107	6.2	78% at 5 yr, 71% at 10 yr following diagnosis
Adolfsson[37] (clinically localized)	1997	122	9.1	90% at 10 yr, 62% at 15 yr following diagnosis
Adolfsson[38] (age < 70 yr)	1991	61	8.0	98% at 5 yr, 92% at 10 yr following diagnosis
Adolfsson[36] (clinical T3)	1999	50	7.75	90% at 5 yr, 74% at 10 yr, 70% at 12 yr following diagnosis

at least 10 years without treatment, is that of tumor progression and eventual death owing to disease.

The percentage of patients dying of prostate cancer, even after 10 years without receiving curative treatment, remains substantial. Sixty-five (13%) of the 514 patients studied by Aus and colleagues survived at least 10 years after diagnosis without receiving curative treatment.[43] In this group, prostate cancer was the cause of death in 63% of the patients. These same authors also examined 490 patients, all of whom survived at least 10 years following prostate cancer diagnosis.[46] These patients represented 16% of all men diagnosed with prostate cancer in Göteborg, Sweden, between 1960 and 1979. Similar to their previous study, prostate cancer accounted for 62% of the deaths in this population, leading these authors to conclude that "early prostate cancer kills if the patient lives long enough."[46]

Prostate cancer also appears to cause an excess mortality in conservatively managed patients who survive at least 10 years following diagnosis. Adolfsson and colleagues identified 1,896 men who were diagnosed with prostate cancer between 1958 and 1983 in Stockholm, Sweden, and who survived at least 10 years following diagnosis.[50] This group represented 15% of all patients with prostate cancer in Stockholm during this time period. These authors determined the relative survival of these patients by dividing their observed survival by the expected survival for age- and time-matched controls in the population. For the entire group, the relative survival continued to decrease for 18 years after diagnosis, after which the decreases in observed and expected survival were equal and relative survival reached a plateau.[50] At approximately 23 years after diagnosis, the observed and expected survivals became equal. Thus, men diagnosed with prostate cancer who survive at least 10 years without curative treatment can expect an excess mortality for approximately 20 years after diagnosis. Similarly, Brasso and colleagues studied 2,570 conservatively treated patients who were diagnosed with prostate cancer in Denmark between 1943 and 1986, all of whom survived at least 10 years following diagnosis.[45] Similar to the other studies, this group represented 15% of all prostate cancer patients reported to the Danish Cancer Registry during that time period. These authors determined that such patients were 1.6 times more likely to die during the study period than age-matched controls.[45] This was equally true for patients 55 to 64 years of age and 65 to 74 years of age at diagnosis, who were 1.7 and 1.5 times more likely to die during the study period than age-matched controls, respectively. When taken together, data from these studies suggest that the natural history of untreated prostate cancer, even in patients with presumed low-grade, low-stage disease at diagnosis, is that of tumor progression and death owing to disease if the patient lives long enough.

NATURAL HISTORY OF PROSTATE CANCER: NEED FOR ADDITIONAL TREATMENT

When examining the natural history of untreated prostate cancer, it is important to consider the need for additional cancer-specific therapy with extended follow-up. Such information provides important insight into the natural history of the disease as treatment in this setting is most often delivered in response to local or distant disease progression.

The risk of receiving additional prostate cancer treatment for patients who are initially untreated is summarized in Table 11–4. Overall, the risk of receiving cancer-specific therapy in these patients ranges from 29 to 60% at 5 years and 57 to 70% at 10 years following diagnosis.[35–37,41,51] The only study in Table 11–4 to include patients receiving immediate treatment was by Rana and colleagues, in which approximately 25% of patients received immediate androgen deprivation.[35]

Table 11–4 includes two studies published by Adolfsson and colleagues.[36,37] It is interesting to compare these studies as they include patients with different stages of disease at diagnosis who were managed on the same surveillance protocol during the same time period. These studies demonstrate that patients with locally advanced disease (stage T3) have a 30% greater chance of receiving additional cancer-specific treatment within 5 years of diagnosis than patients with clinically organ-confined disease (stage T1–T2).[36,37] At 10 years following diagnosis, this difference is not as great.

Table 11–4. NEED FOR ADDITIONAL PROSTATE CANCER TREATMENT IN PATIENTS WHO INITIALLY REMAIN UNTREATED AND THOSE WHO ARE TREATED WITH NONCURATIVE INTENT

Lead Author	Year	N	Follow-up (yr)	Risk of Additional Treatment
Rana[35]	1994	199	4.2	26% required surgical intervention
Warner[41]	1994	75	11.2–13.5	Median interval to treatment = 108 mo
Adolfsson[36] (clinical T3)	1999	50	7.75	60% risk of treatment at 5 yr, 70% risk of treatment at 10 yr
Adolfsson[37] (clinically localized)	1997	122	9.1	29% risk of treatment at 5 yr, 57% risk of treatment at 10 yr
Koppie[51]	2000	329	3.1 yr	52% risk of treatment at 5 yr

The study by Koppie and colleagues included a more contemporary cohort of patients who initially remained untreated after prostate cancer diagnosis.[51] These patients were enrolled in a longitudinal, observational disease registry of patients with prostate cancer who were recruited through a network of community-based and academic urology practices distributed geographically throughout the United States. Given that this was a more contemporary cohort of patients, the most important predictors of additional treatment in this study were young patient age and serum prostate-specific antigen (PSA) at diagnosis.[51] When compared with patients with a serum PSA < 4.0 ng/mL at diagnosis, the relative risk of receiving a secondary cancer treatment for patients with a PSA of 4.1 to 10.0 ng/mL, 10.1 to 20.0 ng/mL and > 20.0 ng/mL at diagnosis was 3.1, 3.7, and 6.9, respectively. Moreover, a change in serum PSA from baseline was also a significant predictor of secondary cancer treatment in a multivariate analysis.

Aus and colleagues described the need for hospital care and palliative treatment in patients with prostate cancer initially treated with noncurative intent.[52] These authors identified 514 patients with prostate cancer, all of whom died between 1988 and 1990, and reported that 61% of the patients who died as a result of prostate cancer required at least one palliative treatment prior to death. Such treatments included TURP, palliative radiation therapy, or upper urinary tract diversion. The need for palliative treatment was significantly higher in patients dying of prostate cancer than in patients who died of other causes. Moreover, for patients with nonmetastatic disease at diagnosis (M0), there was a 58% chance of undergoing TURP, a 35% risk of receiving palliative radiation, and a 22% risk of requiring upper urinary tract diversion. This led to an average of 5 weeks of hospitalization for patients who died as a result of prostate cancer.

PREDICTORS OF DISEASE PROGRESSION AND CANCER-SPECIFIC SURVIVAL

Patient Age at Diagnosis

For patients with prostate cancer who remain untreated or those who receive immediate or delayed androgen deprivation, the relationship between age at diagnosis and disease-specific mortality remains unclear. Egawa and colleagues reported that patient age at diagnosis had no impact on the disease-specific mortality of 107 patients with prostate cancer who remained untreated or were treated with noncurative intent.[34] Chodak and colleagues reported that young age (age < 61) actually had a protective effect on prostate cancer–related death in 828 patients with prostate cancer treated with delayed androgen deprivation.[49] In contrast, most studies to date that have examined the relationship between age at diagnosis and disease-specific mortality in such patients have reported that young age at diagnosis is significantly associated with a higher likelihood of dying from prostate cancer.[43–47] In a study of 6,514 patients with prostate cancer registered in the northern Sweden tumor registry, Gronberg and colleagues demonstrated that the likelihood of dying of prostate cancer increased with decreasing age at diagnosis.[44] Whereas patients less than 60 years of age had a greater than 80% risk of dying from prostate cancer, the risk of prostate cancer–related death was less than 50% in patients over 80 years of age. Similar results were reported by Aus and colleagues and Stattin and colleagues when examining different patient populations.[43,47]

When restricting the analysis only to patients who survive 10 years or longer without receiving curative treatment, patient age at diagnosis continues to have an impact on disease-specific death. Such patients are presumed to have low-grade, low-stage, nonmetastatic disease by virtue of their extended survival despite remaining untreated or receiving palliative treatment only. In a study of 2,570 patients from the Danish Cancer Registry who survived at least 10 years following diagnosis, young age at diagnosis led to a higher risk of prostate cancer–related death.[45] In this series, long-term survivors who were 74 years old or younger had a significantly higher risk of death from prostate cancer than patients who were older than 75 years at diagnosis. Hugosson and colleagues also examined the impact of age at diagnosis on prostate cancer–related death in patients who survived at least 10 years following diagnosis despite receiving noncurative treatment only.[46] These authors also found that prostate cancer as the cause of death increased with lower patient age at diagnosis. The proportional prostate cancer mortality ratio (number of patients dying of prostate cancer/total number of deaths) was 71% for patients age 50 to 60, 66% for patients age 60 to 70, 58% for patients age 70 to 79, and 52% for patients age 80 to 90 at diagnosis.

Clinical Tumor Stage

Clinical tumor stage is a measure of local and distant tumor burden and, as such, should predict outcome for all patients with prostate cancer irrespective of the treatment course that is chosen. However, given the imprecise measures that are available to determine clinical stage, this has not always been the case.[34,53,54] This may be especially true when adjusting for other important factors associated with tumor progression, such as tumor grade.[34] In the study by Egawa and colleagues, patients with clinical stage A1 disease had a significantly better disease-specific survival than patients with more advanced disease at diagnosis.[34] However, when adjusting for tumor grade, stage no longer demonstrated any prognostic significance. McLaren and colleagues reported disease progression in 40% of patients with clinical stage T1 disease and 51% of patients with clinical stage T2 disease at 2 years after prostate cancer diagnosis.[53] After 3 years of follow-up, 60% of the entire group progressed, and clinical stage was no longer a significant predictor of outcome.

In contrast, the majority of studies examining the impact of tumor stage on the natural history of conservatively treated prostate cancer have demonstrated an important association between advanced stage at diagnosis and disease progression.[35–38,40,43,45,47,55] Patients with metastatic disease at the time of diagnosis appear to fare significantly worse than patients with clinically localized disease only. Using data from the Danish Cancer Registry, Brasso and colleagues reported that the median survival was 3.7 years for patients with clinically localized prostate cancer, 1.8 years for patients with regionally advanced disease, and only 1.1 years for patients with metastatic disease at diagnosis.[45] In the subset of patients surviving for at least 10 years after diagnosis, prostate cancer was the direct or contributing cause of death in 61% of patients with clinically localized disease and 76% of patients with advanced disease at diagnosis. Johansson and colleagues examined the outcomes of 642 patients, most of whom were treated with immediate or delayed androgen deprivation.[40] In this study, patients with metastatic disease at diagnosis fared much worse than patients with localized disease, both with respect to tumor progression and corrected survival. Although the 15-year corrected survival was 81% for patients with clinical stage T0–T2 disease and 57% for patients with clinical stage T3–T4 disease at diagnosis, the 15 year corrected survival was only 6% for patients with metastases at diagnosis. In a study of 514 patients with prostate cancer treated with immediate or deferred androgen deprivation, all of whom died between 1988 and 1991, Aus and colleagues reported that the median survival of patients with localized disease at diagnosis was 82 months as compared with only 26 months for patients with metastases at diagnosis.[43]

The extent of local disease also appears to be an important predictor of the natural history of prostate cancer progression. Johansson and colleagues reported that the risk of progression to metastases 15 years after diagnosis was 25% for patients presenting with clinical stage T3–T4 disease as compared with only 13% for patients presenting with clinical stage T0–T2 disease.[40] Similarly, the 15-year corrected survival was lower in patients with locally advanced T3–T4 prostate cancer (57%) when compared with patients with clinically organ-confined disease (81%). Aus and colleagues demonstrated that clinical stage at presentation had an important impact on cause-specific survival and the ultimate risk of death from prostate cancer.[43] These authors reported that 10% of patients with clinical stage T1a disease, 47% with clinical stage T1b disease, 52% with clinical stage T2a disease, 53% with clinical stage T2b–T3 disease, and 70% with clinical stage T4 disease ultimately died of prostate cancer.

Adolfsson and colleagues examined the effect of local tumor stage on prostate cancer progression and disease-specific survival in a series of articles that analyzed patients who initially remained untreated.[36–38,55] All patients were followed at the Karolinska Hospital in Stockholm, Sweden, on a surveillance protocol. When examining patients with clinically localized stage T1–T2 disease, the risk of local progression to clinical stage T3 disease was 72% at 10 years following diagnosis.[38] In these same patients, the likelihood of remaining metastasis free at 10 and 15 years after diagnosis was 77 to 82% and 48%, respectively, and the 10- and 15-year disease-specific survival rates were 90 to 92% and 62%, respectively.[37,38] In contrast, for 50 patients with locally advanced stage T3 disease at presentation, the likelihood of remaining metastasis free was approximately 66% at 10 years, whereas disease-specific survival was only 70 to 74% during this same time period.[36,55] Although these data represent retrospective analyses of patients selected for conservative management of their prostate cancer, the fact that they were treated at the same hospital during the same time period provides some insight into the impact of local tumor stage on the natural history of prostate cancer progression, metastasis, and disease-specific survival. Other authors have also reported a significant association between local tumor stage and disease-specific survival, even after adjusting for other important predictors of outcome, including tumor grade and patient age.[35,47]

Tumor Grade

Histologic tumor grade appears to be the most important factor predicting disease progression and disease-specific survival in patients with prostate cancer who are managed conservatively. In a pooled analysis of 828 patients with prostate cancer from six nonrandomized studies of men treated with observation and delayed androgen deprivation, Chodak and colleagues reported that poorly differentiated disease was the single most important predictor of disease-specific survival.[49] In this study, the likelihood of remaining metastasis free 10 years after diagnosis for patients with well-, moderately, and poorly differentiated tumors was 81%, 58%, and 26%, respectively. Similarly, disease-specific survival 10 years after diagnosis was highly dependent on tumor grade, being 87% for patients with well or moderately differentiated disease and only 34% for patients with poorly differentiated disease.[49] Johansson and colleagues also reported an association between histologic tumor grade and both tumor progression and death from prostate cancer in 642 patients treated with either immediate or delayed androgen deprivation.[40] Local tumor progression and progression to metastases were reported in 22% and 10% of patients, respectively, with well-differentiated disease, 27% and 20% of patients with moderately differentiated disease, and 30% and 31% of patients with poorly differentiated disease. Such increased tumor progression in patients with poorly differentiated disease translated into an increased risk of death from prostate cancer in this group. Only 16% of patients with well-differentiated tumors died of prostate cancer. In contrast, prostate cancer was the cause of death in 38% of patients with moderately differentiated and 68% of patients with poorly differentiated disease.[40] In a study of 6,514 patients with prostate cancer in the northern Sweden regional cancer registry, Gronberg and colleagues reported that the proportion of prostate cancer deaths increased with increasing tumor grade.[44] Forty percent of patients with well-differentiated disease, 54% of patients with moderately differentiated disease, and 72% of patients with poorly differentiated disease died of prostate cancer during the study period.[44] Similar results were seen when restricting the analysis to men less than 70 years of age at diagnosis. Others have reported similar results with respect to disease-specific survival and prostate cancer–related death (Table 11–5).[34,42,43,56] Moreover, authors who

Table 11–5. OUTCOME OF CONSERVATIVE MANAGEMENT OF PROSTATE CANCER ACCORDING TO HISTOLOGIC TUMOR GRADE

Lead Author	N	Follow-up (yr)	Outcome	Well Differentiated (%)	Moderately Differentiated (%)	Poorly Differentiated (%)
Johansson[40]	642	14	Death from prostate cancer	16	38	68
Albertsen[42]	451	15.5	Death from prostate cancer at 15 yrs	9	28	51
Chodak[49]	828	6.6	Disease-specific survival at 10 yrs	87 (well and moderately differentiated)	NS	34
Gronberg[44]	6514	7–23	Number of prostate cancer deaths/ total number of deaths	40	54	72
Albertsen[56]	767	10–20	Probability of death from prostate cancer	4–7	6–11 (Gleason 5) 10–30 (Gleason 6)	42–70 (Gleason 7) 60–87 (Gleason 8)
Egawa[34]	107	6.2	Disease-specific survival at 10 yr	89	87	29
Aus[43]	514	Until death	Risk of prostate cancer–related death	43	48	60

NS = not specified.

have examined tumor grade in multivariate analyses have demonstrated that poorly differentiated disease remains an important predictor of prostate cancer–related death.[34,35,47,49] In these studies, the relative risk of prostate cancer–related death ranges from 2.6 to 3.6 for patients with moderately differentiated disease and 6.1 to 12.9 for patients with poorly differentiated disease when compared to patients with well-differentiated prostate cancer.

Albertsen and colleagues examined the impact of tumor grade on long-term survival among patients with prostate cancer who were treated with either observation or immediate or delayed androgen deprivation.[42,56] In their initial study, these authors reported that tumor grade was highly correlated with death owing to prostate cancer. Nine percent of patients with well-differentiated, 28% of patients with moderately differentiated, and 51% of patients with poorly differentiated disease died as a result of their prostate cancer within 15 years of diagnosis.[42] In fact, the most powerful predictor of survival in this group of patients was histologic tumor grade. These authors also compared the survival of patients with prostate cancer treated conservatively with the expected survival of the general population. Age-adjusted survival for men with tumors with a Gleason score of 2 to 4 was not significantly different from that of the general population. In contrast, the maximum expected loss of life expectancy was 4 to 5 years for men with tumors with a Gleason score of 5 to 7, and 6 to 8 years for men with tumors with a Gleason score of 8 to 10 when compared with the general population.[42] In a subsequent study, Albertsen and colleagues used a competing risk analysis to estimate the probability of dying from prostate cancer in 767 men, age 55 to 74, all of whom remained untreated or received immediate or delayed androgen deprivation only.[56] Similar to the previous study, tumor grade had an important impact on the risk of death from prostate cancer, with 4 to 7% of men with Gleason 2 to 4 disease, 6 to 11% of patients with Gleason 5 disease, 18 to 30% of patients with Gleason 6 disease, 42 to 70% of patients with Gleason 7 disease, and 60 to 87% of patients with Gleason 8 to 10 disease dying of prostate cancer within 15 years of diagnosis.[56]

Serum Prostate-Specific Antigen

Because serum PSA has only been available for routine clinical use since the late 1980s, few studies have examined its ability to predict outcome in patients treated conservatively for their prostate cancer. Serum PSA concentration increases with increasing tumor volume. Thus, it is reasonable to expect that changes in PSA should reflect disease activity in patients who remain untreated. Unfortunately, studies that have examined this serum marker in such patients have reported mixed results.

McLaren and colleagues calculated PSA doubling times (PSAdt) in 113 patients with previously untreated prostate cancer who were prospectively entered into a watchful waiting program.[53] Multivariate analysis demonstrated that PSAdt was significantly correlated with clinical disease progression, stage progression, and time to treatment. With a short PSAdt (less than 18 months), a 50% risk of clinical progression was noted within 6 months of study entry. However, several limitations to this study must be noted. First, there was a very high risk of clinical progression, with 40% of T1 patients and 51% of T2 patients progressing by 2 years and 60% of patients progressing after 3 years of follow-up. In addition, the schedule for performing PSA determinations was variable, and the median follow-up from the time of diagnosis was only 21 months. Nam and colleagues also examined PSA velocity in a group of 141 patients who were initially managed expectantly after prostate cancer diagnosis.[57] All patients received at least two PSA determinations prior to undergoing treatment. Sixty-seven of these 141 patients (48%) eventually underwent radical prostatectomy. Moreover, only 57 patients (40%) had more than three serial PSA measurements with greater than 6 months of follow-up. In this study, 31% of the patients were found to be "rapid risers," defined as patients with a greater than 50% increase in serum PSA over 1 year. However, when restricting the analysis to only those patients with three PSA determinations over at least 6 months, only 14 to 16% of patients were rapid risers. A similar proportion of patients (16%) was found to have a PSAdt less than 2 years. There were no analyses examining the association between PSA velocity and outcome, but PSA velocity was not found to be associated with tumor grade.

Two other studies have examined PSA changes in patients with prostate cancer who remained untreated. Bangma and colleagues performed serial PSA determinations in 29 patients with untreated, organ-confined prostate cancer and correlated PSA changes with clinical outcome.[54] Average follow-up in these patients was 39 months after diagnosis. Although disease progressed locally in 13 patients (45%), neither tumor grade, clinical stage, change in PSA, nor initial PSA level demonstrated a significant association with interval to progression. Gerber and colleagues retrospectively analyzed PSA changes in 49 patients with clinically localized prostate cancer who remained untreated.[58] Mean follow-up while patients remained untreated was 32 months. These authors reported a decrease in serum PSA in 22% of patients during the observation period. In the remaining patients, the mean PSAdt was 56 months, and there was no significant correlation between PSA velocity and age at diagnosis, tumor grade, clinical stage, or initial PSA level. In fact, the short-term change in PSA observed during the first 9 months after diagnosis did not correlate well with overall PSA velocity during the entire follow-up period. This illustrates the importance of adequate follow-up and sufficient PSA determinations when calculating PSA velocity.

The above studies suggest that the variable nature of serum PSA does not allow for accurate measurement of disease activity in patients who remain untreated after diagnosis. Although PSA may accurately monitor disease activity following definitive local therapy, factors such as the growth of BPH may render such measurements less helpful in patients who remain untreated. Other markers of disease progression, such as P53 status and BCL2 expression,[59] have not been extensively studied in patients on watchful waiting. However, Borre and colleagues did examine the association between tumor angiogenesis and outcome in such patients.[60] Angiogenesis, the formation of new blood vessels, is important for tumor growth and metastasis.[61] Microvessel density (a measure of tumor angiogenesis) has been shown to correlate with stage and outcome in a variety of malignancies, including prostate cancer.[62–64] Borre and colleagues retrospectively examined microvessel density in a cohort of 221 patients with prostate cancer who were followed expectantly after diagnosis. Median follow-up in these patients was 15 years.[60] Microvessel density was significantly associated with clinical stage, tumor grade, disease-specific survival, and overall survival for the entire patient population. Microvessel density continued to be a significant predictor of disease-specific survival in a multivariate analysis adjusted for tumor stage and grade. These data demonstrate how molecular markers of disease progression may become useful in predicting the natural history of prostate cancer in patients who remain untreated. Further studies of these markers certainly appear warranted.

REFERENCES

1. Cordon-Cardo C. Mutations of cell cycle regulators. Biological and clinical implications for human neoplasia. Am J Pathol 1995;147:545–60.

2. Landis SH, Murray T, Bolden S, Wingo PA. Cancer statistics, 1999. CA Cancer J Clin 1999;49:8–31.
3. Quinlan DM, Partin AW, Walsh PC. Can aggressive prostatic carcinomas be identified and can their natural history be altered by treatment? Urology 1995;46:77–82.
4. Steinberg GD, Bales GT, Brendler CB. An analysis of watchful waiting for clinically localized prostate cancer. J Urol 1998;159:1431–6.
5. Natarajan N, Murphy GP, Mettlin C. Prostate cancer in blacks: an update from the American College of Surgeons' patterns of care studies. J Surg Oncol 1989;40:232–6.
6. Stamey TA, McNeal JE. Adenocarcinoma of the prostate. In: Walsh PC, Retik AB, Stamey TA, Vaughan ED, editors. Campbell's urology. Philadelphia: WB Saunders; 1992. p. 1159–221.
7. Whitmore WF Jr. Natural history and staging of prostate cancer. Urol Clin North Am 1984;11:205–20.
8. Bumpus HC. Carcinoma of the prostate. Surg Gynecol Obstet 1926;43:150–5.
9. Nesbit RM, Plumb RT. Prostatic carcinoma: a follow-up of 795 patients treated prior to the endocrine era and a comparison of survival rates between these and patients treated by endocrine therapy. Surgery 1946;20:263–72.
10. Nesbit RM, Baum WC. Endocrine control of prostatic carcinoma. JAMA 1950;143:1317–20.
11. Fowler JE Jr, Pandey P, Bigler SA, et al. Trends in diagnosis of stage T1a-b prostate cancer. J Urol 1997;158:1849–52.
12. Epstein JI. Can insignificant prostate cancer be predicted preoperatively in men with stage T1 disease? Semin Urol Oncol 1996;14:165–73.
13. Bridges CH, Belville WD, Insalaco SJ, Buck AS. Stage A prostatic carcinoma and repeat transurethral resection: a reappraisal 5 years later. J Urol 1983;129:307–8.
14. Lowe BA. Management of stage T1a prostate cancer. Semin Urol Oncol 1996;14:178–82.
15. Thompson IM, Zeidman EJ. Extended follow-up of stage A1 carcinoma of prostate. Urology 1989;33:455–8.
16. Matzkin H, Patel JP, Altwein JE, Soloway MS. Stage T1A carcinoma of prostate. Urology 1994;43:11–21.
17. Jewett HJ. The present status of radical prostatectomy for stages A and B prostatic cancer. Urol Clin North Am 1975;2:105–24.
18. Prostate. In: Fleming ID, Cooper JS, Henson DE, et al, editors. AJCC cancer staging manual. Philadelphia: Lippincott-Raven; 1997. p. 219–22.
19. Parfitt HE Jr, Smith JA Jr, Gliedman JB, Middleton RG. Accuracy of staging in A1 carcinoma of the prostate. Cancer 1983;51:2346–50.
20. Paulson DF, Robertson JE, Daubert LM, Walther PJ. Radical prostatectomy in stage A prostatic adenocarcinoma. J Urol 1988;140:535–9.
21. Zincke H, Blute ML, Fallen MJ, Farrow GM. Radical prostatectomy for stage A adenocarcinoma of the prostate: staging errors and their implications for treatment recommendations and disease outcome. J Urol 1991;146:1053–8.
22. Epstein JI, Oesterling JE, Walsh PC. The volume and anatomical location of residual tumor in radical prostatectomy specimens removed for stage A1 prostate cancer. J Urol 1988;139:975–9.
23. Larsen MP, Carter HB, Epstein JI. Can stage A1 tumor extent be predicted by transurethral resection tumor volume, per cent or grade? A study of 64 stage A1 radical prostatectomies with comparison to prostates removed for stages A2 and B disease. J Urol 1991;146:1059–63.
24. Voges GE, McNeal JE, Redwine EA, et al. The predictive significance of substaging stage A prostate cancer (A1 versus A2) for volume and grade of total cancer in the prostate. J Urol 1992;147:858–63.
25. McNeal JE, Price HM, Redwine EA, et al. Stage A versus stage B adenocarcinoma of the prostate: morphological comparison and biological significance. J Urol 1988;139:61–5.
26. Bauer WC, McGavran MH, Carlin MR. Unsuspected carcinoma of the prostate in suprapubic prostatectomy specimens. Cancer 1960;13:370–8.
27. Hanash KA, Utz DC, Cook EN, et al. Carcinoma of the prostate: a 15 year followup. J Urol 1972;107:450–3.
28. Cantrell BB, DeKlerk DP, Eggleston JC, et al. Pathological factors that influence prognosis in stage A prostatic cancer: the influence of extent versus grade. J Urol 1981;125:516–20.
29. Roy CRD, Horne D, Raife M, Pienkos E. Incidental carcinoma of prostate, long-term follow-up. Urology 1990;36:210–3.
30. Epstein JI, Paull G, Eggleston JC, Walsh PC. Prognosis of untreated stage A1 prostatic carcinoma: a study of 94 cases with extended followup. J Urol 1986;136:837–9.
31. Blute ML, Zincke H, Farrow GM. Long-term followup of young patients with stage A adenocarcinoma of the prostate. J Urol 1986;136:840–3.
32. Ingerman A, Broderick G, Williams RD, Carroll PR. Negative repeat transurethral resection of prostate fails to identify patients with stage A1 prostatic carcinoma at lower risk of progression: a long-term study. Urology 1993;42:528–32.
33. Brawn PN. The dedifferentiation of prostate carcinoma. Cancer 1983;52:246–251.
34. Egawa S, Go M, Kuwao S, et al. Long-term impact of conservative management on localized prostate cancer. A twenty-year experience in Japan. Urology 1993;42:520–6; discussion 526–7.
35. Rana A, Chisholm GD, Khan M, et al. Conservative management with symptomatic treatment and delayed hormonal manipulation is justified in men with locally advanced carcinoma of the prostate. Br J Urol 1994;74:637–41.
36. Adolfsson J, Steineck G, Hedlund PO. Deferred treatment of locally advanced nonmetastatic prostate cancer: a long-term followup. J Urol 1999;161:505–8.
37. Adolfsson J, Steineck G, Hedlund PO. Deferred treatment of clinically localized low-grade prostate cancer: actual 10-year and projected 15-year follow-up of the Karolinska series. Urology 1997;50:722–6.
38. Adolfsson J, Carstensen J. Natural course of clinically localized prostate adenocarcinoma in men less than 70 years old. J Urol 1991;146:96–8.
39. George NJ. Natural history of localised prostatic cancer managed by conservative therapy alone. Lancet 1988;1:494–7.
40. Johansson JE, Holmberg L, Johansson S, et al. Fifteen-year survival in prostate cancer. A prospective, population-based study in Sweden. JAMA 1997;277:467–71.
41. Warner J, Whitmore WF Jr. Expectant management of clinically localized prostatic cancer. J Urol 1994;152:1761–5.
42. Albertsen PC, Fryback DG, Storer BE, et al. Long-term sur-

vival among men with conservatively treated localized prostate cancer. JAMA 1995;274:626–31.
43. Aus G, Hugosson J, Norlen L. Long-term survival and mortality in prostate cancer treated with noncurative intent. J Urol 1995;154:460–5.
44. Gronberg H, Damber L, Jonson H, Damber JE. Prostate cancer mortality in northern Sweden, with special reference to tumor grade and patient age. Urology 1997;49:374–8.
45. Brasso K, Friis S, Juel K, et al. Mortality of patients with clinically localized prostate cancer treated with observation for 10 years or longer: a population based registry study. J Urol 1999;161:524–8.
46. Hugosson J, Aus G, Bergdahl C, Bergdahl S. Prostate cancer mortality in patients surviving more than 10 years after diagnosis. J Urol 1995;154:2115–7.
47. Stattin P, Bergh A, Karlberg L, et al. Long-term outcome of conservative therapy in men presenting with voiding symptoms and prostate cancer. Eur Urol 1997;32:404–9.
48. Byar DP, Corle DK. VACURG randomized trial of radical prostatectomy for stages I and II prostate cancer. Urology 1981;17(Suppl):7–11.
49. Chodak GW, Thisted RA, Gerber GS, et al. Results of conservative management of clinically localized prostate cancer. N Engl J Med 1994;330:242–8.
50. Adolfsson J, Rutqvist LE, Steineck G. Prostate carcinoma and long term survival. Cancer 1997;80:748–52.
51. Koppie TM, Grossfeld GD, Miller D, et al. Patterns of treatment in patients with prostate cancer initially managed with surveillance: results from the CaPSURE database. J Urol 2000:164:81–8.
52. Aus G, Hugosson J, Norlen L. Need for hospital care and palliative treatment for prostate cancer treated with noncurative intent. J Urol 1995;154:466–9.
53. McLaren DB, McKenzie M, Duncan G, Pickles T. Watchful waiting or watchful progression? Prostate specific antigen doubling times and clinical behavior in patients with early untreated prostate carcinoma. Cancer 1998;82:342–8.
54. Bangma CH, Hop WCJ, Schroder FH. Serial prostate specific antigen measurements and progression in untreated confined (stages T0 to 3NxM0, grades 1 to 3) carcinoma of the prostate. J Urol 1995;154:1403–6.
55. Adolfsson J. Deferred treatment of low grade stage T3 prostate cancer without distant metastases. J Urol 1993;149:326–8; discussion 328–9.
56. Albertsen PC, Hanley JA, Gleason DF, Barry MJ. Competing risk analysis of men aged 55 to 74 years at diagnosis managed conservatively for clinically localized prostate cancer. JAMA 1998;280:975–80.
57. Nam RK, Klotz LH, Jewett MA, et al. Prostate specific antigen velocity as a measure of the natural history of prostate cancer: defining a 'rapid riser' subset. Br J Urol 1998;81:100–4.
58. Gerber GS, Gornik HL, Goldfischer ER, et al. Evaluation of changes in prostate specific antigen in clinically localized prostate cancer managed without initial therapy. J Urol 1998;159:1243–6.
59. Bauer JJ, Connelly RR, Sesterhenn IA, et al. Biostatistical modeling using traditional variables and genetic biomarkers for predicting the risk of prostate carcinoma recurrence after radical prostatectomy. Cancer 1997;79:952–62.
60. Borre M, Offersen BV, Nerstrom B, Overgaard J. Microvessel density predicts survival in prostate cancer patients subjected to watchful waiting. Br J Cancer 1998;78:940–4.
61. Brem H, Gresser I, Grosfeld J, Folkman J. The combination of antiangiogenic agents to inhibit primary tumor growth and metastasis. J Pediatr Surg 1993;28:1253–7.
62. Weidner N, Carroll PR, Flax J, et al. Tumor angiogenesis correlates with metastasis in invasive prostate carcinoma. Am J Pathol 1993;143:401–9.
63. Silberman MA, Partin AW, Veltri RW, Epstein JI. Tumor angiogenesis correlates with progression after radical prostatectomy but not with pathologic stage in Gleason sum 5 to 7 adenocarcinoma of the prostate. Cancer 1997; 79:772–9.
64. Brawer MK, Deering RE, Brown M, et al. Predictors of pathologic stage in prostatic carcinoma. The role of neovascularity. Cancer 1994;73:678–87.
65. Heaney JA, Chang HC, Daly JJ, Prout GR Jr. Prognosis of clinically undiagnosed prostatic carcinoma and the influence of endocrine therapy. J Urol 1977;118:283–7.
66. Correa RJ Jr, Anderson RG, Gibbons RP, Mason JT. Latent carcinoma of the prostate—why the controversy? J Urol 1974;111:644–6.
67. Lowe BA, Barry JM. The predictive accuracy of staging transurethral resection of the prostate in the management of stage A cancer of the prostate: a comparative evaluation. J Urol 1990;143:1142–5.
68. Zhang G, Wasserman NF, Sidi AA, et al. Long-term followup results after expectant management of stage A1 prostatic cancer. J Urol 1991;146:99–102; discussion 102–3.

12

Radical Retropubic Prostatectomy

PETER R. CARROLL, MD, FACS
MAXWELL V. MENG, MD
TRACY M. DOWNS, MD
GARY D. GROSSFELD, MD, FACS

The case for early detection of prostate cancer is supported by the following: the disease is burdensome, screening for prostate-specific antigen (PSA) improves detection of clinically important tumors without significantly increasing the detection of unimportant tumors, most PSA-detected tumors are curable using current techniques, and there is no cure for metastatic disease.[1] Treatment options for patients with prostate cancer are plentiful.[2] Radical prostatectomy is one option. The rationale supporting radical prostatectomy includes the following: it is likely to be curative for organ-confined cancers and many cancers with limited extracapsular extension, a large number of cancers currently detected are curable using this technique, morbidity associated with radical prostatectomy is limited when performed by experienced surgeons, and adjuvant radiation may be delivered safely and efficiently in selected, high-risk patients.

Radical prostatectomy can be performed through a lower abdominal incision (radical retropubic prostatectomy), through a perineal incision (radical perineal prostatectomy), or laparoscopically. Although early reports suggest that the latter technique is feasible, associated with limited morbidity and acceptable positive margins and biochemical control rates, long-term follow-up in suitable patient populations is not yet available. With the radical retropubic or laparoscopic radical prostatectomy, lymphadenectomy can be performed simultaneously using the same surgical approach. With radical perineal prostatectomy, lymphadenectomy can be performed though a separate incision, laparoscopically, or deleted in those at very low risk of lymph node metastases. Although there are proponents for each technique, the end points for all are similar and include cancer cure and maintenance of acceptable urinary function and, if possible, potency in those potent before the procedure.

PATIENT SELECTION

Radical prostatectomy should be considered in those patients with either organ-confined disease or those with limited extracapsular extension in which a clear surgical margin is possible.[2] Such patients would include those with low- and intermediate-risk cancers defined by T1/T2a disease associated with serum PSA concentrations < 10 ng/mL and no high-grade components (ie, Gleason grade 4 or 5) or those with Gleason grade 7, stage T2b disease associated with serum PSA concentration < 20 ng/mL, respectively. Patients whose cancers have features of more advanced but nonmetastatic disease may also be candidates for the procedure. This would include patients whose cancers are of higher grade, stage T1 to T3a, and are associated with serum PSA concentrations < 20 ng/mL. Low-risk patients should be advised that excellent outcomes might be achieved with a variety of techniques, including watchful waiting in selected patients. Although progression may occur slowly in this patient population, eventual treatment is likely in those who are young or have elevated or rising serum PSA levels.[3] Intermediate-risk patients are challenging as their disease has a high risk of progression if left untreated, and somewhere between 30 and 60 percent may fail on the basis of serial PSA testing, despite standard therapy. More precise markers of progression would be beneficial to better select patients for treatment in this patient population. D'Amico and colleagues tested the hypothesis that the percentage of positive prostate biopsies provides clinically relevant information about early biochemical (PSA) failure following radical prostatectomy.[4] Controlling for the known prognostic factors of pretreatment PSA and cancer grade and stage, they showed that the percentage of positive biopsies (< 34%, 34 to 50%, and > 50%) was an independent predictor of time to PSA failure following surgery. Specifically, the majority of patients (80%) in the intermediate-risk group could be classified as having either a high (86 to 93%) or low (8 to 11%) likelihood of remaining biochemically relapse free. Others have shown that the percentage of prostate biopsies predicts the risk of both extracapsular penetration and biochemical control.[4a, 4b]

Although high-risk patients (T3b; Gleason sum 8, 9, or 10; or serum PSA > 20 ng/mL) can undergo the procedure with acceptable morbidity and excellent rates of local control, long-term cure is less likely, and such patients should be advised that adjuvant therapy may be necessary.[5] Such patients are at high risk of distant failure and should be considered for alternative techniques or adjuvant therapy following surgery. Patients who are to undergo the procedure should be in good physical health and have a long life expectancy.

INDICATIONS FOR PELVIC LYMPHADENECTOMY

Contemporary series of patients with localized prostate cancers suggest that few patients harbor lymphatic disease (4 to 9%), and the risk of lymph node metastases can be quantitated. Although lymphadenectomy is not considered a therapeutic intervention, information gained may alter initial treatment decisions and certainly identifies patients who are at high risk of failure from any local intervention who may be candidates for immediate adjuvant therapy. Whereas patients at intermediate to high risk of lymph node metastases benefit from lymphadenectomy, those at low risk may forgo lymphadenectomy and be treated with radical prostatectomy alone.[6–8] Generally, lymphadenectomy should be considered if the Gleason score is 5 to 6 and the PSA level is 20 ng/mL or greater, or if the Gleason score is 7 or more and the PSA level is 15 ng/mL or greater. Patients with clinical stage C (T3) disease should be considered for the procedure as well. In a thoughtful decision analysis of lymphadenectomy before radical prostatectomy, Meng and Carroll suggested that lymph node dissection is unnecessary in the subset of patients in whom the risk of lymph node involvement is less than 18 percent.[9] The anticipated risk of lymph node metastases can be calculated from the several nomograms or equations currently available.[9a-9c]

RELEVANT SURGICAL ANATOMY

The puboprostatic ligaments anchor the anterior surface of the prostate to the pubis, whereas the posterior surface is flattened against the rectum.[10] The levator ani muscles funnel inferiorly to surround the mid- and apical portions of the prostate. The prostate's anterior and lateral surfaces are covered by the periprostatic fascia, which is formed by the prostatic and levator fasciae. Adjacent to the gland, this layer is called the endopelvic fascia, and it covers both the pelvic floor and important underlying neurovascular structures and the venous plexus of Santorini, a prominent network of veins that overlie the anterior and lateral surfaces of the prostate. This venous plexus serves as the primary venous drainage of the penis. Erectile nerves to the corpora cavernosa travel outside the prostatic capsule posterolaterally in the lateral pelvic fascia between the prostate and the rectum. The cavernous nerves originate in the pelvic plexus and contain both sympathetic and parasympathetic fibers, which supply the corpora cavernosa and the corpus spongiosum. Appreciating these anatomic relationships intraoperatively is essential to avoid unnecessary injury and bleeding (Figure 12–1).[11] The prostatic capsule blends with the anterior lamella of Denonvilliers' fascia on the posterior gland surface. Denonvilliers' fascia is derived from two layers of pelvic peritoneum in the retrovesical space. The anterior lamella of this fascia is adherent to the posterior surface of the prostate and merges laterally with the intermediate layer of the retroperitoneal fascia. This

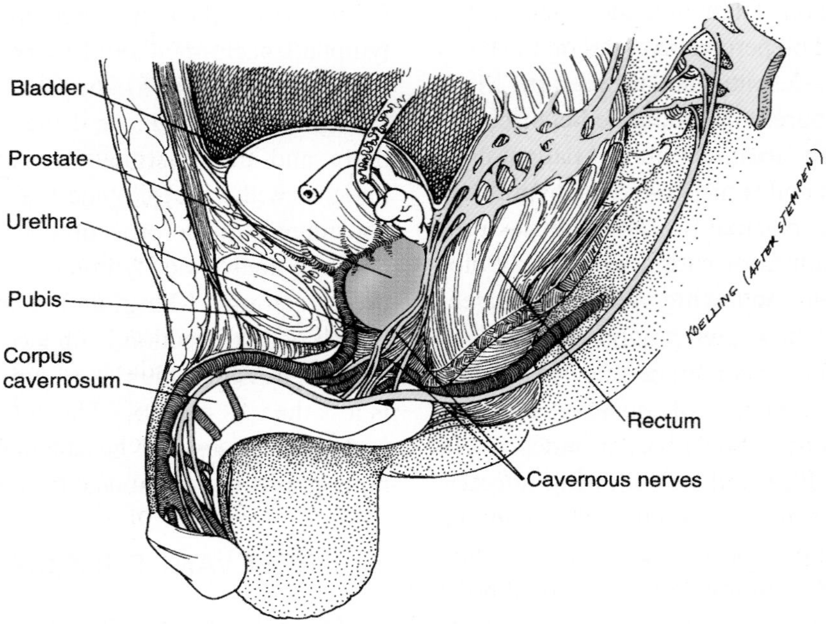

Figure 12–1. Sagittal section through the male pelvis.

layer is continuous with the lateral periprostatic fascia, prostatic sheath, and endopelvic fascia. The posterior lamella of Denonvilliers' fascia covers the anterior and anterolateral surfaces of the rectum. At both the apex and the base, no clear capsule separates the prostate from the striated urethral sphincter or bladder neck, respectively. Prostatic glands can be seen in the substance of the urethral sphincter, and smooth muscle fibers from the detrusor blend with the muscular coat of the prostate.

Whereas voluntary control of voiding begins with relaxation of the striated sphincter in the membranous urethra, smooth muscle components of the bladder neck and prostate contribute to continence in men. Smooth muscle fibers of the preprostatic sphincter are in continuity with the middle circular muscle layer of the bladder and encircle the proximal urethra as the fundus ring. These fibers connect distally with the passive prostatic musculature. The inner longitudinal layer of bladder muscle continues as the inner longitudinal smooth muscle layer of the prostatic urethra. Within the fundus ring is another layer of periurethral muscle fibers that originate in the superficial trigone of the bladder and insert in the musculature of the ejaculatory ducts, near the verumontanum. These elements of the preprostatic sphincter functionally provide resistance to both urine leakage and retrograde seminal ejaculation. The passive prostatic sphincter is located distal to the verumontanum and is closely related to the striated muscle bundles of the adjacent prostatomembranous sphincter.[12] These fibers are semicircular around the verumontanum and encircle the urethra completely as they approach the membranous urethra, located between the inner longitudinal and the prostatic striated sphincter layers.

The prostatic striated sphincter forms a thick muscle layer over the anterior surface of the gland. Distally, these fibers almost completely surround the gland, except for a posterior gap at the apex, and merge with muscles of the membranous urethral sphincter. Fibers of the membranous striated sphincter encircle the urethra, originating at the anterior decussation of the prostatic sphincter and inserting at the perineal body at the level of the perineal membrane. These sphincteric fibers insert broadly over the surface of the prostatic fascia near the apex.[13–15] Steiner has described the external striated sphincter as a unit composed of the following structures acting in an integrated manner: (1) the mucosal infoldings of the urethra, (2) fibroelastic tissue within the urethra, (3) the rhabdosphincter or the striated muscular component of the external sphincter, (4) the puborectalis, and (5) supporting fascial investments, including the pubourethral ligaments anteriorly and the dorsal median fibrous raphe posteriorly.[16]

The primary arterial supply to the prostate comes from the prostatovesical artery that descends inferiorly along the bladder base. The origin of this artery is variable, but it usually comes from the anterior division of the internal iliac artery. The prostatic artery divides at the base of the prostate to give a large posterolateral branch and a smaller anterior branch. The superolateral gland may receive arterial supply from the middle and superior rectal arteries. Urethral branches from the prostatic artery enter the capsule posterolaterally below the bladder neck to supply the transition zone and periurethral glands. Capsular branches, traveling in the neurovascular bundle posterolaterally, enter the capsule to supply the central and peripheral zones. Prostate parenchymal veins, as well as veins draining all deep pelvic structures, intercommunicate with the prostatic venous plexus lying within the periprostatic fascia on the anterior surface of the gland.[14] The deep dorsal vein of the penis emerges beneath the symphysis pubis between the puboprostatic ligaments to join this plexus. The majority of venous blood drains directly into the prostatic and inferior vesical veins to the internal iliac veins.

Preganglionic sympathetic nerves to the preprostatic sphincter and smooth musculature of the prostate gland originate at spinal level L2–3 and pass through the sympathetic chain ganglia to the superior hypogastric plexus. Here they synapse with postganglionic noradrenergic nerves, the cell bodies of which lie in the pelvic plexus lateral to the bladder and prostate. Parasympathetic innervation to the prostatic epithelium originates in the pelvic splanchnic nerves from spinal levels S2–4. These preganglionic neurons synapse in the prostatic plexus, located between the seminal vesicles and the prostate, and send short postganglionic fibers into the prostate stroma. Somatic motor output from the pudendal nerve arises from S1–3 and innervates the external striated sphincter. Some contribution to external sphincter tone may also come from the pelvic nerve.[17–20]

Steiner, on the basis of detailed anatomic studies, suggested that the rhabdosphincter receives somatic innervation via the intrapelvic portion of the pudendal nerve, and the urethral mucosa and smooth muscle receive autonomic innervation via branches of the hypogastric plexus.[16] These nerves enter the urethral sphincter complex at the 5 and 7 o'clock positions.

TECHNIQUE OF RADICAL RETROPUBIC PROSTATECTOMY

Most often, radical prostatectomy is performed using general anesthesia, although use of an epidural catheter alone is feasible. Although some advocate the use of either epidural or spinal anesthesia in addition to a general anesthetic to decrease intraoperative blood loss and improve postoperative pain management, others have advocated the use of general anesthesia with the use of ketorolac tromethamine in the postoperative period.[21–23] A perioperative antibiotic is used by some but may not be necessary. In addition, donation of autologous blood is offered to patients, but given the limited blood loss noted by most experienced surgeons, it may not be necessary.[24–26]

The contemporary technique of radical retropubic prostatectomy has been developed and refined by Walsh and colleagues.[27,28] Patients may be positioned supine or in the very low lithotomy position to facilitate the use of perineal pressure or exposure. All pressure points are well padded. The technique is performed through a lower midline incision. Although the operation has most often been performed using an incision that extended from the symphysis pubis to the umbilicus, a more limited incision of approximately 6 to 8 cm is adequate and more desirable (Figure 12–2). The rectus abdominus muscles are separated in the midline, and the retropubic space is entered. A fixed retractor is placed. Lymphadenectomy may be performed selectively, as described.[9] Lymph node dissection has been modified over the last several years to include lymph node tissue in areas most likely to harbor disease. The limits of dissection, therefore, most often include the obturator nerve posteriorly, the common iliac artery superiorly, the circumflex iliac vein inferiorly, and the internal aspect of the external iliac vein laterally. Exposure to the prostate is facilitated by a "forked" blade, which is used to retract the previously placed Foley catheter superiorly, thereby exposing clearly the endopelvic fascia and anterior surface of the prostate (Figure 12–3).

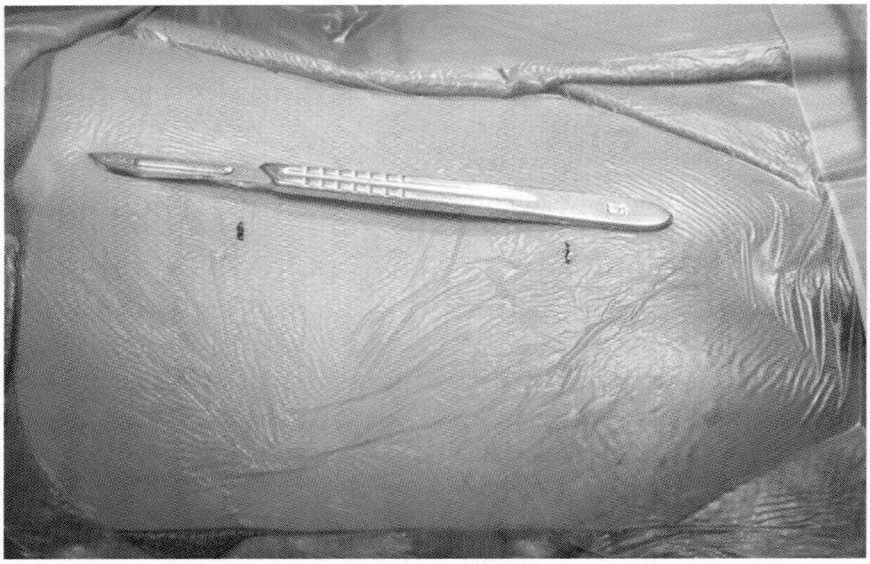

Figure 12–2. Incision. A 6 to 8 cm lower midline incision provides adequate surgical exposure.

Exposure to the prostate when performing a radical retropubic prostatectomy is undertaken by first incising the endopelvic fascia from just lateral to the puboprostatic ligaments along the lateral edge of the prostate (Figure 12–4). A natural fenestration often exists in this area, obviating the need for an incision. The incision is carried parallel to the neurovascular bundles along the lateral surface of the prostate.[29] Fibers of the levator ani are separated from the apex of the prostate. The puboprostatic ligaments, which provide anterior support of the urethra, are left intact over the urethra, but any attachments to the prostate are incised (Figure 12–5). Preservation of the puboprostatic (pubourethral) ligaments may facilitate earlier and more complete return of urinary continence compared with the use of previous tech-

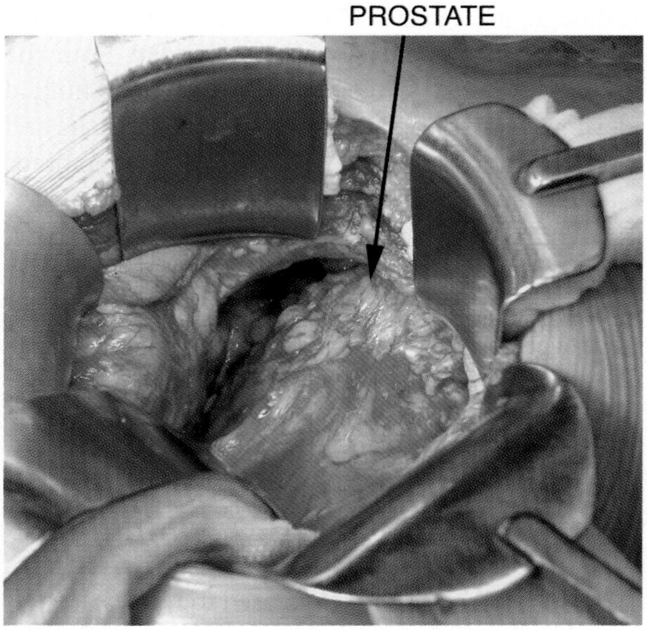

Figure 12–3. Exposure of the prostate. Use of a fixed retractor and malleable retractor blades facilitates exposure of the prostate and regional anatomy (intraoperative photograph).

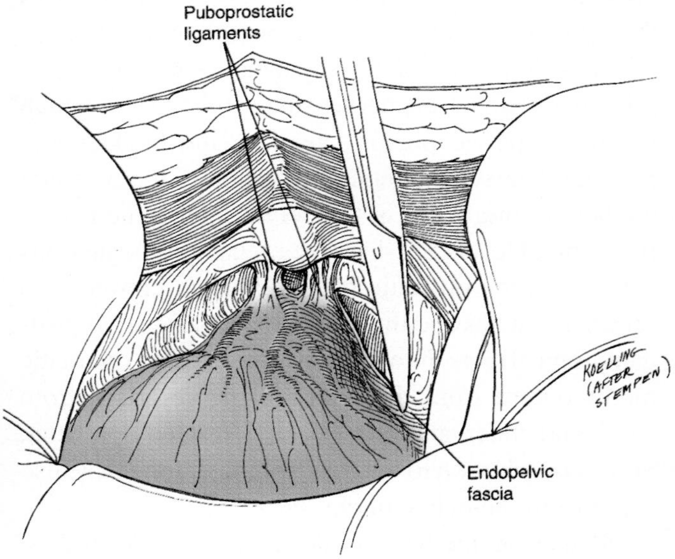

Figure 12–4. Incision in the endopelvic fascia is made just lateral to the puboprostatic ligaments. The incision is continued alongside the lateral edge of the prostate and extends to the base of the prostate proximally.

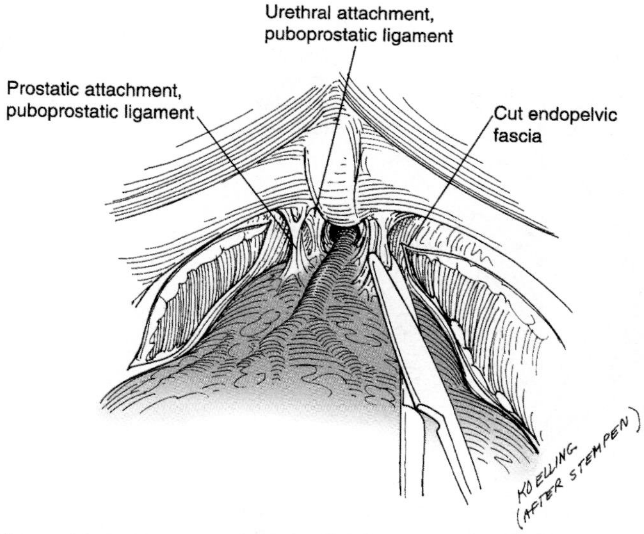

Figure 12–5. The puboprostatic ligaments are cut at their insertion into the anterior surface of the prostate. They are left intact over the urethra.

niques, which incised them over the urethra.[10] Once the puboprostatic ligaments have been incised, the fascia and overlying dorsal vein complex are generally gathered and the suture ligated to facilitate exposure of the prostate, prevent bleeding from the complex once it is cut, and allow clear access to the urethra (Figure 12–6).[30] If a distal suture is placed in the dorsal vein complex at this point, it should include only the overlying dorsal vein complex and not the distal sphincteric continence mechanism or the neurovascular bundles if they are to be spared. A 2-0 or 3-0 absorbable suture may be placed distally at the most anterior portion of the dorsal vein complex and the needle left on the suture. As the dorsal vein is incised, the suture may be used to progressively close the cut end of the dorsal vein complex (Figure 12–7). This maneuver may facilitate hemostasis, allowing clear visualization of the urethra and proper plane of dissection. During nerve-sparing surgery, care should be taken not to draw the neurovascular pedicles medially with either proximal or distal sutures in the dorsal vein complex. Also, care is taken during the apical dissection of the prostate to simultaneously preserve the urethra's distal continence mechanism and excise all prostate tissue. Once the dorsal vein complex has been incised and controlled, the anterior urethral surface is identified.

Penile erection is a neurovascular phenomenon, and the nerves and arterial blood supply (neurovascular bundles) crucial to potency run posterolaterally along either side of the prostate (Figure 12–8). These bundles may be spared during surgery in an effort to preserve potency. However, extracapsular extension, when it does occur, may occur in the region(s) of the neurovascular bundles. These bundles should be preserved cautiously in those at high risk of extracapsular extension. The risk of extracapsular extension can be quantified using pretreatment nomograms or equations, described previously. Such patients include those with multiple positive biopsies on a single side of the prostate, high-volume disease within a biopsy core, induration in the area of the neurovascular bundle, or high-grade disease.

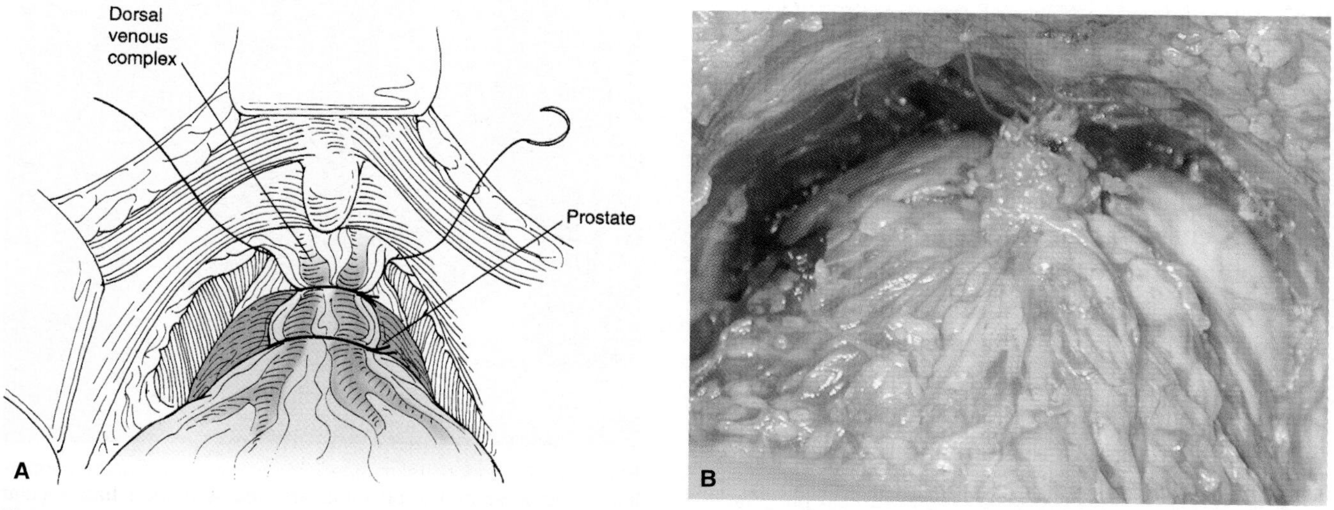

Figure 12–6. *A,* The dorsal vein complex is gathered proximally and distally with 2-0 absorbable suture material. *B,* Intraoperative photograph.

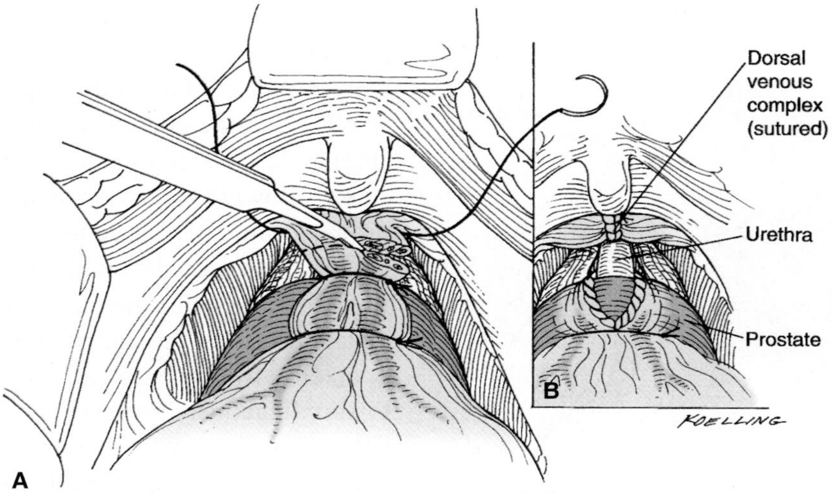

Figure 12–7. *A,* The dorsal vein complex is cut and oversewn distally. This is facilitated by placing a fine, absorbable suture in the complex initially before it is incised. *B,* The suture can be advanced posteriorly as the incision is carried to the urethral surface.

In addition, return of potency following a nerve-sparing radical prostatectomy is not only a function of technique but also of patient age and preoperative sexual function. Older patients and those with poor preoperative potency may not benefit from a nerve-sparing approach.

The neurovascular bundles can be located using anatomic landmarks. During nerve-sparing radical prostatectomy, the lateral prostatic fascia should be incised anterior to the bundles and the neurovascular bundles should be separated from the prostatic capsule before the urethra is incised. The neurovascular bundles run deep to the lateral prostatic fascia at approximately the 5 and 7 o'clock positions along the posterolateral surface of the prostate. The incision in the lateral prostatic fascia is best made not at the apex of the prostate but more proximally near the midportion of the prostate (Figure 12–9).[29] The fascial incision can be carried both proximally and distally, allowing the bundles to be pushed posteriorly. Small vascular branches to the prostate may be taken using small clips or 4-0 or 5-0 absorbable sutures. The use of right-angled instruments (scissors, clamps, and clip appliers) facilitates preservation of the bundles and dissection of the prostate. The neurovascular bundles are at the most risk for damage at the time of urethral dissection and transection, ligation of the lateral pedicles, and dissection of the seminal vesicles.

Recent studies have suggested that intraoperative frozen section (IFS) analysis may be used to better determine the status of the surgical margin in patients undergoing nerve-sparing radical prostatecotmy. Cangiano and colleagues used IFS analysis of inked mar-

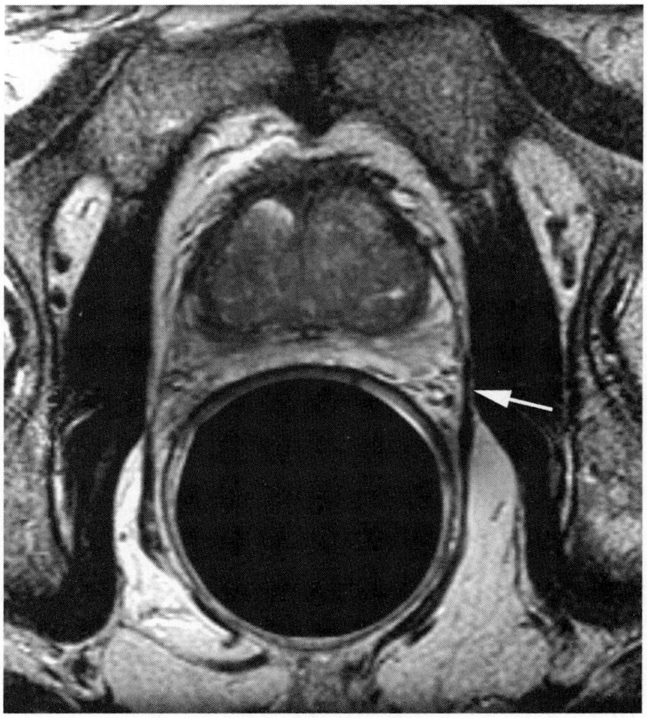

Figure 12–8. Endorectal magnetic resonance image at the midportion of the prostate. The posterolateral course of the neurovascular bundles is noted (*arrows*).

gins in 48 men who underwent nerve-sparing radical prostatectomy.[31] If tumor was seen at the inked margin, the ipsilateral neurovascular bundle was resected and submitted separately to the pathologist. Nine patients had disease at the inked margins on frozen sections. However, no tumor was seen in any of the resected bundles when IFS was positive. In the 39 patients (82%) with negative frozen sections, the neurovascular bundles were preserved. Potency rates were noted to be significantly improved in patients with the nerve-sparing procedure compared with those who had excision of the neurovascular bundles.

We recently examined the use of IFS analysis in 101 patients undergoing nerve-sparing radical prostatectomy at the University of California, San Francisco (UCSF). Clinical disease stage was T1 in 20 patients, and T2a in 35 patients, and T2b in 46 patients. Mean serum PSA prior to surgery was 7.2 ng/mL. Sixty-two, 28, and 11 patients had Gleason scores of 2 to 6, 7, and 8 to 10, respectively. Intraoperative frozen section analysis was performed on the surgical margin thought to be at risk for tumor involvement based on the results of systematic prostate biopsy, transrectal ultrasonography, or intraoperative inspection. If the frozen section was positive, additional tissue (including the neurovascular bundle when appropriate) was subsequently removed. Frozen section results were compared with those on the final, permanent tissue section as well as to the status of the additionally resected tissue.

Intraoperative frozen section results were identical to those obtained on the final, permanent section in 92 of the 101 (91%) cases. Of the 15 patients with positive frozen section diagnosis, 11 had identical findings on the permanent pathologic sections. Of the 86 patients with negative frozen section diagnosis, 81 had negative permanent sections. The positive and negative predictive values for IFS technique were 73 and 94 percent, respectively. Of the 15 patients with positive IFS, 12 (80%) had no evidence of tumor in additionally resected tissue. Prostate-specific antigen recurrence was noted in 7 percent of the study population. The risk of recurrence in patients with either positive or negative IFS findings was similar. These data suggest that IFS may be applied during radical prostatectomy to spare the neurovascular bundles in select patients.

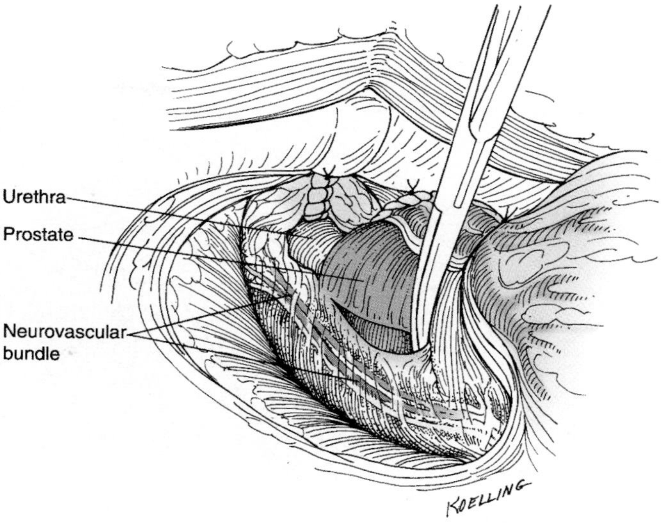

Figure 12–9. The lateral prostatic fascia is incised and the neurovascular bundle(s) is gently dropped posteriorly away from the prostatic capsule.

Once the neurovascular bundles have been separated unilaterally or bilaterally from the prostatic capsule (in cases of nerve-sparing surgery), the urethral incision can be performed. An anterior incision is made, and the Foley catheter is grasped and pulled into the wound before being cut distally (Figure 12–10). Care should be taken not to pull the catheter up under tension as this may shear portions of the prostatic capsule at the apex of the gland. In addition, the sphincter should not be put under tension ("telescoped") as this may tear the sphincter from its fascial attachments. The posterior portion of the urethra can be incised sharply under direct vision with care being taken to either include or exclude the neurovascular bundles depending on the extent of surgery in individual cases (Figure 12–11). Once the posterior portions of the urethra and sphincter have been cut, Denonvilliers' fascia and the rectourethralis muscle are identified.[16] These later structures can be cut sharply, avoiding the neurovascular bundles. These posterior incisions should be carried distally and posteriorly enough to include all prostate tissue and Denonvilliers' fascia in the midline, respectively, to ensure complete cancer excision.

Use of a nerve stimulation device during surgery may facilitate identification and preservation of the neurovascular bundles.[32,33] Electrical stimulation may result in smooth muscle relaxation of penile

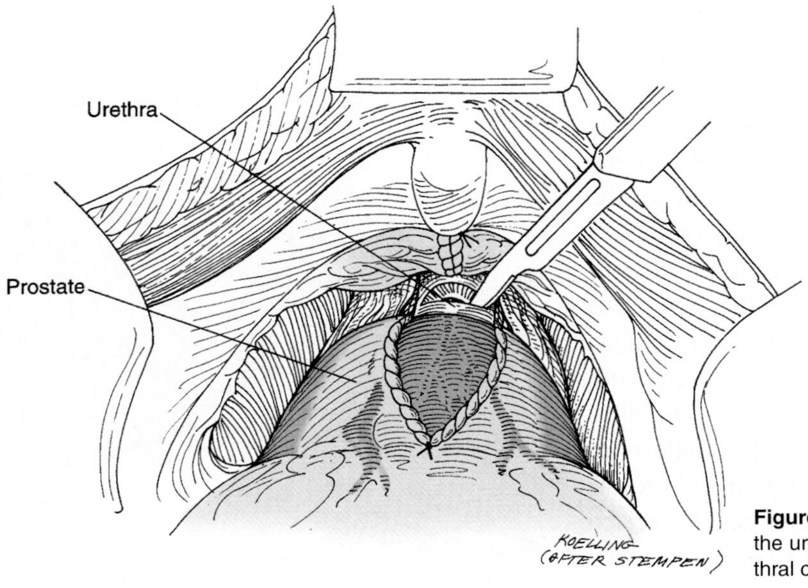

Figure 12–10. The anterior surface of the urethra is incised, exposing the urethral catheter, which is grasped and cut.

tissue and expansion of corporal sinusoids, resulting in increased penile blood flow, girth, and length. Either intracavernous pressure or penile circumference monitoring can note such changes. Early experience using a commercially available intraoperative, nerve stimulation device and continuous monitoring of penile circumference during stimulation suggests that its use may allow for better preservation of erectile function. However, others have failed to show that the results of intraoperative monitoring correlate well with postoperative return of sexual function.

The lateral pedicles and branches of the prostatic and rectal arteries are lighted alongside the prostate. In those cases in which the neurovascular bundles are to be preserved, care should be taken to ligate them anterior to the bundles. Dissection proceeds superiorly or cranially, exposing Denonvilliers' fascia over the seminal vesicles and ampullae of the vas deferens (Figure 12–12). The fascia is incised, the ampullae

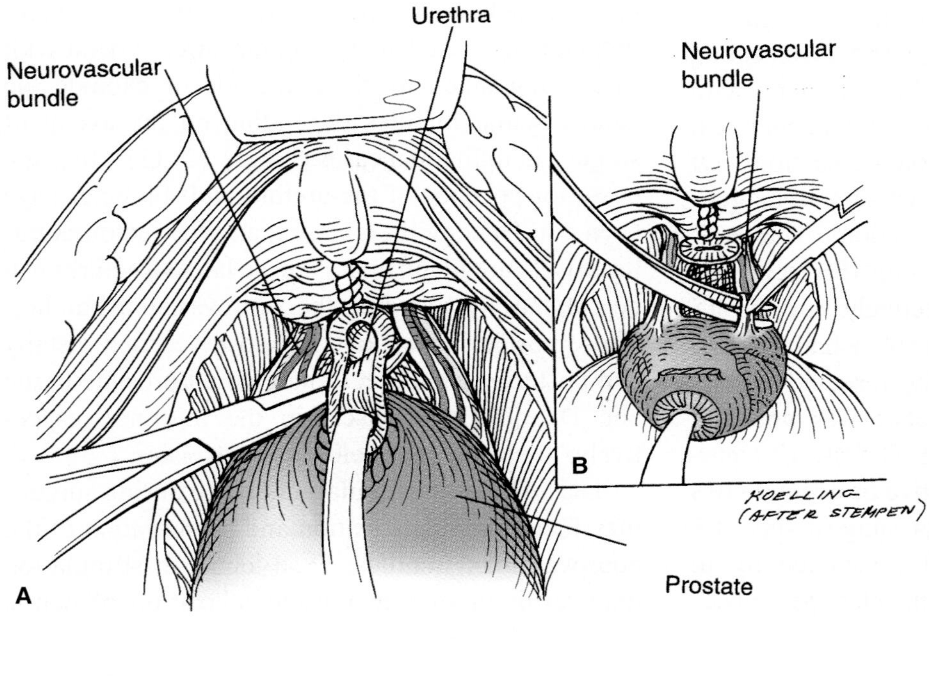

Figure 12–11. *A,* The posterior surface of the urethra is cut under direct vision, with care being taken to avoid inadvertent injury to the neurovascular bundles or incomplete excision of the posterior apex of the prostate, which often travels more distally than its anterior aspect. *B,* Small vessels are cut or ligated as they enter the prostate.

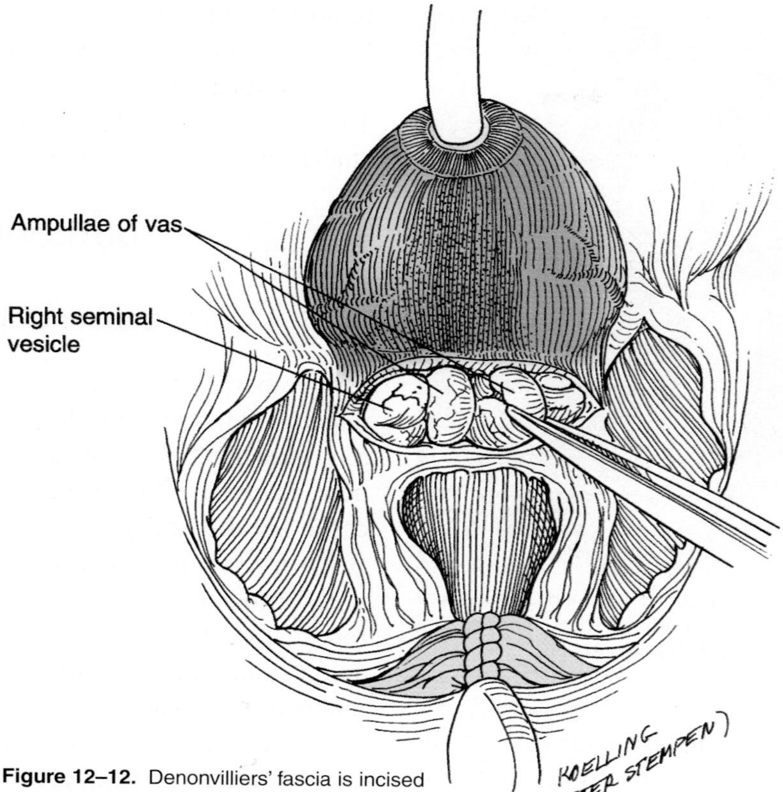

Figure 12–12. Denonvilliers' fascia is incised over the seminal vesicles and ampullae of the vas deferens.

are clipped or tied before being cut, and each seminal vesicle is excised in its entirety. Dissection should proceed just alongside the seminal vesicle to avoid injury to the neurovascular bundles as the pelvic nerve plexus lies very close to the seminal vesicles. The prostate is then separated from the bladder neck circumferentially. In select cases in which the risk of cancer extension at the bladder neck is minimal, the circular fibers of the bladder neck can be preserved. Bladder neck preservation may allow for earlier and more complete return of urinary continence compared with techniques whereby the bladder neck is excised more extensively.[34] In addition, the risk of a bladder neck contracture may be reduced. Rarely is the bladder neck a site of a positive margin, suggesting that bladder neck preservation is not likely to result in cancer recurrence.[34a] However, Lepor and associates found that bladder neck preservation might be associated with preservation of benign prostatic tissue in this area. Such residual tissue may give rise to a detectable serum PSA. In those cases whereby more extensive dissection at the bladder neck is necessary, the bladder neck is closed to a smaller size; 3-0 or 4-0 absorbable suture material is used to evert the bladder mucosa anteriorly and laterally. The bladder neck can be narrowed in a "racket handle" fashion, if necessary, using a continuous 4-0 or 3-0 absorbable suture.

The bladder neck is sutured to the urethra using interrupted 3-0 or 4-0 suture material over a 16 or 18F urethral catheter. Generally, six to eight interrupted sutures are placed (Figure 12–13). Care is taken when placing these sutures posterolaterally to avoid injury to the autonomic and somatic innervation of the external urinary sphincter and the neurovascular bundles.[16] The sutures should include only the cut end of the urethra and not the levator musculature or nerve fibers. A closed drainage system is placed, and the wound is closed. The fascia is generally closed using a running 1-0 or 0 suture. The skin is approximated and closed. As patients are hospitalized for only 2 to 3 days, it may be best to close the skin using fine running subcuticular sutures rather than staples to avoid an early return visit for staple removal.

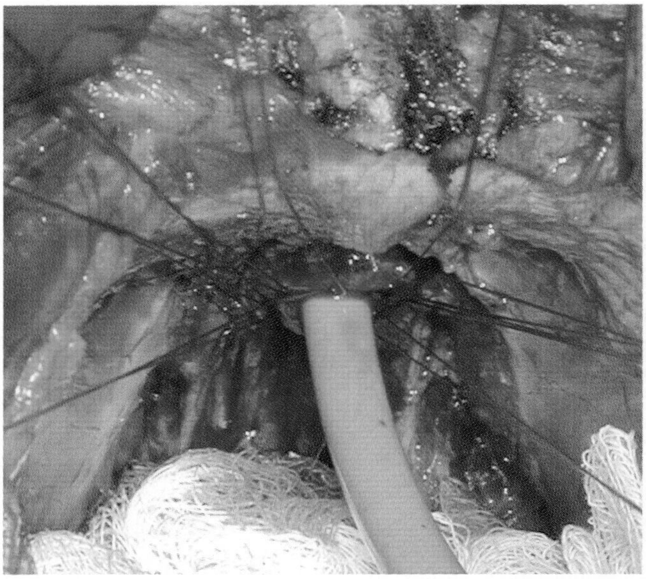

Figure 12–13. The distal sphincteric continence mechanism is well preserved, and eight absorbable sutures on round needles are placed for the anastomosis (intraoperative photograph).

Patients thought to be at an increased risk of postoperative urinary incontinence (ie, advanced age, previous radiation, cancer at the apex requiring wide excision) may be candidates for autologous fascial sling placement at the time of radical prostatectomy. On making a lower abdominal midline incision, the rectus fascia is sharply incised. A strip of rectus fascia measuring approximately 1 × 8 cm is harvested. This piece of fascia is trimmed of all fat, and the ends of the fascia are plicated with 2-0 absorbable or nonabsorbable suture, the ends of which were left long. This fascial piece is placed in normal saline while the remainder of the radical prostatectomy is carried out as described. After the vesicourethral anastomosis is completed, the sling is carefully placed underneath the anastomosis using a right-angled clamp (Figure 12–14). Care is taken to position the sling at the level of the anastomosis and external sphincter and not more proximally. The free suture ends are placed through the ipsilateral rectus fascia. The rectus fascia is closed inferiorly using interrupted absorbable suture material and the sling sutures are tied loosely, without tension, on the rectus fascia. Closure is then completed.

Hospitalization is limited to 2 days in most situations. The drain is removed when drainage is minimal, usually by hospital day 2. The urethral catheter is removed generally between 5 and 10 days following the procedure.[35] Those who undergo placement of a urethral sling have their catheters removed between 10 and 14 days following the procedure. Contrast studies are not necessary before catheter removal.

OUTCOMES

Cancer Control

Contemporary methods of radical prostatectomy for patients with clinically localized disease are generally associated with excellent outcomes. Survival may be reported in several ways: overall survival, cause-specific survival, and biochemical relapse-free survival. In a series of over 600 men treated with prostatectomy, Trapasso and colleagues reported a 10-year crude survival rate of 86 percent and a cause-specific survival of 94 percent.[36] In an independent analysis of men treated at the Mayo Clinic, Zincke and colleagues reported crude and cause-specific survival rates of 75 and 90 percent, respectively.[37,38] The crude survival rates at 10 and 15 years after surgery were similar to those of age-matched men from the general population without prostate cancer.

However, between 22 and 50 percent of patients thought to have organ-confined prostate cancer at

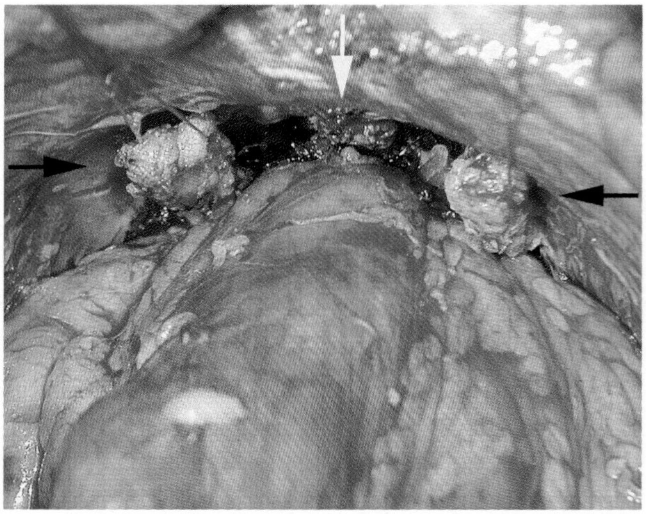

Figure 12–14. The rectus fascial sling is carefully placed underneath the vesicourethral anastomosis using a right-angled clamp. *Black arrows* point toward the ends of the rectus fascial sling, and a *white arrow* points toward the urethrovesical anastomosis.

the time of surgery are later found to have disease beyond the prostate based on careful review of the surgical specimen.[39–42] Given the protracted nature of prostate cancer and the fact that residual and/or recurrent disease may respond to salvage or secondary therapy such as radiation or androgen deprivation, postoperative follow-up with serum PSA testing has become an important end point in follow-up. Biochemical failure is defined as either the persistence of a detectable PSA after surgery or the development of a detectable PSA in those with a previously undetectable postoperative level. Total serum PSA has a half-life of 2 to 3 days, and its clearance follows first-order elimination kinetics; thus, the duration between surgery and PSA nadir generally takes several weeks and varies as a function of the patient's preoperative PSA.[43] Indeed, virtually all recurrent clinical and metastatic disease is preceded by a rising PSA, and only a few sporadic cases of recurrence have been reported in the absence of a detectable serum PSA level. Therefore, follow-up after surgery is relatively straightforward and usually consists of symptom assessment and measurement of serum PSA. The frequency of testing varies depending on the risk of recurrence and the time since surgery. In general, serum PSA is measured every 3 to 4 months for the first year, biannually for the second year and third years, and annually thereafter. What constitutes a detectable serum PSA varies among investigators, and the use of ultra- or hypersensitive PSA assays improves the lead time for early detection of recurrence.[44,45] Whereas biochemical disease-free survival is defined by an undetectable serum PSA following surgery, clinical disease-free survival refers to freedom from detectable local or metastatic disease as assessed by physical examination and the selective use of imaging and biopsy techniques.

In two contemporary prostatectomy series from the Cleveland Clinic and Johns Hopkins Hospital totaling more than 2,000 patients, not one patient showed signs of clinical disease in the absence of PSA failure.[39,46] Following biochemical (PSA) failure, up to 68 percent of men will progress to detectable clinical disease at a median follow-up of 19 months. With adjuvant therapy such as radiation or androgen deprivation at the time of PSA failure, the rate of progression to clinical disease is reportedly lower at 21 percent.[39] Metastatic disease following PSA failure occurs in 34 percent of patients without adjuvant or salvage therapy, and investigators have reported a median actuarial time to metastases of 8 years from the time of PSA failure.[46] For those who develop metastatic disease, the median actuarial time to death in one series was 5 years from the date of metastasis.[46]

Radical prostatectomy is associated with overall 5- and 10-year actuarial biochemical progression-free survival rates ranging from 59 to 83 percent and 47 to 74 percent, respectively (Table 12–1).[36,37,39,46–50] The variability in outcomes most likely reflects differences in patient selection and definition of biochemical failure and, to a lesser extent, variations in surgical technique. Reflecting the natural history of disease progression, clinical disease-free rates are considerably higher at 84 to 86 percent (5 years) and 72 to 78 percent (10 years).

The risk of disease progression varies directly with increasing pathologic disease stage, preoperative serum PSA levels, Gleason scores, and surgical

Table 12–1. BIOCHEMICAL RELAPSE-FREE SURVIVAL FOLLOWING RADICAL PROSTATECTOMY

Institution	N	5 Years, %	10 Years, %	Outcome	Follow-up, yr
Washington University[47]	925	78	61	PSA < 0.6 ng/mL	2.3 (mean)
Duke[49]	1,319	65–70	—	PSA < 0.5 ng/mL	4.0 (median)
Baylor[48]	500	77	74	PSA < 0.4 ng/mL	2.7 (median)
University of California, Los Angeles[36]	601	69	47	PSA < 0.4 ng/mL	2.8 (median)
		86	78	Clinically free of disease	
Mayo Clinic[37]	3,170	70	52	PSA < 0.2 ng/mL	5.0 (mean)
		85	72	Clinically free of disease	
Cleveland Clinic[39]	423	59	—	PSA < 0.2 ng/mL	4.3 (median)
		84	—	Clinically free of disease	
Johns Hopkins[50]	1,623	80	68	PSA < 0.2 ng/mL	5.0 (mean)
University of California, San Francisco	666	78	—	PSA < 0.2 ng/mL	3.1 (median)

margin status. At the UCSF, patients with pathologically confined disease (ie, ≤ pT2, and for all grades) have a 5-year PSA progression-free actuarial survival rate of 80 percent compared with 57 percent in those with non–organ-confined disease (stages T3a and b and node-positive disease). Similarly, pretreatment serum PSA correlates with outcome. For patients stratified into risk groups according to pretreatment PSA values of ≤ 4 ng/mL, 4.1 to 10 ng/mL, 10.1 to 20 ng/mL, and > 20 ng/mL, 5-year PSA progression-free rates are 83, 78, 65, and 37 percent, respectively. Those patients found to have relatively well-differentiated cancers are more likely to do well compared with those with poorly differentiated cancers. For all stages and serum PSA levels, those with Gleason sums ≤ 6 have a 77 percent biochemical progression-free rate, compared with 67 percent for those with Gleason sums of 7 (generally Gleason scores of 3/4 or 4/3) and 40 percent for those with Gleason sums of 8 to 10. Indeed, low-risk patients as defined by stage (< T2a), serum PSA (< 10 ng/mL), and grade (no Gleason score 4 or 5) appear to have a PSA relapse-free survival of approximately 92 percent.

The kinetics of biochemical recurrence correlate with the pattern of relapse. Patel and colleagues found that patients with PSA doubling times of 6 months or greater had an 80 percent clinically disease-free rate at a mean follow-up of 58 months as compared with 64 percent in those with PSA doubling times of less than 6 months.[51] Furthermore, patients who progressed to aggressive distant metastatic disease had a shorter median PSA doubling time than those with only biochemical failure or local disease recurrence (4.3 versus 11.7 months, respectively).[52]

Complications

Contemporary methods of radical prostatectomy are associated with limited morbidity. Perioperative mortality is exceedingly rare, at approximately 0.2 percent.[37,53] The perioperative mortality rate at UCSF is 0.13 percent. Intraoperative rectal injury and the need for a colostomy have decreased from 1 and 0.2 percent, respectively, prior to 1988 to 0.6 and 0.06 percent currently. The rectal injury rate at UCSF is 0.13 percent, and no patient has required a colostomy. Similarly, complications such as myocardial infarction (0.1 to 0.4%), deep venous thrombosis (1.1%), pulmonary embolism (0.75%), blood transfusions (< 5%), anastomotic stricture (4%), inguinal hernia (1%), and incisional hernia (0.6%) are becoming more uncommon. In the series by Catalona and colleagues, the incidence of stricture decreased with surgical experience from 6.0 percent for the first 1,000 patients treated to 1.1 percent in the last 870 patients.[53] Complication rates are likely to decrease further with further experience and refinements in technique.[54]

For the most part, only biomedical end points, death, physical disability, or cure, have been assessed following the diagnosis and treatment of prostate cancer. Relatively little effort has been placed on assessing the impact of this disease, its diagnosis and subsequent treatment, and health-related quality of life.[55] Although the annual death rate from prostatic cancer is high, several studies have noted that progression may occur slowly in selected patients with clinically localized cancers left untreated. Treatment is associated with a well-defined risk of morbidity. Therefore, the compromise between disability and cure is especially troublesome for many patients with prostate cancer and their physicians. Greater emphasis on the more common disease-specific complications has occurred. The most common disease-specific domains likely to be affected by focal treatment (ie, surgery or radiation) include sexual, urinary, and bowel function and bother.[56]

As described earlier, urinary continence is maintained by the bladder neck, prostatic smooth muscle, and external striated sphincter. After radical prostatectomy, immediate postoperative incontinence may occur in up to 80 percent of patients. More contemporary series report a much lower rate of immediate incontinence.[53,57] Fortunately, the majority of patients, 86 to 92 percent, recover urinary continence within the first 12 months after surgery. However, depending on patient age, definition of incontinence, method of assessment, and surgical technique, incontinence rates at 1 year vary from 3 to 36 percent.[58–60] Approximately 90 percent of men who undergo radical prostatectomy will be continent at 1 year when continence is defined as no regular use of pads and/or no leakage with moderate exercise. In a multivariate analysis of risk factors for urinary incontinence, Eastham and colleagues reported that decreasing age, preservation of both neurovascular bundles, an absence of an anastomotic stricture, and careful preservation of the external striated urinary sphincter were independently associated with preservation of continence.[61] Severe and persistent incontinence defined as leakage with normal activity or the need for three or more pads per day occurs in 1 to 6 percent of patients. Such patients may be candidates for use of an artificial sphincter or collagen injection.[62]

At UCSF, a contemporary cohort of patients (n = 217) underwent radical retropubic prostatectomy between 1999 and 2000 by a single surgeon. Each patient was surveyed anonymously using a detailed questionnaire, which included the University of California, Los Angeles/Rand Prostate Cancer Index quality-of-life urinary domain questions. Overall continence 1 year after radical prostatectomy was 98 percent, as defined above. Average time to continence was 2 to 4 weeks. Immediate continence was achieved in 23 percent of men. Over half (55%) of the men were continent by 1 month. In terms of continence satisfaction, 77 percent were "delighted" or "pleased," whereas only 4% rated their satisfaction as "unhappy" or "terrible." Additionally, patients were asked how big a problem urinary function was after radical prostatectomy. Eighty-one percent felt that there was either "no problem" or a "very small problem." Only 3 percent of patients felt that this was a "big" problem. Patients with increased risk factors for urinary incontinence such as advanced age, previous radiation, increased body mass index, and wide extent of apical dissection also underwent a simultaneous urethral sling procedure using autologous rectus fascia (n = 52). Interestingly, this high-risk group of patients also had a similar average continence profile. Twenty percent were continent immediately, whereas 61 percent were continent by 1 month, a statistically significant increase in the rapidity of return to continence. In this group, the vast majority of continence return occurred in the first 2 months, with continence in 84 percent of patients who received simultaneous urethral sling placement. This is in contrast to the nonsling patient cohort who continued to achieve continence but at later time points. It may be true that the use of the urethral sling confers an earlier return to continence, as well as increases the incidence of continence in a cohort of patients especially at risk for postoperative urinary incontinence. Fecal incontinence is rare following radical retropubic prostatectomy but may occur more often following perineal prostatectomy.

Return of potency after radical prostatectomy is dependent on many factors, including preoperative potency status, cancer stage, patient age, and whether one or both neurovascular bundles are spared. With the advent of the nerve-sparing approach to radical retropubic prostatectomy, selected patients treated by an experienced surgical team can anticipate return of potency without sacrificing cancer control.[28,53] High rates of postoperative potency are not reported by all investigators.[60,63] In general, physicians underestimate the degree of disability encountered by patients. Catalona and colleagues reported recovery of potency in 68 and 47 percent of preoperatively potent men treated with bilateral or unilateral nerve-sparing surgery, respectively.[53] Furthermore, younger patients reported superior outcomes. With a follow-up period of at least 18 months, 90 percent of men between age 40 and 49 were potent compared with 80, 60, and 47 percent of their counterparts in their fifties, sixties, and seventies, respectively. Rabbani and colleagues studied 314 consecutive men managed with radical prostatectomy to determine predictors of the recovery of sexual function following surgery.[64] Patient age, preoperative potency status, and extent of neurovascular bundle preservation were predictive of potency recovery. At 3 years following the operation, 76, 56, and 47 percent of those ages < 60, 60 to 65, and > 65 years were potent. Not surprisingly, men with only partial erections preoperatively and those who underwent unilateral nerve-sparing surgery were less likely to recover potency, 47 and 25 percent, respectively. All studies suggest that the patients most likely to benefit from nerve-sparing surgery are those who are young, potent, and sexually active and have focal disease. It also appears that return of spontaneous erections following nerve-sparing surgery may be improved with early use of either sildenafil or intracavernous injection therapy.[65–67] Sural nerve grafting at the time of radical prostatectomy in those patients for whom resection of the neurovascular bundle is necessary to achieve adequate surgical margins has been described.[68] However, given the considerable stage migration that has occurred, most patients currently undergoing radical prostatectomy are candidates for preservation of their neurovascular bundles, which is likely to result in better preservation of sexual function than the use of sural nerve grafts.

Potency following radical prostatectomy can be restored in a variety of ways. Men who have undergone nerve-sparing surgery who have not regained erections adequate for vaginal penetration may be excellent candidates for the use of sildenafil. Approximately 43 to 75 percent of such patients may respond favorably to this drug.[65–67] The most common side effects include headache, flushing, visual disturbances, and nasal congestion. For those who do not respond to sildenafil or are not candidates for it, use of either intraurethral or intracorporeal therapy will likely result in adequate return of potency. Vacuum erection devices and, less commonly, insertion of a penile prosthesis are other alternatives.

NEOADJUVANT AND ADJUVANT THERAPY

A significant number of men who undergo standard local treatment for prostate cancer will experience biochemical recurrence, which may herald the development of clinical recurrence in some. A recent analysis of patients enrolled in a disease registry of prostate cancer patients demonstrated that 22 percent of patients who received initial treatment with radical prostatectomy, radiation therapy, or cryotherapy required a second form of prostate cancer treatment within 3 years of initial therapy.[69] The risk of biochemical and clinical recurrence is related to cancer stage, volume and grade, preoperative serum PSA, and surgical margin status.

Kattan and colleagues developed both pre- and postoperative nomograms for disease recurrence following radical prostatectomy.[70,71] For those who have undergone radical prostatectomy, several models have been proposed to identify patients at very high risk for relapse.[72–74] From the above information, one can broadly identify patients who would be at high risk of relapse for whom adjuvant therapy following radical prostatectomy may be of most benefit. High-risk patients would be those having the following clinical and pathologic findings: (1) positive seminal vesicles; (2) Gleason score 6 and PSA > 18 ng/mL; (3) Gleason score 7 and PSA > 14 ng/mL; (4) Gleason score 8, 9, or 10 and any PSA; and (5) those with positive surgical margins. Several strategies have been evaluated to decrease or lengthen the time to disease recurrence.

Neoadjuvant Androgen Deprivation

Some investigators have tested the hypothesis that recurrence rates following radical prostatectomy could be reduced by neoadjuvant androgen deprivation. Such therapy could decrease the likelihood of positive surgical margins leading to a decrease in local recurrence rates. Every randomized trial performed to date has shown that neoadjuvant androgen deprivation significantly decreases the rate of positive surgical margins. The rates of positive surgical margins were decreased by approximately 40 to 60 percent with neoadjuvant androgen deprivation in several series.[75–86] To date, neoadjuvant androgen deprivation has not been associated with improvements in clinical or biochemical control rates.[86a] Klotz and colleagues recently reported the results of a trial sponsored by the Canadian Urologic Oncology Group. A total of 213 patients with localized prostate cancer were randomized to radical prostatectomy alone (101) or 12 weeks of cyproterone acetate followed by surgery (112).[81] The probability of biochemical progression at 36 months was similar for the groups treated by surgery alone or cyproterone acetate followed by surgery, 30.1 versus 40.2 percent ($p = .3233$), respectively. This and similar trials are ongoing, and failure to demonstrate a small but significant benefit to neoadjuvant therapy may be owing to insufficient follow-up, short duration of androgen deprivation, insufficient power of some trials to demonstrate a benefit, or inclusion of large numbers of either very low- or high-risk patients in such trials. Most trials reported to date have used 3 months of androgen deprivation before surgery. Some suggest that extending the length of time of neoadjuvant androgen deprivation before surgery may translate into improved outcomes.[87, 88, 88a] Further improvements in serum PSA and prostate tumor volume occur with longer duration of treatment. Any potential improvement in outcome may be confined to patients with adverse pretreatment characteristics such as high cancer grade or serum PSA. It is clear, however, that neoadjuvant androgen deprivation cannot substitute for careful preoperative risk assessment and meticulous surgical technique.

Adjuvant Systemic or Radiation Therapy

Optimal treatment for patients with adverse disease characteristics, as well as the timing of such treatment, remains controversial. Standard second treatment options following radical prostatectomy include radiation therapy with or without androgen deprivation or androgen deprivation alone. Adjuvant treatment, if given, can be tailored to the risk of relapse and to the pattern of suspected relapse, local versus distant. Distant relapse may be more likely in those with high-grade disease, lymph node metastasis, and very high pretreatment PSA as well as those patients who fail to have their serum PSA fall to undetectable levels immediately after surgery. Patients at high risk for distant relapse are also ideal candidates for experimental adjuvant, systemic therapy.

The impact of positive surgical margins on outcome is a matter of controversy. Between 14 and 41 percent of patients undergoing radical prostatectomy have tumor extending to the surgical margin on final pathologic analysis, with 33 to 62 percent of these patients ultimately failing based on detectable serum PSA levels.[48,89–94] Radiation therapy may be given following surgery based on adverse disease characteristics such as positive surgical margins (adjuvant radiation) or after a documented disease recurrence (therapeutic radiation) based on either biopsy-proven recurrence or biochemical failure alone.[95–100] Proponents of adjuvant radiation argue that treatment is more effective when the local tumor burden is minimal and that series to date show that patients who undergo adjuvant radiation achieve and maintain an undetectable serum PSA 77 to 94 percent of the time. However, despite improved local tumor control, no survival advantage has been demonstrated with adjuvant radiation, between 42 and 70 percent of patients with positive surgical margins will maintain undetectable serum PSA levels without adjuvant therapy, and radiation for biochemical recurrence, if given early, may still be efficacious. Pathologic factors such as the location, extent, and number of positive margins may have an impact on the likelihood of disease recurrence in this setting. Certainly, those with multiple positive biopsies are at an increased risk of recurrence compared with those with a single, focal margin positive for disease. Some have demonstrated that a positive margin at the bladder neck was associated with a shorter time to biochemical recurrence than a positive margin at the apex.[91] Others have failed to show such a difference.[90] Recently, Leibovich and colleagues retrospectively evaluated the records of a nested matched cohort of 76 patients with pathologic stage T2N0 prostate cancer and a single positive margin who underwent adjuvant radiation therapy within 3 months of radical prostatectomy.[101] These patients were matched one to one with 76 controls who did not receive adjuvant radiation therapy. Patients and controls were matched for the margin site, age, preoperative serum PSA, Gleason score, and DNA ploidy. They identified a significant improvement in those who received adjuvant radiation. Those who received adjuvant radiation had a 5-year clinical and biochemical progression-free survival rate of 88 ± 5 percent compared with 59 percent for those who did not receive radiation following surgery. A benefit to radiation was seen in those with positive margins at both the base and the apex.

Prospective randomized trials of surveillance versus adjuvant radiation following radical prostatectomy in high-risk patients are not available. The Southwest Oncology Group has completed a randomized trial examining this question, but the results of this study are not yet available. A decision to give adjuvant radiation is based on the (1) likelihood of cancer recurrence with adjuvant radiation, (2) the likelihood of cancer recurrence with surveillance alone, (3) the efficacy of radiation when given for biochemical recurrence (efficacy of therapeutic radiation), and (4) the morbidity of radiation. Grossfeld and colleagues at UCSF created and tested a decision analysis model to help determine the preferred management of a positive surgical margin(s) following radical prostatectomy.[89] The model suggested that immediate radiation may be the preferred course of management for patients with a positive surgical margin(s) and a high likelihood of recurrent local, rather than distant, disease. Such patients included those with low- to intermediate-grade disease (Gleason score < 8), multiple positive margins, and no evidence of seminal vesicle invasion. Surveillance was still recommended for patients with a preoperative PSA < 15 ng/mL and those with a single positive margin. However, the authors stressed that their model was based on literature and institution-based estimates of the efficacy of adjuvant and delayed radiation. The model may be most useful to physicians and patients who can use individualized probability estimates and utility values to determine their preferred course of management after surgery.

Patients with high-risk features, other than positive surgical margins, may be candidates for adjuvant systemic therapy. The risk and timing of recurrence can be estimated using a variety of models, as defined earlier.[73,74] The timing and type of systemic therapy following radical prostatectomy in high-risk patients remain controversial. Most such patients who have undetectable serum PSA levels following surgery are candidates for surveillance, with delayed treatment if necessary or immediate adjuvant therapy. Such patients may be ideal candidates for clinical trials. Trials are currently under way examining the potential benefit of a variety of agents in such patients.

Whereas neoadjuvant and adjuvant androgen deprivation appears to be of value when combined with radiation therapy in high-risk patients, it is unclear whether such therapy improves outcomes in combination with surgery compared to surveillance with delayed therapy only in those who manifest cancer recurrence based on PSA testing.[101a] Messing and colleagues studied 98 men who underwent radical prostatectomy and pelvic lymphadenectomy and who were found to have nodal metastases.[102] These patients were randomly assigned to receive immediate androgen deprivation therapy, with either an agonist of gonadotropin-releasing hormone or bilateral orchiectomy, or to be followed until disease progression. After a median of 7.1 years of follow-up, 7 of 47 men who received immediate androgen deprivation had died, as compared with 18 of 51 men in the observation group ($p = .02$). The cause of death was prostate cancer in 3 men in the immediate-treatment group and in 16 men in the observation group ($p = .01$). At the time of the last follow-up, 36 men in the immediate-treatment group (77%) and 9 men in the observation group (18%) were alive and had no evidence of recurrent disease, including undetectable serum PSA levels ($p < .001$). In the observation group, the disease recurred in 42 men; 13 of the 36 who were treated had a complete response to local treatment or hormonal therapy (or both), 16 died of prostate cancer, and 1 died of another disease. Their conclusion that immediate androgen deprivation therapy after radical prostatectomy and pelvic lymphadenectomy improves survival and reduces the risk of recurrence in patients with node-positive prostate cancer has been questioned by some. However, early androgen deprivation may benefit those with minimal metastatic disease. The exact timing of such therapy remains to be determined.

SUMMARY

In summary, radical prostatectomy is a safe operation and an effective procedure for properly selected patients. Major complications are rare and decrease with the surgeon's experience. With current refinements in technique, significant urinary incontinence is rare and preservation of potency is possible in selected patients. Patients most likely to benefit from this approach are those who have long life expectancies and have either organ-confined disease or limited extracapsular extension, which can be excised completely. Adjuvant therapy in selected patients may further improve long-term cause-specific and biochemical relapse-free survival.

REFERENCES

1. Walsh PC. Prostate cancer kills: strategy to reduce deaths Urology 1994;44:463–6.
2. Thompson IM. Counseling patients with newly diagnosed prostate cancer. Oncology (Huntingt) 2000;14:119–26, 131; discussion 135–6.
3. Koppie TM, Grossfeld GD, Miller D, et al. Patterns of treatment of patients with prostate cancer initially managed with surveillance: results from the CaPSURE database. Cancer of the Prostate Strategic Urological Research Endeavor. J Urol 2000;164:81-8.
4. D'Amico AV, et al. Clinical utility of the percentage of positive prostate biopsies in defining biochemical outcome after radical prostatectomy for patients with clinically localized prostate cancer. J Clin Oncol 2000;18:1164–72.

4a Grossfeld GD, Chang JJ, Broering JM, et al. Under staging and under grading in a contemporary series of patients undergoing radical prostatectomy: results from the Cancer of the Prostate Strategic Urologic Research Endeavor database. J Urol 2001;165:851-6.
4b Grossfeld GD, Latini DM, Lubeck DP, et al. Predicting disease recurrence in intermediate and high-risk patients undergoing radical prostatectomy using percent positive biopsies: results from CaPSURE. Urology 2002;59:560-5.
5. Amling CL, et al. Primary surgical therapy for clinical stage T3 adenocarcinoma of the prostate. Semin Urol Oncol 1997;15:215–21.
6. Bishoff JT, et al. Pelvic lymphadenectomy can be omitted in selected patients with carcinoma of the prostate: development of a system of patient selection. Urology 1995:45:270–4.
7. Narayan P, et al. Utility of preoperative serum prostate-specific antigen concentration and biopsy Gleason score in predicting risk of pelvic lymph node metastases in prostate cancer. Urology 1994:44;519–24.
8. Partin A, et al. Combination of prostate-specific antigen, clinical stage, and Gleason score to predict pathological stage of localized prostate cancer. A multi-institutional update. JAMA 1997;277:1445–551.
9. Meng MV, Carroll PR. When is pelvic lymph node dissection necessary before radical prostatectomy? A decision analysis. J Urol 2000;164:1235–40.
9a Kattan MW, Stapleton AM, Wheeler TM, Scardino PT. Evaluation of a nomogram used to predict the pathologic stage clinically localized prostate carcinoma. Cancer 1997;79:528-37.
9b Polascik TJ, Pearson JD, Partin AW. Multivariate models as predictors of pathological stage using Gleason score, clinical stage, and serum prostate-specific antigen. Semin Urol Oncol 1998;16:160-71.
9c Penson DF, Grossfeld GD, Li YP, et al. How well does the Partin nomogram predict pathological stage after radical prostatectomy in a community based population? Results of the cancer of the prostate strategic urological research endeavor. J Urol 2002;167:1653-7.
10. Steiner MS. The puboprostatic ligament and the male urethral suspensory mechanism: an anatomic study. Urology 1994;44:530–4.
11. Di Lollo S, et al. The morphology of the prostatic capsule with particular regard to the posterosuperior region: an anatomical and clinical problem. Surg Radiol Anat 1997;19:143–7.
12. Light JK, Rapoll E, Wheeler TM. The striated urethral sphincter: muscle fibre types and distribution in the prostatic capsule. Br J Urol 1997;79:539–42.
13. Burnett AL, Mostwin JL. In situ anatomical study of the male urethral sphincteric complex: relevance to continence preservation following major pelvic surgery. J Urol 1998;160:1301–6.
14. Myers RP. Anatomical variation of the superficial preprostatic veins with respect to radical retropubic prostatectomy. J Urol 1991;145:992–3.
15. Myers RP. Male urethral sphincteric anatomy and radical prostatectomy. Urol Clin North Am 1991;18:211–27.
16. Steiner MS. Anatomic basis for the continence-preserving radical retropubic prostatectomy. Semin Urol Oncol 2000;18:9–18.
17. Shafik A, Doss D. Surgical anatomy of the somatic terminal innervation to the anal and urethral sphincters: role in anal and urethral surgery. J Urol 1999;161:85–9.
18. Strasser H, et al. Anatomy and innervation of the rhabdosphincter of the male urethra. Prostate 1996;28:24–31.
19. Vaalasti A, Hervonen A. Autonomic innervation of the human prostate. Invest Urol 1980;17:293–7.
20. Zvara P, et al. The detailed neuroanatomy of the human striated urethral sphincter. Br J Urol 1994;74:182–7.
21. Frank E, et al. Postoperative epidural analgesia following radical retropubic prostatectomy: outcome assessment. J Surg Oncol 1998;67:117–20.
22. Gottschalk A, et al. Preemptive epidural analgesia and recovery from radical prostatectomy: a randomized controlled trial. JAMA 1998;279:1076–82.
23. Reinhart DI. Minimising the adverse effects of ketorolac. Drug Saf 2000;22:487–97.
24. Goad JR, et al. Radical retropubic prostatectomy: limited benefit of autologous blood donation. J Urol 1995;154:2103–9.
25. O'Hara JF Jr, et al. Use of preoperative autologous blood donation in patients undergoing radical retropubic prostatectomy. Urology 1999;54:130–4.
26. Noldus J, Gonnermann D, Huland H. Autologous blood transfusion in radical prostatectomy: results in 263 patients. Eur Urol 1995;27:213–7.
27. Walsh PC. Radical prostatectomy: a procedure in evolution. Semin Oncol 1994;21:662–71.
28. Walsh PC, Partin AW, Epstein JI. Cancer control and quality of life following anatomical radical retropubic prostatectomy: results at 10 years. J Urol 1994;152(5 Pt 2):1831–6.
29. Ghavamian R, Zincke H. An updated simplified approach to nerve-sparing radical retropubic prostatectomy. BJU Int 1999;84:160–3.
30. Koch MO. Management of the dorsal vein complex during radical retropubic prostatectomy. Semin Urol Oncol 2000;18:33–7.
31. Cangiano TG, et al. Intraoperative frozen section monitoring of nerve sparing radical retropubic prostatectomy. J Urol 1999;162(3 Pt 1):655–8.
32. Klotz L. Neurostimulation during radical prostatectomy: improving nerve-sparing techniques. Semin Urol Oncol 2000;18:46–50.
33. Klotz L. Intraoperative cavernous nerve stimulation during nerve sparing radical prostatectomy: how and when? Curr Opin Urol 2000;10:239–43.
34. Soloway MS, Neulander E. Bladder-neck preservation during radical retropubic prostatectomy. Semin Urol Oncol 2000;18:51–6.
34a Lepor H, Chan S, Melamed J. The role of bladder neck biopsy in men undergoing radical retropubic prostatectomy with preservation of the bladder neck. J Urol 1998;160:2435-9.
35. DeMarco RT, Bihrle R, Foster RS. Early catheter removal following radical retropubic prostatectomy. Semin Urol Oncol 2000;18:57–9.
36. Trapasso JG, et al. The incidence and significance of detectable levels of serum prostate specific antigen after radical prostatectomy. J Urol 1994;152(5 Pt 2):1821–5.

37. Zincke H, et al. Long-term (15 years) results after radical prostatectomy for clinically localized (stage T2c or lower) prostate cancer. J Urol 1994;152(5 Pt 2):1850–7.
38. Zincke H, et al. Radical prostatectomy for clinically localized prostate cancer: long-term results of 1,143 patients from a single institution. J Clin Oncol 1994;12:2254–63.
39. Kupelian PA, et al. Stage T1-2 prostate cancer: a multivariate analysis of factors affecting biochemical and clinical failures after radical prostatectomy. Int J Radiat Oncol Biol Phys 1997;37:1043–52.
40. Partin AW, et al. Combination of prostate-specific antigen, clinical stage, and Gleason score to predict pathological stage of localized prostate cancer. A multi-institutional update [published erratum appears in JAMA 1997;278: 118]. JAMA 1997;277:1445–51.
41. Badalament RA, et al. An algorithm for predicting nonorgan confined prostate cancer using the results obtained from sextant core biopsies with prostate specific antigen level. J Urol 1996;156:1375–80.
42. Grossfeld GD, et al. Does the completeness of prostate sampling predict outcome for patients undergoing radical prostatectomy?: data from the CAPSURE database. Urology 2000;56:430–5.
43. Sokoll LJ, Chan DW. Prostate-specific antigen. Its discovery and biochemical characteristics. Urol Clin North Am 1997;24:253–9.
44. Haese A, et al. Supersensitive PSA-analysis after radical prostatectomy: a powerful tool to reduce the time gap between surgery and evidence of biochemical failure. Anticancer Res 1999;19:2641–4.
45. Yu H, et al. Ultrasensitive assay of prostate-specific antigen used for early detection of prostate cancer relapse and estimation of tumor-doubling time after radical prostatectomy. Clin Chem 1995;41:430–4.
46. Pound CR, et al. Natural history of progression after PSA elevation following radical prostatectomy. JAMA 1999;281: 1591–7.
47. Catalona WJ, Smith DS. 5-year tumor recurrence rates after anatomical radical retropubic prostatectomy for prostate cancer. J Urol 1994;152(5 Pt 2):1837–42.
48. Ohori M, et al. Prognostic significance of positive surgical margins in radical prostatectomy specimens. J Urol 1995; 154:1818–24.
49. Iselin CE, et al. Surgical control of clinically localized prostate carcinoma is equivalent in African-American and white males. Cancer 1998;83:2353–60.
50. Partin AW, et al. Serum PSA after anatomic radical prostatectomy. The Johns Hopkins experience after 10 years. Urol Clin North Am 1993;20:713–25.
51. Patel A, et al. Recurrence patterns after radical retropubic prostatectomy: clinical usefulness of prostate specific antigen doubling times and log slope prostate specific antigen. J Urol 1997;158:1441–5.
52. Partin AW, et al. Evaluation of serum prostate-specific antigen velocity after radical prostatectomy to distinguish local recurrence from distant metastases. Urology 1994;43: 649–59.
53. Catalona WJ, et al. Potency, continence and complication rates in 1,870 consecutive radical retropubic prostatectomies. J Urol 1999;162:433–8.
54. Thompson IM, et al. Have complication rates decreased after treatment for localized prostate cancer? J Urol 1999;162: 107–12.
55. Lubeck DP, et al. Changes in health-related quality of life in the first year after treatment for prostate cancer: results from CaPSURE. Urology 1999;53:180–6.
56. Litwin MS, et al. Quality-of-life outcomes in men treated for localized prostate cancer. JAMA 1995;273:129–35.
57. Goluboff ET, et al. Urinary continence after radical prostatectomy: the Columbia experience. J Urol 1998;159:1276–80.
58. Kerr LA, Zincke H. Radical retropubic prostatectomy for prostate cancer in the elderly and the young: complications and prognosis. Eur Urol 1994;25:305–11.
59. Heathcote PS, et al. Health-related quality of life in Australian men remaining disease-free after radical prostatectomy. Med J Aust 1998;168:483–6.
60. Stanford JL, et al. Urinary and sexual function after radical prostatectomy for clinically localized prostate cancer: the Prostate Cancer Outcomes Study. JAMA 2000;283:354–60.
61. Eastham JA, et al. Risk factors for urinary incontinence after radical prostatectomy. J Urol 1996;156:1707–13.
62. Wahle GR. Urinary incontinence after radical prostatectomy. Semin Urol Oncol 2000;18:66–70.
63. Talcott JA, et al. Patient-reported impotence and incontinence after nerve-sparing radical prostatectomy. J Natl Cancer Inst 1997;89:1117–23.
64. Rabbani F, et al. Factors predicting recovery of erections after radical prostatectomy. J Urol 2000;164:1929–34.
65. Zippe CD, et al. Role of Viagra after radical prostatectomy. Urology 2000;55:241–5.
66. Zippe CD, et al. Sildenafil citrate (Viagra) after radical retropubic prostatectomy: pro [editorial]. Urology 1999;54:583–6.
67. Blander DS, et al. Efficacy of sildenafil in erectile dysfunction after radical prostatectomy. Int J Impot Res 2000;12: 165–8.
68. Kim ED, et al. Interposition of sural nerve restores function of cavernous nerves resected during radical prostatectomy. J Urol 1999;161:188–92.
69. Grossfeld GD, et al. Use of second treatment following definitive local therapy for prostate cancer: data from the caPSURE database. J Urol 1998;160:1398–404.
70. Kattan MW, et al. A preoperative nomogram for disease recurrence following radical prostatectomy for prostate cancer. J Natl Cancer Inst 1998;90:766–71.
71. Kattan MW, Wheeler TM, Scardino PT. Postoperative nomogram for disease recurrence after radical prostatectomy for prostate cancer. J Clin Oncol 1999;17:1499–507.
72. D'Amico AV, et al. Utilizing predictions of early prostate-specific antigen failure to optimize patient selection for adjuvant systemic therapy trials. J Clin Oncol 2000;18: 3240–6.
73. D'Amico AV, et al. Assessment of outcome prediction models for patients with localized prostate carcinoma managed with radical prostatectomy or external beam radiation therapy. Cancer 1998;82:1887–96.
74. Partin A, et al. Selection of men at high risk for disease recurrence for experimental adjuvant therapy following radical prostatectomy. Urology 1995;45:831–8.

75. Fair WR, et al. Use of neoadjuvant androgen deprivation therapy in clinically localized prostate cancer. Clin Invest Med 1993;16:516–22.
76. Fair WR, et al. The indications, rationale, and results of neoadjuvant androgen deprivation in the treatment of prostatic cancer: Memorial Sloan-Kettering Cancer Center results. Urology 1997;49(3A Suppl):46–55.
77. Fair WR, Scher HI. Neoadjuvant hormonal therapy plus surgery for prostate cancer. The MSKCC experience. Surg Oncol Clin N Am 1997;6:831–46.
78. Gleave ME, et al. Neoadjuvant androgen withdrawal therapy decreases local recurrence rates following tumor excision in the Shionogi tumor model. J Urol 1997;157:1727–30.
79. Goldenberg SL, et al. Randomized, prospective, controlled study comparing radical prostatectomy alone and neoadjuvant androgen withdrawal in the treatment of localized prostate cancer. Canadian Urologic Oncology Group. J Urol 1996;156:873–7.
80. Hennenfent BR. Pathological staging and biochemical recurrence after neoadjuvant androgen deprivation therapy in combination with radical prostatectomy in clinically localized prostate cancer. Br J Urol 1998;82:166.
81. Klotz LH, et al. CUOG randomized trial of neoadjuvant androgen ablation before radical prostatectomy: 36-month post-treatment PSA results. Canadian Urologic Oncology Group. Urology 1999;53:757–63.
82. Labrie F, et al. Downstaging by combination therapy with flutamide and an LHRH agonist before radical prostatectomy. Cancer Surv 1995;23:149–56.
83. Meyer F, et al. Neoadjuvant hormonal therapy before radical prostatectomy and risk of prostate specific antigen failure. J Urol 1999;162:2024–8.
84. Soloway MS, et al. Randomized prospective study comparing radical prostatectomy alone versus radical prostatectomy preceded by androgen blockade in clinical stage B2 (T2bNxM0) prostate cancer. The Lupron Depot Neoadjuvant Prostate Cancer Study Group. J Urol 1995;154 (2 Pt 1):424–8.
85. Van Poppel H, et al. Neoadjuvant hormonal therapy before radical prostatectomy decreases the number of positive surgical margins in stage T2 prostate cancer: interim results of a prospective randomized trial. The Belgian Uro–Oncological Study Group. J Urol 1995;154(2 Pt 1):429–34.
86. Witjes WP, Schulman CC, Debruyne FM. Preliminary results of a prospective randomized study comparing radical prostatectomy versus radical prostatectomy associated with neoadjuvant hormonal combination therapy in T2–3 N0 M0 prostatic carcinoma. The European Study Group on Neoadjuvant Treatment of Prostate Cancer. Urology 1997;49(3A Suppl):65–9.
86a Soloway MS, Pareek K, Sharifi R, et al. Neoadjuvant androgen ablation before radical prostatectomy in cT2bNxMo prostate cancer: 5-year results. J Urol 2002;167:112-6.
87. Gleave ME, et al. Optimal duration of neoadjuvant androgen withdrawal therapy before radical prostatectomy in clinically confined prostate cancer. Semin Urol Oncol 1996;14(2 Suppl 2):39–45; discussion 46–7.
88. Gleave ME, et al. Long-term neoadjuvant hormone therapy prior to radical prostatectomy: evaluation of risk for biochemical recurrence at 5-year follow–up. Urology 2000; 56:289–94.
88a Gleave ME, Goldenberg SL, Chin JL, eg al. Randomized comparative study of 3 versus 8-month neoadjuvant hormonal therapy before radical prostatectomy: biochemical and pathological effects. J Urol 2001;166:500-6.
89. Grossfeld GD, et al. Management of a positive surgical margin after radical prostatectomy: decision analysis. J Urol 2000;164:93–9; discussion 100.
90. Grossfeld GD, et al. Impact of positive surgical margins on prostate cancer recurrence and the use of secondary cancer treatment: data from the CaPSURE database. J Urol 2000;163:1171–7; quiz 1295.
91. Obek C, et al. Positive surgical margins with radical retropubic prostatectomy: anatomic site-specific pathologic analysis and impact on prognosis. Urology 1999;54:682–8.
92. Watson RB, Civantos F, Soloway MS. Positive surgical margins with radical prostatectomy: detailed pathological analysis and prognosis. Urology 1996;48:80–90.
93. Wieder JA, Soloway MS. Incidence, etiology, location, prevention and treatment of positive surgical margins after radical prostatectomy for prostate cancer. J Urol 1998;160: 299–315.
94. Epstein JI. Incidence and significance of positive margins in radical prostatectomy specimens. Urol Clin North Am 1996;23:651–63.
95. McCarthy JF, Catalona WJ, Hudson MA. Effect of radiation therapy on detectable serum prostate specific antigen levels following radical prostatectomy: early versus delayed treatment. J Urol 1994;151:1575–8.
96. Petrovich Z, et al. Radiotherapy following radical prostatectomy in patients with adenocarcinoma of the prostate. Int J Radiat Oncol Biol Phys 1991;21:949–54.
97. Zietman AL, et al. Adjuvant irradiation after radical prostatectomy for adenocarcinoma of prostate: analysis of freedom from PSA failure. Urology 1993;42:292–9.
98. Coetzee LJ, Hars V, Paulson DF. Postoperative prostate-specific antigen as a prognostic indicator in patients with margin-positive prostate cancer, undergoing adjuvant radiotherapy after radical prostatectomy. Urology 1996;47:232–5.
99. Gibbons RP, et al. Adjuvant radiotherapy following radical prostatectomy: results and complications. J Urol 1986; 135:65–8.
100. Syndikus I, et al. Postoperative radiotherapy for stage pT3 carcinoma of the prostate: improved local control. J Urol 1996;155:1983–6.
101. Leibovich BC, et al. Benefit of adjuvant radiation therapy for localized prostate cancer with a positive surgical margin. J Urol 2000;163:1178–82.
101aZincke H, Lau W, Bergstralh E, Blute ML. Role of early adjuvant hormonal therapy after radical prostatectomy for prostate cancer. J Urol 2001;166:2208-15.
102. Messing EM, et al. Immediate hormonal therapy compared with observation after radical prostatectomy and pelvic lymphadenectomy in men with node-positive prostate cancer. N Engl J Med 1999;341:1781–8.

13

Radical Perineal Prostatectomy

VERNON E. WELDON, MD

The burden of prostate cancer for men in the United States is similar to that of breast cancer for women: 15% will be clinically affected, 3% will die of it, and it is the second leading cause of cancer deaths.[1] As there is no curative treatment for advanced prostate cancer, enhanced detection of clinically organ-confined cancer that can be cured with available technology is the main strategy for reducing prostate cancer mortality rates.

The use of serum levels of prostate-specific antigen (PSA) since 1987 for screening and early detection of prostate cancer has been largely successful in shifting prostate cancer to lower stages on detection.[2] In populations under continuous PSA surveillance for several years, over 80% of cases are now detected when clinically localized, and in those cases, occult lymph node metastases have almost disappeared.[3,4] With enchanced early detection and the availability of effective treatment for localized disease, prostate cancer mortality in the United States decreased for the first time at an average of −1.6% per year during 1990 to 1996.[1]

Both radical prostatectomy and radiation therapy can be effective treatment for localized prostate cancer, but only surgical removal of the prostate can reliably eliminate all of the cancer that is confined within the treated area as it does not rely on clonal susceptibility to induction of apoptosis for effectiveness. Because control of localized cancer by radical prostatectomy[3,5–8] is unsurpassed by any other treatment, substantial efforts have been devoted to refining surgical techniques and minimizing any adverse impact on the quality of life. The perineal approach to radical prostatectomy offers several advantages in achieving this goal. It is truly minimally invasive, providing access to the prostate through a small incision at its most superficial location just beneath the perineal subcutaneous tissue. The apex of the prostate is easily accessible, usually only 5 cm beneath the perineal skin. Since no muscles pull on the incision, pain is minimal, and the usual total hospital stay is 1 or 2 days. With this approach, blood loss is sufficiently low that fewer than 2% of cases require transfusion, and routinely having blood available for transfusion is unnecessary. In this author's series of more than 500 cases, no perioperative deaths have occurred and the serious complication rate is 2%, whereas 95% are continent and 70% of a select group are potent.[9]

HISTORIC DEVELOPMENT

The early lithotomists discovered the morbidity and survival advantages of the perineal approach to the lower genitourinary tract, and Celsus,[10] in the first century AD, described a curvilinear perineal incision for removing bladder stones. In 1852, Demarguay[11] described a perineal approach to stones in the prostatic urethra that is identical to the current approach for radical prostatectomy, including semicircular incision anterior to the anus, division of the rectourethralis muscle, and blunt dissection of the rectum from the prostate. Küchler,[12] in 1866, first described the potential use of the perineal route for partial excision of the prostate for prostate cancer, and it was performed by Bilroth[13] in 1867. Leisrink[14] must be credited with performing the first total perineal prostatectomy for prostate cancer in 1883, including anastomosis of the bladder neck to the membranous urethra. He also removed part of the anterior rectal wall, and the patient died within a few days.

Young's[15,16] study of perineal enucleation of prostatic hyperplasia in 1903 led to his classic technique of radical perineal prostatectomy, which he described in 1905. This remains the basis of the modern technique, but with two important modifications. First, additional wide excision of the adjacent periprostatic fascia was attributed to Dillon by Weyrauch in 1959.[17] Second, after Walsh and Donker[18] described preservation of the cavernous nerves and potency with radical retropubic prostatectomy, Weldon and Tavel[19] adapted those same conservations to radical perineal prostatectomy in 1988. We also further delineated the anatomy of the alternative extended dissection of the periprostatic fascia with excision of the neurovascular bundle, thereby achieving wider margins.[19,20] Modern radical perineal prostatectomy should always selectively include one of these modifications on each side.

PATIENT SELECTION

Radical prostatectomy is an appropriate treatment for men with adenocarcinoma clinically confined within the prostate who are likely to live long enough to benefit from it. With occasional exceptions, this restricts radical prostatectomy to men with tumors in clinical stages T1 and T2, N0, M0[21] who are not older than 75 years and who have no other disease limiting their time at risk from their cancer to less than 10 years. Healthy men at age 75 have a mean survival of 10.5 years.[22,23] Initially localized prostate cancer usually progresses relatively slowly and without symptoms. It may soon progress to an incurable stage, but it is unlikely to cause significant morbidity or mortality before 8 to 10 years.[24,25] Men undergoing radical prostatectomy accept immediate risks to avoid symptomatic bony metastases and cancer death several years later. Those with a more advanced tumor stage, life-limiting comorbidity, or more advanced age generally have a risk versus benefit analysis that favors palliative treatment.

Attempts to enhance clinical staging with imaging beyond transrectal ultrasonography, including computed tomography and magnetic resonance imaging with body and rectal coils, have not had sufficient predictive value to determine treatment.[26] However, radical prostatectomy can be excluded in men with high-grade or high-volume tumor located at the base of the prostate when selective sonographically guided transrectal biopsy of the seminal vesicles demonstrates extraprostatic extension.[27]

Within the clinical stage limitations, the risks of understaging and PSA relapse after radical prostatectomy are directly related to five preoperative parameters: increasing clinical substage (T2b, T2c), biopsy Gleason score, PSA level,[28] volume of tumor in systematic biopsy cores,[29,30] and the presence of perineural space invasion in the biopsy specimen.[31] No single adverse factor prohibits radical prostatectomy, but increasing extent and number of adverse factors increase the risk of failure. High-grade but low-volume tumors with PSA levels under 10 ng/mL are optimally treated by radical prostatectomy.[32,33] However, no man in our series with a PSA level greater than 30 ng/mL had either pathologically specimen-confined disease on 3-mm step-section analysis or an undetectable PSA 5 years after surgery alone.[34] The risks of extraprostatic extension and PSA relapse are over 50% when 50% or more of the total number of systematic biopsy cores or 25% or more of the total length of biopsy cores contain cancer.[29,30] However, there is substantial overlap, and even when 100% of the cores are positive, 29% of these tumors are organ confined.[30] Patients with perineural space invasion on biopsy have twice the PSA relapse rate of those without.[31] Patient age is also a relevant factor as young men with high-risk tumors have more to gain from attempted curative surgery because of the total years of life that can be saved despite diminished cure rates.

Tables developed by Partin and colleagues[28] correlating multiple risk factors with probable pathologic stage have been used to counsel men about radical prostatectomy. However, those tables have at least three serious limitations. The estimates often have wide 95% confidence intervals. Pathologic stage is not an optimal surrogate end point since it predicts excessive failure rates. As many as 60% of patients with extracapsular extension do not have detectable PSA at 7 years after surgery.[3] Also, those tables are currently outdated since stage migration with advancing time in the PSA era is an independent variable that reduces the risk of advanced pathologic stage and lymphatic metastases.[3,35]

At the earlier end of the disease spectrum, it is desirable to avoid unnecessary treatment of likely clinically insignificant tumors. The concept of insignificant prostate cancer is a major factor in explaining the observation that 30% of men older than 50 years undergoing autopsy have prostate cancer, but only 15% of men are clinically affected. Other contributing factors are the direct relationship between advancing age and the rate of acquisition of prostate cancer, the generally slow growth rate of prostate cancer, and the many competing causes of death at advanced age. The hypothesis that insignificant cancers have low to medium grade and a volume less than 0.5 mL[36] is generally accepted. Initially, it was proposed that finding only focal cancer in systematic prostate biopsies might indicate the discovery of insignificant cancer.[37] However, we found that focal cancer on biopsy in men with an elevated PSA level or from an area of palpable abnormality was very likely only a sampling artifact, and it correlated with significant cancer in 94%.[38] If biopsy is restricted to men with either of these risk factors, which control for a high prevalence of significant cancer, thus taking Bayes's theorum into account, the risk of discovering and treating insignificant cancer is very low. Only 1% of our radical prostatectomy series had insignificant cancer.[34]

Low-volume, well-differentiated prostate cancer incidentally discovered on transurethral resection of the transition zone and involving less than 5% of the specimen is more likely to be insignificant, at least within 15 years. Most of these clinical stage T1a tumors can be followed with serial PSA determinations and selected repeat systematic biopsies, with intervention reserved for those with documented progression.

Ultimately, every treatment decision must be individualized, factoring the chance of cure with the number of years at risk and the patient's own values concerning immediate versus long-term risks.

PELVIC LYMPHADENECTOMY

The chief limitation of the perineal approach has been the inability to sample the pelvic lymph nodes through the same incision. However, even early in the PSA era, it was evident that the absence of lymph node metastases could be predicted by a combination of multiple risk factors.[28] By 1993, we found that men with impalpable prostate cancer or cancer palpably confined to one lobe (T1–T2b), a Gleason score less than 7, and a PSA level less than 11 ng/mL had a node-negative predictive value of 99%.[34] Men at risk underwent concomitant pelvic lymphadenectomy, and nodal metastases were found in 6% of all men undergoing radical prostatectomy.[34] Since then, with the full impact of stage migration during advancing time in the PSA era, lymph node metastases have become rare.[3] Concomitant mini-lap pelvic lymphadenectomy is now reserved for the fewer than 10% of cases with high-grade tumor (Gleason scores 8 through 10) or the occasional case still presenting with high stage or high PSA levels, and the rate of lymph node metastases is now 1%.[3] With this current low incidence, any regular use of pelvic lymphadenectomy is difficult to rationalize. When pelvic lymphadenectomy is omitted, the rare patient with detectable PSA immediately after surgery has at least gained better local disease control and can be assumed to have metastatic disease and be treated with androgen deprivation.

ANATOMY

Pelvic Fascia

A clear understanding of the pelvic fascia is required to perform radical perineal prostatectomy with modern nerve-sparing or extended radical modifications. The pelvic fascia is a single continuous layer of fibroareolar and fatty tissue around all of the pelvic organs above the levator ani muscle. Previously described visceral and parietal layers are never seen in surgical disssection. Embryologically, the fascia is derived from the adjacent visceral mesenchyme.[39] Denonvilliers' membrane, the single fibrous membrane that he called the prostatoperitoneal membrane[40] (colloquially called the anterior layer of Denonvilliers' fascia), is derived from the embryonic fusion of the most caudal portion of the peritoneal sac within the pelvis (Figure 13–1).[41] It is interposed between the rectum and the prostate and extends caudally from the peritoneal cul-de-sac for a variable distance, but often down to the apex of the prostate. Its lateral margins extend to the neurovas-

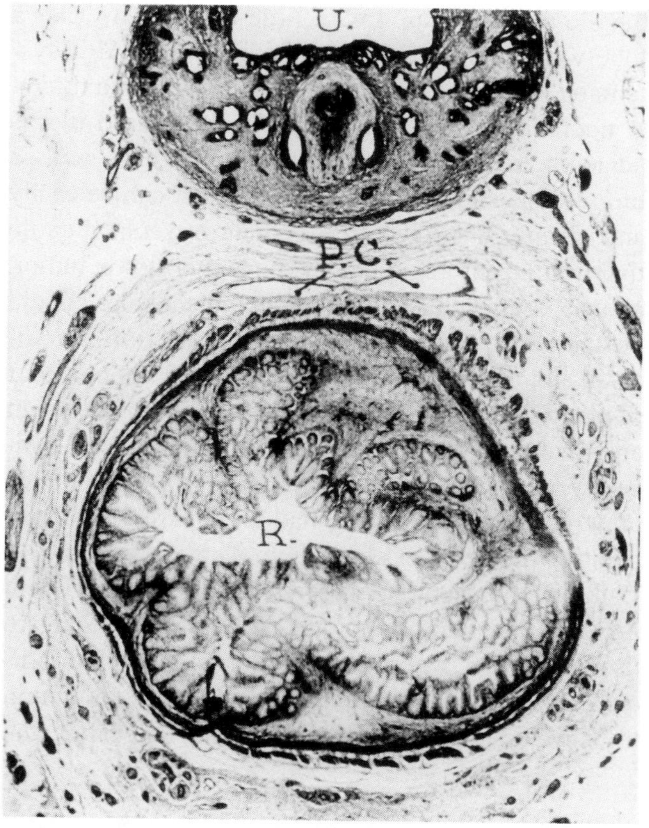

Figure 13–1. Histologic transverse section through the pelvis of a 161.4-mm human embryo, with the prostate and its urethra (*U.*) superior and the rectum (*R.*) inferior. The caudal extension of the peritoneal cavity (*P.C.*) is located between these organs. Note the large neural fibers in the lateral rectal fascia extending to the posterolateral prostate that constitute the fetal neurovascular bundles. (Reproduced with permission from Tobin CE, Benjamin JA. Anatomical and surgical restudy of Denonvilliers' fascia. Surg Gynecol Obstet 1945;80:373–88.)

cular bundles on each side.[42,43] It loosely covers the dorsal surface of the seminal vesicles but is densely adherent to the dorsal prostatic capsule. It is separated from the rectum by the ventral rectal fascia (colloquially called the posterior layer of Denonvilliers' fascia), the portion of the continuous pelvic fascia that extends in a frontal plane across the pelvis to join the lateral portions of the pelvic fascia on each side (Figures 13–2 and 13–3).

Neurovascular Bundles

The cavernous nerves originate in the pelvic nerve plexuses that are located within the lateral rectal fascia on each side of the rectum in a parasagittal plane and at the level of the tips of the seminal vesicles.[43] The cavernous nerves course caudally and ventrally as part of the neurovascular bundles with branches of the middle rectal artery and vein. They lie within the lateral pelvic fascia at its junction with the ventral rectal fascia (see Figure 13–3) and over the dorsolateral aspects of the prostate and membranous urethra. The nerve and vascular structures of the bundles are embedded in a variable amount of fat that increases their bulk and allows them to be easily identified visually. The nerves penetrate the urogenital diaphragm to reach the corpora cavernosa. Nerve branches to the prostate from the neurovascular bundles are concentrated into short inferior apical pedicles and longer and broader superior basal pedicles.

Related Rectal Anatomy

The three taenia coli, the bands of longitudinal muscle of the intra-abdominal colon, become concentrated beneath the peritoneal reflection on the rectum into two broad anterior and posterior bands. Some fasicles of the anterior longitudinal muscle band insert into the perineal body (the midline junction of the transverse perineal and bulbocavernosus muscles), forming the rectourethralis muscle.[44]

Caudal to the rectourethralis muscle, some fibers of the medial portion of the levator ani, the puborectalis muscle, insert onto the anterior rectal wall, whereas most of this muscle forms a sling around the rectum posteriorly. The striated external anal sphincter is innervated by branches of the internal pudendal nerves that cross the ischiorectal fossae and enter at 3 and 9 o'clock. They can be jeopardized by excessive posterior extensions of the incision.

NERVE-SPARING VERSUS EXTENDED DISSECTION

The modern era of radical prostatectomy is defined by the description of the paired neurovascular bundles and their relevance to postoperative impotence[18] and the local spread of prostate cancer.[45] Perineal nerve sparing can preserve spontaneous potency in 70% of selected men, and even unilateral nerve sparing can succeed in 68%.[9] However, the primary route of cancer penetration of the prostatic capsule is through the perineural spaces, the areas of anatomic vulnerability created by the penetrating

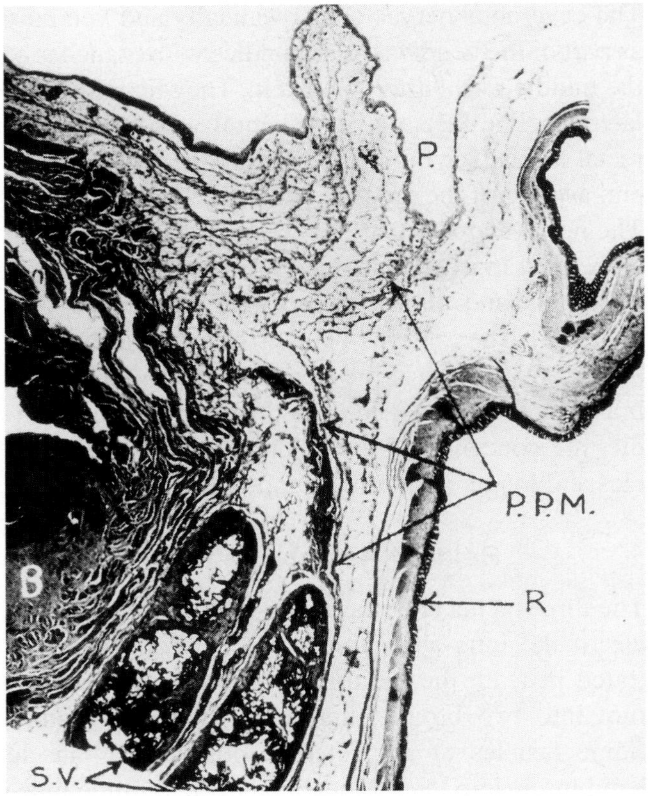

Figure 13–2. Histologic sagittal section through an adult male rectovesical peritoneal cul-de-sac (*P.*). Seminal vesicle (*S.V.*) and ampulla of vas deferens at left and rectum (*R.*) at right. Note Denonvilliers' prostatoperitoneal membrane (*P.P.M.*) extending from the cul-de-sac "dimple" over the dorsal wall of the seminal vesicle. Also note the areolar ventral rectal fascia between Denonvilliers' membrane and the rectal wall. (Reproduced with permission from Tobin CE, Benjamin JA. Anatomical and surgical restudy of Denonvilliers' fascia. Surg Gynecol Obstet 1945;80:373–88.)

nerves from the neurovascular bundles.[45] Up to 18% of all radical prostatectomy specimens have small-volume capsular penetration only in the area of the neurovascular bundle.[34] In those cases, ipsilateral nerve sparing would create a positive specimen margin, whereas an extended dissection sacrificing that bundle would leave negative margins, with a 15% advantage in the long-term freedom from PSA relapse rate for the negative margin group.[3]

There are reasonable strategies for potent men that account for these facts and are unlikely to compromise cancer cure, while also minimizing unnecessary potency loss. Clinical stage T1b tumors without significant peripheral zone involvement and T1c tumors with low PSA levels, medium grade, and limited volume on systematic biopsy are often ideal cases for bilateral nerve sparing. A neurovascular bundle may be spared with little risk if it overlies a lobe with no clinically detectable tumor and if systematic biopsy of that lobe reveals little or no tumor. A neurovascular bundle may also be spared if it is adjacent to a small palpable tumor (T2a) with a biopsy Gleason score 6 or less and if it can be easily and cleanly dissected free. A neurovascular bundle that is adjacent to any larger- or higher-grade tumor, or that is unusually adherent to the capsule, should be sacrificed. Bilateral extended dissection is indicated for all impotent men, those who consider potency unimportant, and those unwilling to accept any discretionary risk in the treatment of their cancer. With this selective approach, 7% of patients undergoing nerve sparing had an apparently related positive margin, but all of them were only focal.[34]

It is important to understand the two different dissection planes within the pelvic fascia that are used for either a nerve-sparing or an extended radical dissection. The initial approach is always within the envelope of the perirectal fascia. Thereafter, the

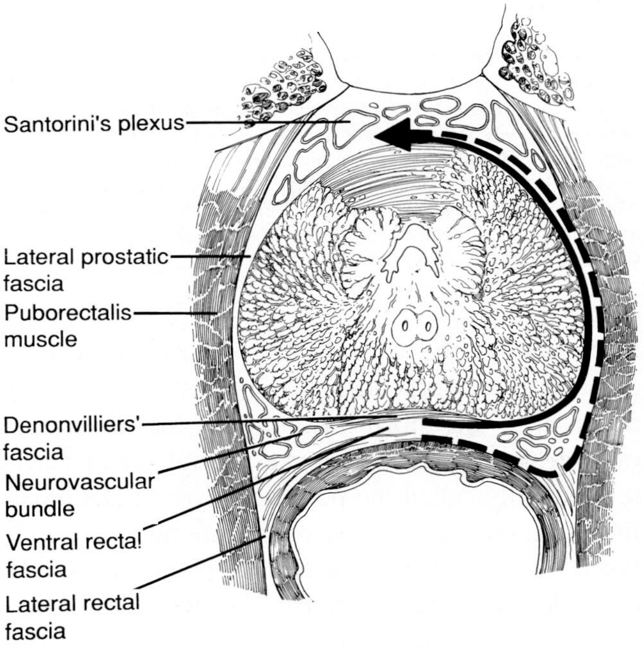

Figure 13–3. Transverse section through the prostate at the level of the verumontanum. Note the continuous nature of the pelvic fascia. The lateral prostatic fascia and the lateral rectal fascia comprise the lateral pelvic fascia. The *solid line* indicates the nerve-sparing dissection plane on Denonvilliers' membrane and the prostatic capsule. The *broken line* indicates the extended radical dissection plane excising the neurovascular bundle and the periprostatic fascia. (Reproduced with permission from Weldon VE. Radical perineal prostatectomy. In: Das S, Crawford ED, editors. Cancer of the prostate. New York: Marcel Dekker, 1993. p. 225–66.)

decision to proceed through or around the ventral rectal fascia determines the type of dissection. When an extended radical dissection with wide excision of the adjacent periprostatic fascia and the enclosed neurovascular bundle is planned, the dissection plane is around the ventral rectal fascia and on the rectal wall. It extends laterally around the neurovascular bundle and through the lateral rectal fascia onto the medial levator ani, the puborectalis muscle. It then turns ventrally on this muscle outside the lateral prostatic fascia and then onto the plane of the anterior prostatic capsule beneath Santorini's venous plexus. This dissection achieves margins on the rectal wall and the levator ani muscle (see Figures 13–3 and 13–4).

When potency sparing with preservation of the neurovascular bundle is planned, the dissection plane is through the ventral rectal fascia onto Denonvilliers' membrane. It continues ventrally on the prostatic capsule inside the lateral prostatic fascia and beneath Santorini's venous plexus (see Figure 13–3). Either of these dissection planes may be used on each side.

PREOPERATIVE PREPARATION

Although the incidence of inadvertent proctotomy in our series was only 1% and had no sequela,[9] division of the rectourethralis muscle and the modern operative modifications require extensive dissection on the rectal wall. Therefore, bowel preparation and antibiotic prophylaxis appropriate for colorectal operations are advisable. Preliminary cystoscopy after induction of anesthesia helps to avoid unusual but potentially troublesome surprises from bladder stones and tumors and urethral strictures. Special instruments are helpful but not required. The most useful are the prostatic tractors designed by Lowsley and Young (Figure 13–5) and a self-retaining retractor (Figure 13–6). Retractor or head-mounted lights facilitate the deeper dissection of the seminal vesicles.

OPERATIVE PROCEDURE

Patient Position

The exaggerated lithotomy position is required (Figure 13–7). To avoid neuropathy from stretching the sciatic and femoral nerves, proper position of the pelvis should be achieved by placing supporting pads under the sacrum rather than by using rotational forces on the legs. Position requirements exclude some patients

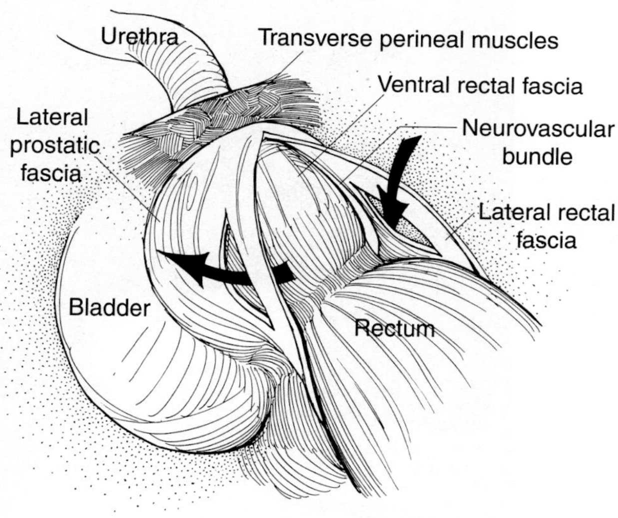

Figure 13–4. Initial approach within the envelope of the perirectal fascia reveals the prostate within the pelvic fascia. A bilateral extended dissection (*arrows*) excises all of this fascia and the enclosed neurovascular bundles with the prostate.

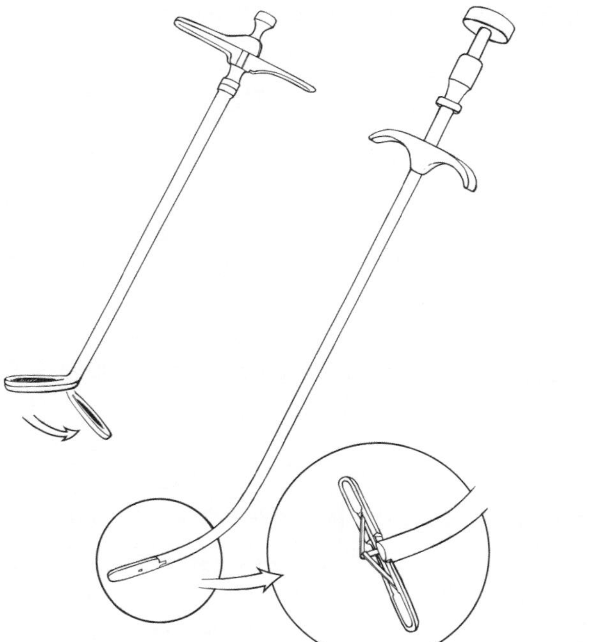

Figure 13–5. Prostatic tractors of Young (*left*) and Lowsley (*right*) closed for transurethral passage and opened for specimen traction. (Reproduced with permission from Weldon VE. Radical perineal prostatectomy. In: Crawford ED, Das S, editors. Current genitourinary cancer surgery. 2nd ed. Baltimore: Williams and Wilkins; 1997. p. 258–87.)

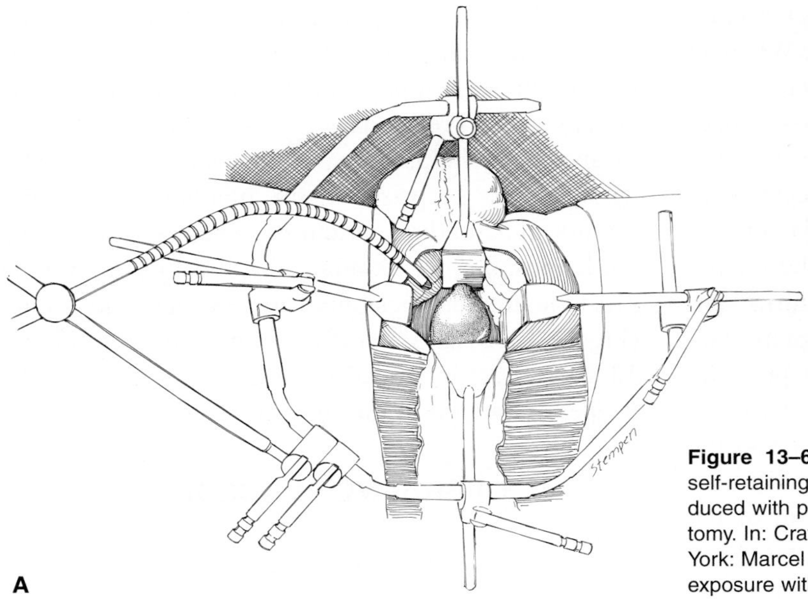

A

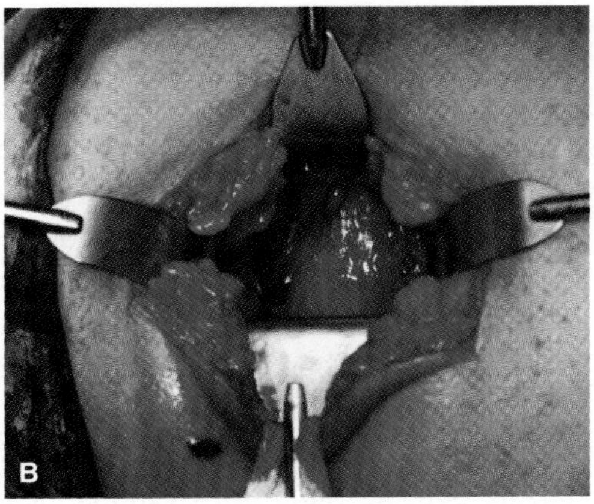

Figure 13–6. Table-mounted Omni-Tract Surgical mini-crescent self-retaining retractor. *A*, With retractor mounted fiber-light. (Reproduced with permission from Weldon VE. Radical perineal prostatectomy. In: Crawford ED, Das S, editors. Cancer of the prostate. New York: Marcel Dekker; 1993. p. 225–66.) *B*, Retractor maximizes the exposure with the minimal incision.

from the perineal approach, including those with severe ankylosis of the hips or spine or such extreme obesity that the weight on the diaphragm requires excessive ventilatory pressure that restricts cardiac filling. The common degenerative spine and disk problems are not a contraindication since the flexed position is often beneficial for them.

Incision

With an empty and prepared rectum, no special draping to isolate the anus is required. An inverted U incision is made outside the anal sphincter and inside the ischial tuberosities as described by Young[16] (Figure 13–8). The subsphincteric approach of Belt[46] pro-

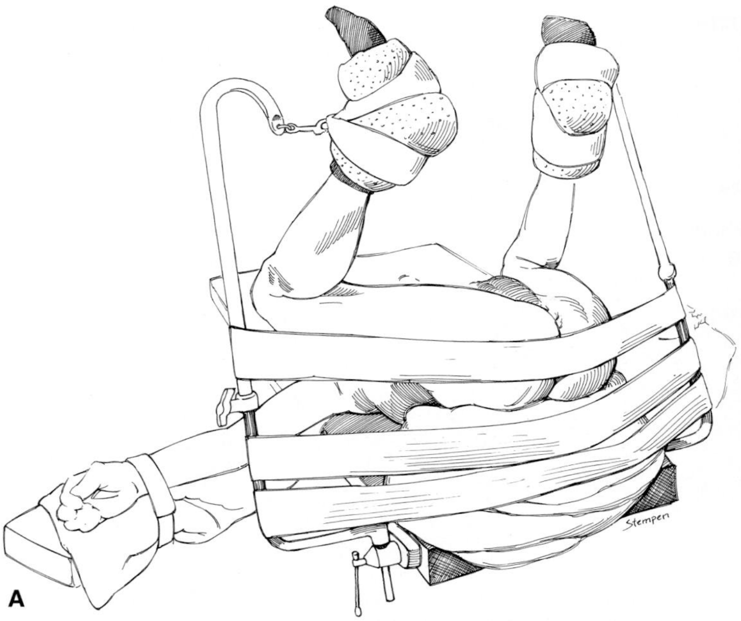

A

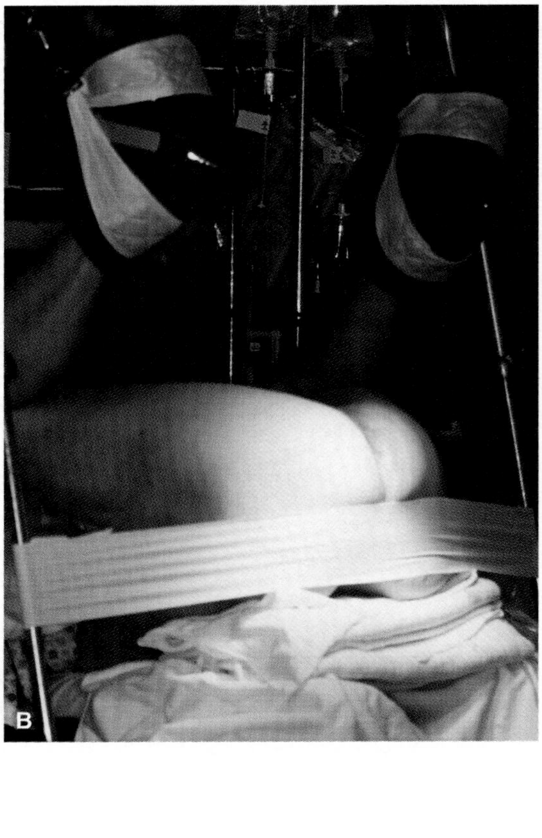

Figure 13–7. Exaggerated lithotomy position. *A* and *B,* All weight is borne on the folded cotton flannel sheets under the sacrum. *(A,* Reproduced with permission from Weldon VE. Radical perineal prostatectomy. In: Crawford ED, Das S, editors. Cancer of the prostate. New York: Marcel Dekker, 1993.)

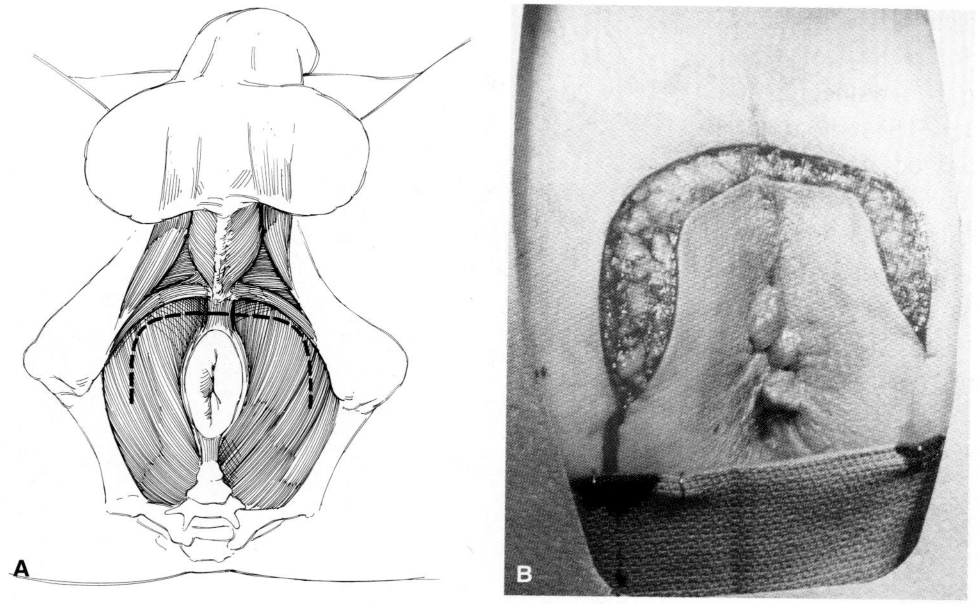

Figure 13–8. *A*, The perineal body, located in the center of the perineum, is the site of attachment of the transverse perineal muscles laterally, the bulbocavernosus muscle ventrally, and the central tendon dorsally. The *broken line* indicates the position of the skin incision and the site of division of the central tendon. (Reproduced with permission from Weldon VE. Radical perineal prostatectomy. In: Crawford ED, Das S, editors. Cancer of the prostate. New York: Marcel Dekker. 1993.) *B*, The skin incision.

vides more restricted exposure. The vertical limbs of the incision should not extend posteriorly beyond the 3 and 9 o'clock positions relative to the anus to avoid damaging the nerves to the external anal sphincter.

This small, minimally invasive exposure may limit the access to very large prostates. However, no patient in this author's experience has, so far, ever been excluded from this approach because of prostate size, and intact prostates up to 180 g have been removed.

Full development of the incision requires transecting the central tendon of the perineum, opening the ischiorectal fossae, and exposing the ventral rectal wall. The central tendon is the vertical, midline, anterior striated muscle extension of the external anal sphincter that attaches it to the perineal body. Lateral incisions through the subcutaneous fascia allow digital development of the fossae and the plane between the rectal wall and the central tendon (Figure 13–9).

Rectal Mobilization

Dissection on the longitudinal smooth muscle of the rectal wall leads to the rectourethralis muscle, which connects the rectum to the perineal body. The rec-

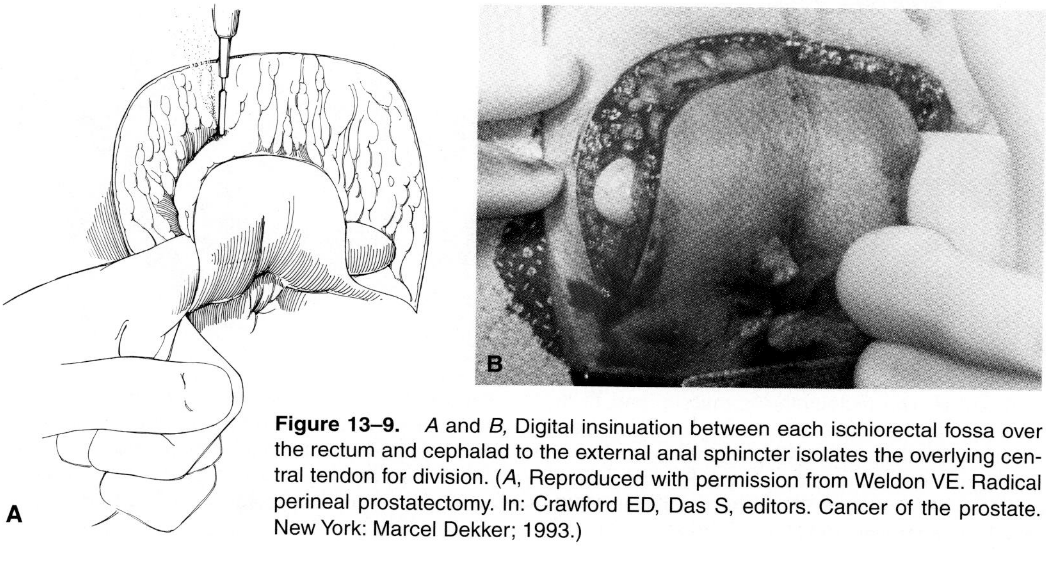

Figure 13–9. *A* and *B,* Digital insinuation between each ischiorectal fossa over the rectum and cephalad to the external anal sphincter isolates the overlying central tendon for division. (*A*, Reproduced with permission from Weldon VE. Radical perineal prostatectomy. In: Crawford ED, Das S, editors. Cancer of the prostate. New York: Marcel Dekker; 1993.)

tourethralis muscle must be visualized as a strap suspending the tent of the anterior rectal wall (Figure 13–10). Skeletonizing this strap and placing it on tension assists in safe transection. The rectourethralis muscle must be completely divided. Any broad and indefinite remnant is best divided after penetrating it and spreading in the midline (Figure 13–11).

Complete transection of the rectourethralis muscle gives entry to the key space between the rectum and its ventral fascia (Figure 13–12). The plane of dissection now turns at a right angle from the hori-

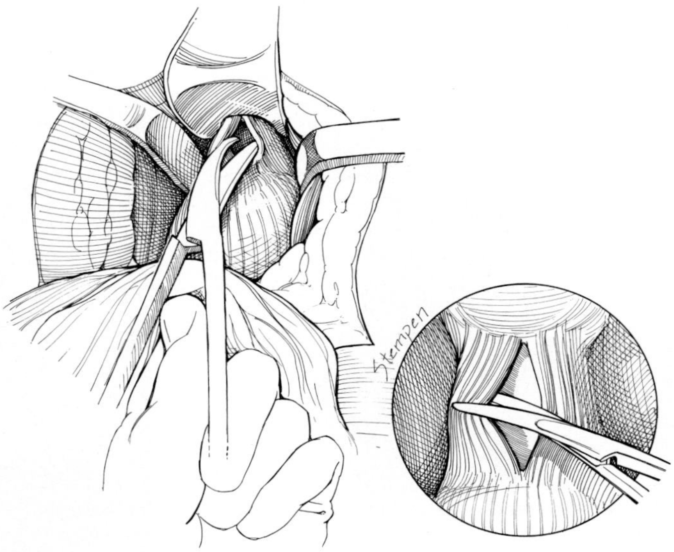

Figure 13–11. Complete division of the rectourethralis muscle. After any discrete central or lateral edge is divided, any remaining broad and indefinite muscle is completely penetrated and split longitudinally by scissors-spreading in the midline. *Inset:* Each remaining half is then completely incised beginning at the newly created medial edge and extending laterally. (Reproduced with permission from Weldon VE. Radical perineal prostatectomy. In: Crawford ED, Das S, editors. Current genitourinary cancer surgery. 2nd ed. Baltimore: Williams and Wilkins; 1997. p. 258–87.)

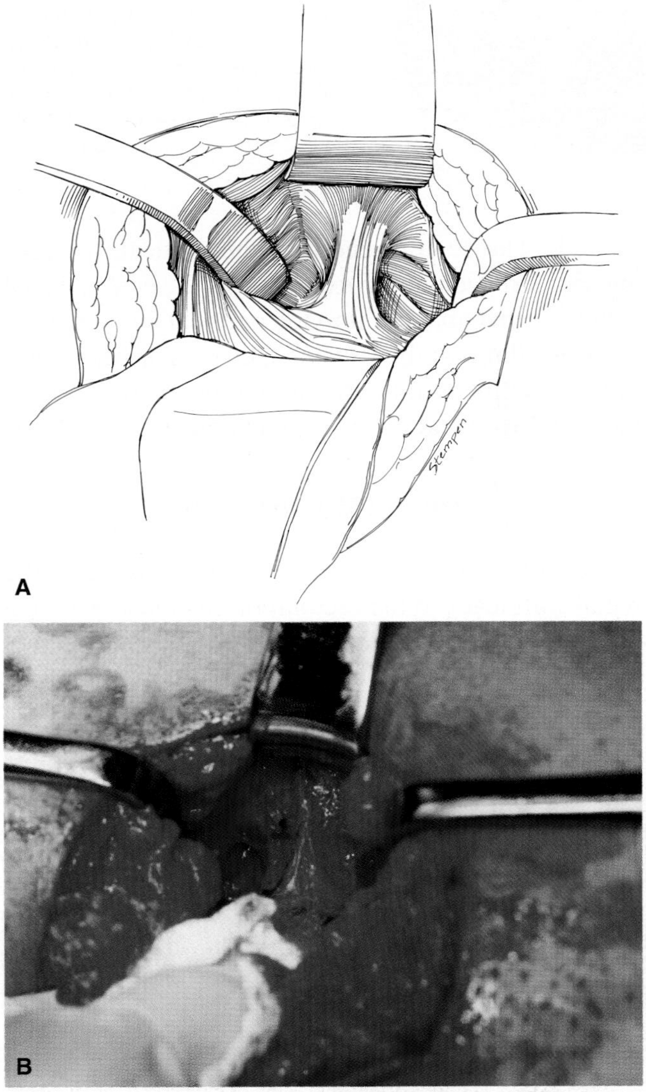

Figure 13–10. *A* and *B,* The rectourethralis muscle, part of the anterior band of longitudinal smooth rectal muscle that connects the rectum to the perineal body, is isolated in preparation for division. (*A,* Reproduced with permission from Weldon VE. Radical perineal prostatectomy. In: Das S, Crawford ED, editors. Cancer of the prostate. New York: Marcel Dekker; 1993.)

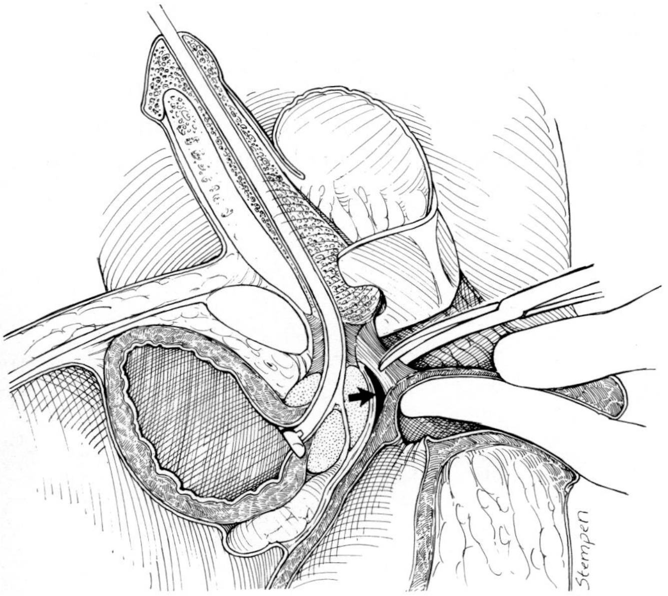

Figure 13–12. After sharp transection of the rectourethralis muscle, the key space (*arrow*) between the rectal wall and its ventral fascia is entered. (Reproduced with permission from Weldon VE. Radical perineal prostatectomy. In: Crawford ED, Das S, editors. Current genitourinary cancer surgery. 2nd ed. Baltimore: Williams and Wilkins; 1997.)

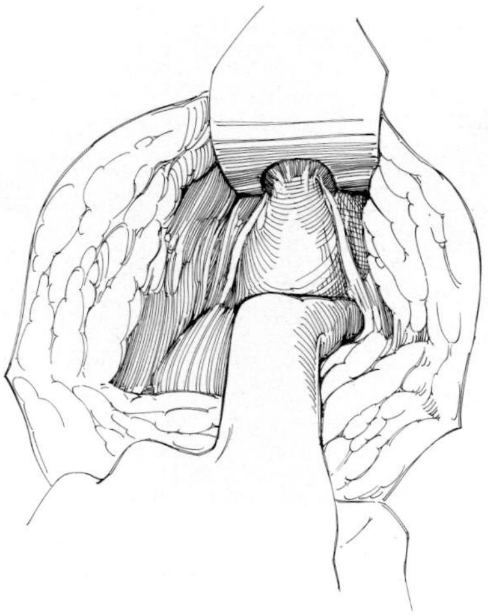

Figure 13–13. Digital dissection develops the vertical plane between the rectal wall and its ventral rectal fascia. The neurovascular bundles are within the lateral aspects of the fascia. (Reproduced with permission from Weldon VE. Radical perineal prostatectomy. In: Das S, Crawford ED, editors. Cancer of the prostate. New York: Marcel Dekker; 1993.)

zontal to the vertical, and this space is best developed by blunt, digital, cephalad, and lateral dissection while keeping the fingernail on the prostate (Figure 13–13). The space is opened down to the level of the prostatic base, and the rectal wall is retracted with a padded retractor to expose all of the ventral rectal fascia and both laterally located neurovascular bundles. Variable amounts of fatty infiltration of the bundles contribute to their visual prominence, allowing easy, direct identification (Figure 13–14).

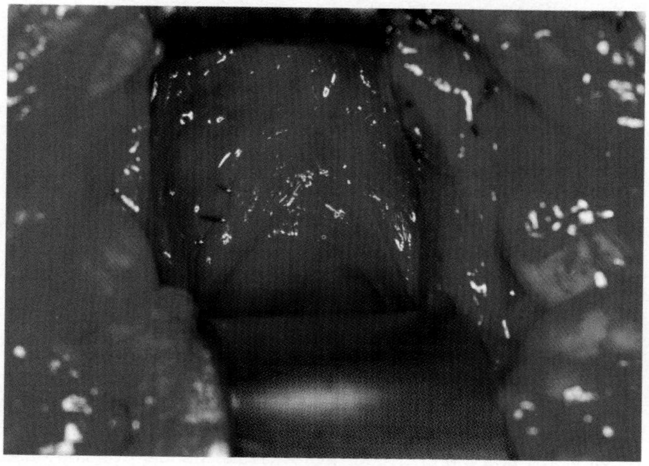

Figure 13–14. Rectum retracted, exposing the ventral rectal fascia and the enclosed bilateral neurovascular bundles. Note the prominent bulge of the neurovascular bundles forming an inverted V, resulting from their oblique course on each side from their most lateral position at the base of the prostate to a more medial position at its apex.

The ventral rectal fascia is the key to modern nerve-sparing and extended radical modifications. Thus far, the operation has proceeded within the envelope of the perirectal fascia. To escape this envelope, further dissection on each side must proceed either through the ventral rectal fascia for a nerve-sparing dissection or around it for an extended dissection.

Nerve-Sparing Dissection

The ventral rectal fascia is incised vertically, medial to the neurovascular bundle. A midline incision is used for a bilateral nerve-sparing dissection (Figure 13–15). This fascia and the enclosed neurovascular bundle are carefully separated from the prostatic capsule. The main areas of attachment of the neurovascular bundles are the inferior and superior

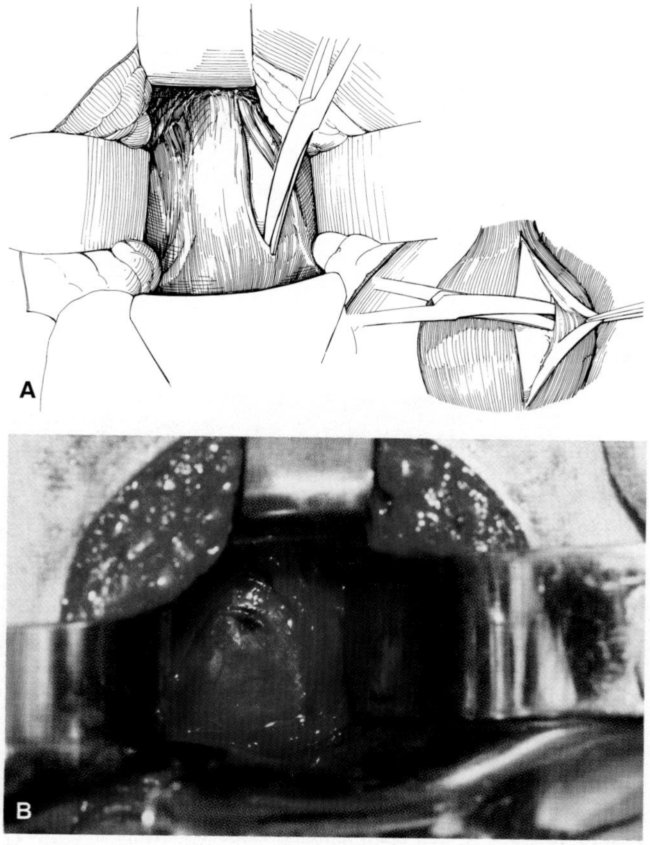

Figure 13–15. *A* and *B*, Vertical incision of the ventral rectal fascia medial to the neurovascular bundles exposes Denonvilliers' membrane. *A*, *inset:* beginning mobilization of the left neurovascular bundle at the lateral edge of Denonvilliers' membrane. (Reproduced with permission from Weldon VE. Radical perineal prostatectomy. In: Das S, Crawford ED, editors. Cancer of the prostate. New York: Marcel Dekker; 1993.)

neural pedicles located at the apex and base. They must be divided sharply, with hemoclip control of the superior pedicle to avoid bleeding (Figure 13–16). The neurovascular bundles must be mobilized at least 1 cm over the membranous urethra and sufficiently proximal at the base to allow them to slip to the side and avoid stretching during removal of the prostate (Figure 13–17).

Extended Radical Dissection

The ventral rectal fascia and neurovascular bundle remain on the prostate, and the thin lateral rectal fascia is opened vertically just lateral to the bundle, exposing the levator ani muscle (Figure 13–18). Blunt

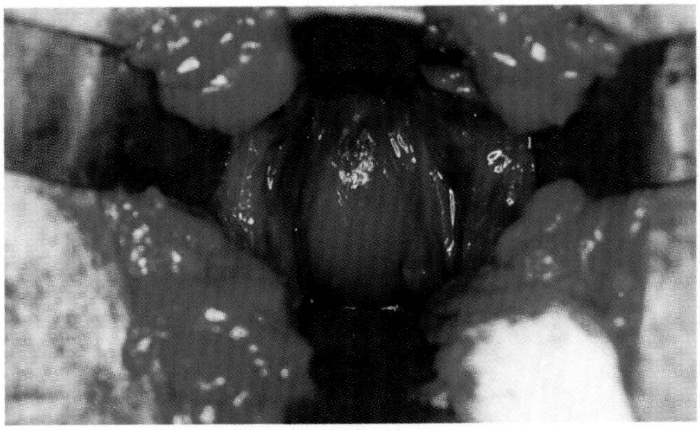

Figure 13–17. After complete mobilization, the neurovascular bundles slip to the side where they are situated vertically lateral to the prostate.

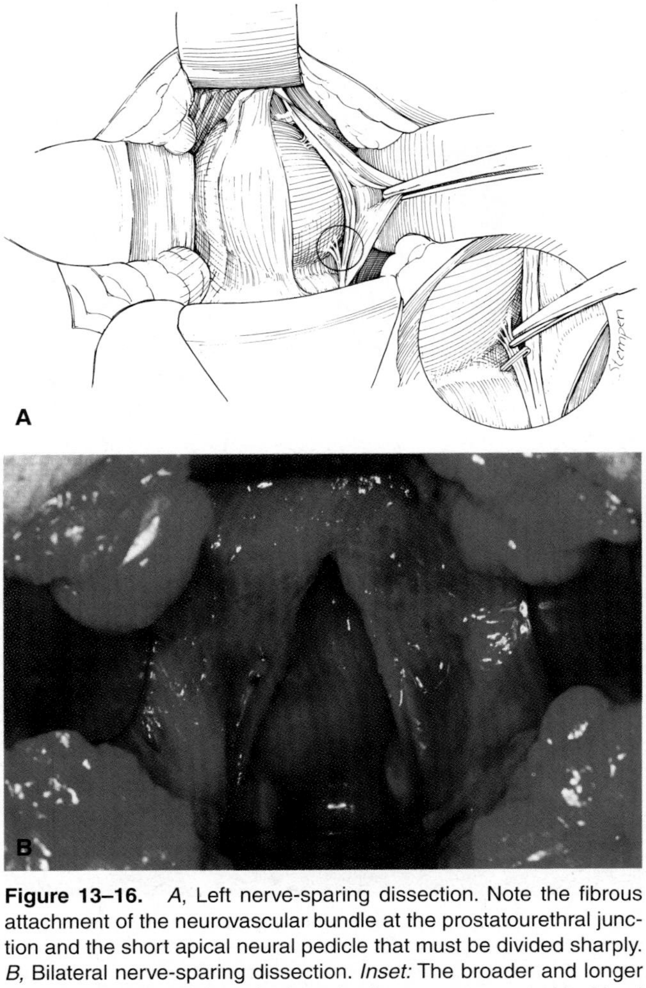

Figure 13–16. *A,* Left nerve-sparing dissection. Note the fibrous attachment of the neurovascular bundle at the prostatourethral junction and the short apical neural pedicle that must be divided sharply. *B,* Bilateral nerve-sparing dissection. *Inset:* The broader and longer superior neural pedicle at the base is always accompanied by blood vessels that must be clipped. (Reproduced with permission from Weldon VE. Radical perineal prostatectomy. In: Das S, Crawford ED, editors. Cancer of the prostate. New York: Marcel Dekker; 1993.)

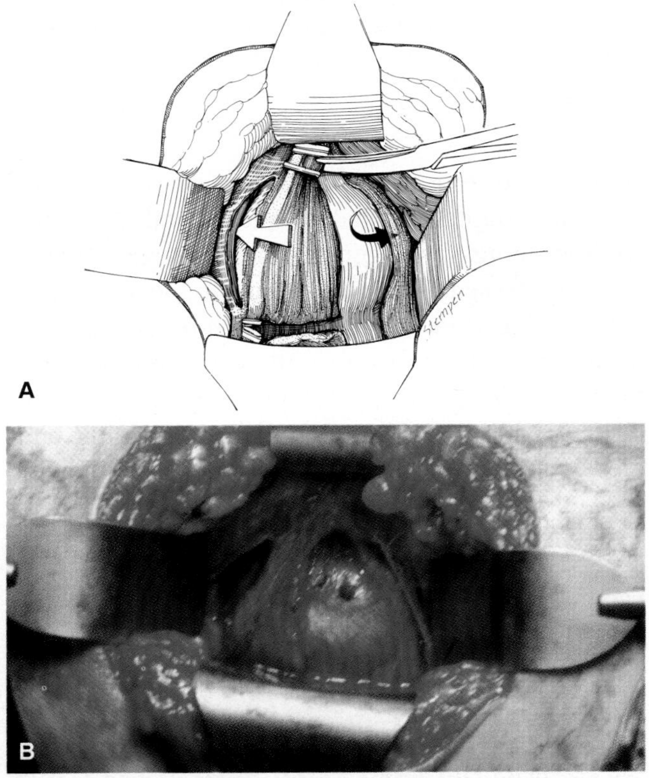

Figure 13–18. *A* and *B,* Vertical incision of the ventral rectal fascia with a left nerve-sparing and a right extended radical dissection. The left ventral rectal fascia and neurovascular bundle have been mobilized off the prostate. The right ventral rectal fascia and neurovascular bundle remain on the prostate, and the right lateral rectal fascia lateral to the bundle has been opened. *A,* The *black arrow* demonstrates the nerve-sparing dissection plane between the prostate capsule and the lateral prostatic fascia on the patient's left side. On the patient's right side, an extended radical dissection divides the ventral rectal fascia and the enclosed neurovascular bundle over the base and apex of the prostate. The *white arrow* demonstrates the extended radical dissection plane betwen the levator ani muscle and the lateral prostatic fascia. (Reproduced with permission from Weldon VE. Radical perineal prostatectomy. In: Das S, Crawford ED, editors. Cancer of the prostate. New York: Marcel Dekker; 1993.)

digital dissection ventrally then completely develops the avascular plane between the levator muscle and the lateral prostatic fascia. The ventral rectal fascia and the enclosed neurovascular bundle are transected transversely at the level of the base and apex of the prostate. The lateral prostatic fascia also remains on the prostate, and it is later incised around the bladder neck.

Early Vascular Pedicle Division

The vascular pedicles, entering the base of the prostate just lateral to the seminal vesicles, are also adjacent to the proximal neurovascular bundles but in a deeper plane. The bundles can be injured at this point. With a bilateral nerve-sparing dissection, it is advisable to delay dividing the vascular pedicles until the prostate is fully mobilized and can be pulled away to more easily and safely isolate the vascular pedicles. However, with a bilateral extended dissection or on the side of a unilateral extended dissection, and always with very large prostates, early division of the vascular pedicles is useful in reducing blood loss and severing the main structures that restrict specimen mobilization.

The space between the remaining cuff of the ventral rectal fascia and the underlying Denonvilliers' membrane is developed cephalad before dividing Denonvilliers' membrane transversely over the seminal vesicles. Dissection on the lateral margin of the seminal vesicle isolates the adjacent vascular pedicle for division and proximal ligation (Figure 13–19). There is little back-bleeding from the pedicle stump on the specimen. The dissection of the vesicles and vasal ampullae can be accomplished through this posterior access (Figure 13–20) or can be deferred until the bladder neck is circumcised to allow both anterior and posterior access.

Apical Dissection

The focus of the operation now moves from the base of the prostate to its apex. The junction of the membranous urethra with the prostatic apex is isolated and divided precisely (Figures 13–21 and 13–22). Easy perineal access to the apex just 5 cm beneath the perineal skin facilitates precise dissection with both optimal membranous urethral preservation and avoidance of inadvertent incisions into the prostate.[34]

Puboprostatic Ligament Division

The prostate is rotated dorsally, exposing the anterior prostatic capsule and the puboprostatic ligaments beneath Santorini's venous plexus. These ligaments must be sharply divided rather than avulsed to reduce the risk of a positive margin if there is tumor in the transition zone[34] (Figure 13–23).

Bladder Neck Division

The anterior base of the prostate is palpable lateral and cephalad to the puboprostatic ligaments. After the ligaments are divided, Santorini's venous plexus

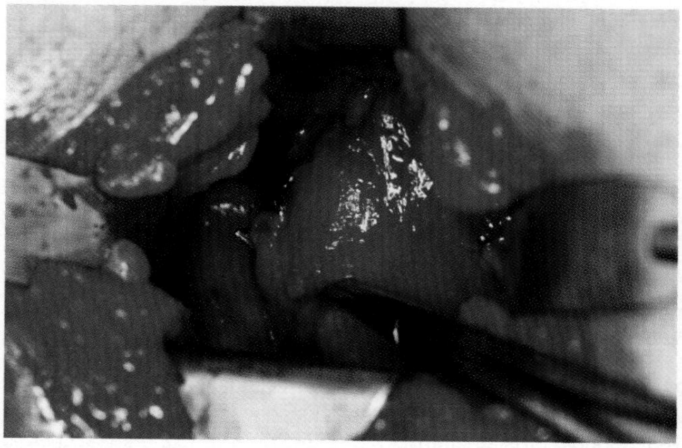

Figure 13–19. Isolation of the right vascular pedicle of the prostate. After Denonvilliers' membrane is incised transversely over the base of the seminal vesicles, a right-angle forceps inserted lateral to the seminal vesicle "hooks" the pedicle.

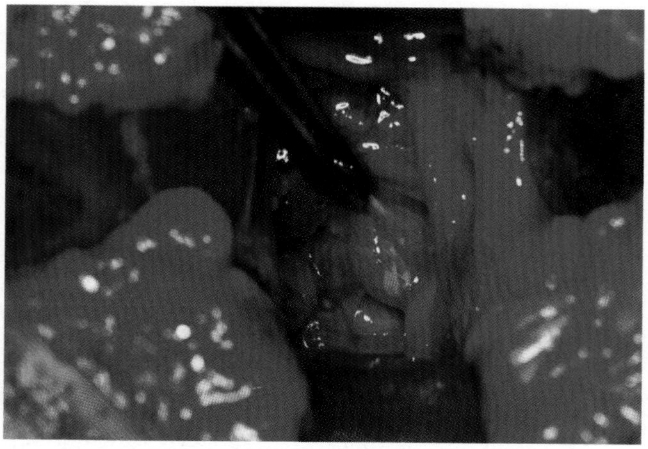

Figure 13–20. Left seminal vesicle grasped by forceps after the left vascular pedicle has been divided. In this case, the vertical, laterally adjacent left neurovascular bundle has been preserved.

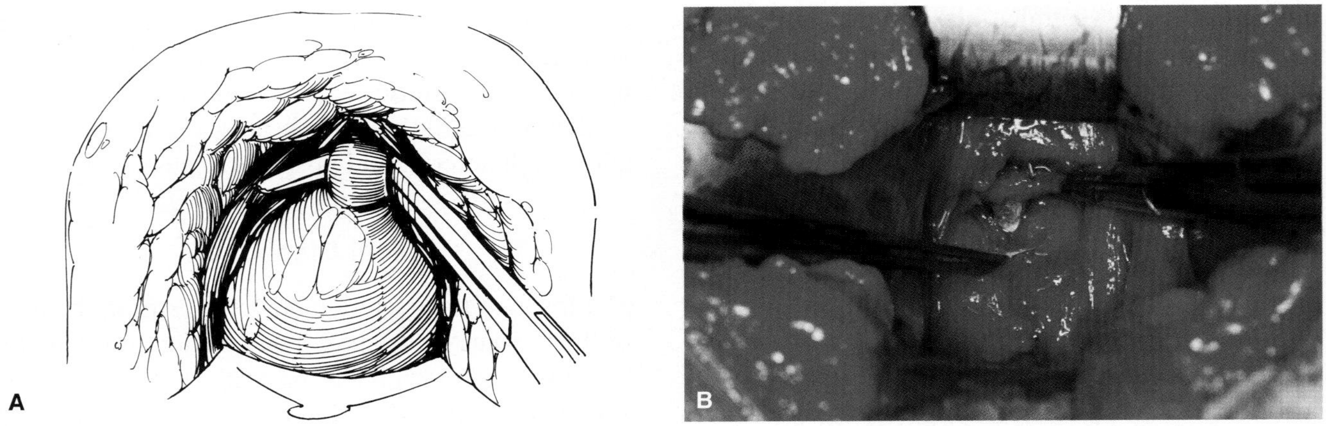

A B

Figure 13–21. Isolation of the junction of the prostatic apex and the membranous urethra during a bilateral nerve-sparing dissection. A right-angle forceps encircles the proximal membranous urethra. *A,* The urethra is shelled out between the laterally displaced neurovascular bundles. (Reproduced with permission from Weldon VE, Tavel FR. Potency-sparing radical perineal prostatectomy: anatomy, surgical technique and initial results. J Urol 1988;140:559–62.) *B,* The dorsal urethral wall has been incised precisely at its junction with the prostate, exposing the intraurethral metal shaft of Lowsley's tractor. Note the vertical neurovascular bundles on each side.

can be pushed cephalad in the midline, where the bladder neck muscularis is then separated from the prostate (Figure 13–24). This dissection preserves most of the bladder neck, although it will be trimmed later. Routine wide excision of the bladder neck is both unnecessary and futile since cancer invasion of the bladder neck is unusual (3%) and when it occurs and it is a marker for large tumor volume that is always accompanied by a positive margin at another site.[34] If an extended dissection has been performed on either side, the lateral prostatic fascia on that side is now incised around the bladder neck (see Figure 13–23, A).

The anterior bladder neck mucosa is then opened, and further specimen traction is provided by a 0.5 in Penrose drain looped through the prostatic urethra around the anterior lobe (Figure 13–25). If not previously accomplished, the vascular pedicles must now be divided to allow complete circumcision of the bladder neck (Figures 13–26 and 13–27). If a pedunculated prostatic middle lobe impedes visualization of the posterior bladder neck mucosa, risking

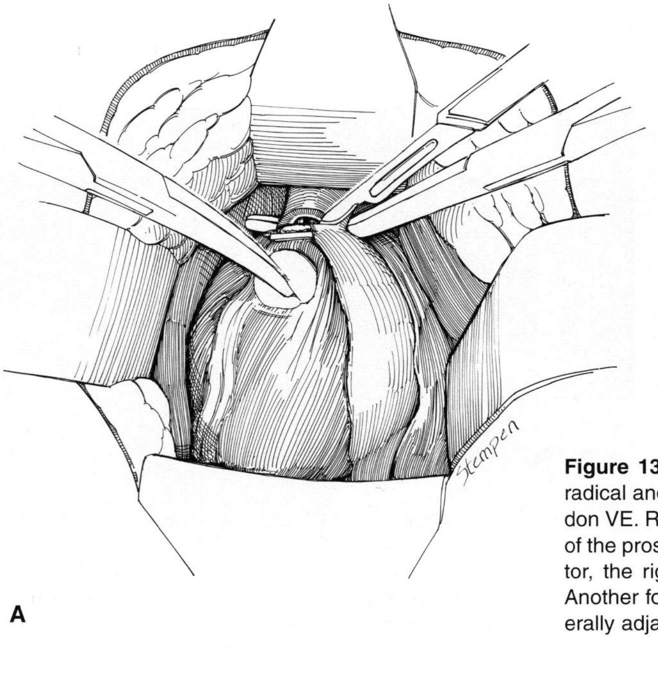

A

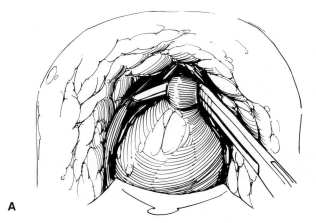

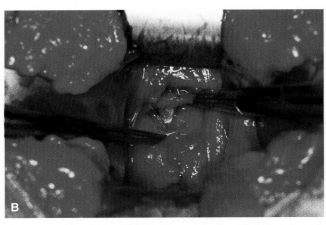

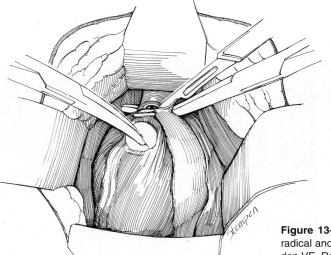

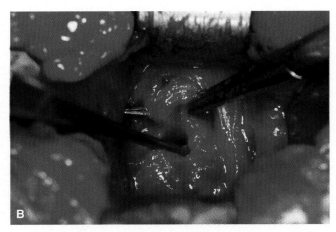

B

Figure 13–22. *A,* Division of the dorsal urethral wall during a right extended radical and left nerve sparing dissection. (Reproduced with permission from Weldon VE. Radical perineal prostatectomy. In: Das S, Crawford ED, editors. Cancer of the prostate. New York: Marcel Dekker; 1993.) *B,* After removing Lowsley's tractor, the right-angle forceps isolates the intact ventral urethral wall for division. Another forceps opens the lumen of the apical urethra. Note the vertical and laterally adjacent left neurovascular bundle.

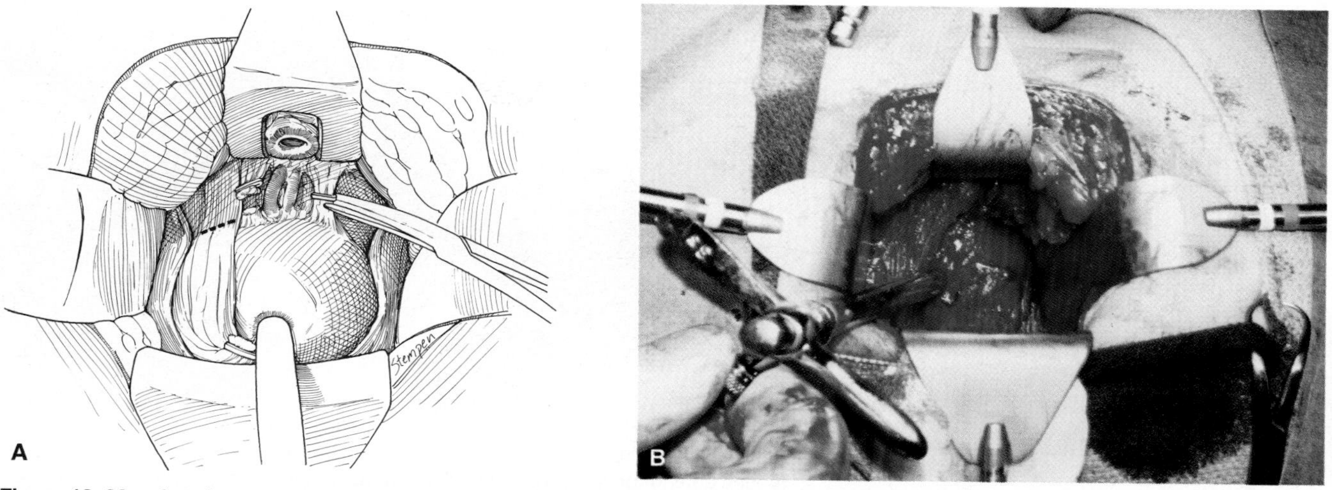

Figure 13–23. Anterior prostate dissection, with Young's short prostatic tractor entering the apical urethra and rotated dorsally. *A*, Sharp dissection of the puboprostatic ligaments, with a left nerve-sparing and a right extended radical dissection. The *broken line* indicates the site of division of the right lateral pelvic fascia at the bladder neck. Note the clipped right neurovascular bundle at the prostatic apex. (Reproduced with permission from Weldon VE, Tavel FR, Neuwirth H, Cohen R. Patterns of positive specimen margins and detectable prostate specific antigen after radical perineal prostatectomy. J Urol 1995;153:1565–9.) *B*, Anterior dissection while sparing the right neurovascular bundle situated vertically.

injury to the ureteral orifices, it can be grasped by a single-toothed uterine tenaculum and pulled out to allow safe incision behind it.

Seminal Vesicle Dissection

If not accomplished earlier, complete dissection of the seminal vesicles and division of the vasal ampullae are now performed, securing small arteries with hemoclips (Figures 13–28 and 13–29). This completely frees the specimen.

Vesicourethral Anastomosis

The bladder neck is inspected and trimmed. Bladder neck preservation does not enhance continence, but it reduces anastomotic tension and contributes to the very low incidence of anastomotic strictures.[9] How-

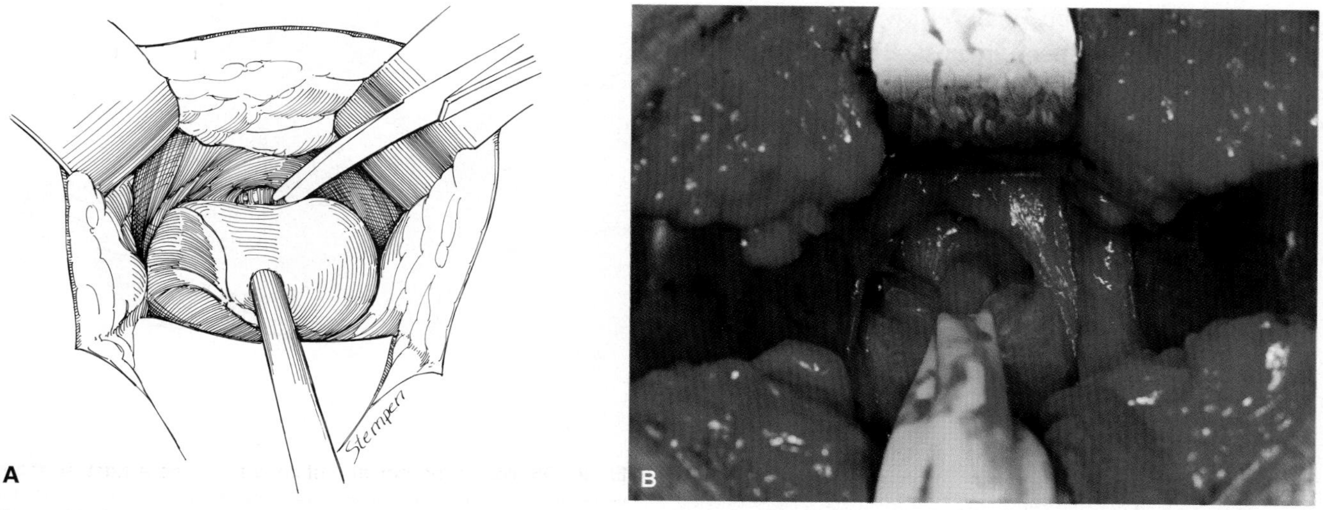

Figure 13–24. Anterior bladder neck–sparing dissection. Circular bladder neck muscle is completely separated from the prostate, exposing the mucosa. *A,* Right extended radical dissection with tractor through prostatic urethra. (Reproduced with permission from Weldon VE. Radical perineal prostatectomy. In: Das S, Crawford ED, editors. Cancer of the prostate. New York: Marcel Dekker; 1993.) *B*, Bilateral nerve-sparing dissection with Penrose drain looped through the prostatic urethra and through a small opening in the intact cylinder of bladder neck mucosa, around the anterior prostate. Note the laterally displaced bilateral neurovascular bundles situated vertically.

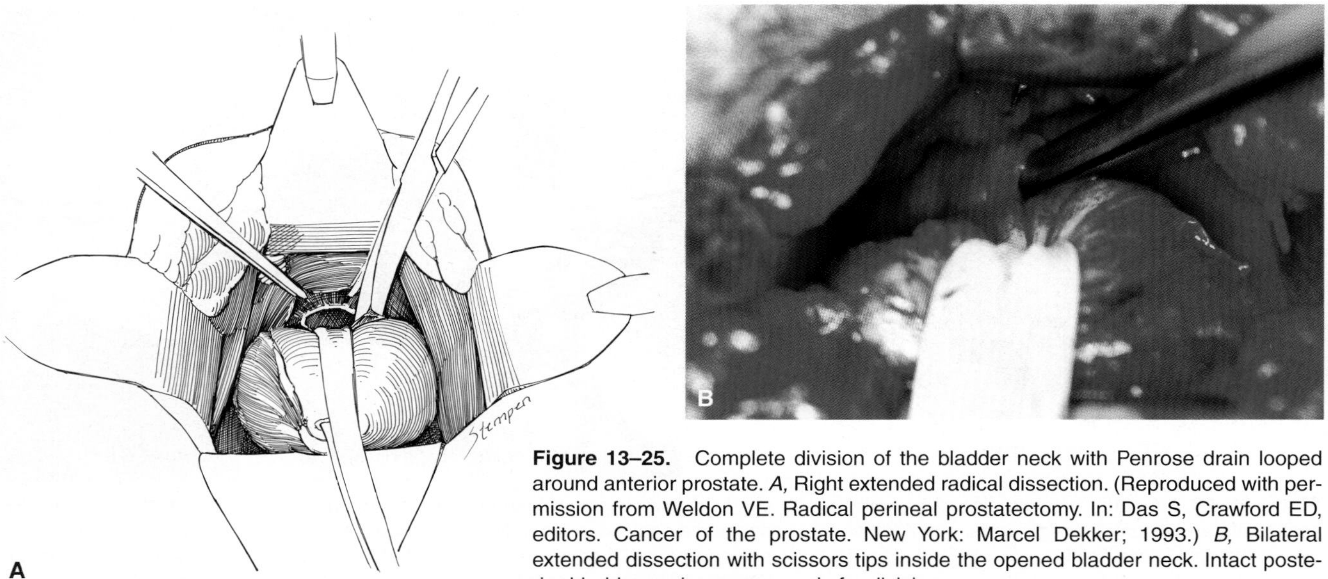

A

Figure 13–25. Complete division of the bladder neck with Penrose drain looped around anterior prostate. *A,* Right extended radical dissection. (Reproduced with permission from Weldon VE. Radical perineal prostatectomy. In: Das S, Crawford ED, editors. Cancer of the prostate. New York: Marcel Dekker; 1993.) *B,* Bilateral extended dissection with scissors tips inside the opened bladder neck. Intact posterior bladder neck mucosa ready for division.

ever, microscopic benign prostatic glands are retained on 44% of preserved bladder necks,[47,48] and trimming the neck will reduce the risk of a benign source of detectable PSA postoperatively. It also provides enhanced microscopic assessment of the most proximal margin.

The anastomosis of the anterior bladder neck to the membranous urethra is accomplished around a 20-Ch Foley catheter with 9 or 10 interrupted, synthetic, absorbable 2-0 sutures (Figures 13–30 and 13–31). Because of the easy perineal access, precise mucosal approximation can be achieved without separately everting the bladder neck mucosa. The anterior bladder neck is approximated around the urethra without attempting to tighten it. Any redundant posterior bladder neck is closed vertically as a "racquet handle."

Closure

The rectum is inspected prior to closure. Any proctotomy is meticulously closed in two layers with synthetic, absorbable sutures. The anterior band of longitudinal muscle usually provides a secure second layer. A 0.25" Penrose is placed with its center looped into the wound, and each end is separately brought though the opposite corners of the incision and sutured to the skin. A drain placed in this manner will not be pulled out with friction when the patient is sitting.

The perineal wound is closed in two layers, with continuous absorbable subcutaneous and intradermal skin sutures (Figure 13–32). This closure will adequately resist the shearing forces associated with sitting.

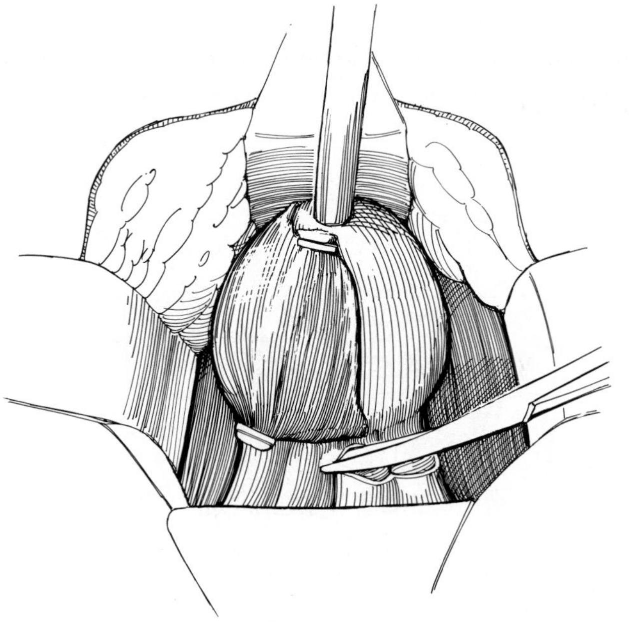

Figure 13–26. If not accomplished in the early dissection, transverse incision of Denonvilliers' membrane is performed over the base of the seminal vesicles, giving access to the laterally located vascular pedicles. Right extended radical dissection shown with clipped right neurovascular bundle. (Reproduced with permission from Weldon VE. Radical perineal prostatectomy. In: Das S, Crawford ED, editors. Cancer of the prostate. New York: Marcel Dekker; 1993.)

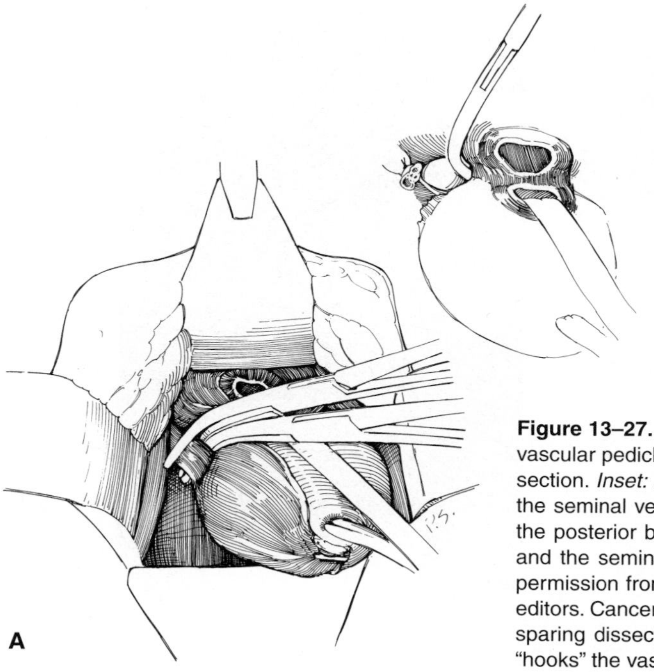
A

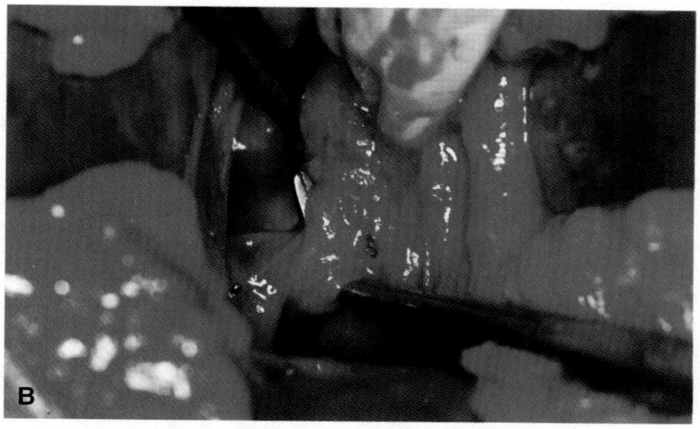
B

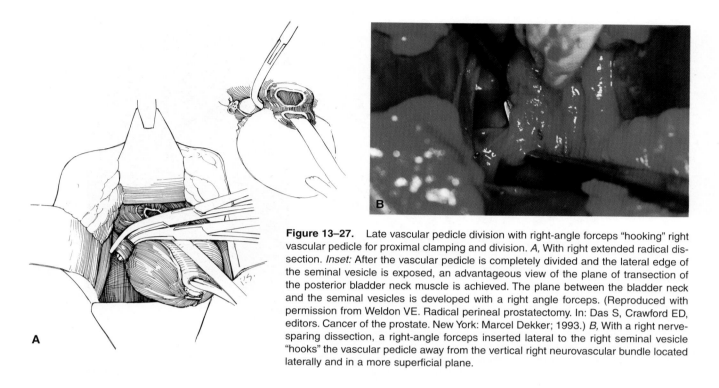

Figure 13–27. Late vascular pedicle division with right-angle forceps "hooking" right vascular pedicle for proximal clamping and division. *A,* With right extended radical dissection. *Inset:* After the vascular pedicle is completely divided and the lateral edge of the seminal vesicle is exposed, an advantageous view of the plane of transection of the posterior bladder neck muscle is achieved. The plane between the bladder neck and the seminal vesicles is developed with a right angle forceps. (Reproduced with permission from Weldon VE. Radical perineal prostatectomy. In: Das S, Crawford ED, editors. Cancer of the prostate. New York: Marcel Dekker; 1993.) *B,* With a right nerve-sparing dissection, a right-angle forceps inserted lateral to the right seminal vesicle "hooks" the vascular pedicle away from the vertical right neurovascular bundle located laterally and in a more superficial plane.

The specimen (Figure 13–33) is fixed overnight in formalin in preparation for detailed pathologic analysis, preferably with a 3-mm step-section technique.[34]

POSTOPERATIVE CARE

Full ambulation and a regular diet are resumed on the first postoperative day. With the usual minimal urinary extravasation, the perineal drain is removed on the first day. Regular administration of nonsteroidal anti-inflammatory agents for the initial 48 hours provides most of the necessary analgesia. Additional patient-controlled doses of narcotics are available on the first night. Most patients are ready for discharge on the first day, and the rest the second day. The catheter is removed at 1 week with a negative cystogram, or at 2 weeks without one.

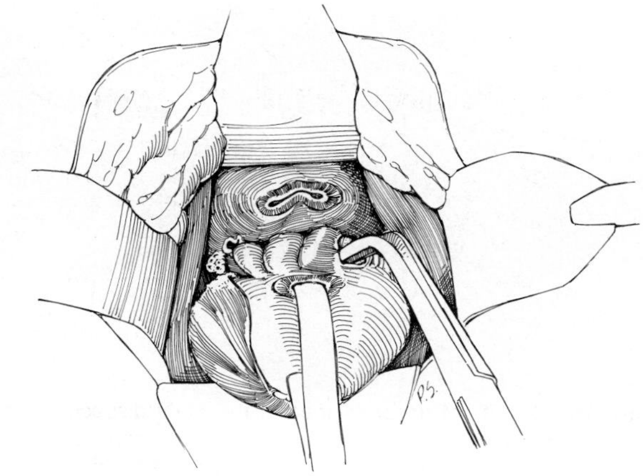
A

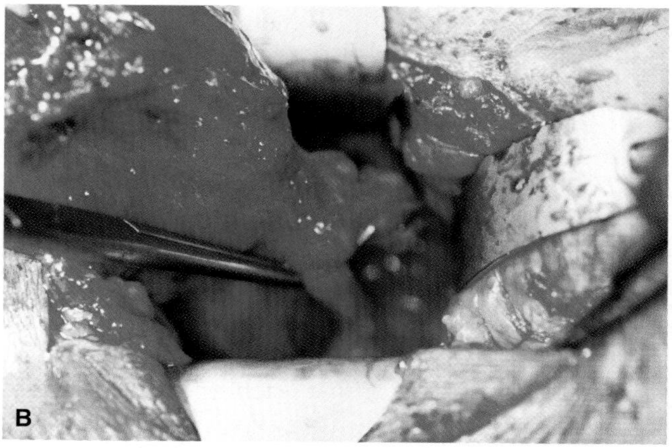
B

Figure 13–28. *A,* Anterior seminal vesicle dissection during right extended radical dissection. Right-angle forceps opens the cleft between the left seminal vesicle and the ampulla of the left vas deferens. (Reproduced with permission from Weldon VE. Radical perineal prostatectomy. In: Das S, Crawford ED, editors. Cancer of the prostate. New York: Marcel Dekker; 1993.) *B,* Posterior dissection with right-angle forceps hooking the ampulla of the left vas deferens for division. Mobilized left seminal vesicle is located laterally.

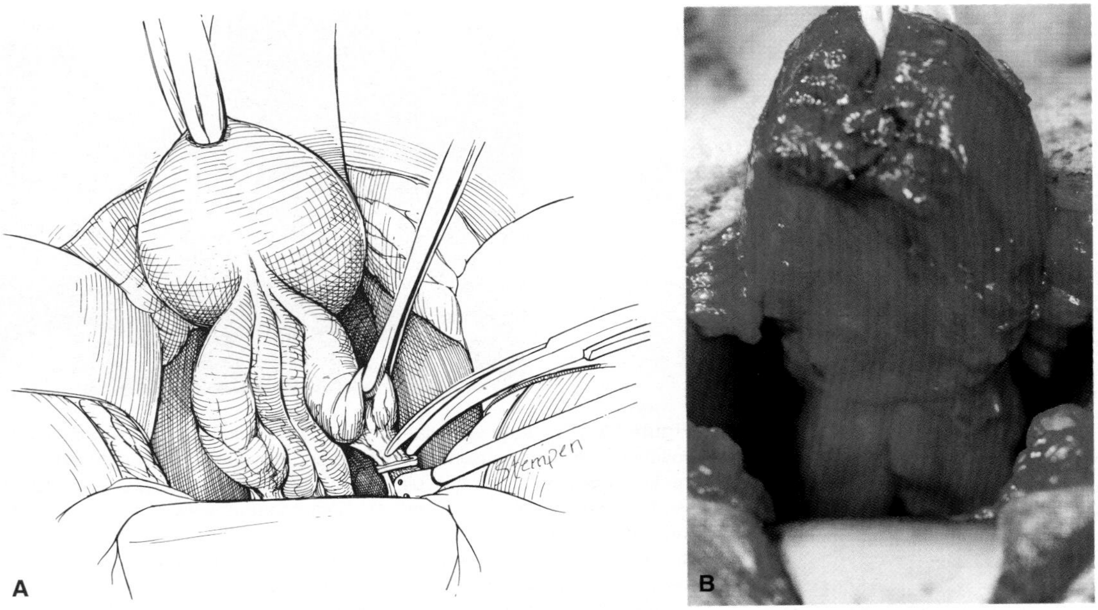

Figure 13–29. *A,* Complete bilateral seminal vesicle excision is performed, using traction and counter traction to isolate, clip, and divide the numerous small arteries. (Reproduced with permission from Weldon VE. Radical perineal prostatectomy. In: Das S, Crawford ED, editors. Cancer of the prostate. New York: Marcel Dekker; 1993.) *B,* Specimen freed by completing the seminal vesicle dissection bilaterally. Note the abundant periprostatic fascia around the apex of the prostate, giving wide margins with a bilateral extended dissection.

COMPLICATIONS

Morbidity

Complications that occurred in this author's initial 220 cases are listed in Table 13–1. There have been no deaths. Serious complications, including venous thrombosis or embolism, myocardial infarction, and necrotizing pancreatitis, occurred in 2%.[9] Venous thrombosis or embolism occurred only in men who underwent concomitant pelvic lymphadenectomy. Blood loss in these cases (rounded to the nearest 100 mL) is shown in Figure 13–34. Median operative blood loss was 600 mL (mean 645). Maximum blood loss was 2,000 mL, and 95% lost 1,200 or less.[9]

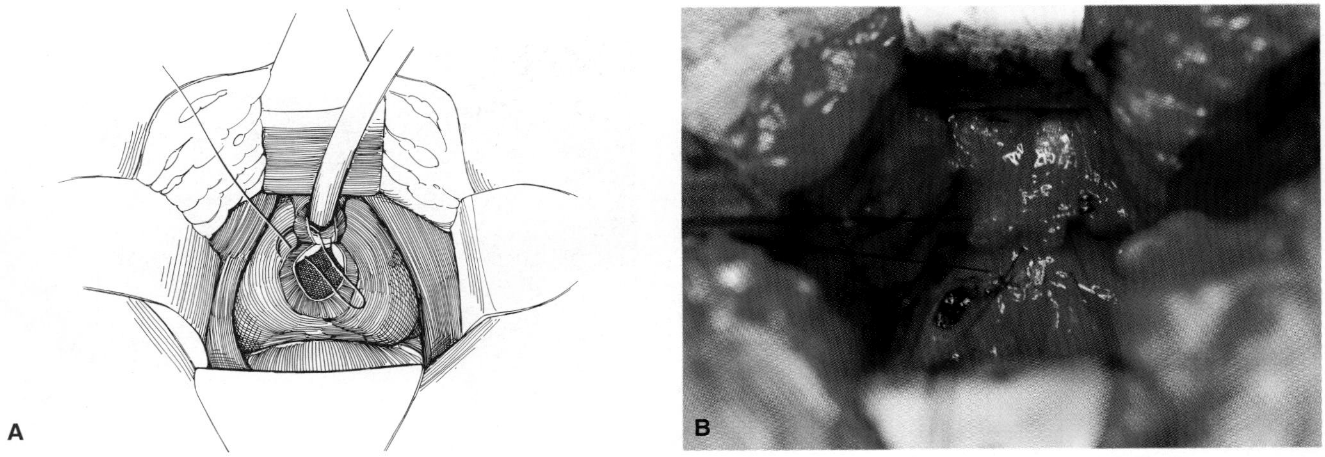

Figure 13–30. Anastomosis of the anterior bladder neck to the anterior membranous urethra with the 3 initial sutures. *A,* With the catheter pulled through the urethra and lifted up to expose the anterior urethral wall. (Reproduced with permission from Weldon VE. Radical perineal prostatectomy. In: Das S, Crawford ED, editors. Cancer of the prostate. New York: Marcel Dekker; 1993.) *B,* With the catheter tip pushed through and then withdrawn into the urethra to identify its anterior wall.

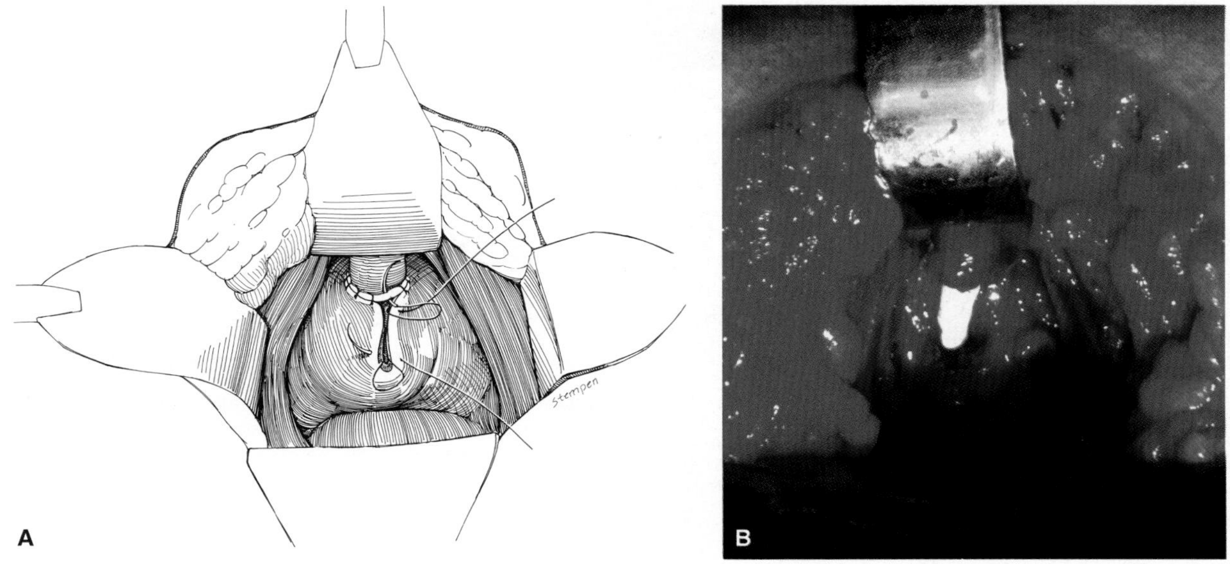

Figure 13–31. *A* and *B,* After the catheter tip is placed into the bladder, the anterior bladder neck is approximated around the stump of the membranous urethra. Any redundant posterior bladder neck is closed vertically. (*A,* Reproduced with permission from Weldon VE. Radical perineal prostatectomy. In: Das S, Crawford ED, editors. Cancer of the prostate. New York: Marcel Dekker, 1993.) The anterior bladder neck is approximated around the stump of the membranous urethra. Any redundant posterior bladder neck is closed vertically.

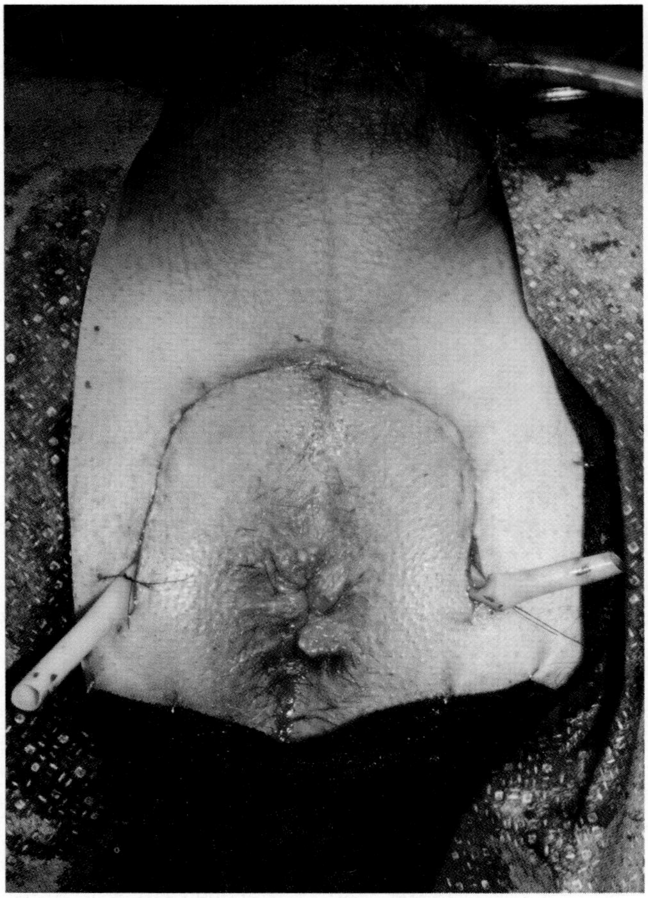

Figure 13–32. The closed incision with the drain.

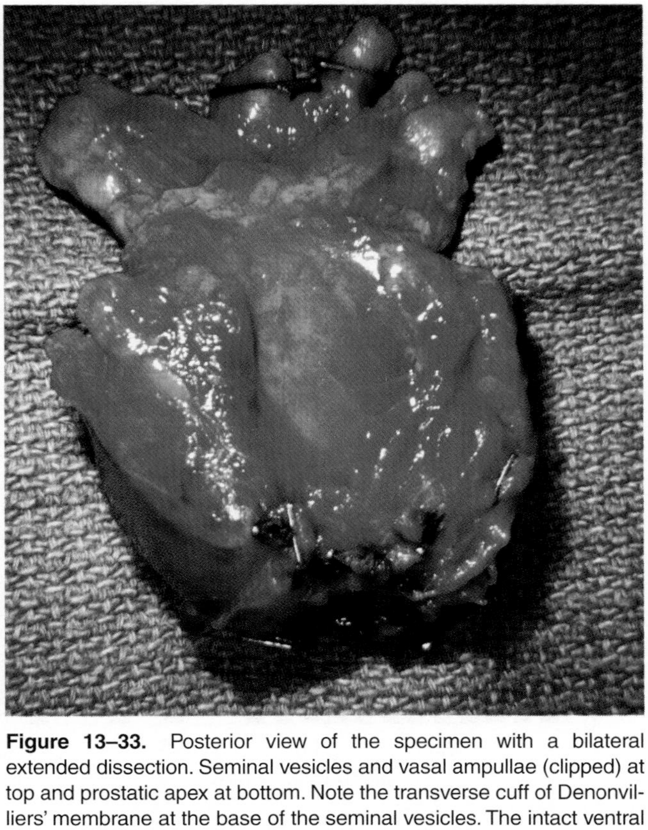

Figure 13–33. Posterior view of the specimen with a bilateral extended dissection. Seminal vesicles and vasal ampullae (clipped) at top and prostatic apex at bottom. Note the transverse cuff of Denonvilliers' membrane at the base of the seminal vesicles. The intact ventral rectal fascia overlies this membrane from the base of the prostate to its apex. The posterolaterally enclosed neurovascular bundles are very prominent owing to marked fatty infiltration in this specimen. Note the clips on the transected neurovascular bundles at the apex.

Table 13–1. COMPLICATIONS AFTER RADICAL PERINEAL PROSTATECTOMY IN 220 CONSECUTIVE PATIENTS

	No. of Pts	%
Anastomotic stricture	3	1
Inadvertent proctotomy	3	1
Pulmonary embolus	2	1
Deep venous thrombosis only	1	0.5
Necrotizing pancreatitis	1	0.5
Myocardial infarction	1	0.5
Atrial fibrillation	2	1
Transient peripheral neuropathy	4	2
Prolonged urinary extravasation	4	2
Prolonged lymph drainage*	4	2
Transient genital edema*	3	1
Lymphocele*	5	3
Clostridium difficile colitis	2	1
Obstructed catheter	1	0.5
Perineal cellulitis	3	1
Pneumonia	1	0.5
Total	40	18

Adapted from Weldon et al.[9]
Pts = patients
*Concomitant pelvic lymphadenectomy in 181 patients.

Continence

Continence (no daily pads) in these patients, related to postoperative time, is shown in Figure 13–35. After 10 months, 95% were continent. Of the 5% who were incontinent, 25% had mild (one pad daily), 42% had moderate (two to three pads daily), and 33% had severe (four to six pads daily) incontinence. None were totally incontinent. Poor bladder compliance or instability ameliorated by anticholinergic medication was a major factor in 17% of the incontinent men. Patient age was the only significant related variable. All incontinent men were age 69 or older. Collagen injections for sphincteric insufficiency have been very helpful, and they may be more effective after the perineal approach since incontinence was never total and the precise apical dissection and anastomosis leaves a relatively long and pliable supradiaphragmatic urethral segment that more easily accepts the injected material.[9] Table 13–2 lists the number of patients and incontinence rates in our series at Marin General Hospital,[9] and the other reported contemporary, large, and consecutive radical perineal and retropubic prostatectomy series that used regular pad use as the criterion.[48–54]

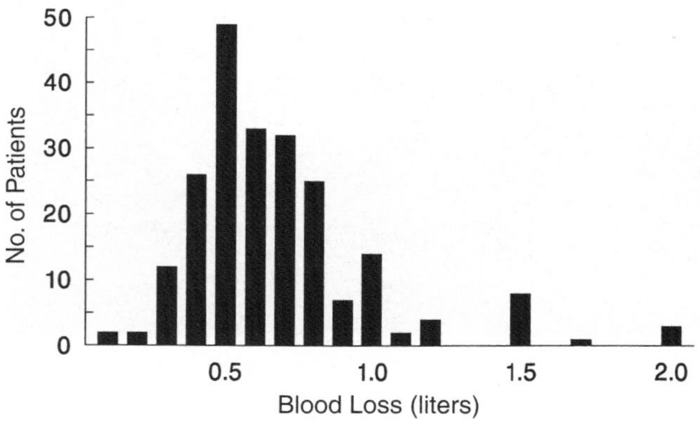

Figure 13–34. Operative blood loss during radical perineal prostatectomy in 220 consecutive patients. (Reproduced with permission from Weldon VE, Tavel FR, Neuwirth H. Continence, potency, and morbidity after radical perineal prostatectomy. J Urol 1997;158:1470–5.)

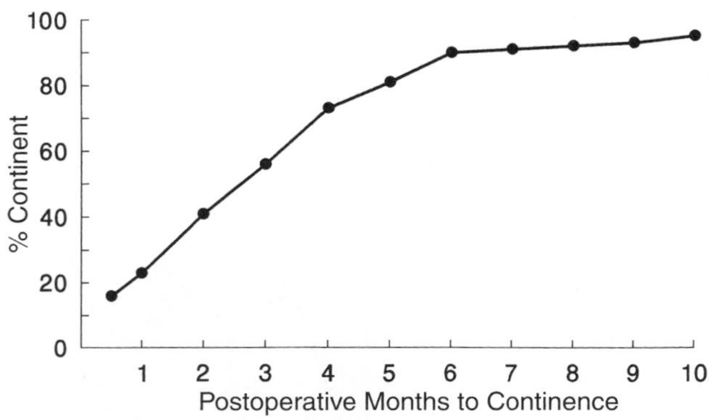

Figure 13–35. Cumulative postoperative continence as a function of time after radical perineal prostatectomy in 220 consecutive patients. (Reproduced with permission from Weldon VE, Tavel FR, Neuwirth H. Continence, potency, and morbidity after radical perineal prostatectomy. J Urol 1997;158:1470–5.)

Potency

Potency (unassisted, repeated, and prolonged vaginal penetration) related to postoperative time in the initial

Table 13–2. INCIDENCE OF INCONTINENCE AFTER RADICAL PERINEAL AND RETROPUBIC PROSTATECTOMY

Institution	No. of Pts	% Incontinent
Perineal		
Marin General[9]	220	5
Duke[49]	122	4
Mason Clinic[50]	207	8
Retropubic		
Johns Hopkins[51]	593	8
Washington University[52]	435	6
Baylor[53]	581	9
Stanford[54]	481	20

Adapted from Weldon et al.[9]
Pts = patients.

50 patients (who had good preoperative potency a minimum of 18 months follow-up and who were otherwise candidates for nerve sparing) is shown in Figure 13–36. After 2 years, 70% are potent without any assistance. Again, patient age was the only related variable. Potency returned in all men younger than age 50 but in only 29% age 70 or older. Bilateral nerve sparing was successful in 73% and unilateral in 68%.[9] This high success rate with unilateral nerve sparing may be unique to the perineal approach. In this posterior approach, the posterolaterally located neurovascular bundles are more easily and directly seen and can be precisely preserved. However, the specimen must be removed from between the bundles, and there is a greater risk of stretching them. With unilateral perineal nerve sparing, the single remaining neurovascular bundle is optimally preserved and removal of the contralateral bundle provides more space, thus reducing the risk of stretching the remaining bundle. Table 13–3 lists the number of patients and potency preservation rates in our series at Marin General Hospital[9] and the other reported contemporaneous and consecutive radical perineal and retropubic prostatectomy series with adequate follow-up.[49,52,55,56]

Table 13–3. INCIDENCE OF POTENCY PRESERVATION AFTER RADICAL PERINEAL AND RETROPUBIC PROSTATECTOMY

Institution	No. of Pts	% Potent
Perineal		
Marin General[9]	50	70
Duke[49]	22	77
Retropubic		
Johns Hopkins[55]	503	68
Washington University[52]	295	59
Stanford[56]	213	20

Adapted from Weldon et al.[9]
Pts = patients.

CANCER CONTROL

Pathologic status on 3-mm step-section analysis and postoperative PSA status provide a basis for comparing the effectiveness of disease control with the perineal and the retropubic approaches to radical prostatectomy. We compared the margin status and early PSA outcomes of our initial 220 patients with those in Walsh's contemporaneous landmark retropubic series from Johns Hopkins reported by Partin and colleagues[57] and Epstein and colleagues[58] (Table 13–4). Despite a substantially greater fraction of high-risk patients in our perineal cohort, the outcomes were very similar.[34] Analysis of our positive margins (Figure 13–37) revealed a lower incidence of solitary positive apical margins with the perineal as compared with the retropubic approach (Table 13–5).[34,58–60] This appears to be a durable difference,[61] related to the difference in access to the apex between the two approaches. Now that most retropubic surgeons have changed their approach to the apex by detaching the puboprostatic ligaments at the prostate and dissecting beneath Santorini's venous plexus,[62] which replicates the anterior perineal dis-

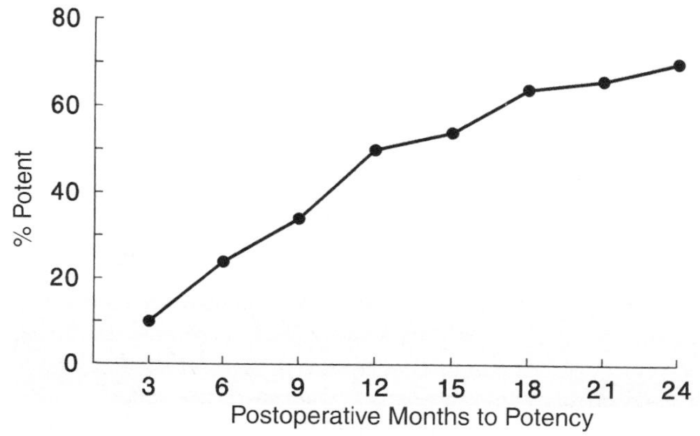

Figure 13–36. Cumulative postoperative potency as a function of time after nerve-sparing radical perineal prostatectomy in 50 patients. (Reproduced with permission from Weldon VE, Tavel FR, Neuwirth H. Continence, potency, and morbidity after radical perineal prostatectomy. J Urol 1997;158:1470–5.)

Table 13–4. COHORT CHARACTERISTICS AND OUTCOMES AFTER RADICAL RETROPUBIC AND PERINEAL PROSTATECTOMY

	Retropubic (Johns Hopkins[57,58])	Perineal (Marin General[34])
Cohort characteristics		
Preoperative PSA		
Normal (%)	42	11
Mean ng/mL	7.5	12.2
Clinical stages T2b–c (%)	33	45
Outcomes		
Organ confined (%)	40	41
Negative margins (%)	59	56
Detectable postoperative PSA (%)	19	21

PSA = prostate-specific antigen.
Adapted from Weldon et al.[34]

37. Terris MK, McNeal JE, Stamey TA. Detection of clinically significant prostate cancer by transrectal ultrasound-guided systematic biopsies. J Urol 1992;148:829–32.
38. Weldon VE, Tavel FR, Neuwirth H, Cohen R. Failure of focal prostate cancer on biopsy to predict focal prostate cancer: the importance of prevalence. J Urol 1995;154:1074–7.
39. Tobin CE, Benjamin JA, Wells JC. Continuity of the fasciae lining the abdomen, pelvis and spermatic cord. Surg Gynecol Obstet 1946;83:575–96.
40. Denonvilliers CPD. Anatomie du périnée. Bull Soc Anat Paris 1836;11:105–7.
41. Tobin CE, Benjamin JA. Anatomical and surgical restudy of Denonvilliers' fascia. Surg Gynecol Obstet 1945;80: 373–88.
42. Villers A, McNeal JE, Freiha F, et al. Invasion of Denonvilliers' fascia in radical prostatectomy specimens. J Urol 1993;149:793–8.
43. Lepor H, Gregerman M, Crosby R, et al. Precise localization of the autonomic nerves from the pelvic plexus to the corpora cavernosa: a detailed anatomical study of the adult male pelvis. J Urol 1985;133:207–12.
44. Woodburne RT. The pelvis. In: Essentials of human anatomy. New York: Oxford University Press; 1957. p. 477.
45. Villers A, McNeal JE, Redwine EA, et al. The role of perineural space invasion in the local spread of prostatic adenocarcinoma. J Urol 1989;142:763–8.
46. Belt E. Radical perineal prostatectomy in early carcinoma of the prostate. J Urol 1942;48:287–97.
47. Weldon VE, Neuwirth H, Bennett PM. Bladder neck sparing during radical perineal prostatectomy risks preserving benign prostate glands. Abstracts of the Western Section AUA Annual Meeting 1998;37.
48. Lepor H, Chan S, Melamed J. The role of bladder neck biopsy in men undergoing radical retropubic prostatectomy with preservation of the bladder neck. J Urol 1998;160:2435–9.
49. Frazier HA, Robertson JE, Paulson DF. Radical prostatectomy: the pros and cons of the perineal versus retropubic approach. J Urol 1992;147:888–90.
50. Gibbons RP, Correa RJ Jr, Brannen GE, Mason JT. Total prostatectomy for localized prostate cancer. J Urol 1984;131:73–6.
51. Steiner MS, Morton RA, Walsh PC. Impact of anatomical radical prostatectomy on urinary continence. J Urol 1991;145:512–5.
52. Catalona WJ, Basler JW. Return of erections and urinary continence following nerve-sparing radical retropubic prostatectomy. J Urol 1993;150:905–7.
53. Eastham JA, Kattan MW, Rogers E, et al. Risk factors for urinary incontinence after radical prostatectomy. J Urol 1996;156:1707–13.
54. Geary ES, Dendinger TE, Freiha FS, Stamey TA. Incontinence and vesical neck strictures following radical retropubic prostatectomy. Urology 1995;45:1000–6.
55. Walsh PC, Partin AW, Epstein JI. Cancer control and quality of life following anatomical radical retropubic prostatectomy: results at 10 years. J Urol 1994;152:1831–6.
56. Geary ES, Dendinger TE, Freiha FS, Stamey TA. Nerve sparing radical prostatectomy: a different view. J Urol 1995;154:145–9.
57. Partin AW, Pound CR, Clemens JQ, et al. Serum PSA after anatomic radical prostatectomy. The Johns Hopkins experience after 10 years. Urol Clin North Am 1993;20:713–25.
58. Epstein JI, Pizo G, Walsh PC. Correlation of pathologic findings with progression after radical retropubic prostatectomy. Cancer 1993;71:3582–3.
59. Stamey TA, Villers AA, McNeal JE, et al. Positive margins at radical prostatectomy: importance of the apical dissection. J Urol 1990;143:1166–73.
60. Rosen MA, Goldstone L, Lapin S, et al. Frequency and location of extracapsular extension and positive surgical margins in radical prostatectomy specimens. J Urol 1992;148:331–7.
61. Weldon VE. Letter to the editor: Re: prognostic implications of a positive apical margin in radical prostatectomy specimens. J Urol 1998;159:2105.
62. Lowe BA. Preservation of the anterior urethral ligamentous attachments in maintaining post-prostatectomy urinary continence: a comparative study. J Urol 1997;158:2137–41.
63. Weldon VE. Letter to the editor. Re: radical prostatectomy for prostate cancer: the perineal approach increases the risk of surgically induced positive margins and capsular incisions. J Urol 1999;161:1287.
64. Polascik TJ, Pound CR, DeWeese TL, Walsh PC. Comparison of radical prostatectomy and iodine 125 interstitial radiotherapy for the treatment of clinically localized prostate cancer: a 7-year biochemical (PSA) progression analysis. Urology 1998;51:884–90.
65. Lu-Yao GL, Yao SL. Population-based study of long term survival in patients with clinically localized prostate cancer. Lancet 1997;349:906–10.

14

Laparoscopic Radical Prostatectomy

CHRISTOPHER J. KANE, MD
MARSHALL L. STOLLER, MD
GARY D. GROSSFELD, MD, FACS
PETER R. CARROLL, MD, FACS

Radical prostatectomy is a common form of treatment for localized prostate cancer.[1] Widespread use of serum prostate-specific antigen (PSA) screening has resulted in downward stage migration and a greater proportion of patients presenting with lower-stage disease[2] who are therefore candidates for curative local therapy. Although the morbidity, complications, and outcomes of radical retropubic prostatectomy and radical perineal prostatectomy have improved substantially, there is constant refinement being made on surgical techniques to improve outcomes. The application of laparoscopy to radical prostatectomy was inevitable with the increasing penetration of laparoscopic surgery in urology. The first report of laparoscopic radical prostatectomy (LAPRP) by Schuessler and colleagues in 1997 demonstrated the feasibility of the procedure.[3] Over a period of more than 4 years, they performed nine LAPRPs with an average operative time of 9 hours, average hospitalization of 7.3 days, including two postoperative complications of cholecystitis and pulmonary embolism. Although a technical accomplishment, they concluded that there was no benefit, at that time, over open radical retropubic prostatectomy.

Based on their experience, the technical challenge of the procedure, and the perceived minimal benefit over conventional radical prostatectomy, there was little enthusiasm in the United States for LAPRP. Raboy and colleagues published a series of two LAPRPs performed extraperitoneally in 1998 with encouraging results and operative times between 4 and 5.5 hours.[4]

Interest in LAPRP exploded in 1999 and 2000 based on the pioneering work of two French groups. Guillonneau and colleagues reported the results of 40 patients who had LAPRP performed at the Institut Mutualiste Montsouris in Paris.[5] Their operative time averaged 4.5 hours, catheter time was 7.6 days, and transfusion rate was 17.5%. They reported a 17.5% positive margin rate with 89.7% undetectable serum PSA at 1 month of follow-up. Jacob and colleagues also reported the results of 20 patients undergoing LAPRP at Hospital Henri-Mondor in Creteil, France. Their operative time averaged 6.4 hours, catheter time was 10.7 days, and transfusion rate was 10%. They reported that all patients maintained an undetectable PSA with a mean follow-up of 6 months.[6] Abbou and colleagues reported their experience after 43 patients and decreased their operative time to 4.3 hours and the transfusion rate to 4.3%. Although their positive margin rate was 27.9%, all of their patients had an undetectable serum PSA with 1-month follow-up. Continence, defined as no leakage and assessed using a patient-administered questionnaire, was 84%.[7] Similarly, Guillonneau and Vallancien updated their experience with 120 LAPRPs and reduced their operative times to an average of 4 hours, blood loss to 402 mL, transfusion rate to

10%, and positive margin rate to 15%. With a mean follow-up of 2.2 months, the undetectable PSA rate was 94.7%. Continence 6 months following surgery was reported in 72% of patients, and 45% of their last 20 patients who were potent preoperatively regained potency following surgery.[8]

Rassweiler and colleagues recently reported the Heilbronn, Germany, experience of LAPRP in 180 patients with a different technique. They use a six-port technique and approach the space of Retzius initially, incise the endopelvic fascia, control the dorsal vein with sutures, and divide the urethra. They then perform the prostatectomy in a retrograde fashion, similar to open prostatectomy. They approach the vas deferens and seminal vesicles after the bladder neck division and then perform a vesicourethral anastomosis with an interrupted technique. Their mean blood loss was 1,200 mL, with a 31% transfusion rate. Their positive margin rate was 16%, and 95% of their patients had an undetectable serum PSA at 1 year.[9]

Long follow-up is unavailable for current LAPRP series, and few data concerning postoperative sexual function exist. A well-conducted, confidential, patient-completed questionnaire study of urinary continence after LAPRP was recently published.[10] Olsson and colleagues distributed 115 questionnaires before surgery and then at 1, 3, 6, and 12 months postoperatively. No pad use was reported by 18, 58, 69, and 78% of patients at 1, 3, 6, and 12 months, respectively, although only 37 patients completed the 12-month questionnaire.[10] Although continence data vary widely in the literature and are sensitive to the method of questioning,[11] this compares favorably with large open prostatectomy series.

Updated results from currently available series of LAPRP are outlined in Table 14–1.[3,4,7–9,12–14] If a series is available only in abstract form, it is included in Table 14–1; however, if a series is in abstract and published manuscript form, the published manuscript data are preferentially included.

Numerous centers worldwide are now performing LAPRP; however, the benefits of LAPRP over standard radical prostatectomy are not clear. The potential benefit of more precise dissection owing to the magnification and illumination of the laparoscope exists but must be realized by improved oncologic and functional outcomes. The outcomes that must be equivalent or superior to open radical prostatectomy prior to strong positive recommendation are oncologic outcomes (biochemical and cancer-specific survival), urinary continence and quality of life, sexual function and quality of life, perioperative morbidity and pain and return to normal activity, and, finally, cost. Although proponents of LAPRP claim equivalence or superiority in many of these areas, larger series, with more robust follow-up and standardized assessments of outcomes with comparison to standard techniques, will be required before the promise of LAPRP is objectively confirmed.

DESCRIPTION OF PROCEDURE

The preoperative preparation of the patient includes informed consent in which the risks, benefits, and complications of radical prostatectomy are reviewed as well as the complications that are unique to LAPRP, including the possibility of open conversion and a longer operative time. Most surgeons recom-

Table 14–1. SUMMARY OF LAPRP SERIES

Lead Author	N	Time (hours)	EBL (mL)	Transfusion Rate (%)	Conversion (%)	Positive Margin (%)	Continence (%)	Potency with B Nerve Sparing (%)	Hospitalization (days)
Schussler[3]	9	9.4	640	0	0	11	67	50	7.3
Raboy[4]	2	4.8	500	50	0	50	NA	NA	2.5
Guillonneau[8]	120	4.0	402	10	5.8	15	72	45	6.6
Abbou[7]	43	4.3	NA	4.7	0	27.9	84	14	7.2
Van Velthoven[12]	22	6.7	490	31	23	23	NA	NA	NA
Rassweiler[9]	180	4.5	1,230	31	4.4	16	97 (12 mo)	NA	10
Tuerk[13]	152	4.4	185	1.3	0	23.4	92	NA	NA
Zippe[14]	50	5.4	225	2	2	20	76	31	1.6

LAPRP = laparoscopic radical prostatectomy; NA = not available; EBL = estimated blood loss (CC).

mend a preoperative mechanical bowel preparation with oral magnesium citrate. Perioperative intravenous antibiotics, usually a first-generation cephalosporin, and prophylaxis for thromboembolic complications with either lower-extremity sequential compression devices or low-molecular-weight heparin are administered.

We place adhesive foam padding on the patient's back, which prevents the sliding that may occur from the exaggerated Trendelenburg's position. After induction of general anesthesia, an orogastric tube is placed to be removed immediately following surgery, and the patient is placed in the supine or low lithotomy position with the legs spread to allow rectal or perineal access. The surgical preparation extends from the upper abdomen to the mid-thighs including the patient's penis, scrotum, and perineum. An 18 French urethral catheter is placed. We use a five-port technique, with the first being a 12 mm placed infraumbilically. The ports are placed in a fan distribution with two 12-mm ports lateral to the rectus abdominus muscles in a line 2 to 5 cm inferior to the infraumbilical port and two 5-mm ports 3 cm medial to the anterior superior iliac spines (Figure 14–1). The primary surgeon works from the patient's left side through the left iliac and pararectus ports while the assistant stands on the right and works through the corresponding right-sided ports. The camera operator stands on the left toward the patient's head. Alternatively, the camera operator can sit at the head of the operating table. If available, the camera can be held by a voice-operated robot, creating more space for the surgeon and assistant. A single large monitor is placed at the foot of the operating table.

The patient is placed in Trendelenburg's position and a transverse peritoneal incision is made in the pouch of Douglas (Figure 14–2). Each vas deferens is identified, clipped, and transected. Hemostasis throughout the operation can be achieved with bipolar electrocautery, monopolar electrocautery, or the harmonic scalpel. Alternatively, endoscopic clips may be required at times to assist with hemostasis. Each seminal vesicle is carefully dissected circumferentially, with the assistant providing anterior and posterior retraction and suction where needed. A transverse incision is made in Denonvilliers' fascia

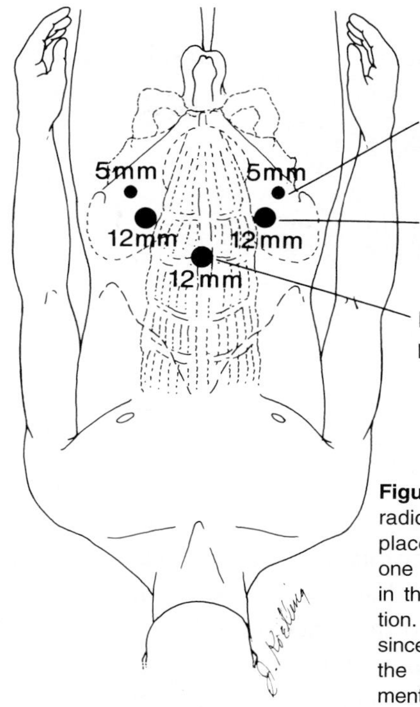

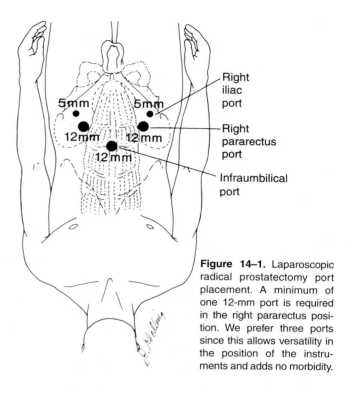

Figure 14–1. Laparoscopic radical prostatectomy port placement. A minimum of one 12-mm port is required in the right pararectus position. We prefer three ports since this allows versatility in the position of the instruments and adds no morbidity.

at the seminal vesicle–prostate junction, allowing access between the fascia and the anterior perirectal fat (Figure 14–3). This plane is opened with blunt dissection to the level of the apex of the prostate.

The bladder is then instilled with 200 mL of sterile water. A peritoneal incision is made in the ante-

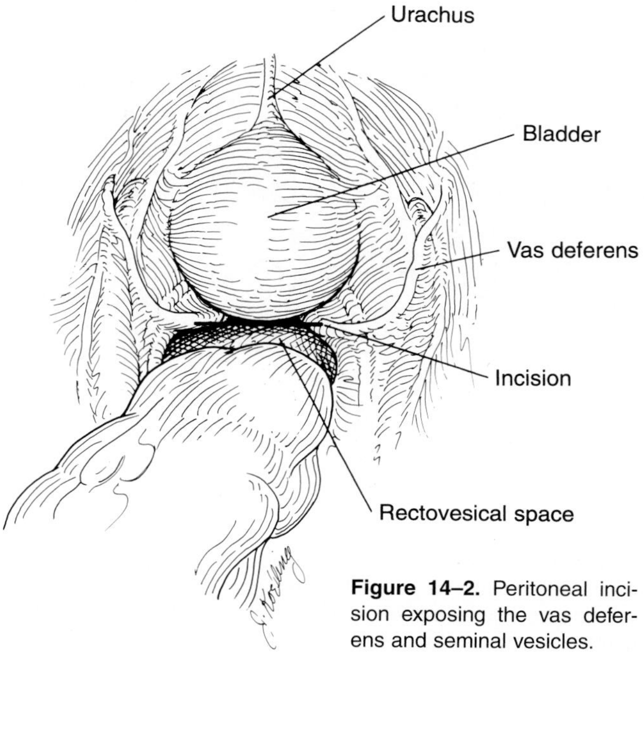

Figure 14–2. Peritoneal incision exposing the vas deferens and seminal vesicles.

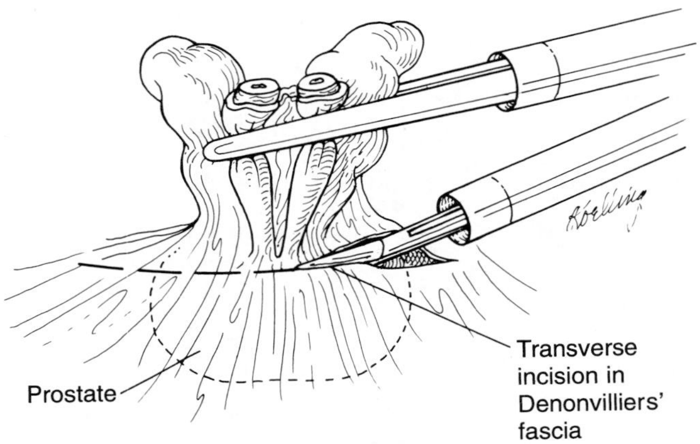

Figure 14–3. Transverse incision in tented leaflet of Denonvilliers' fascia, allowing access between the prostate and rectum.

rior abdominal peritoneum starting lateral to one obliterated umbilical artery, across the urachus and extending lateral to the other umbilical artery (Figure 14–4). The space of Retzius is bluntly entered, taking care to avoid bladder injury. The prostate and endopelvic fascia are visualized and the fat overlying the anterior surface of the prostate and endopelvic fascia is cleared. The endopelvic fascia is incised, preserving the puboprostatic ligaments. We place an endoscopic Babcock clamp using the left pararectus port and transfer the camera to the

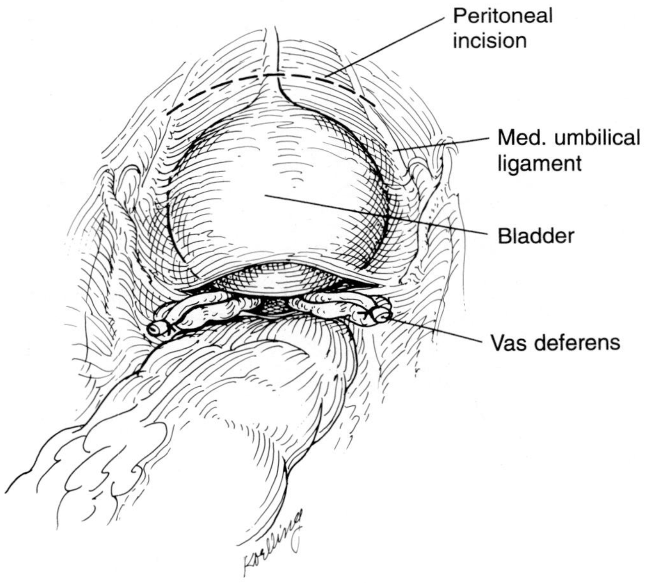

Figure 14–4. Anterior peritoneal incision allowing access to the space of Retzius. This incision is performed quite anterior to avoid creating an anterior peritoneal flap, which can interfere with subsequent dissection and suturing.

right pararectus port so that an articulating endoscopic gastrointestinal anastomotic stapler (Endo-GIA, U.S. Surgical, Norwalk, CT) can be applied through the midline 12-mm port (Figure 14–5). This is placed as distal as possible on the dorsal vein, and care is taken not to include the urethra in the stapler. Since the staples and cutting device do not reach the distal 6 mm of the instrument, there is little risk of urethral injury if the device is applied cautiously. Alternatively, the dorsal vein complex can be controlled with intracorporally placed distal and proximal sutures as described by the French centers with the greatest experience, or even incised with the harmonic scalpel. In cases in which bleeding is encountered from the dorsal vein complex, a figure of eight suture can be placed in a manner similar to open retropubic surgery to obtain control.

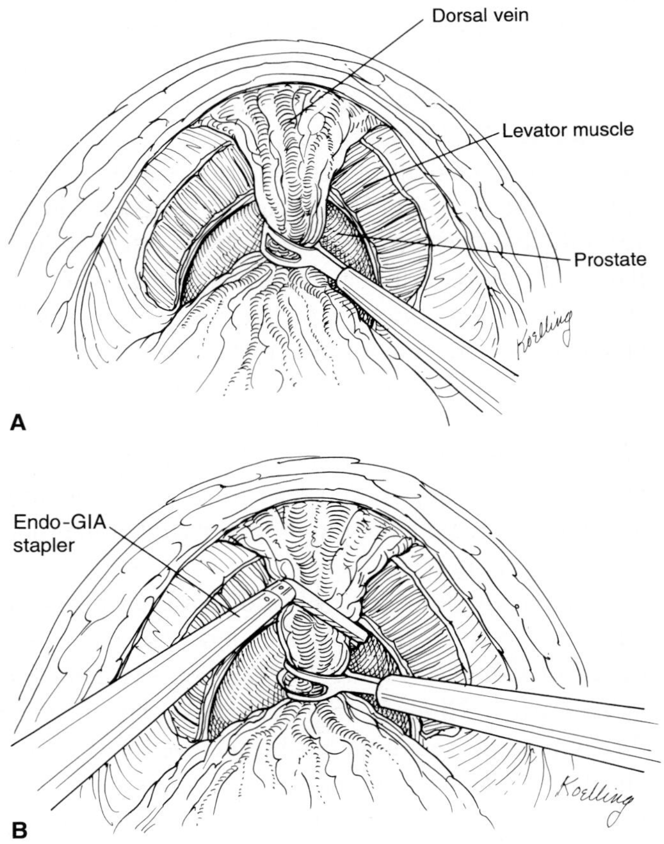

Figure 14–5. *A,* After incision of the endopelvic fascia bilaterally, the dorsal vein is gathered in an endoscopic Babcock clamp. This facilitates distal suture control or endoscopic gastrointestinal anastomotic stapler placement. *B,* Distal placement of the endoscopic gastrointestinal anastomotic stapler on the dorsal vein places two parallel lines of three rows of staples and divides between them. The articulating stapler is ideal since it allows vertical placement of the device.

The bladder neck dissection is then performed with the assistant placing anterior traction on the prostate and the surgeon incising the prostatovesical junction to identify circumferential bladder neck fibers (Figure 14–6). The anterior bladder neck mucosa is incised, and the Foley catheter balloon is deflated so that the tip can be grasped and brought anteriorly. The posterior bladder neck is then dissected and transected. If the bladder neck is large, interrupted 6 o'clock sutures can be placed at this point, completing a tennis racket closure, or an anterior tennis racket closure can be completed at the end of the anastomosis. The dissection then proceeds posteriorly, through the remaining posterior bladder neck fibers, into the previously dissected seminal vesicle space.

Anterior and contralateral traction on a seminal vesicle helps to visualize the ipsilateral prostatic pedicle. If a non–nerve-sparing procedure is planned, the articulating Endo-GIA can be applied to each pedicle (Figure 14–7). For a nerve-sparing procedure, the lateral prostatic fascia can be visualized and incised antegrade so that the neurovascular bundle can be visualized. Dissection can be carried out with clips and bipolar cautery or harmonic scalpel close to the posterolateral prostate, releasing the specimen from its pedicle.

The prostate is then retracted posteriorly and the apical dissection is performed. Any remaining dorsal vein is transected with electrocautery until the anterior surface of the urethra is identified. Great care is taken to maximize urethral preservation. The neurovascular bundles can be dissected from the dorsolateral apex at this juncture to facilitate preservation if desired. The anterior urethra is sharply divided, and the catheter is withdrawn and gently lifted by the assistant, allowing the posterior portion of the urethra to be visualized and transected. With cranial retraction on the prostate, the rectourethralis attachments are divided and the remaining attachments between the prostate and prostatic pedicles or Denonvilliers' fascia are divided. The free specimen is placed in the left lower abdomen for retrieval at the end of the case.

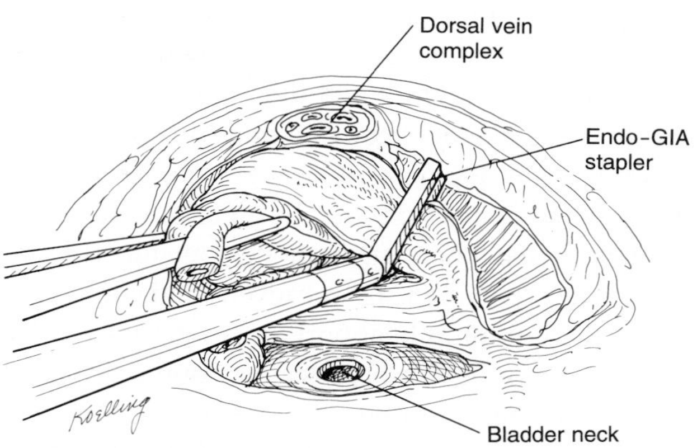

Figure 14–7. With contralateral retraction on the seminal vesicle, the ipsilateral prostatic pedicle is identified and divided with either a harmonic scalpel or the endoscopic gastrointestinal anastomotic stapler. If nerve sparing is desired, the neurovascular bundles should be identified distally and dissected prior to the antegrade division of the pedicle close to the posterolateral prostate.

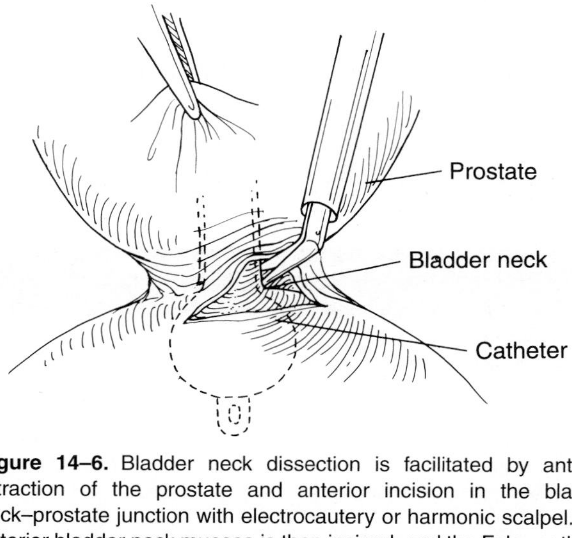

Figure 14–6. Bladder neck dissection is facilitated by anterior retraction of the prostate and anterior incision in the bladder neck–prostate junction with electrocautery or harmonic scalpel. The anterior bladder neck mucosa is then incised, and the Foley catheter is withdrawn and its tip grasped by the assistant and lifted anteriorly to facilitate the posterior bladder neck incision.

The vesicourethral anastomosis is then performed. This is the most challenging portion of the case and requires training and practice to complete. Either a running anastomosis as described by Abbou and colleagues[7] or an interrupted anastomosis as described by Guillonneau and colleagues[5] can be employed. In the running anastomosis, the initial suture is placed outside in on the bladder neck in the 3 o'clock position and then inside out on the urethra in a corresponding location. The knot is tied, and then the suture is run across the posterior anastomosis using the left iliac port and the right pararectus port with the assistant following. The suture is secured and another suture is used to run the anterior anastomosis after placing a urethral catheter. For the interrupted technique, the initial sutures are placed in the posterior anastomosis, with the suture passing inside out on the urethra and then outside in on the corresponding bladder neck and the knots tied within the lumen. After the posterior layer is completed, the Foley catheter is inserted, and the anterior sutures are placed with the knots tied on the outside (Figure 14–8). The specimen is retrieved and delivered through the infraumbilical port, enlarging it to allow specimen removal. A closed suction drain is placed using one of the 5-mm ports. Subcuticular skin closure is performed, and small dressings are placed.

The patient's diet is advanced from clear liquids the evening of surgery to a regular diet postoperative day 1. Early ambulation is encouraged. Intravenous ketorolac is used every 6 hours for the first 24 hours and then converted to oral pain medication when tolerating a regular diet. The target for discharge is the evening of postoperative day 1, although 2 or 3 days may be required depending on patient factors and resumption of bowel activity.

COMPLICATIONS

A summary of complications of LAPRP from six European centers was recently presented.[15] It reviews the work of 13 surgeons in six centers over the initial 32 months of performing transperitoneal LAPRPs. The average operative time was 4.4 hours, with a transfusion rate of 3.5%. The specific complications are reviewed in Table 14–2. There were no deaths; an open conversion rate of 2% and a reoperation rate of 1.9% were reported. It must be emphasized, however, that early in a surgeon's experience, long operative times, in the 8-hour range, and a higher conversion rate and overall complication rate may be encountered. For example, the Institut Mutualiste Montsouris group reported a 14% (5/35) open conversion rate early in their experience.[5] In addition, 3 patients (8.5%) had their anastomosis completed via small Pfannenstiel's incisions. In spite of the longer operative times and higher conversion rates early in their experiences, the outcomes of even the early patients appear favorable. The technical challenge of the procedure has been difficult to surmount for some, leading to discontinuation of LAPRP prior to mastery of the procedure. Weber and colleagues discontinued LAPRP after a series of nine patients demonstrated high operative times, high positive margins (78%), and a high conversion rate (44%).[16]

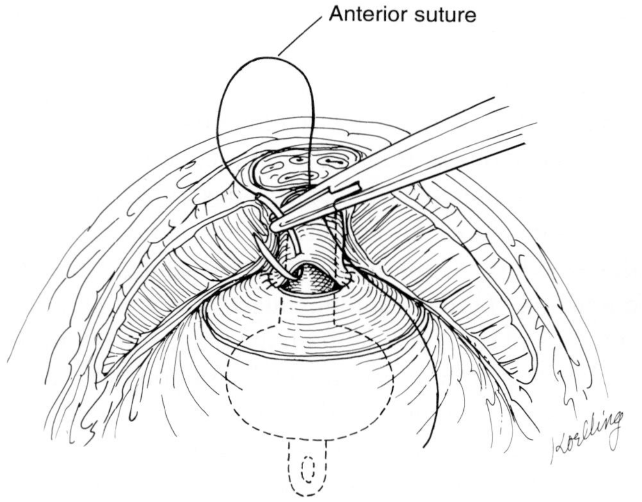

Figure 14–8. Interrupted absorbable sutures are placed in the vesicourethral anastomosis. Typically, 8 to 10 sutures are placed, beginning posteriorly. If there is redundant bladder neck, it is closed with interrupted anterior sutures, creating an inverted "tennis raquet."

SUMMARY

Transperitoneal laparoscopic prostatectomy can be performed safely by experienced laparoscopic surgeons who perform a significant volume of these procedures. The outstanding magnification and illumination of laparoscopy allow excellent intraoperative visualization of anatomic structures. Areas in which LAPRP may improve on results from standard open prostatectomy include early postoperative pain, time to return to full activities, blood loss, and transfusion rate. Factors with which LAPRP may achieve similar results to standard open radical

Table 14–2. COMPLICATIONS OF LAPRP FROM 6 EUROPEAN CENTERS

Transfusion rate	3.5%	(44/1,248)
Urinary retention	3.4%	(43/1,248)
Open conversion	2.0%	(26/1,248)
Rectal or bowel injury	1.2%	(15/1,248)
Ureteral injury	1.0%	(12/1,248)
Reoperation	1.9%	(23/1,248)
Thromboembolic complications	0.2%	(2/1,248)
Death	0.0%	(0/1,248)

Adapted from Sulser et al.[15]

LAPRP = laparoscopic radical prostatectomy.

prostatectomy are cancer control, urinary continence, and potency preservation, although larger series of patients with longer follow-up will be required to establish this with certainty. It is unlikely that LAPRP will compete with standard open prostatectomy with respect to operative time, operating room charges, or total cost of hospitalization. Catheter time, which surgeons performing LAPRP have decreased significantly, also can be limited after standard open radical prostatectomy as long as the anastomosis is watertight and of good quality.[17] This practice change has been motivated in part by the analysis of LAPRP series with short catheterization times. Prospective studies with objectively assessed outcomes comparing LAPRP to open radical prostatectomy are needed to evaluate whether the results of LAPRP will justify the enthusiasm surrounding the procedure.

REFERENCES

1. Potosky AL, Harlan LC, Stanford JL, et al. Prostate cancer practice patterns and quality of life: the Prostate Cancer Outcomes Study. J Natl Cancer Inst 1999;91:1719–24.
2. Amling CL, Blute ML, Lerner SE, et al. Influence of prostate-specific antigen testing on the spectrum of patients with prostate cancer undergoing radical prostatectomy at a large referral practice. Mayo Clin Proc 1998;73:489–90.
3. Schuessler WW, Schulam PG, Clayman RV, Kavoussi LR. Laparoscopic radical prostatectomy: initial short-term experience. Urology 1997;50:854–7.
4. Raboy A, Albert P, Ferzli G. Early experience with extraperitoneal endoscopic radical retropubic prostatectomy. Surg Endosc 1998;12:1264–7.
5. Guillonneau B, Cathelineau X, Barrett E, et al. Laparoscopic radical prostatectomy: technical and early oncological assessment of 40 operations. Eur Urol 1999;36:14–20.
6. Jacob F, Salomon L, Hoznek A, et al. Laparoscopic radical prostatectomy: preliminary results. Eur Urol 2000;37: 615–20.
7. Abbou CC, Salomon L, Hoznek A, et al. Laparoscopic radical prostatectomy: preliminary results. Urology 2000;55: 630–4.
8. Guillonneau B, Vallancien G. Laparoscopic radical prostatectomy: the Montsouris experience. J Urol 2000;163:418–22.
9. Rassweiler J, Sentker L, Seeman O, et al. Laparoscopic radical prostatectomy with the Heilbronn technique: an analysis of the first 180 cases. J Urol 2001;166;2101–8.
10. Olsson LE, Salomon L, Nadu A, et al. Prospective patient reported continence after laparoscopic radical prostatectomy. Urology 2001;58:570–2.
11. Litwin MS, Lubeck DP, Henning JM, Carroll PR. Differences in urologist and patient assessments of health related quality of life in men with prostate cancer: results of the CaPSURE database. J Urol 1998;159:1988–92.
12. VanVelthoven R, Peltier A, Hawaux E, Vendewalle J. Transperitoneal laparoscopic anatomic radical prostatectomy, preliminary results [abstract]. J Urol 2000;163 Suppl:141.
13. Tuerk I, Degar S, Winkelman B, Loening S. Laparoscopic radical prostatectomy—the Berlin experience [abstract]. J Urol 2001;165 Suppl:326.
14. Zippe CD, Meraney AM, Sung GT, Gill IS. Laparoscopic prostatectomy in the USA: Cleveland Clinic series of 50 patients [abstract]. J Urol 2001;165 Suppl:326.
15. Sulser T, Guillonneau B, Vallancien G, et al. Complications and initial experience with 1228 laparoscopic radical prostatectomies at 6 European centers. J Urol 2001;165 Suppl:150.
16. Weber HM, Eschholz G, Gunnewig M, et al. Laparoscopic radical prostatectomy?—not for us [abstract]. J Urol 2001; 165 Suppl:150.
17. Lepor H, Neider AM, Fraiman MC. Early removal of urinary catheter after radical retropubic prostatectomy is both feasible and desirable. Urology 2001;58:425–9.

15

Radiobiology: Old, Present, Future, and Practical Considerations

ALEXANDER R. GOTTSCHALK, MD, PHD
MACK ROACH III, MD

GENERAL RADIOBIOLOGY

Radiobiology is the study of the response of tumor and normal tissue to radiation therapy. This multifactorial field includes analysis of cell survival, dose response, dose fractionation, dose rate, oxygenation, temperature, cell cycle distribution, radiation sensitizers, and molecular abnormalities and predicting acute and late complications. In this chapter, we first discuss some general radiobiologic principles. We then refer to radiobiologic considerations specific to prostate cancer. Finally, we discuss how radiobiology can be inferred from clinical trials and how knowledge of radiobiology may alter current therapies.

Survival Curves

Early radiobiology investigated the proportion of cells that survived after a given dose of radiation was delivered. After a cell is radiated it may die, it may remain viable, unable to divide, or it may continue proliferating. Only continuously growing cancer cells contribute to the morbidity and mortality of the patient. Therefore, radiation biologists have developed clonogenic survival assays to examine only that fraction of cells that will continue to divide after radiation is delivered. Clonogenic survival curves are generated from established cell lines actively growing in vitro. These cells are collected, counted, and irradiated with different doses of radiation. These cells are then plated in dishes and incubated for 1 to 2 weeks. Cells that survive and grow will form macroscopic colonies. The number of colonies is counted and adjusted for the plating efficiency (PE), which is the percentage of cells forming colonies in the absence of radiation. The PE is often in the range of 50 to 90%. Surviving fractions are then calculated by the formula:

$$\text{surviving fraction} = \frac{\text{colonies counted}}{(\text{cells seeded}) \times \text{PE}}$$

The process is repeated over a dose range (Figure 15–1). Then the surviving fraction is plotted against dose on a semilog scale (Figure 15–2). The majority of radiobiology that follows deals with the ability to alter this survival curve to gain a therapeutic advantage.

The initial part of the survival curve is flat (slope close to 0). The flat part of the radiation survival curve is often referred to as the shoulder of the curve. The broader the shoulder, the higher dose of radiation needed to obtain cell death. The shape of the shoulder varies depending on cell types. Lymphocytes have a very small shoulder and in turn are very sensitive to small doses of radiation. Neural tissue has a large shoulder and is relatively resistant to radiation. Prostate epithelium has an intermediate sensitivity.

Response of Tissue to Radiation

The shape of the survival curve can be expressed as a linear quadratic formula:

$$S = e^{-\alpha D - \beta D^2}$$

where S is the fraction of cells surviving a dose D and α and β are constants. The shape of the survival curves differs between normal tissue and tumor. Radiobiologic principles attempt to exploit the difference in the survival curves of tumor and normal tissue. The difference in survival curves is partly attributable to the growth rate of the cells. Rapidly growing normal tissue (eg, intestinal mucosa, oral mucosa, and bone marrow) shows survival curves similar to tumor cells. These rapidly dividing tissues are considered early response tissue because they show the effects of radiation in days to weeks. In contrast, slowly dividing tissues (eg, muscle, bone, and nerves) are considered late responding and show the effects of radiation after months to years. These different tissue types can be described by the ratio α/β. Acute-responding tissue has a high α/β ratio of 10 or higher, whereas late-responding tissue has a low α/β ratio in the range of 3 to 4 (1.5 to 2 for central nervous system tissue).

Fractionation

Based on the different α/β ratios for tumor and normal tissue, distinct survival curves can be calculated for normal tissue and for tumor. Fractionated radiotherapy has developed to take advantage of the difference between early and late responding tissues. As the number of fractions increases, the survival curves for early and late responding tissues separate, causing a therapeutic gain. Therefore, decreasing the dose per fraction and increasing the total dose allows for sparing normal tissue while keeping the effect on the tumor constant. This fractionation becomes the basis of modern-day radiotherapy.

The difference in the response of normal tissue and tumor is in part owing to their differential ability to repair DNA damage caused by the radiation. The proportion of radiation damage that is repairable is greater in the slowly growing normal tissues than in the faster growing tumors. Therefore, allowing time to elapse between radiation fractions will first allow for DNA damage to be repaired within normal cells. If the time between fractions increases beyond a certain length, DNA repair may occur within the tumor cells; however, tumors often have impaired ability to repair damaged DNA. In addition, certain cellular

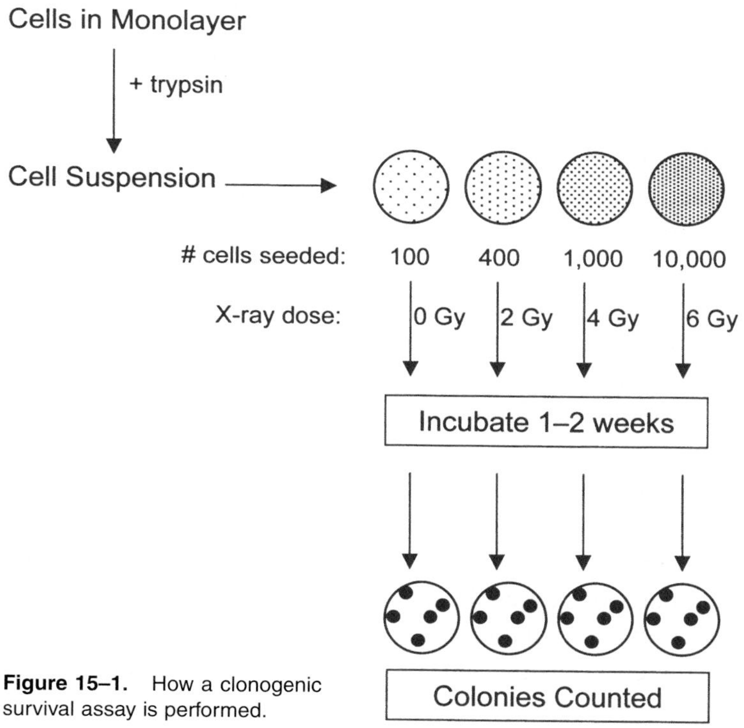

Figure 15–1. How a clonogenic survival assay is performed.

allows for inappropriate activation of signaling pathways and leads to cell growth and/or survival.

Although many gene mutations have been found in prostate cancer, the exact role of each gene is highly debated and currently the focus of investigation. It is safe to say that multiple genetic events must occur before prostate cancer develops. Similar to the mutations that lead to the development of cancer, additional mutations may contribute to a tumor's resistance to therapy. Therefore, much investigation surrounds blocking the abnormal signaling pathways in cancer cells to increase their sensitivity to traditional chemotherapy and/or radiation.

PROSTATE-SPECIFIC RADIOBIOLOGY

Fractionated Radiotherapy for Prostate Cancer

Radiation therapy for prostate cancer is usually delivered in 1.8 to 2.0 Gy fractions over 7 to 8 weeks. The development of any radiotherapy treatment plan takes into account the balance of local tumor control and normal tissue side effects. Although a biologically equivalent dose of radiation can be given over a shorter period of time (3 to 6 weeks), this accelerated treatment would require higher doses of radiation per day and, in turn, increase the risk of normal tissue side effects. Because of increased side effects, higher dose per fraction of radiation is not used in the clinical treatment of prostate cancer outside an experimental protocol setting.

The normal tissues that are of most concern in radiation therapy for prostate cancer are the rectum, bladder, urethra, and bulb of the penis. Much attention is given to the amount of radiation received by these organs in an attempt not to exceed their tolerance. Although it is well accepted that a dose of 60 Gy, in 2-Gy fractions, to the entire rectum results in a 5% chance of a serious complication, it is also well understood that a smaller volume of rectum can receive much higher doses of radiation. With the development of computer-based conformal treatment planning, smaller volumes of normal tissues are within the radiation field, allowing for high total doses to be tolerated. Higher doses of radiation theoretically lead to better local tumor control. Whether higher doses of radiation result in a better clinical outcome (freedom from progression or overall survival) is currently highly debated.

Proliferation Rate of Prostate Cancer

Prostate cancer is among the slowest growing of all human cancers. The proliferation rate of prostate cancer correlates highly with the Gleason score. High-grade tumors (Gleason score 8 to 10) are much faster growing than the low-grade tumors (Gleason score 6 or less). The most common form of prostate cancer is the slow-growing, low-grade tumor. This slow rate of growth implies that repopulation and redistribution do not play major roles in the radiobiology of prostate cancer. Although hyperfractionated (twice per day) radiotherapy has been shown to be advantageous in rapidly growing tumors (eg, small cell lung cancer and squamous cell carcinoma in the head and neck region),[1,2] it is unlikely to be of any benefit in slow-growing prostate cancer.

Because prostate tumors often are so slow growing, their response to fraction size might be more similar to late-responding normal tissues than that of rapidly proliferating tumors (ie, have a low α/β ratio). If this is so, the smaller doses of radiation per fraction, which spare normal tissue in most other types of tumors, might not provide such an advantage in prostate cancer. In this scenario, it would be logical to hypothesize that higher doses per fraction (hypofractionation) might obtain better clinical outcomes. This theory would argue that brachytherapy with HDR iridium 192 source could provide improved tumor control. Unfortunately, there is no clinical evidence that a HDR brachytherpy provides any advantage to permanent seed (low-dose rate) brachytherapy or external beam radiation therapy. Additional details regarding the low α/β ratio and hypofractionated radiotherapy will be discussed later.

Dose Rate

Both total dose and dose rate may play a role in the treatment of prostate cancer. The total dose of radiation therapy with external beam treatments is in the neighborhood of 70 Gy. The total dose delivered with brachytherapy using iridium 125 or palladium 103 is approximately 145 and 100 Gy, respectively.

Although these total doses seem much higher than those delivered with external beam radiation, it is important to remember that the dose from permanent seed brachytherapy is delivered over a much longer time period. The half-lives of iodine 125 and palladium 103 are 60 and 17 days, respectively. Three-quarters of the total dose is given in two half-lives and 87.5% in three half-lives. Low dose rate brachytherapy with iodine 125 equates to the lowest possible dose per fraction (of external beam radiation therapy) and therefore requires treatment to higher doses than 70 Gy in 1.8 to 2 Gy fractions. As the dose rate of radiation decreases, a larger total dose is required to have an equivalent effect to higher dose rates. The higher total dose is needed because low dose rate theoretically allows for more repair of DNA damage during the time of radiation.

Hormones

The prostate is an androgen-dependent organ requiring these hormones for its development and maintenance. Similarly, prostate cancer is known to use endogenous androgens as growth factors. Manipulation of these hormones plays an important role in the biology of prostate cancer. In the laboratory, withdrawing androgens from prostate cancer cell lines inhibits their growth. In addition, the sensitivity of cell lines to radiation is increased in the absence of androgens. Although not all laboratory findings have corresponding clinical applications, androgen suppression plays a major role in the treatment of prostate cancer. Although it is true that androgen suppression allows for decreased growth of human prostate cancer, androgen suppression alone is never curative, and disease progression invariably occurs. Disease progression occurs by the acquisition of androgen-independent growth. The molecular basis of androgen-independent growth may involve mutations in the androgen receptor, associated proteins, or target genes. More common than androgen suppression alone, androgen suppression is used in conjunction with radiation therapy for locally advanced and high-grade prostate cancer. A number of clinical trials have shown that total androgen suppression plus radiation therapy is superior to radiation therapy alone in patients with high-risk disease.[7–9]

Molecular Basis of Viral Therapy

Adenoviruses are being investigated as a new method of delivering targeted gene therapy. Adenoviruses can infect a wide variety of epithelial cells, including prostate epithelium. Once inside the cell, the virus uses the cell's normal proteins to produce and package more virus particles. The virus then lyses and kills the cell, exposing neighboring cells to new virus particles. Nonreplicating adenoviruses have limited clinical application as they would require that every single tumor cell be infected with the virus. Currently, there are no methods of delivery that allow for infection of every tumor cell. Therefore, replicating adenoviruses that have been modified to gain a therapeutic advantage are currently being investigated. One approach is an engineered virus that is specific for prostate cancer. By placing prostate-specific antigen (PSA) and probasin regulatory elements (eg, promoters and enhancers) in key locations within the adenovirus genome, scientists have developed an adenovirus that will replicate only within PSA-producing cells. Therefore, although this modified adenovirus may infect many different cell types, it only replicates and kills prostate cells. This prostate-specific adenovirus has been used clinically in patients who have local failures after radiation therapy and has produced PSA responses.[10] In addition, laboratory experiments have shown synergy between radiation therapy and this prostate-specific adenovirus.[11] In the long term, this virus may be used in conjunction with more traditional therapies such as surgery or radiation therapy.

A second viral approach is to generate an adenovirus that can replicate only in cancer cells that have mutations in *P53*. *P53* mutations are common in a wide variety of cancers. Interestingly, *P53* mutations are not very common in prostate cancer and probably occur late in prostate cancer pathogenesis. In this molecular approach, the *E1B* gene is deleted from the adenovirus genome. E1B is a viral protein that binds to and inhibits P53. Inactivation of P53 is critical for viral replication. Since the viral *E1B* gene is deleted, this modified virus will only replicate in cells deficient in P53 or the P53 pathway (P53, MDM2, or P19^{arf}).[12,13] These other members within the P53 pathway have not been fully investigated in prostate cancer; therefore, the effectiveness of this viral approach in prostate cancer is still uncertain. Abnormalities within the P53 pathway are probably more common than initially appreciated. This viral approach is currently being investigated in colorectal and head and neck cancers with interesting success.

Other Novel Therapeutic Strategies

As scientists investigate the pathogenesis of cancer, new specific molecular mutations are being discovered. As an understanding of the biochemical functions of the protein becomes available, companies are generating a class of drugs that will inhibit these specific proteins. Unlike traditional chemotherapy, this new class of drugs has the unique properties of killing only cancer cells with little to no toxicity to normal cells. Recently, STI-571 has made news for its unique cancer-specific design. STI-571 inhibits the bcr-abl mutant protein, a mutation found in 95% of patients with CML. Although the bcr-abl translocation is not found in prostate cancer, there are other mutations that may be targeted in patients with prostate cancer.

The *EGFR* is another example of a molecular abnormality that can be specifically targeted. *EGFR* is overexpressed or mutated on many different tumors, including prostate cancer. Several different approaches have been used to target *EGFR*.[14] Monoclonal antibodies against *EGFR* (such as C225) bind to and block signal through the receptor. Antisense oligonucleotides directed against *EGFR* may bind to the messenger ribonucleic acid and prevent protein expression. Finally, small molecule inhibitors (OSI-774, ZD 1839) bind and inhibit the tyrosine kinase activity of *EGFR*. ZD 1839 (Iressa) has been used with patients with prostate cancer in phase I clinical trials. Initially, these novel approaches are used as single-agent therapy; eventually, they will be used in combination with traditional therapy such as chemotherapy, hormonal therapy, and radiation therapy. There is great belief that using a targeted therapy, such as *EGFR* blockade, will increase the sensitivity of the tumor cell to radiation.

Although molecular abnormalities as possible prognostic markers or targets of therapy are of extreme interest to biologists, they are not without their own set of difficulties. Prostate cancer is not necessarily a uniform disease. Scientists have identified prostate cancer as a multifocal disease process (Table 15–1).[15] Although molecular abnormalities may be identified in a single prostate biopsy or part of the prostatecomy specimen, the multifocal nature of prostate cancer suggests that several different molecular abnormalities may be present within different areas of the prostate gland and therefore complicate the routine use of molecular markers for prognosis or therapy.

CLINICAL CONSIDERATIONS AND PRACTICAL APPLICATIONS OF THE RADIOBIOLOGY OF PROSTATE CANCER: CRITIQUE OF THE MYSTIQUE OF α/β RADIOBIOLOGY

The background provided above summarizes many of the issues that are considered to be relevant to understanding basic radiobiologic aspects of prostate cancer radiotherapy. Some of the most respected radiobiologists in the world recently came to the conclusion that prostate cancer has a very low α/β ratio.[16–19] Based on this conclusion, they appear to be convinced that regimens that include hypofractionated treatment schedules such as HDR might be the best way to treat prostate cancer. Table 15–2 summarizes some of the recent studies making this point.[16,18,20–24] For example, Brenner and Hall used two retrospective data sets (one using EBRT and the other permanent prostate implant [PPI]) using PSA-based end points to assess tumor control for prostate cancer.[16] The linear-quadratic model was used for the analysis to assess the impact of fractionation on out-

Table 15–1. PROSTATE CANCER IS A MULTIFOCAL DISEASE PROCESS

Tumors/Patient	No. of Patients (%)	No. of Tumors	Mean Tumor Volume (cc)
1	66 (43.7)	66	6.52
2	47 (31.1)	94	1.48
3	25 (16.6)	75	1.01
4	8 (5.3)	32	0.59
5	4 (2.6)	20	0.40
6	1 (0.7)	6	0.22
Total	151 (100)	293	

Table 15–2. SELECTED RECENT PUBLICATIONS ADDRESSING RADIOBIOLOGIC ASPECTS OF PROSTATE CANCER

Authors (Year)	Study Design	Conclusions from Authors
Brenner and Hall (1999)[16]	Two retrospective data sets (one using EBRT and the other PPI) using PSA-based end points were used to assess tumor control for prostate cancer. The linear-quadratic model was used for the analysis to assess the impact of fractionation on outcome.	Prostatic cancers appear to be more sensitive to changes in fractionation than most other cancers. The estimated α/β value was 1.5 Gy (0.8, 2.2), reflecting the relationship between cellular proliferative status and sensitivity to fraction size. HDR brachytherapy/external beam regimens (using larger fractions) could be designed to be as efficacious as low dose rate. Hypofractionation schemes would be expected to maintain current tumor control and late effects, but with less acute morbidity. Owing to the logistic and financial advantages of fewer numbers of fractions, this type of approach may be preferred.
Fowler et al (2001)[18]	Seventeen papers published from 1995 to 2000 were used to estimate bNED using EBRT, ^{125}I, or ^{103}Pd PPI. This analysis focused on intermediate-risk patients. Three methods of estimating α/β were employed. Two high-dose boost doses were analyzed using 2-year bNED data.	Using the two methods, the α/β ratios ranged from 1.4 to 1.9 Gy, and if mean or median doses were used instead of the prescribed dose, the estimate of α/β would be substantially below 1 Gy. The third method, although based on early follow-up, was consistent with low values of α/β in the region of 2 Gy or below. All of the estimates point toward low values of α/β, at least as low as the estimates of Brenner and Hall[16] and possibly lower than the expected values of about 3 Gy for late complications. Hypofractionation trials for intermediate-risk prostatic cancer appear to be indicated.
Camphausen et al (2001)[20]	Surgical removal of a primary tumor can result in the rapid growth of metastases (via loss of angiogenesis inhibitors produced by the primary tumor). This study evaluates the impact of radiotherapy on distant metastases from a Lewis lung carcinoma (a known producer of an inhibitor of angiogenesis). Fifty Gy in five fractions were compared to no EBRT.	Complete response of the primary tumor was seen in 25 of 35 (71%) mice. Examination of their lungs revealed > 46 (range, 46 to 62) surface metastases in the treated animals compared with 5 (range, 2 to 8) in the untreated animals. The average number of surface metastases increased from five per lung (range, 2 to 13) in the control animals to 53 per lung (range, 46 to 62) in the irradiated animals ($p < .001$). Administration of recombinant angiostatin prevented the growth of the metastases after the treatment of the primary. In this model, the use of radiation to eradicate a primary tumor resulted in the growth of previously dormant lung metastases and suggests that combining angiogenesis inhibitors with radiation therapy may control distant metastases.
Speight et al (2001)[21]	A total of 927 patients treated with external beam radiotherapy alone were studied.	Patients with intermediate-risk disease defined as risk of lymph node involvement between 15 and 35% benefited the most by higher doses, but there appeared to be a plateau in the dose-response curve.
Kupelian et al (2001)[22]	Radiation dose response as determined by biochemical relapse-free survival in patients with favorable localized prostate cancers was studied.	Patients receiving ≥ 72 Gy, the 5-year bRFS rates were both 95% versus 77% for patients receiving < 72 Gy, $p = .010$. For patients receiving 74 Gy, the 4-year bRFS rate was 94% versus 96% for patients receiving 78 Gy; $p = .90$. A multivariate analysis for factors affecting bRFS rates using Cox proportional hazards demonstrated that there was a clear radiation dose response in patients with favorable localized prostate cancers (ie, stage T1–T2, biopsy Gleason score ≤ 6, and iPSA ≤ 10 ng/mL) but no apparent benefit to the use of doses above 74 Gy.
Vicini et al (2001)[23]	Retrospective analysis of data from articles were identified through the MEDLINE database, CancerLit database, and reference lists of relevant articles assessing the impact of increasing RT dose on outcomes.	Twenty-two reports involving in excess of 11,000 patients were identified. Patients with poor risk features (eg, PSA ≥ 10, Gleason score ≥ 7, or tumor stage ≥ T2b) were most likely to benefit from increasing doses of radiation. However, the optimal RT dose and the magnitude of benefit of dose escalation remains to be defined.
Roach et al (2001)[24]	A total of 1,323 men with prostate cancer randomized to WP RT + NHT, PO RT + NHT, WP RT + AHT, and PO RT + AHT. LH-RH and an antiandrogen were given 2 months before and during RT (NHT) or for 4 months following RT (AHT).	NHT and WP RT experienced a 4-year PFS of ~60% compared with 45% when treated with PO RT ($p = .001$). However, patients treated with AHT experienced a similar PFS with WP or PO RT. Prophylactic WP RT and NHT reduced the risk of disease progression for patients with high-risk prostate cancer. However, NHT combined with RT was no more effective than AHT when only the prostate was irradiated, and WP RT was no more effective than PO RT without NHT.

EBRT = external beam radiation therapy; PPI = permanent prostate implant; PSA = prostate-specific antigen; HDR = high-dose rate; bNED = biochemical, no evidence of disease; bRFS = biochemical relapse-free survival; iPSA = pretreatment prostate-specific antigen; RT = radiation therapy; WP = whole pelvis; NHT = neoadjuvant hormonal therapy; PO = prostate only; AHT = adjuvant hormonal therapy; LH-RH = luteinizing hormone–releasing hormone; PFS = progression-free survival.

come. They concluded that prostate cancers appear to be more sensitive to changes in fractionation than most other cancers. The estimated α/β value was approximately 1.5 Gy, reflecting the relationship between cellular proliferative status and sensitivity to fraction size. They also concluded that HDR brachytherapy/external beam regimens (using larger fractions) could be designed to be as efficacious as low dose rate and hypofractionation schemes. Such regimens would be expected to maintain current tumor control and late effects, but with less acute morbidity. Owing to the logistic and financial advantages of fewer numbers of fractions, they felt that this could well become the preferred approach.

Similarly, Fowler and colleagues reviewed 17 papers published from 1995 to 2000 estimating biochemical, no evidence of disease [bNED] rates using EBRT, iodine 125, or palladium 103 PPI.[18] This analysis focused on intermediate-risk patients. Three methods of estimating α/β were employed. Two high-dose boost doses were analyzed using 2-year bNED data. They concluded that using the two methods, the α/β ratios ranged from 1.4 to 1.9 Gy, and if mean or median doses were used instead of the prescribed dose, the estimate of α/β would be substantially below 1 Gy. The third method, although based on early follow-up, was consistent with low values of α/β in the region of 2 Gy or below. All of the estimates point toward very low values of α/β, at least as low as the estimates of Brenner and Hall. Again, they concluded that hypofractionation trials for intermediate-risk prostate cancer appear to be indicated. More recently, King and Fowler reached similar conclusions about prostate α/β ratios.[19]

How accurate are the assumption made by the group of radiobiologists described above? It is likely that given available data, their estimates are reasonably accurate if the data are as robust as assumed. Unfortunately, it is likely that the control rates are significantly overestimated for some populations of patients and the complication rates underestimated for all populations. The latter point is made by comparing patient-versus physician-reported rates of complications.[25] The major reasons for concluding that the control rates are overly optimistic relate to the inadequacy of follow-up. Although the follow-up was described as "mature" in the article by Brenner and Hall, in fact, the data were not. Although the follow-up extended to 5 years, the median follow-up for the study reported by Brenner and Hall was only 32 months for brachytherapy patients. A closer look at the primary source for the brachytherapy data reveals that the patients receiving doses > 140 Gy (who did the best) had substantially shorter follow-up than those who received lower doses.[26] In the report by Fowler and colleagues, the 2-year bNED was used.[18] Using the conventional definitions for PSA failure, outcomes appear to be very sensitive to the duration of follow-up. For example, Vicini and colleagues reported that, using the American Society for Therapeutic Radiology and Oncology (ASTRO) consensus definition, an accurate outcome required follow-up 2 years beyond the median follow-up.[27] Investigators from the University of Chicago have similarly reported a critical dependence of follow-up on accurately assessing outcome.[28] Thus, the dose-response curve was biased (because of shorter follow-up) in favor of those receiving higher doses, and the dose-response curve is likely to be less steep.

Also of concern was the use of PSA failure as the major end point for determining success. Although, posttreatment PSA has been widely adopted as an acceptable end point by many practicing physicians, it has not been proven to be a surrogate for survival. In an analysis of patients treated in Radiation Therapy Oncology Group (RTOG) trials, Roach and colleagues previously demonstrated that Gleason score was the most important predictor of death caused by prostate cancer.[29] In a contemporary group of patients with a median follow-up of 5 years, Roach and colleagues confirmed this observation.[30] In the study by Fowler and colleagues, so-called intermediate-risk patients were chosen to investigate the impact of fraction size.[18] Unfortunately, our data suggest that this risk group stratification scheme is flawed, and PSA failure is inadequate to assess survival. The point is that since Gleason score is the most important predictor of survival and a high Gleason score is associated with a short survival and more rapidly dividing tumors, the conclusions reached by our esteemed radiobiologists may underestimate the α/β ratios. Their assumptions are probably most accurate for patients with a Gleason score < 7, many of whom may not require any treatment.

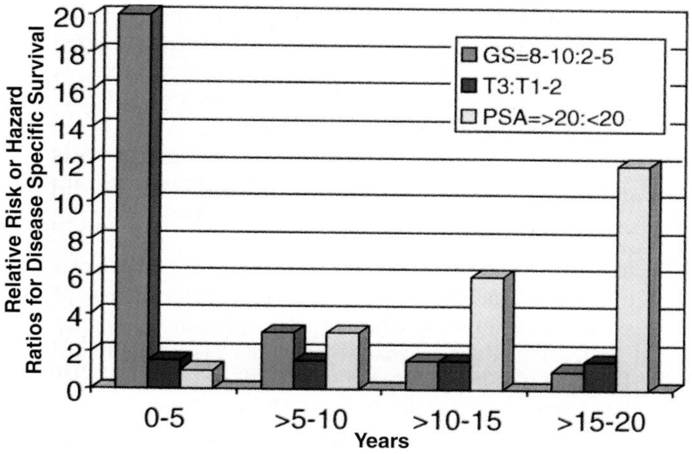

Figure 15–3. Hazard ratio model for the impact of Gleason score (GS), tumor stage, and prostate-specific antigen (PSA) on survival from prostate cancer.[29,30]

Figure 15–3 provides a theoretic view of prostate cancer biology based on recent clinical data and the data from the RTOG risk groups.[24,25]

An additional consideration is the fact that the practice of medicine frequently reflects practical considerations that supersede radiobiologic considerations. For example, a rather broad practical clinical question currently confronting the radiation oncologist and patients is "How should the type, dose, and volume irradiated be influenced by a patient's clinical stage, Gleason score, PSA, or other prognostic factors (eg, number + biopsies, gland size, symptom status)?" An example as to how practical considerations may negate the theoretical biologic issues proposed concerning the value of hypofractionation comes from the results of a recent phase III prospective randomized trial reported by the RTOG.[24] In this study, Roach and colleagues demonstrated that patients with an estimated risk of lymph node involvement > 15 percent benefit from elective nodal radiotherapy in combination with neoadjuvant hormonal therapy. Since the gut is not tolerant of large fractions and 5 weeks of external beam therapy would be required anyway, if HDR is no more effective than conventional fractionated radiotherapy, how much cost saving is there likely to be if 2 to 3 more weeks are replaced with anesthesia and one or more HDR treatments? Of further concern is the assumption that complications would be the same or less with hypofraction. To date, rates of stricture and incontinence (> 5% for both) appear to be higher in patients treated with HDR than seen in patients treated with three-dimensional conformal radiation therapy (3DCRT).[31,32]

In summary, the dose-response curve is likely to be flatter than many of the radiobiologists assume, and hypofractionation may be more morbid. The prostate cancers we are most concerned about are those with higher Gleason scores. These tumors are likely to be the ones with the highest α/β ratios among prostate cancers because of the shorter survival intervals associated with them.[30] These patients usually will benefit from pelvic nodal radiotherapy, which is not well suited to hypofractionation.[24] Our data and that of others suggest that we are nearing the flat portion of the dose-response curve and would benefit from bringing more biology and less radiation into our future therapies.[21–23]

REFERENCES

1. Turrisi AT 3rd, Kim K, Blum R, et al. Twice-daily compared with once-daily thoracic radiotherapy in limited small-cell lung cancer treated concurrently with cisplatin and etoposide. N Engl J Med 1999; 340:265–71.
2. Fu KK, Pajak TF, Trotti A, et al. A Radiation Therapy Oncology Group (RTOG) phase III randomized study to compare hyperfractionation and two variants of accelerated fractionation to standard fractionation radiotherapy for head and neck squamous cell carcinomas: first report of RTOG 9003. Int J Radiat Oncol Biol Phys 2000;48:7–16.
3. Vernon CC, Hand JW, Field SB, et al. Radiotherapy with or without hyperthermia in the treatment of superficial localized breast cancer: results from five randomized controlled trials. International Collaborative Hyperthermia Group. Int J Radiat Oncol Biol Phys 1996;35:731–44.
4. Overgaard J, Gonzalez Gonzalez D, Hulshof MC, et al. Randomised trial of hyperthermia as adjuvant to radiotherapy for recurrent or metastatic malignant melanoma. European Society for Hyperthermic Oncology. Lancet 1995; 345:540–3.
5. Shah NP, Sawyers CL. Recent success with the tyrosine kinase inhibitor STI-571—lessons for targeted therapy of cancer. Curr Opin Investig Drugs 2001;2:422–3.
6. Mughal TI, Goldman JM. Chronic myeloid leukaemia. STI 571 magnifies the therapeutic dilemma. Eur J Cancer 2001;37:561–8.
7. Pilepich MV, Winter K, John MJ, et al. Phase III Radiation Therapy Oncology Group (RTOG) trial 86-10 of androgen deprivation adjuvant to definitive radiotherapy in locally advanced carcinoma of the prostate. Int J Radiat Oncol Biol Phys 2001;50:1243–52.
8. Lawton CA, Winter K, Murray K, et al. Updated results of the phase III Radiation Therapy Oncology Group (RTOG) trial 85–31 evaluating the potential benefit of androgen suppression following standard radiation therapy for

unfavorable prognosis carcinoma of the prostate. Int J Radiat Oncol Biol Phys 2001;49:937–46.
9. Bolla M, Gonzalez D, Warde P, et al. Improved survival in patients with locally advanced prostate cancer treated with radiotherapy and goserelin. N Engl J Med 1997;337: 295–300.
10. DeWeese TL, van der Poel H, Li S, et al. A phase I trial of CV706, a replication-competent, PSA selective oncolytic adenovirus, for the treatment of locally recurrent prostate cancer following radiation therapy. Cancer Res 2001;61: 7464–72.
11. Chen Y, DeWeese T, Dilley J, et al. CV706, a prostate cancer-specific adenovirus variant, in combination with radiotherapy produces synergistic antitumor efficacy without increasing toxicity. Cancer Res 2001;61:5453–60.
12. McCormick F. Interactions between adenovirus proteins and the p53 pathway: the development of ONYX-015. Semin Cancer Biol 2000;10:453–9.
13. McCormick F. ONYX–015 selectivity and the p14ARF pathway. Oncogene 2000;19:6670–2.
14. Barton J, Blackledge G, Wakeling A. Growth factors and their receptors: new targets for prostate cancer therapy. Urology 2001;58:114–22.
15. Miller GJ, Cygan JM. Morphology of prostate cancer: the effects of multifocality on histological grade, tumor volume and capsule penetration. J Urol 1994;152:1709–13.
16. Brenner DJ, Hall EJ. Fractionation and protraction for radiotherapy of prostate carcinoma. Int J Radiat Oncol Biol Phys 1999;43:1095–101.
17. Duchesne GM, Peters LJ. What is the alpha/beta ratio for prostate cancer? Rationale for hypofractionated high-dose-rate brachytherapy [editorial]. Int J Radiat Oncol Biol Phys 1999;44:747–8.
18. Fowler J, Chappell R, Ritter M. Is alpha/beta for prostate tumors really low? Int J Radiat Oncol Biol Phys 2001; 50:1021–31.
19. King CR, Fowler JF. A simple analytic derivation suggests that prostate cancer alpha/beta ratio is low. Int J Radiat Oncol Biol Phys 2001;51:213–4.
20. Camphausen K, Moses MA, Beecken WD, et al. Radiation therapy to a primary tumor accelerates metastatic growth in mice. Cancer Res 2001;61:2207–11.
21. Speight JL, Weinberg VK, McLaughlin PW, Sandler HM. 3D conformal radiotherapy improves PSA failure rates for intermediate risk patients at conventional doses. Paper presented at: Proceeding of the American Society for Therapeutic Radiology and Oncology. San Antonio, TX, 1999.
22. Kupelian PA, Buchsbaum JC, Reddy CA, Klein EA. Radiation dose response in patients with favorable localized prostate cancer (stage T1-T2, biopsy Gleason < or = 6, and pretreatment prostate-specific antigen < or = 10). Int J Radiat Oncol Biol Phys 2001;50:621–5.
23. Vicini FA, Abner A, Baglan KL, et al. Defining a dose-response relationship with radiotherapy for prostate cancer: is more really better? Int J Radiat Oncol Biol Phys 2001;51:1200–8.
24. Roach M, Lu JD, Lawton C, et al. A phase III trial comparing whole-pelvic (WP) to prostate only (PO) radiotherapy and neoadjuvant to adjuvant total androgen suppression (TAS): preliminary analysis of RTOG 9413. Int J Radiat Oncol Biol Phys 2001;51:(3S1):3.
25. Joly F, Brune D, Couette JE, et al. Health-related quality of life and sequelae in patients treated with brachytherapy and external beam irradiation for localized prostate cancer. Ann Oncol 1998;9:751–7.
26. Stock R, Stone N, Tabert A, et al. A dose-response study for I-125 prostate implants. Int J Radiat Oncol Biol Phys 1998;41:101–8.
27. Vicini FA, Kestin LL, Martinez AA. The importance of adequate follow-up in defining treatment success after external beam irradiation for prostate cancer. Int J Radiat Oncol Biol Phys 1999;45:553–61.
28. Connell PP, Ignacio L, McBride RB, et al. Caution in interpreting biochemical control rates after treatment of prostate cancer: length of follow-up influences results. Urology 1999;54:875–9.
29. Roach M, Lu J, Pilepich MV, et al. Four prognostic groups predict long term survival from prostate cancer following radiotherapy alone on Radiation Therapy Oncology Group clinical trials. Int J Radiat Oncol Biol Phys 2000; 47:609–15.
30. Roach M, Weinberg V, McLaughlin P, Sander H. Death due to prostate cancer following radiotherapy (XRT) alone: defining candidates for early "salvage" trials. Proceedings of American Society of Clinical Oncology, San Francisco, May 2001;20:176a.
31. Stromberg J, Martinez A, Gonzalez J, et al. Ultrasound-guided high dose rate conformal brachytherapy boost in prostate cancer: treatment description and preliminary results of a phase I/II clinical trial. Int J Radiat Oncol Biol Phys 1995;33:161–71.
32. Mate TP, Gottesman JE, Hatton J, et al. High dose-rate afterloading 192Iridium prostate brachytherapy: feasibility report. Int J Radiat Oncol Biol Phys 1998;41:525–33.

16

External Beam Radiation Therapy

JOYCELYN L. SPEIGHT, MD, PhD
MACK ROACH III, MD

In 2002, an estimated 189,000 new cases of prostate cancer were diagnosed, leading to 30,200 deaths in American men.[a] The availability of widespread screening in the latter quarter of the twentieth century undoubtedly led to increases in diagnosis. External beam radiotherapy (EBRT) has been used for more than 30 years in the management of localized prostate cancer; however, the more recent increases in the use of radiotherapy as a primary management strategy probably result from long-term survival rates that appear to be equivalent to those achieved with radical prostatectomy when patients are matched by T stage and Gleason score (GS).[1–7] Several options exist for delivering EBRT, including three-dimensional conformal radiotherapy (3DCRT), "conventional" radiotherapy (non-3DCRT), intensity-modulated radiotherapy (IMRT), and proton and neutron beam irradiation. An in-depth discussion of the nuances of each of these last two external radiotherapy techniques is beyond the scope of this text; however, we highlight some of their pertinent features. Several excellent sources of information are available elsewhere.[7a-c]

Interstitial implantation of radioactive sources or brachytherapy is another very popular and efficacious management option for selected patients with localized prostate cancer. Several studies have suggested that low-risk patients (stage ≤ T2a, prostate-specific antigen [PSA] < 10 ng/mL, GS ≤ 6) treated with radioactive seed implantation have equivalent PSA control rates to patients treated with EBRT.[8–10] Biochemical control rates for intermediate- and high-risk patients (stage ≥ T2b, PSA ≥ 10 ng/mL, GS ≥ 7) have been reported in some studies to be higher when patients were treated with the addition of EBRT compared to implant alone.[10–12] A discussion of brachytherapy can be found in Chapter 17.

No clear consensus exists, either among physicians or patients, as to which treatment option is best. It is clear that certain patients may be better suited for one or another of these modalities. This may be true because not all patients have an equal risk of death owing to prostate cancer by virtue of differences in their age, pathologic stage of disease, and tumor histology (GS).[13] In the remainder of this chapter, we attempt to provide an overview of current techniques, uses, and treatment outcomes for the management of prostate adenocarcinoma with EBRT.

GENERAL PRINCIPLES OF RADIOTHERAPY

The initial active agents in therapeutic radiation treatments are packets of high energy x-rays or photons. The effects of EBRT on tumor cells (the "target") are mediated through the induction of unrepaired double-strand breaks in deoxyribonucleic acid (DNA), caused directly via electrons set in motion by photons or indirectly via free hydroxyl radicals, generated via electron disruption of water molecules.[14] High linear energy transfer radiation (heavy particles) primarily produce direct DNA damage. The expression of radiation damage is seen when the target cells enter mitosis and attempt to divide. Typically, tissues with low mitotic activity, such as the heart and spinal cord, exhibit radiation effects much later than cells with a high growth fraction, such as epithelial or tumor cells. In addition to this classic mechanism, radiation has also been shown to induce programmed cell death or apoptosis.[15] Normal tissues are also susceptible to radiation damage and are the dose-limiting structures in a radiotherapy treatment plan. Table 16–1 summarizes the classic tissue tolerance levels to radiation for normal tissues of interest during fractionated radiotherapy of prostate cancer.[16]

Historically, the unit of radiation dose was the rad, or radiation absorbed dose. The contemporary unit of measurement is the Gray (Gy). One Gy is equal to 100 rads. Standard fractionation refers to the delivery of single daily treatment fractions of 180 centigray (cGy; 1.8 Gy) or 200 cGy (2.0 Gy). Monotherapy radiation typically requires cumulative doses of at least 70 to 72 Gy for local control of gross prostate tumors. Prophylactic radiotherapy for presumed microscopic disease, such as might exist within lymph nodes, requires doses in the range of 45 to 50 Gy. A comprehensive discussion of radiobiology can be found in Chapter 15.

CONVENTIONAL VERSUS CONFORMAL EXTERNAL BEAM RADIOTHERAPY

Conventional EBRT (non-3DCRT), a technique popularized by Bagshaw and associates in the 1970s and 1980s for definitive treatment of prostate cancer, delivers the dose to the prostate gland using a small 6 × 6 to 8 × 8 cm "four-field box" or a whole-pelvis field, followed by a cone down boost to the prostate gland[17] (Figure 16–1A, and B). Custom blocking is not commonly used; instead, corner blocks are used to shape the treatment fields, which are based on bony anatomic landmarks. Dose distributions are calculated in one plane, with the dose prescribed to isocenter and normalized to an isodose line chosen by the physician. Treatment fields so designed, or based on the location of Foley catheter balloons or bladder and rectal contrast, result in inadequate coverage of the clinical target volume (CTV) in 20 to 40 percent of patients.[18–20] Large-size glands or cases of advanced disease necessitating coverage of the seminal vesicles were often partially treated when small fields were used. The use of whole-pelvis fields encompassed the target; however, more normal tissue (bladder or rectum) was unnecessarily irradiated. In addition to total dose and dose per fraction, the volume of normal tissue receiving radiation influences the probability of radiation-induced normal tissue injury.

Further compounding the problem of poor target delineation are inadequate radiation dose, inaccurate assessment of GS, and understaging, which may have contributed to high local failure rates reported at 10 and 15 years following conventional EBRT, even for patients predicted to have the lowest risk of relapse. Several studies have suggested a correlation between dose and local control, with tumor control probability increasing with increasing dose. Higher doses than those deliverable with non-3DCRT are necessary to overcome tumor cell resistance to radiation.[21–23] Non-3DCRT treatment plans are limited by normal tissue toxicity (bladder and rectum), vis à vis their inability to safely deliver doses above 70 Gy, mainly owing to inadequate treatment planning tools.

Advanced imaging modalities such as computed tomography (CT), used in conjunction with computer algorithms that allow accurate three-dimensional delineation of target volumes and rapid dose calculations at all points within the outlined tissue volumes, led to the development of three-dimensional treatment-planning systems (3DCRT). The first 3D CRT planning system received US Food and Drug Administration approval in the mid-1980s. Three-dimensional conformal radiotherapy uses a sophisticated image-based approach with more precise anatomic definition of the target and normal tissue volumes, which allows smaller treatment margins and delivery of higher radiation doses.[24] Multiple radiation beams focused on the target reduce the integral dose received

Table 16–1. WHOLE-ORGAN RADIATION TOLERANCE DOSES FOR FRACTIONATED RADIATION THERAPY

Organ	TD5/5* (cGy)	TD 5/50† (cGy)	Clinical End Point
Small intestine	5,000	6,000	Ulcer
Colon	5,500	6,500	Ulcer
Bladder	6,500	7,500	Ulcer
Urethra	6,500	8,000	Stricture
Rectum	6,000	8,000	Ulcer

Modified from Rubin P, Constine LS, Nelson DF.[16]
*The radiation dose associated with a 5% risk of occurrence of the clinical end point at 5 years.
†The radiation dose associated with a 50% risk of occurrence of the clinical end point at 5 years.

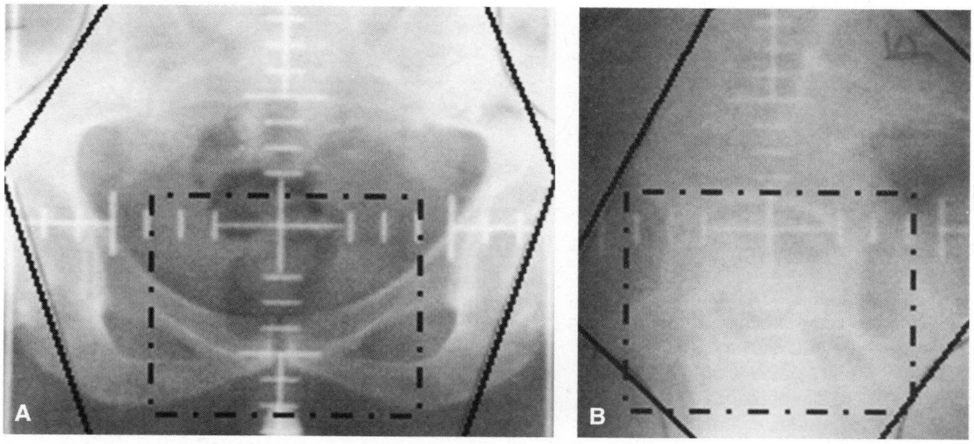

Figure 16–1. *A,* An anteroposterior and *B,* left lateral simulation film for a whole-pelvis treatment. The *heavy black lines* represent corner blocks that might typically be drawn. The *inset dashed line box* represents an 8 × 8 cm field. No blocking is used with smaller fields.

by surrounding normal tissue. Incident beam angles and the shape of the treatment field are designed using a beam's eye view (BEV—a vantage point from the radiation source looking out along the axis of the photon beam toward the CTV) (Figure 16–2). The use of multiple noncoplanar beams that conform to the shape of the target, allows for the use of smaller margins that include less of the adjacent normal tissues in the treatment field than is possible with non-3DCRT. The shape of the high-dose region of the dose distribution conforms to the contour of the CTV. The amount of normal tissue in the high-dose region is minimized, allowing the dose to the CTV to be increased while resulting in decreased acute and chronic toxicity.[25–33] Visual representations of the dose received by the target or normal tissue volumes, called dose volume histograms, aid in the quantitative and qualitative analysis of a three-dimensional treatment plan (Figure 16–3). Figure 16–4, A shows an example of a BEV of an anterior treatment field from a 3DCRT plan. Figure 16–4, B shows an example of a BEV of a left lateral treatment field from a 3DCRT plan. Figure 16–4, C shows coronal, sagittal, and axial views of a dose distribution obtained from a seven-field 3DCRT plan.

Owing to its advantages, 3DCRT is considered the "standard of care" for the management of prostate cancer when using EBRT. Despite this, as of the late 1990s, conformal radiotherapy techniques were currently used in only approximately 15 to 20 percent of radiotherapy centers (Jean Owen, Radiation Therapy Oncology Group [RTOG] headquarters, personal communication).

DOSE

Many of the technical problems associated with non-3DCRT radiotherapy have been resolved with conformal planning systems (Table 16–2). In addition to reduction in toxicity, conformal techniques have facilitated attempts to establish a dose response. An improvement in local control, PSA

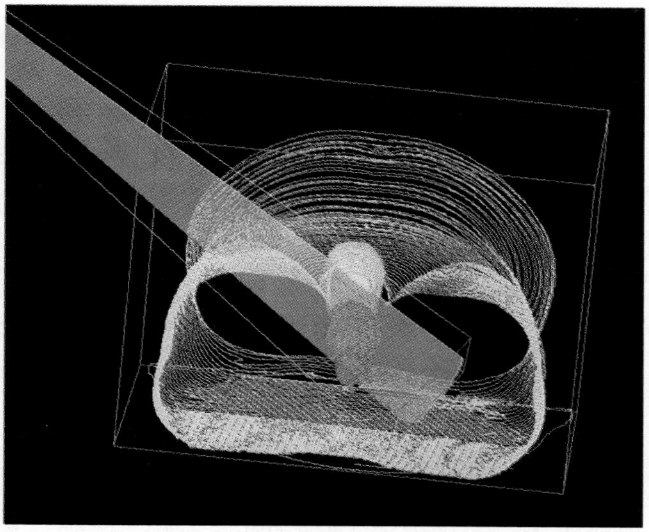

Figure 16–2. A room view of a three-dimensional treatment plan showing a right anterior oblique noncoplanar beam and the bladder (*yellow*), prostate gland (*purple*), and rectum (*brown*). These images are a computer-generated recontruction of the pelvic anatomy created from a computed tomographic scan.

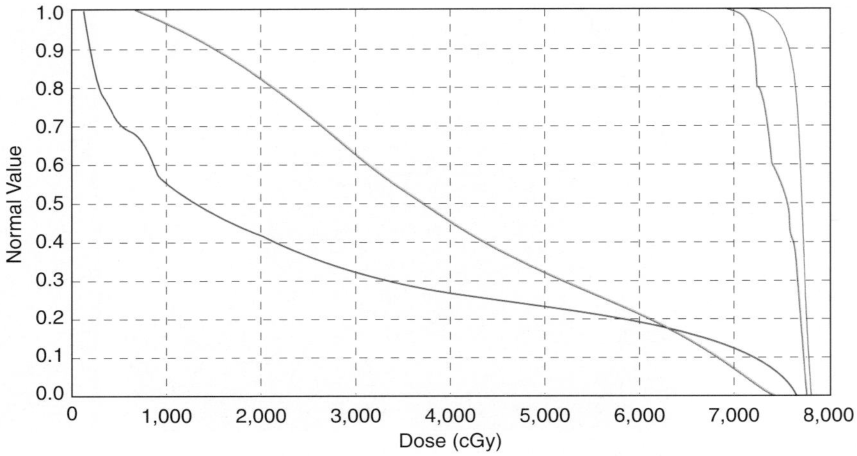

Figure 16–3. A dose volume histogram that incrementally quantifies the dose received by volume for the prostate (*pink line*), bladder (*blue line*), rectum (*green line*), and seminal vesicles (*red line*). In this plan, the prostate gland and the seminal vesicles are the clinical target volume; they both receive 100% of the prescription dose (7,200 cGy). Fifty percent of the bladder receives only 18% of the prescription dose (1,400 cGy) and 50% of the rectum receives approximately 3,600 cGy.

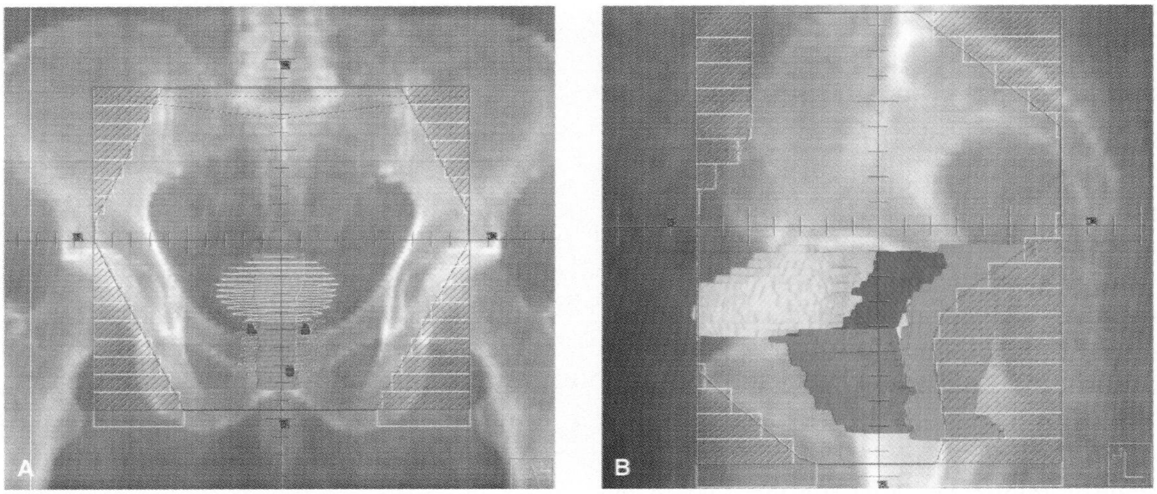

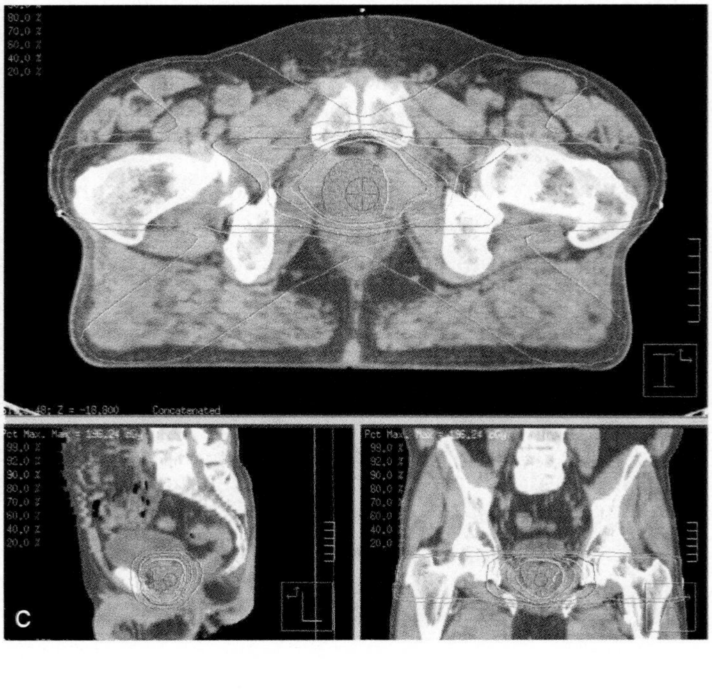

Figure 16–4. *A,* An example of a beam's eye view of an anterior treatment field with wire outline reconstruction of the prostate gland (*pink*) and bladder (*yellow*) and volume reconstruction of the rectum (*brown*). The *rectangles with hatched lines* indicate areas of beam blocking. The treatment field is the unblocked area in the center of the image. *B,* An example of a beam's eye view of a left lateral treatment field with volume reconstructions of the prostate gland (*pink*), seminal vesicles (*red*), bladder (*yellow*), and rectum (*brown*). The *rectangles with hatched lines* indicate areas of beam blocking. The treatment field is the unblocked area in the center of the image. *C,* Axial, sagittal, and coronal views of the dose distribution obtained from a seven-field conformal plan taken at the isocenter. The prostate gland is represented in pink. The prostate with margin is encompassed within the 92% isodose line (*blue*). Other isodose lines are shown (*the legend in the upper left corner*). In this plan, note the minimal amount of anterior rectal wall within the full-treatment dose region. In this plane, less than half of the rectum receives 50% of the prescribed dose and the femoral heads receive 40% of the prescribed dose.

Table 16–2. CONVENTIONAL VERSUS CONFORMAL RADIOTHERAPY AND POST-EBRT LOCAL FAILURE

Issue	Conventional (Non-3D) EBRT	Conformal (3D) EBRT	Benefit of 3D EBRT
Target definition	Inaccurate field size Incorrect field placement Larger margins Generic blocks (corner) Two to four coplanar fields or arcs	Field size and location based on CT reconstruction and BEV Fields conform to CTV Margins based on CTV Accurate, custom blocking Multiple noncoplanar fields	Accurate target definition; no marginal miss Less normal tissue radiated; decreased tissue toxicity Lower integral dose to normal tissues
Dose	Dose calculated in single plane Dose limited by technique and normal tissue tolerance	Dose calculated at all points/all planes High-dose region conforms to CTV Conformal plans	Higher treatment doses possible Less dose to normal tissue; decreased toxicity

EBRT = external beam radiotherapy; 3D = three-dimensional; CT = computed tomography; BEV = beam's eye view; CTV = clinical target volume.

response, freedom from PSA failure, and disease-free survival can be seen with increasing radiotherapy doses; however, the dose needed to achieve a maximal PSA response has yet to be defined[9,34–42] (Table 16–3). Only one randomized dose escalation trial has been completed, comparing the rate of biochemical control achieved with 70 versus 78 Gy. An initial report showed significant improvement in 4-year actuarial NED rates (no evidence of disease) for patients with pretreatment PSA > 10 ng/mL treated with 78 Gy.[43] However, with additional follow-up (median 51.98 months), no bNED (no evidence of disease by biochemical [PSA] failure) benefit was seen with the higher dose.[44]

The common theme of the results from the various studies is that higher doses than those deliverable with non-3DCRT are needed for biochemical control. Post-treatment biopsy data corroborate suboptimal tumor eradication with conventional radiotherapy doses.[45] The radiotherapy dose required for maximal

Table 16–3. RADIOTHERAPY DOSE RESPONSE/DOSE ESCALATION STUDIES

Institution (Lead Author, Year)	Groups	Comments
UCSF (Roach, 1996[36])	GS 8–10, PSA < 20 ng/mL	Doses > 71.5 Gy improved outcomes
MDAH (Pollack, 1997[38])	All groups, except PSA ≤ 4 ng/mL	Dose response better > 77 Gy
Fox Chase (Hanks, 1998[40])	Patients with PSA > 10 ng/mL	Doses > 76 Gy improved 5-year bNED
MSKCC (Zelefsky, 1998[9])	Intermediate- and high-risk patients	Doses ≥ 75.6 Gy improved local control
MDAH (Pollack, 1999[43])	Patients with PSA > 10 ng/mL	Dose = 77 Gy improved biochemical control
UCSF (Speight, 1999[37])	Essentially all lymph node risk groups	Doses ≥ 69 Gy improved freedom from PSA failure; no benefit to dose > 77 Gy Significantly improved PSA control for intermediate-risk patients with 3DCRT
UAB (Fiveash, 2000[97])	Stage T1–T2, Gleason score 8–10	Doses > 70 Gy yielded better results
Fox Chase (Hanks, 2000[81])	Unfavorable, PSA < 10 ng/mL, unfavorable PSA = 10–19.9 ng/mL, and favorable PSA > 20 ng/mL	Doses of 75–80 Gy yield improved 5-year bNED rates for unfavorable patients with PSA < 20 ng/mL and favorable patients with PSA levels > 20 ng/mL
CC (Kupelian, 2000[98])	Essentially all subgroups	Doses ≥ 72 Gy associated with improved biochemical and disease-free survival
MDAH (Pollack, 2000[44])	Stage T1–T2, PSA > 10 ng/mL	Doses > 67–77 Gy associated with improved biochemical control; no benefit to doses > 77 Gy
CAV (Bey, 2000[41])		Doses > 74 Gy yield higher probability of achieving PSA nadir ≤ 1 ng/mL
TJCC (Valicenti, 2000[23])	GS 8–10	Doses > 66 Gy improve DSS and OS

UCSF = University of California San Francisco; MDAH = M.D. Anderson Hospital; Fox Chase = Fox Chase Cancer Center; MSKCC = Memorial Sloan-Kettering Cancer Center; UAB = University of Alabama; CC = Cleveland Cinic; CAV = Centre Alexis Vautrin; TJCC = Thomas Jefferson Cancer Center; GS = Gleason score; PSA = prostate-specific antigen; bNED = no evidence of disease by biochemical (PSA) failure; DSS = disease-specific survival; OS = overall survival; 3DCRT = three-dimensional conformal radiotherapy; Gy = Gray.

PSA suppression will probably vary with risk as determined by pretreatment prognostic variables such as PSA, GS, and T stage. Once available, the results of RTOG 9406, a prospective randomized dose escalation trial, should help answer this question.

LOCAL CONTROL RATES FOLLOWING RADIOTHERAPY

Estimated rates of post-EBRT local control range from 70 to 90 percent.[17,46] These clinical assessments have tended to underestimate failure, primarily owing to the presence of occult disease. The reported rate of positive biopsies following radiotherapy treatment ranges from 21 to 93 percent in various series,[47–53] significant because post-treatment biopsy status at 24 to 36 months is an independent predictor of outcome.[45] Because of the potential morbidity of biopsies taken after high-dose EBRT, post-treatment PSA levels are accepted as a surrogate to assess treatment efficacy,[45,54,55] and an undetectable or low PSA nadir is considered a significant predictor of outcome.

However, two issues complicate the use of PSA as a measure of treatment efficacy. First, PSA has not been validated as a reliable predictor of overall or disease-specific survival. An additional problem has been the nonuniform definition of biochemical failure, which has influenced reported estimates of failure.[56–58] The current standard defines postradiotherapy biochemical failure as three consecutive increases in the PSA once the nadir has been reached. The time of failure is taken as the time point halfway between the first and second PSA rises.[59]

Given the long natural history of prostate cancer, another important end point to evaluate treatment success is disease-specific survival. Three analyses have reported the long-term outcome of EBRT alone in men with clinically localized prostate cancer treated in phase III RTOG trials.[5,23,60] Multivariate analysis showed that centrally reviewed GS, clinical stage, and pathologic lymph node status correlated with disease-specific survival and overall survival. Using these clinical features, four distinct prognostic subgroups were defined. Each group and their 5-, 10-, and 15-year disease-specific survival rates following radiotherapy are summarized in Table 16–4. These data provide a useful estimate of a patient's risk of death from prostate cancer over time, and a guide to the relative efficacy of EBRT alone.

ALTERNATIVE RADIOTHERAPY TECHNIQUES

Intensity-Modulated Radiation Therapy (IMRT)

The development of computer-driven optimization programs has allowed the development of the next "generation" of three-dimensional planning systems; IMRT. In general, two basic IMRT approaches exist: fixed fields delivered with a dynamic multileaf collimator ("step and shoot") or rotational fields delivered in a slice-by-slice manner (serial tomotherapy). Intensity-modulated radiation therapy can be "forward" or "backward" planned.

At its most sophisticated level (at this time), IMRT incorporates an inverse or "backwards" planning approach to generate nonuniform beam profiles, with varying radiation intensity across the photon beam (intensity modulation). As with 3DCRT, treatment planning commences with the delineation of the target and normal tissue volumes and definition of the dose to be delivered to the treatment volume. Unlike 3DCRT, the dose distribution is chosen

Table 16–4. DISEASE-SPECIFIC SURVIVAL BY RTOG RISK GROUP FOR TREATMENT WITH RADIOTHERAPY ALONE

RTOG Risk Group	No of Deaths/No. of Patients	5-Year DSS,* %	10-Year DSS,* %	15-Year DSS,* %
1	53/363	96 (94–98)	86 (82–90)	72 (62–83)
2	84/232	94 (92–97)	75 (70–81)	61 (51–72)
3	92/338	83 (79–87)	62 (55–70)	39 (26–60)
4	154/324	64 (58–70)	34 (27–42)	27 (20–37)

*95% confidence intervals in parentheses.
Group 1 = Gleason score (GS) 2–6 and T1–2Nx; Group 2 = GS 2–6, T3Nx or N+, or GS 7, T1–2Nx; Group 3 = GS 7, T3Nx, or N+, or GS 8–10, T1–2Nx; Group 4 = GS 8–10, T3Nx, or N; DSS = disease-specific survival; RTOG = Radiation Therapy Oncology Group.
Modified from Roach et al.[60]

ieve the spec-
ne constraints
interest, and
normal tissues (ie, bladder, rectum, bulb of the penis). Associated with each constraint is a "penalty" that characterizes the relative importance of each constraint and thus dose/volume limit. Once these parameters are defined, a complex composite plan, consisting of hundreds to thousands of small radiation beams or "beamlets" of different intensity and angles, is generated to deliver a homogeneous dose distribution to the treatment volume. The intensity profile of each beam can be iteratively adjusted, using the computer optimization algorithm, to satisfy the predetermined dose specifications. The use of IMRT can provide higher radiotherapy doses, often with more conformity, to the planning volume, without an increase in normal tissue toxicity.[61,62]

Particle Beam Radiotherapy

Particle beam radiation is an alternate form of EBRT. This type of radiotherapy uses heavy particles (neutrons or protons), with different physical characteristics than those of photons, that are believed to allow the delivery of higher dose equivalents of radiation.

Neutrons

Neutrons are uncharged, heavy atomic particles. The postulated benefit of neutron-based radiotherapy is their relative lack of oxygen dependence, which makes them better suited to killing hypoxic tumor cells, and resistance to the repair of sublethal radiation damage, which denotes a larger relative biologic effect on slow-growing tumors such as prostate cancer.[14] The RTOG conducted a randomized trial comparing treatment outcomes in patients treated with photons to those treated with photons and neutrons.[62] A statistically significant improvement in local control (58 versus 70%; $p = .04$) and overall survival (26 versus 46%; $p = .04$) was seen at 10 years. Another trial comparing photon to neutron therapy showed significantly better 10-year local control rates with the latter (53 versus 78%; $p = .0007$) but no difference in survival. Of note was the significant increase in grade 3 to 4 late gastrointestinal toxicity associated with neutron treatment.[63]

Protons

Protons are similar to neutrons except protons possess a positive charge. The hypothesized advantage of proton therapy is that protons deposit the majority of their energy at the end of their path length. A sharp drop-off in dose to nearly zero occurs beyond this point. This results in more conformal dose distributions since the high-dose area can be confined to the tumor volume, with limited dose going to adjacent tissues.[64] The results of a randomized trial from Massachusetts General Hospital (MGH) showed a significant improvement in local control but no difference in disease-free, relapse-free, or overall survival in patients with GS 7 to 10 tumors who were treated with mixed photon and proton beam irradiation compared with patients treated with photons alone. No benefit was seen in other groups of patients, and 5-year actuarial rates of rectal bleeding were significantly higher after mixed beam therapy ($p = .002$).[65,66] Investigators at Loma Linda University Medical Center reported 4-year bNED rates with mixed beam irradiation that were comparable to those for surgery and 3DCRT and lower toxicity rates than those seen in the MGH study.[67]

Summary

Retrospective and prospective studies support the efficacy of radiotherapy as a treatment for prostate cancer. Three-dimensional conformal radiotherapy is an appropriate treatment option for patients with prostate cancer who choose a nonsurgical option, as well as for those patients for whom surgery is not an optimal treatment. Conformal radiotherapy has measurable treatment benefits as compared to non-3DCRT techniques in terms of tumor control probability and diminished toxicity and should be considered the standard of care (see Table 16–2). The magnitude of the benefits in terms of disease control may vary with a patient's risk of death from prostate cancer. Some intermediate and virtually all high-risk patients have not fared well with any single-modality treatment. Adjunctive therapies such as hormone ablative therapy are probably required, as are discussed in the following section.

COMBINED MODALITY THERAPY

Hormone Therapy and External Beam Radiation Therapy

Since the demonstration of the responsiveness of prostate carcinoma to hormone deprivation,[68] androgen ablation has been used in the management of locally advanced and metastatic disease. The basis for combining hormone therapy with EBRT is derived from experimental and clinical data showing a reduction in the volume of hormone-sensitive tumor cells in vivo, cessation of cell division in vitro, and a decrease in the radiation dose required for cell killing both in vivo and in vitro.[69,70] These findings suggest a synergism between the effects of androgen deprivation and radiation therapy, which leads to increased local and regional cell killing.[69–71] Proposed mechanisms for these effects include reduction in cell clone number, induction of apoptosis, and shifting of cells into more radiosensitive phases of the cell cycle.

Several retrospective evaluations have been completed that compare some form of androgen deprivation given in conjunction with radiotherapy to radiotherapy alone for patients with clinically localized prostate cancer. Most have noted significant improvements in local control and disease-free survival; however, an overall survival benefit has not been consistently demonstrated. The effect of adjuvant and neoadjuvant hormone suppression has also been evaluated in prospective randomized trials (Table 16–5). Radiation Therapy Oncology Group protocol 8531 evaluated the effect of long-term goserelin monotherapy ("long-term" hormone therapy [LTHT]) started during the last week of radiotherapy or at the time of relapse. A significant improvement in local control and biochemical control and a decline in the rate of distant metastases were demonstrated for patients treated with early hormone ablation. A significant absolute and cause-specific survival advantage was seen for GS 8 to 10 patients treated with early hormone therapy (66 versus 55%; $p = .03$).[72–74] Radiation Therapy Oncoloy Group protocol 8610, which evaluated the use of 4 months of neoadjuvant and concurrent hormone ablation with goserelin and flutamide ("short-term" hormone therapy [STHT]), initially reported improvements only in local control, biochemical control, and distant metastasis-free survival at 5 years.[75] With longer follow-up, a significant improvement in absolute survival was seen for patients with GS 2 to 7 tumors (72 versus 52%, $p = .015$).[75] A Canadian

Table 16–5. RANDOMIZED TRIALS: RT + ANDROGEN ABLATION VERSUS RT ALONE

Lead Author (Year)	Arms	Comment
Pilepich[72] (1997) Pilepich[73] (2000)	RT + aHT vs RT alone (HT at relapse)	RTOG 8531: improved LC and bNED and decreased DM with aHT; improved OS and CSS for GS 8–10 patients
Pilepich[74] (1995) Pilepich[74,75] (2000)	naHT × 2 mo then HT + RT vs RT alone	RTOG 8610: improved LC, PFS, and lower DM with naHT at 5 yr; greatest OS benefit to GS 2–7 patients at 8 yr
Laverdiere[76] (1997)	naHT × 3 mo then RT vs naHT + RT then aHT × 6 mo vs RT alone	Decreased positive biopsy rates and median PSA at 12 mo with naHT; greatest benefit with LTHT
Bolla[77] (1997)	RT + HT × 1 mo then HT × 3 yr vs RT alone	EORTC 22863; improved LC, time to progression, DFS, and OS at 5 yr with HT
Granfors[78] (1998)	Orchiectomy + RT vs RT alone for pT1–4, N0–3, M0 patients	Improved CSS, DFS, and OS for orchiectomy + RT in node-positive patients
Hanks[99] (2000)	4 mo naHT/concurrent HT + RT with vs without 2 yr aHT	RTOG 9202: improved bNED, decreased DM rate DFS and OS with LTHT; increased DSS and OS for GS 8–10
Roach[80] (2001)	4 arms: 4 mo naHT/concurrent HT + RT vs RT then aHT × 4 mo and WRPT vs PORT	RTOG 9413: no benefit to aHRT with WPRT or PORT or to naHT with PORT; improved local control with naHT with WPRT at 5 yr

RT = external beam radiotherapy; aHT = adjuvant hormone therapy; HT = hormone therapy; RTOG = Radiation Therapy Oncology Group; LC = local control; bNED = no evidence of disease by biochemical (PSA) failure; DM = distant metastases; OS = overall survival; CSS = cause-specific survival; GS = Gleason score; naHT = neoadjuvant hormone therapy; PFS = progression-free survival; PSA = prostate-specific antigen; LTHT = long-term hormone therapy; EORTC = European Organization for Research and Treatment of Cancer; DFS = disease-free survival; WPRT = whole-pelvis radiotherapy; PORT = prostate-only radiotherapy.

trial reported a 65% incidence of positive biopsies at 2 years post-treatment following radiotherapy alone compared with a 28 percent positive biopsy rate when 3 months of neoadjuvant hormonal therapy was given prior to radiotherapy. More impressive still was the 5 percent lower incidence of positive biopsies when hormonal ablation therapy was continued following the completion of radiotherapy, for a total of 10 months.[76] The European Organization for Research and Treatment of Cancer (EORTC) trial demonstrated that 1 month of neoadjuvant androgen blockade prior to radiotherapy followed by 3 years of adjuvant hormone blockade yielded statistically significant improvements in local control, disease-free survival, and overall survival at 5 years[77] compared with patients treated with radiotherapy alone.

Androgen ablation also benefits lymph node–positive patients. A Swedish study randomized surgically staged patients (pT1–4,N0–3,M0) to EBRT plus orchiectomy or EBRT alone. At a median follow-up of 9.3 years, disease-free (69 versus 39%) and cause-specific survival (73 versus 56%) were higher in the combined therapy group. When stratified by nodal status, no survival benefit was seen in node-negative patients.[78] Subset analysis of node-positive patients treated on RTOG 8531 also showed improved bNED (no biochemical evidence of disease). Control rates and freedom from metastatic progression with adjuvant hormone ablation; no differences in disease-specific survival or overall survival were noted.[79]

The RTOG has systematically evaluated the strategy of androgen blockade in conjunction with EBRT, and the benefit of LTHT in locally advanced disease has been convincingly demonstrated. A more recent area of investigation is evaluating the potential role of hormone manipulation in low-risk (T1–2, PSA $\leq$ 10 ng/mL, GS $\leq$ 6 or lymph node risk < 15%) and intermediate-risk (T1–2, PSA $\leq$ 10 ng/mL, GS > 6 or PSA > 10 ng/mL, PSA $\leq$ 6 or T3, PSA $\leq$ 10 ng/mL, GS $\leq$ 6 or lymph node risk $\geq$ 15%) prostate cancer. A meta-analysis of earlier RTOG hormone plus radiotherapy trials suggested that patients with large-volume (5×5 cm^3), GS 2 to 6 tumors benefited in terms of local control and overall survival from STHT. This finding was subsequently corroborated by the 8-year report from RTOG 8610.[73] An on going trial, RTOG 9408, which evaluates STHT in well-differentiated (GS 2 to 6) tumors, will provide additional information.

Radiation Therapy Oncology Group protocol 9413, which addresses short-term androgen ablation in intermediate-risk tumors, has been published in abstract form. This four-arm randomized prospective trial evaluates the effect of 4 months of neoadjuvant versus 4 months of adjuvant hormone ablation (STHT) on patients with intermediate-risk prostate cancer as defined by an estimated risk of lymph node involvement of greater than 15 percent based on GS and PSA. The effect of whole-pelvis radiation therapy (WPRT) versus prostate-only radiation therapy (PORT) was also evaluated.[80] Preliminary analysis demonstrated that patients treated with neoadjuvant STHT experienced a higher 4-year progression-free survival than patients treated with adjuvant STHT. Patients treated with WPRT had a significantly improved progression-free survival than patients treated with PORT (56 versus 46%; $p = .014$). When all four arms were compared, patients treated with neoadjuvant hormone ablation and WPRT had a highly significant advantage for progresson-free survival over all other treatment groups (61 versus 45, 49, and 47%; $p = .005$). No significant overall survival difference was reported at a median follow-up of 59.3 months. Longer follow-up is anxiously awaited to confirm these results and also to determine if a survival advantage becomes evident, as has occurred with previous trials.

Hormone Summary

Neoadjuvant and adjuvant hormone suppression combined with radiotherapy improves local control, prolongs disease-free survival, delays the time to the development of metastatic disease, and prolongs cause-specific survival and overall survival in some patient subsets (see Table 16–5). The data are sufficiently compelling, and it is common practice to recommend long-term hormone ablation for patients who have a high risk for biochemical failure. Based on the meta-analysis of RTOG trials and RTOG 9413, short-term hormone suppression may see more widespread use in intermediate-risk patients in conjunction with whole-pelvis radiation.[60,72–74,76,77,80,81]

Treatment Toxicity

Treatment-related toxicity can occur during and/or after EBRT and is classified as early (acute) or late (chronic). Total dose, dose per fraction, and the volume of normal tissue irradiated influence the probability of radiation-induced injury, as do preexisting comorbid conditions such as inflammatory bowel disease, previous treatment with chemotherapy, or previous urologic surgery. Complications that occur in the course of the treatment for prostate cancer primarily affect the intestinal tract, the genitourinary tract, and sexual function. Treatment sequelae in each of these areas has an influence on quality of life.

The severity of intestinal sequelae is directly related to the volume of bowel within the treatment field. In RTOG trials using non-3DCRT methods, side effects were noted in 0.4 to 1.6 percent of patients. Diarrhea and proctitis are easily controlled with antidiarrheal medicines or dietary modification. Chronic injury including persistent diarrhea, rectal hypermotility and cramping, rectal ulceration or bleeding, stricture, and bowel obstruction or perforation were reported in 0.4 to 1.7 percent of patients after non-3DCRT. Urinary irritability is probably the most frequently reported side effect during therapy. Most patients experience temporary, acute urinary symptoms during radiation treatment including frequency, nocturia, and dysuria. Urinary incontinence is uncommon and appears to be related to prior transurethral resection of the prostate procedures.[82,83]

Erectile dysfunction or impotence is perhaps the most worrisome side effect of radiotherapy, with post-treatment erectile dysfunction reported by 30 to 50 percent of men who were potent prior to treatment.[84–87] Several confounding variables appear to influence the likelihood of potency preservation including age, comorbid vascular disease (ie, diabetes, hypertension), and pre-existing erectile dysfunction,[85,88] as do treatment technique and dose[89–95] and androgen ablation therapy.[9,96] The multitude of confounding variables makes the accurate assessment of post-EBRT potency extremely difficult.

CONCLUSION

The management of prostate cancer continues to evolve, within each modality and between modalities, and some patients will be better treated with combined therapy. Points of controversy have shifted somewhat to include not only who needs to be treated but also what the treatment should be. Prospective randomized trials will continue to play a pivotal role in resolving these controversies and should be actively supported. Furthermore, several novel therapies including vaccines, immunotherapy, and growth receptor inhibitors loom on the horizon and may assume greater importance, particularly in the management of minimal or recurrent disease.

Radiotherapy, in its various forms, remains a mainstay in the treatment of patients with prostate cancer, as does androgen ablation for selected patients. New technology has significantly improved radiotherapy treatments, yet there remains room for further development, not only in the arena of more sophisticated technology but also in the expansion of the use of 3DCRT techniques beyond the 10 to 20 percent of centers where it is currently the standard. What is evident is that all prostate cancer is not equal. Treatment plans need to be individualized and evidence based, and, ultimately, the most appropriate therapy will probably be dictated by a combination of clinical variables, including the GS, the PSA, the number of positive biopsies, and perhaps other, as yet unidentified factors.

REFERENCES

a. A cancer journal for clinicians. American Cancer Society. 2001;51:35–75

1. Hanks GE, Buzydlowski, JW, Perez CA, et al. The 10-year outcome of pathologic and imaging node positive patients treated with irradiation in Radiation Therapy Oncology Group (RTOG)-7506. J Urol 1996;155 Suppl:611A.
2. Iselin CE, Robertson JE, Paulson. Radical prostatectomy: oncological outcome during a 20 year period. J Urol 1999; 161:163–8.
3. Jacobson SJ, Bergstrahl EJ, Zincke H, et al. Population based study of comorbidity and survival following a diagnosis of prostate cancer. J Urol 1996;155 Suppl:324A.
4. Lu J, Yao G, Yao, SL. Population based study of long-term survival in patients with clinically localized prostate cancer. Lancet 1997;349:9906–18.
5. Roach M, Lu J, Pilepich MV, et al. Long-term survival years after radiotherapy alone: RTOG prostate cancer trials. J Urol 1999;161,
6. Pound CR, Partin AW, Epstein JI, et al. PSA following anatomical radical retropubic prostatectomy: an interim report. Urol Clin North Am 1997;24:395–406.
7. Hanks GE, Hanlon AL, Schultheiss TE, et al. Conformal external beam treatment of prostate cancer. Urology 1997; 50:87–92.

7a. Laramore GE, Krall JM, Thomas FJ, et al. Fast neutron radiotherapy for locally advanced prostate cancer. Final report of a Radiation therapy Oncology Group randomized clinical trial. Am J Clin Oncol 1993;16:164-7.

7b. Slater JD, Yonemoto LT, Rossi CJ Jr, et al. Conformal proton therapy for prostate carcinoma. Int J Radiat Oncol Biol Phys 1998;42:299-304.

7c. De Meerleer GO, Vakaet L, Dr Gersem W, et al. Radiotherapy of prostate cancer with or without intensity modulated beams: a planning comparison. Int J Radiat Oncol Biol Phys 2000;47:639-48.

8. Zelefsky MJ, Hollister T, Raben A. Five-year biochemical outcome and toxicity with transperineal CT-planned permanent I-125 implantation for patients with localized prostate cancer. Int J Radiat Oncol Biol Phys 2000;47:1261–6.

9. Zelefsky MJ, Leibel SA, Gaudin PB, et al. Dose escalation with three-dimensional conformal radiation therapy affects the outcome in prostate cancer. Int J Radiat Oncol Biol Phys 1998;41:491–500.

10. Brachman DG, Thomas T, Hilbe J, et al. Failure free survival following brachytherapy alone or external beam irradiation alone for T1-2 prostate tumors in 2227 patients: results from a single practice. Int J Radiat Oncol Biol Phys 2000;48:111–7.

11. D'Amico AV, Schultz D, Loffredo M. Biochemical outcome following external beam radiation therapy with or without androgen suppression therapy for clinically localized prostate cancer. JAMA 2000;284:1280–3.

12. Grado GL, Larson TR, Balch, et al. Actuarial disease-free after prostate cancer brachytherapy using interactive techniques with biplane ultrasound and fluoroscopic guidance. Int J Radiat Oncol Biol Phys 1998;42:289–98.

13. Albertsen PC, Hanley JA, Gleason DF, et al. Competing risk analysis of men aged 55-74 years at diagnosis managed conservatively for clinically localized prostate cancer. JAMA 1998;280:975–80.

14. Hall E. Radiobiology for the radiologist. 5th ed. Lippincott Williams and Wilkins; 2000.

15. Allan DJ. Radiation induced apoptosis: its role in a MANcaT (mitosis-apoptosis-differentiation-calcium-toxicity) scheme of cytotoxicity mechanisms. Int J Radiat Oncol Biol Phys 1992; :145.

16. Rubin P, Constine LS, Williams JP. Late effects of cancer treatment: radiation and drug toxicity. In: Perez CA, Brady LW, editors. Principles and practice of radiation oncology. 3rd ed. Lippincott-Raven; 1998.

17. Bagshaw MA, Cox RS, Ray GR. Status of prostate cancer at Stanford University. Monogr Natl Cancer Inst 1998;7:47.

18. Ten Haken RK, et al. Boost treatment of the prostate using shaped, fixed fields. Int J Radiat Oncol Biol Phys 1989; 6:193.

19. Ten Haken RK, et al. Treatment planning issues related to prostate movement in response to differential filling of the rectum and bladder. Int J Radiat Oncol Biol Phys 1991; 20:1317.

20. Roach M, et al. The role of the urethrogram during simulation for localized prostate cancer. Int J Radiat Oncol Biol Phys 1993;25:299.

21. Malaise EP, Deschavanne PJ, Malaise B. The relationship between potentially lethal damage repair and intrinsic radiosensitivity of human cells. Int J Radiat Oncol Biol Phys 1989;56:597–604.

22. Porter EH. The statistics of dose/cure relationships for irradiated tumours. Part II. Br J Radiol 1980;53:336–45.

23. Valecenti R, Lu J, Pilepich MV, et al. Survival advantage from higher-dose radiation therapy for clinically localized prostate cancer treated on the Radiation Therapy Oncology Group. J Clin Oncol 2000;18:2740–6.

24. Roach M, Pickett B, Phillips TL. An analysis of the advantages as well as the physical and clinical limitations of three-dimensionally (3D) based co-planar conformal external beam irradiation (XRT) in the treatment of localized prostate cancer. In: Minet P, editor. Three-dimensional treatment planning. Liege; 1993.

25. Dearnaley DP, Khoo VS, Norman A, et al. Reduction of radiation proctitis by conformal radiotherapy techniques in prostate cancer: a randomized trial. Lancet 1999;353:267.

26. Koper PCM, Stroom JC, Van Putten WLJ, et al. Acute morbidity reduction using 3DCRT for prostate carcinoma: a randomized study. Int J Radiat Oncol Biol Phys 1999;43: 727–34.

27. Nguyen LN, Pollack A, Zagars GK. Late effects after radiotherapy for prostate cancer in a randomized dose-response study: results of a self-assessment. Urology 1998;51:991.

28. Tait DM, Nahum AE, Meyer LC, et al. Acute toxicity in pelvic radiotherapy: a randomized trial of conformal versus conventional treatment. Radiother Oncol 1997;42:121–36.

29. Schultheiss. Late GI and GU complications in the treatment of prostate cancer. Int J Radiat Oncol Biol Phys 1997;37:3–11.

30. Michaelski JM, et al. Preliminary report of toxicity following 3D radiation therapy for prostate cancer on 3DOG/RTOG 9406. Proceedings of the American Society for Therapeutic Radiology and Oncology 40th annual meeting. Int J Radiat Oncol Biol Phys 1998;42 Suppl:142.

31. Roach M, et al. Treatment of 100 consecutive patients by using six-field conformal radiation therapy: acute and short term toxicity. Radiology 1993;189 Suppl:183.

32. Michalski JM, Purdy JA, Winter K, et al. Preliminary report of toxicity following 3D radiation for prostate cancer on 3DOG/RTOG 9406. Int J Radiat Oncol Biol Phys 2000; 46:391–402.

33. Michalski JM, Winter K, Purdy JA, et al. Update of toxicity following 3D radiation for prostate cancer on RTOG 9406. Int J Radiat Oncol Biol Phys 2000;48(3 Suppl):228.

34. Hanks GH, et al. Conformal technique dose escalation for prostate cancer: biochemical evidence improved cancer control with higher doses in patients with pretreatment prostate specific antigen < 10 ng/ml. Int J Radiat Oncol Biol Phys 1996;35:861.

35. Hanks GH, et al. Dose escalation in the conformal treatment of prostate cancer: optimization is made possible by understanding the dose responses for control of cancer and late morbidity. Int J Radiat Oncol Biol Phys 1996;36 Suppl 1:99.

36. Roach M, et al. Radiotherapy for high grade clinically localized adenocarcinoma of the prostate. J Urol 1996;156: 1719–23.

37. Speight JL, Weinberg VK, McLaughlin PW, et al. 3D conformal radiotherapy improves PSA failure rates or intermediate risk patients at conventional doses. In: Cox J, editor. Proceedings of the American Society for Therapeutic Radiology and Oncology. San Antonio, TX, 1999. p. 346.

38. Pollack A, Zagars GK. External beam radiotherapy dose response of prostate cancer. Int J Radiat Oncol Biol Phys 1997;39:1011–18.
39. Zelefsky MJ, Leibel SA, Kutcher GK, et al. The feasibility of dose escalation with three-dimensional conformal radiotherapy in patients with prostatic carcinoma. Cancer J Sci Am 1995;1:142–50.
40. Hanks GE, Hanlon AL, Schultheiss TE, et al. Dose escalation with 3D conformal treatment: five years outcomes, treatment optimization, and future directions Int J Radiat Oncol Biol Phys 1998;41:501–10.
41. Bey P, Carrie C, Beckendorf V, et al. Dose escalation with 3DCRT in prostate cancer: French study of dose escalation with conformal 3D radiotherapy I prostate cancer—preliminary analysis. Int J Radiat Oncol Biol Phys 2000;48: 513–7.
42. Pinover WH, Hanlon AL, Horwitz et al. Defining the appropriate radiation dose for pretreatment PSA ≤ 10 ng/ml prostate cancer. Int J Radiat Oncol Biol Phys 2000;47: 649–54.
43. Pollack A, Zagars GK, Smith LG, et al. Preliminary results of a randomized dose—escalation study comparing 70 Gy to 78 Gy for the treatment of prostate cancer. Int J Radiat Oncol Biol Phys 1999;45 3 Suppl:146.
44. Pollack A, Smith LG, Von Eschenbach AC. External beam radiotherapy dose response characteristics of 1127 men with prostate cancer treated in the PSA era. Int J Radiat Oncol Biol Phys 2000;48:507–12.
45. Crooks J, Malone S, Perry G, et al. Postradiotherapy biopsies: what do they really mean? Results for 498 patients. Int J Radiat Oncol Biol Phys 2000;48:355–67.
46. Hanks GE, Martz KL, Diamond J. The effect of dose on local control of prostate cancer Int J Radiat Oncol Biol Phys 1988;5:1299.
47. Crooks J, Robertson S, Collin G, et al. Clinical relevance of trans-rectal ultrasound, biopsy and serum prostate specific antigen following external beam radiotherapy for carcinoma of the prostate. Int J Radiat Oncol Biol Phys 1993; 27:31–7.
48. Babain RJ, Kojima M, Saitoh M, et al. Detection of residual prostate cancer after external radiotherapy. Cancer 1995; 75:2153–8.
49. Miller EB, Ladaga LE, El-Mahdi AM, et al. Reevaluation of prostate biopsy after definitive radiation therapy: frequency and prognostic significance of positive results of post-irradiation biopsy after definitive radiation therapy. Urology 1993;41:311–6.
50. Scardino PT. The prognostic significance of biopsies after radiotherapy for prostatic cancer. Semin Urol 1983;1: 243–52.
51. Scardino PT, Wheeler TM. Local control of prostate cancer with radiotherapy: frequency and prognostic significance positive results of post-irradiation biopsy. Monogr Natl Cancer Inst 1988;7:95–103.
52. Schelhammer PF, El-Mahdi AM, Higgins EM, et al. Prostate biopsy after definitive treatment by interstitial 125-iodine implant or external beam radiation therapy. J Urol 1987; 137:897–901.
53. Kuban DA, El-Mahdi AM, Schelhammer PF. The significance of post-irradiation prostate biopsies with long term follow up. Int J Radiat Oncol Biol Phys 1992;24:409–14.
54. Shipley WU, Thames H, Sandler HM, et al. Radiation therapy for clinically localized prostate cancer: a multi-institutional pooled analysis. JAMA 1999;218:1598–604.
55. Hanlon A, Hanks GE. Scrutiny of the ASTRO consensus definition of biochemical failure in irradiated prostate cancer patients demonstrates its usefulness and robustness. Int J Radiat Oncol Biol Phys 2000;46:559–566.
56. Horowitz E, Vicini F, Ziaja E, et al. Assessing the variability of outcome for patients treated with localized prostate irradiation using different definitions of biochemical control. Int J Radiat Oncol Biol Phys 1996;36:565–71.
57. Vicini F, Kestin LL, Martinez FA. The importance of adequate follow-up in defining treatment success after external beam irradiation for prostate cancer. Int J Radiat Oncol Biol Phys 1999;45:553–61.
58. Horowitz EH, Vicini FA, Ziaja EM. The correlation between the ASTRO Consensus Panel definition of biochemical failure and clinical outcome for patients with prostate cancer treated with external beam irradiation. American Society of Therapeutic Radiology and Oncology. Int J Radiat Oncol Biol Phys 1998;41:267–72.
59. American Society for Therapeutic Radiology and Oncology Consensus Panel. Consensus statement: guidelines for PSA following radiotherapy. Int J Radiat Oncol Biol Phys 1997;37:1035–41.
60. Roach M, Lu J, Pilepich MV. Four prognostic subgroups predict long-term survival from prostate cancer following radiotherapy alone on Radiation Therapy Oncology Group trials. Int J Radiat Oncol Biol Phys 2000;47:609–15.
61. Shu HKG, Lee TT, Vigneault, et al. Toxicity following high dose three-dimensional radiation therapy and intensity modulated radiation therapy for clinically localized prostate cancer. Urology 2001;57:102–7.
62. Pirzkall A, Carol M, Lohr F, et al. Comparison of intensity-modulated radiotherapy with conventional conformal radiotherapy for complex-shaped tumors. Int J Radiat Oncol Biol Phys 2000;48:1371-80.
63. Forman JD, Duclos M, Sharma R, et al. Conformal mixed neutron and photon irradiation in localized and locally advanced prostate cancer: preliminary estimate of the therapeutic ratio. Int J Radiat Oncol Biol Phys 1995;35:259–66.
64. Lee M, et al. A comparison of proton and megavoltage x-ray treatment planning for prostate cancer. Radiother Oncol 1984;33:239.
65. Shipley WU, Verhey LJ, Munzenrider JE, et al. Advanced prostate cancer: the results of a randomized comparative trial of high dose irradiation boosting with conformal protons compared with conventional dose irradiation using photons alone. Int J Radiat Oncol Biol Phys 1995;32:3–12.
66. Slater JD, Yonemoto LT, Rossi CJ Jr, et al. Conformal proton therapy for prostate carcinoma. Int J Radiat Oncol Biol Phys 1998;42:299–304.
67. Rossi CJ, et al. Particle beam radiation therapy in prostate cancer: is there an advantage? Semin Radiat Oncol 1998; 8:115.
68. Huggins C, Hodges CV. Studies of prostate cancer: I. The effects of castration, of estrogen and of androgen injection on serum phosphatases in metastatic carcinoma of the prostate. Cancer Res 1941;1:293–7.
69. Sklar G. Combined anti-tumor effect of suramin plus irradiation I prostate cancer cells: the role of apoptosis. J Urol 1993;150:1526–32.

70. Zeitman AL, Nakfoor BM, Prince EA, et al. The effect of androgen deprivation and radiation therapy on an androgen-sensitive murine tumor: an in vitro and in vivo study. Cancer J Sci Am 1997;3:31–6.
71. Widmark A, Damber JE, Berg A, et al. Estramustine potentiates the effects of irradiation on the Dunning (R3327) rat prostatic adenocarcinoma. Prostate 1994;24:73–83.
72. Pilepich MV, Caplan R, Byhardt RW, et al. Phase III trial of androgen suppression using goserelin in unfavorable prognosis carcinoma of the prostate treated with definitive radiotherapy: report of Radiation Therapy Oncology Group Protocol 85-31. J Clin Oncol 1997;15:1013–21.
73. Pilepich MV, Winter K, Byhardt RW, et al. Androgen ablation adjuvant to definitive radiotherapy in carcinoma of the prostate: year 2000 update of RTOG phase III studies 8610 and 8531. Int J Radiat Oncol Biol Phys 2000:114.
74. Pilepich MV, Sause WT, Shipley WU, et al. Androgen deprivation with radiation therapy compared with radiation therapy alone for locally advanced prostatic carcinoma: a randomized comparative trial of the Radiation Therapy Oncology Group. Urology 1995;45:616–23.
75. Pilepich MV, Winter K, Roach M, et al. Phase III Radiation Therapy Oncology Group (RTOG) trial 86-10 of androgen deprivation before and during radiotherapy in locally advanced carcinoma of the prostate. Int J Radiat Oncol Biol Phys 1998;42:177.
76. Laverdiere J, Gomez JL, Cusan L, et al. Beneficial effect of combination hormonal therapy administered prior and following external beam irradiation therapy in localized prostate cancer. Int J Radiat Oncol Biol Phys 1997;37: 247–52.
77. Bolla M, Gonzalez D, Warde P, et al. Improved survival in patients with locally advanced prostate cancer treated with radiotherapy and goserelin. N Engl J Med 1997;337: 295–300.
78. Granfors T, Modig H, Damber JE, et al. Combined orchiectomy and external beam radiotherapy versus radiotherapy alone for non-metastatic prostate cancer with or without pelvic lymph node involvement: a prospective randomized study. J Urol 1998;159:2030–4.
79. Lawton CA, Winter K, Byhardt R, et al. Androgen suppression plus radiation vs. radiation alone for patients with D1 (pN+) adenocarcinoma of the prostate (results based on a national prospective randomized trial RTOG 85-31). Int J Radiat Oncol Biol Phys 1997;38:931–9.
80. Roach M, Lu JD, Lawton C, et al. A phase III trial comparing whole pelvic (WP) to prostate only (PO) radiotherapy and neoadjuvant to adjuvant total androgen suppression (TAS). Preliminary analysis of RTOG 9413. 2001;51 Suppl 1:3.
81. Hanks GE, Hanlon AL, Pinover WH, et al. Dose selection for prostate cancer patients based on dose comparison and dose response studies. Int J Radiat Oncol Biol Phys 2000; 46:823–32.
82. Lawton CA. Long-term treatment sequelae following external beam irradiation for adenocarcinoma of the prostate: analysis of RTOG studies 7506 and 7706. Int J Radiat Oncol Biol Phys 1991;21:935–9.
83. Lawton CA, et al. Evaluation of significant late morbidity from external beam irradiation for adenocarcinoma of the prostate (analysis from RTOG studies 7506 and 7706 [abstract]). Proceedings of the 32nd Annual ASTRO Meeting. Int J Radiat Oncol Biol Phys 1997;19 Suppl 1:1190.
84. Chinn D, Holland J, Crownover R, et al. Potency following high dose three-dimensional conformal radiotherapy and the impact of prior major urologic surgical procedures in the patients treated for prostate cancer. Int J Radiat Oncol Biol Phys 1995;33:15–22.
85. Mantz CA, Song P, Farhabgi E, et al. Potency probability following conformal megavoltage radiotherapy using conventional doses for localized prostate cancer. Int J Radiat Oncol Biol Phys 1997;37:551–7.
86. Lilleby W, Fossa S, Waehre H, et al. Long-term morbidity and quality of life in patients with localized prostate cancer undergoing definitive radiotherapy or radical prostatectomy. Int J Radiat Oncol Biol Phys 1999;43:735–43.
87. Litwin MS, Flanders SC, Pasta DJ, et al. Sexual function and bother after radical prostatectomy or radiation for prostate cancer: multivariate quality of life analysis from CaPSURE. Urology 1999;54:503–8.
88. Zelefsky MJ, Eid JF. Elucidating the etiology of erectile dysfunction after definitive therapy for prostate cancer. Int J Radiat Oncol Biol Phys 1998;40:129–33.
89. Vijayakumar S, Myrianthopoulis LC, Dabrowski J, et al. In the radiotherapy of prostate cancer, technique determines the doses to penile structures. Br J Radiol 1999;72:882–8.
90. Weil MD, Crawford ED, Cornish P, et al. Minimal toxicity with 3-FAT radiotherapy of prostate cancer. Semin Urol Oncol 2000;18:127–132.
91. Weil MD, Pickett B, Kuerth S, et al. A three field arc technique (3-FAT) for treating prostate cancer. Int J Radiat Oncol Biol Phys 1998;40:733–8.
92. Zelefsky MJ, Wallner KE, Ling CC, et al. Comparison of the 5-year outcome and morbidity of three-dimensional conformal radiotherapy versus transperineal permanent iodine-125 implantation for early stage prostate cancer. J Clin Oncol 1999;17:517–22.
93. Beard CJ, Propert KJ, et al. Complications after treatment with external beam irradiation in early-stage prostate cancer patients: a prospective multi-institutional outcomes study. J Clin Oncol 1997;15:223–9.
94. Beard CJ, Lamb C, et al. Radiation associated morbidity in patients undergoing small-field external beam irradiation for prostate cancer. Int J Radiat Oncol Biol Phys 1998;41:257–62.
95. Pickett B, Fisch BM, Weinberg VK, et al. Dose to the bulb of the penis is associated with the risk of impotence following radiotherapy for prostate cancer. Int J Radiat Oncol Biol Phys 1997;35(3 Suppl):1011.
96.
97. Fiveash JB, Hanks GE, Roach MR, et al. 3D conformal radiation therapy (3DCRT) for high-grade prostate cancer: a multi-institutional review. Int J Radiat Oncol Biol Phys 2000;47:335–342.
98. Kupelian PA, Mohan DS, Lyons J, et al. Higher than standard radiation doses ($\geq$ 72 Gy) with or without androgen deprivation in the treatment of localized prostate cancer. Int J Radiat Oncol Biol Phys 2000;46:567–74.
99. Hanks GE, Lu JD, Machtay M, et al. RTOG protocol 92-02: a phase III trial of the use of long term total androgen suppression following neoadjuvant hormonal cytoreduction in locally advanced carcinoma of the prostate. Int J Radiat Oncol Biol Phys 2000;48 Suppl 1:112.

17

Brachytherapy

I-CHOW HSU, MD
MACK ROACH III, MD

The term brachytherapy is derived from the Greek root "brachy," which means short distance. Brachytherapy refers to techniques of delivering radiation by placing radioactive sources (usually in the form of seeds or wires) in close proximity to or directly into the tumor. Shortly following the discovery of radium in 1898, brachytherapy became an important part of cancer therapy. Effective chemotherapy and surgical techniques were in their infancy when brachytherapy established a track record for the treatment of a variety of tumor types.

Brachytherapy is generally reserved for well-defined lesions that can be accessed by direct visualization or with assistance using sophisticated imaging (ultrasonography, computed tomography [CT], or magnetic resonance imaging [MRI]). The unique physical advantages associated with the use of brachytherapy result from the fact that the radioactive sources are located within the treatment volume; thus, the amount of normal tissue the radiation has to travel through to reach its target is minimized. Deep-seated tumors can be treated without radiating the skin or other dose-limiting organs. The second advantage is attributable to the "inverse square" law. The intensity of the radiation decreases proportionally to the inverse of the square of the distance between the source and the target. Because of this exponential attenuation of radiation intensity, the dose decreases at a much greater rate near the radioactive source. This intrinsic dose heterogeneity can be a double-edged sword. If the sources are properly placed, very high doses can be delivered to the tumor, and a minimum dose is given to the normal structures located near the tumor, the opposite is true if a source(s) is improperly placed. Understanding this principle is the key to successful application of brachytherapy.

The application of brachytherapy to treat prostate cancer dates back to the beginning of the twentieth century, decades before the development of high-energy external beam radiotherapy (EBRT) and prior to the development of the modern radical prostatectomy.[1–3] However, it was not until the 1970s, when the radioactive seeds became available and an open implant technique was developed by Whitmore and Hilaris at Memorial Hospital that this approach could be applied routinely.[4] This technique involved retropubic exposure of the prostate and the "freehand" insertion, from anterior to posterior, of needles loaded with radioactive iodine 125 (Figure 17–1). The needles were inserted based on visual inspection and palpation of the needle tips in the rectum. The needles were then withdrawn, leaving the radioactive seeds in the prostate. The number of seeds needed was determined from a nomogram based on the estimated size of the gland and the activity of the radioactive seeds. Unfortunately, it is now known that, using this technique, the resulting radiation dose distributions were inferior to what is currently possible using computerized planning and ultrasonography. Analysis of the postoperative images from these early cases showed the limited consistency and accuracy in the placement of the seeds. This led to frequent underdosing of the tumor and overdosing of the normal structures leading to local failures and

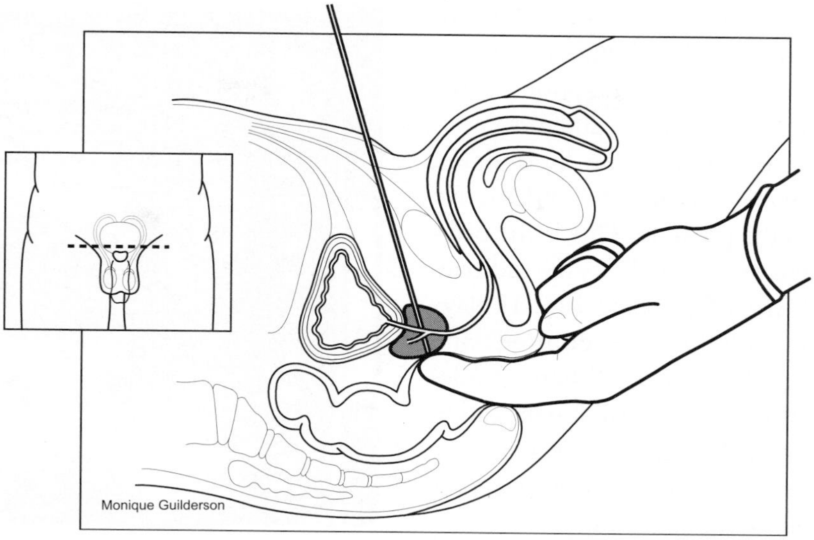

Figure 17–1. Retropubic freehand approach for permanent seed implant.

complications. With the development of the megavoltage linear accelerator, the nerve-sparing radical prostatectomy, and the accompanying reports of success with these approaches, the interest in prostate brachytherapy waned.[2,5–9]

Important lessons were learned from these early experiences with prostate brachytherapy. Prostate brachytherapy requires consistent and accurate placement of the radioactive sources. Since the dose varies steeply around the source, small errors in placement of the source can lead to suboptimal dosimetry. Clearly, better planning, imaging, and guidance were needed. In 1983, Holms and colleagues developed a transperineal implant technique with transrectal ultrasonography (TRUS) guidance.[10] Using TRUS guidance, a real-time image of the implant volume could be seen and the position of each implant needle adjusted to ensure accurate placement (Figures 17–2 and 17–3). This led to improvements in the quality and reproducibility of prostate brachytherapy and a resurgence of interest in prostate brachytherapy. Most investigators believe that as a result of a TRUS-based approach, there has been a substantial reduction in perioperative morbidity. Unfortunately, the only formal comparison published to date failed to substantiate this belief.[11]

In this review, we do not discuss the controversies surrounding the various definitions of prostate-specific antigen (PSA) or biochemical failure. Many excellent reviews have been published, and still there is no consensus.[12] We have attempted to provide enough information to the reader so that the definition used by the authors is at least reasonable. Most will agree that a low nonrising or undetectable PSA is a good definition of treatment success, but only longer follow-up will allow us to make more definitive statements about this important end point.

MODERN PROSTATE BRACHYTHERAPY

The TRUS-guided implant technique is the backbone of modern prostate brachytherapy. Whether it

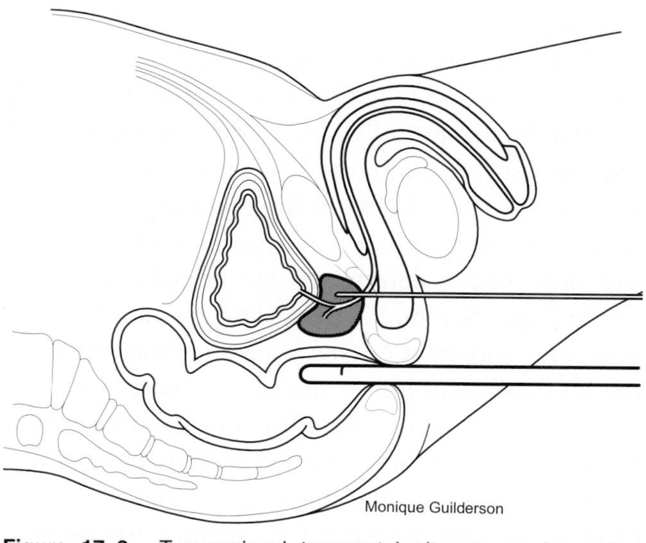

Figure 17–2. Transperineal transrectal ultrasonography–guided approach for permanent seed implant.

is permanent or temporary, high-dose rate (HDR), or low-dose rate (LDR), modern brachytherapy uses a similar technique of transperineal insertion of the seed-bearing needle or after-loading catheters.

As implied from its name, the permanent prostate implant involves leaving the radioactive sources permanently in the prostate. This is the original technique described by Holms.[10] As the radioactive sources decay (60 days for iodine 125, 17 days for palladium 103), radiation is emitted and absorbed by the surrounding tissue. When an adequate amount of radiation is delivered, it can lead to sterilization of all tumor cells. After more than five half-lives have passed, the source activity becomes similar to the background radiation level.

In the temporary prostate implant, the radioactive sources are loaded in the after-loading catheters for the duration of the treatment. A single fraction or multiple fractions of treatments can be delivered using the same after-loading catheter. After a predetermined dose is delivered, the sources and the catheters are removed. The catheters can be loaded manually with ribbons containing evenly spaced radioactive seeds. Most commonly, a remote after-loading approach under robotic control is used to deliver treatments. Besides minimizing the radiation exposure to operating personnel, this type of remote after-loading system provides greater flexibility for delivering custom dose distributions by moving a single radioactive source along the after-loading catheters in a fashion that can be optimized using inverse planning.

Brachytherapy can be categorized based on the rate at which the radiation is delivered. High dose rate brachytherapy delivers > 1 Gy to the treated volume in just a few minutes. On the other end of the spectrum is the LDR brachytherapy, which can include both temporary and permanent implants. The dose rate is determined by the half-life of the isotope and its initial activity. For a given dose, the dose rate and fraction size can dramatically affect the biologic response of the tumor and normal tissue. Over the last two decades, a better understanding of the radiobiology has led to new theories and models.[13–15] However, clinical trials validating these models are just beginning to mature, so debates about the merits of the different models continue.

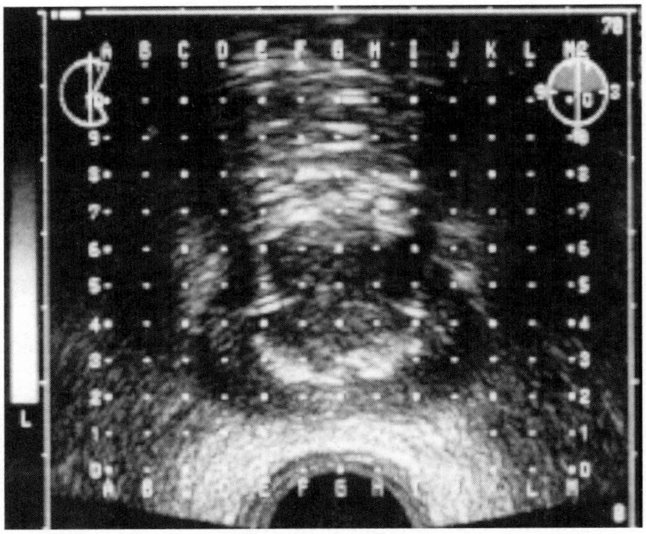

Figure 17–3. Transrectal ultrasonography improved the quality of implant by guiding the insertion of radioactive seeds. Proper operation of the equipment and familiarity with ultrasonography imaging are prerequisites for effective brachytherapy.

PERMANENT SEED IMPLANT

The dosimetric goal of brachytherapy is to accurately place radioactive seeds into the prostate delivering a relatively homogeneous high dose to the target volume while sparing the surrounding normal structures and the urethra. Generally, this involves three steps: pretreatment planning, the operative implant procedure, and postimplant evaluation. During the preplanning study, 5-mm transverse images of the prostate gland from its apex to base are obtained using TRUS placed on a "stepper." The stepper is a stabilization device that allows the probe to move along its long axis precisely in small increments creating axial images. These axial images are then transferred into the brachytherapy treatment planning system. The proper loading and spacing of radioactive seeds in implant needles are determined using the planning software.

At the time of the implant procedure, the implant needles are loaded with appropriate activity isotope according to the plan. A guiding template is placed on the stepper and needles are inserted to the proper location and depth with guidance from the template and ultrasonography. The TRUS probe is inserted into the patient's rectum using the stepper. The probe is positioned so that it best reproduces the image obtained at the time of preplanning. With help from fast planning software and specialized needle loaders or dispensing devices, some brachytherapy specialists have chosen to use intraoperative planning (real time) rather than the preplanning approach. This approach basically combines the preplanning and the implant procedure into one visit to the operating room.[16] In fact, currently no permanent implant technique incorporates true real-time-dosimetry because this would require that the precise location of all seeds is known and that planning software can account for this information immediately. From a practical standpoint, all implants are real time intraoperative because adjustments can be made in the needle position as clinical judgment dictates.

The most commonly used radioisotope for permanent seed prostate implant is radioactive iodine 125. This isotope has a half-life of 60 days and average energy of 28 KeV. It is commonly supplied in a titanium-encapsulated form. When used as monotherapy (without EBRT), the usual dose is approximately 144 Gy or 14,400 rads. When combined with EBRT, the usual dose is 108 Gy. Older literature quoted dose prescriptions of 160 Gy and 120 Gy, respectively. This difference is owing to a change in the conversion factors used to measure doses and does not reflect a real change in desired dose. It is important to be aware that a number of different vendors are currently providing iodine 125 seeds, and because of design differences, they cannot be used interchangeably.[17] Thus, preplanning software must include the unique dosimetric data associated with each vendor's product in order that accurate pre- and post-treatment plans are generated.

The other commonly used isotope is palladium 103. This isotope has a half-life of 17 days and average energy of 21 KeV. Based on theoretical calculations, palladium 103 may be preferable for the treatment of high-grade tumors. This is based on the assumption that high-grade tumors have a shorter doubling time and thus need to be treated quickly before they can repopulate.[18] Clinical results thus far have not demonstrated a difference in outcome compared to iodine 125.[19] Palladium 103 may be associated with a shorter duration of acute urinary symptoms, but the greater cost associated with this isotope may more than offset this potential benefit.

Once the radioactive seeds are implanted (released from the needle) into the prostate, their position cannot be adjusted. Thus, it is very important to ensure that physicians can consistently and reliably place radioactive seeds precisely where they are intended. To demonstrate that this is the case, it is important to systematically evaluate and document the implant quality. This is done by obtaining a postimplant CT scan. Based on these CT images, the position of the radioactive seeds and their relationship to the critical structures can be measured and doses to these structures can be calculated. Studies have shown that prostate volume can change over time after implant and can lead to significant variation in the dose delivered; thus, these scans are usually done 3 to 4 weeks following the implant.[20–22] There appears to be a relationship between treatment failure and the calculated volume of prostate that received the prescribed dose.[23] Stock and colleagues were the first to demonstrate that the dose that was delivered to 90% of the gland (D90) could have a critical impact on the subsequent risk of PSA failure.[23] However, short follow-up and evidence of a learning curve complicated their analysis of this dose-response curve. For example, in their analysis, the patients who received lower doses tended to be patients treated when the brachytherapists were less experienced, and they also tended to have longer follow-up for these patients. Potters and colleagues have also recently reported similar findings concerning the need to adequately irradiate the prostate delivering a D90 $\geq$ 90%.[24] Interestingly, the rule of thumb concerning the dose-response curve did not appear to hold true for patients receiving EBRT in conjunction with the implant.

TEMPORARY IMPLANT

The technique of temporary prostate implant has also become a TRUS-based procedure. During the implant procedure, the after-loading catheters are inserted under TRUS guidance. The catheters are typically secured in position using a perineal template. The location of the catheters is determined using orthogonal radiography or a CT scan. Each catheter's position is then transferred into a computer, and using the treatment planning software, the optimal loading is determined. Each catheter is then loaded with radioactive ribbons or seeds. Iridium 192 is the most commonly used source for temporary implants. The radioactive sources are removed after a predetermined dose is delivered. The amount of time the radioactive sources remain in the implant depends on the activity of the source and total dose delivered. This can range from hours to days in LDR treatments and minutes in HDR treatments. After the treatment is completed, the after-loading catheters are removed before the patient is sent home. Since radioactive sources are loaded outside of the operating room, the exposure to personnel is minimized. Temporary prostate implants are usually administered using multiple fractionated treatments delivered over one or two inpatient stays or one to three outpatient visits.

Prior to the widespread availability of computer-controlled remote after-loading technology, temporary implants were loaded manually. Modern after-loading machines are based on computer-driven stepping motors that control the placement of a high-activity iridium 192 source located at the end of a cable. The newer sources have high specific activity and are small and flexible. This allows them to travel through narrow and tortuous catheters. The combination of the ability to after-load the sources and computer-controlled placement of the radioactive source gives HDR brachytherapy unprecedented flexibility and control. By controlling the amount of time the source spends at points along the catheter (dwell time), a variety of intensity, dose patterns, and volumes can be generated to fit the clinical needs. The modern treatment planning software also allows the dwell time to be optimized to produce better coverage of the implant volume with less dose heterogeneity and minimizes the dose to critical normal structures (Figures 17–4 and 17–5).[25,26]

The linear-quadratic model provides a mathematical basis for estimating the clinical effects of alternative fractionation schemes. In this model, the response of tissue to altered fractionation is determined by the tissue's α/β ratio. Tissue with a higher α/β ratio is less sensitive to a high dose per fraction or hypofractionated radiotherapy. In clinical practice, most tumors have a high α/β ratio; therefore, these tumors are treated with standard fractionated or hyperfractionated radiotherapy. Conversely, tumors with a lower α/β ratio can be treated effectively with a higher dose per fraction radiotherapy or hypofractionated radiotherapy. The α/β value commonly used for acute responding tissue and tumor is 10 to 12. Recent studies estimating the α/β value for prostate carcinoma have shown that prostate cancer might have an exceptionally low α/β ratio of 1.5.[27–29] This suggests that there is a rationale for treating prostate cancer using HDR radiotherapy.[30–32] Based on this principle, trials were designed to test the feasibility of HDR monotherapy. Preliminary reports suggest that HDR monotherapy may be well tolerated and feasible.[33,34] If this approach proves to be equally effective and no more morbid than other forms of

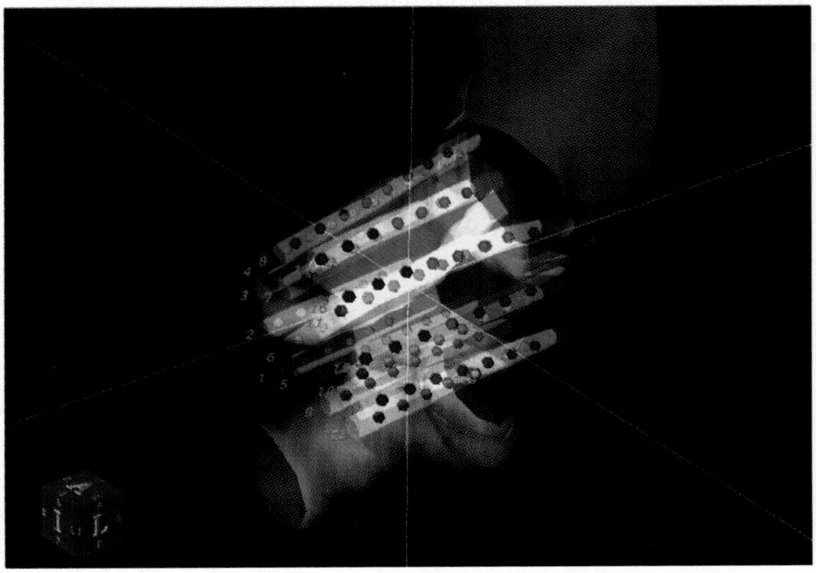

Figure 17–4. Three-dimensional brachytherapy planning system is an important part of modern brachytherapy. Critical organs such as the urethra, rectum, and bladder are contoured during the treatment planning process, and doses delivered to the critical organs can be accurately controlled.

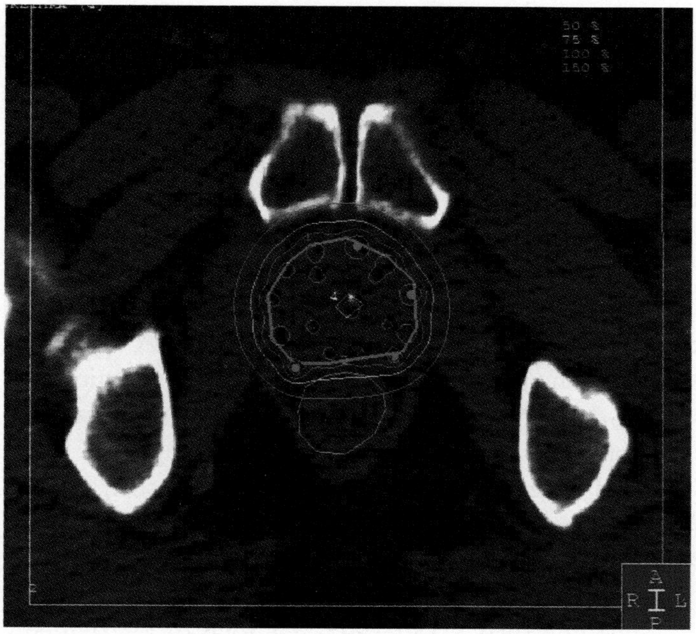

Figure 17–5. Very conformal dose distribution can be delivered to the prostate using a modern brachytherapy treatment system. A steep dose fall-off outside of the implant volume decreases the dose and volume of radiated normal structures.

radiotherapy, it could substantially reduce the cost and may establish a new standard to which other therapy is compared.

PATIENT SELECTION

The permanent prostate seed implantation (PPI) has been used both as a monotherapy and in combination with EBRT. Patients with a relatively low risk of extracapsular extension and lymph node involvement are ideal candidates for permanent seed implant alone. Patients interested in permanent seed implant but with one or more adverse risk factors (PSA > 10 ng/mL, Gleason score > 6 or a ≥ bulky T2b disease) are frequently treated with EBRT for 5 weeks before or after the implant. Despite these general guidelines, some expert brachytherapists believe that as long as an adequate margin is applied there is no need for EBRT, whereas other experts routinely recommend the use of external beam in combination with PPIs.[24,35,36]

Prior transurethral resection of the prostate (TURP) is a relative contraindication to PPI, especially if there is a large residual defect, tumor was found in the TURP specimen, or continence is marginal. A high International Prostate Symptom Score (IPSS > 15) may also be a relative contraindication to PPI as it is thought to be a risk factor for acute urinary retention after implantation. Other relative contraindications to PPI include prostate size greater than 50 cc and pubic arch interference. Pubic arch interference is assessed by measuring the widest portion of the prostate and the narrowest portion of the pelvic inlet on CT scan. Patients with large prostates (> 50 cc) may be implanted with or without downsizing using hormonal therapy.[37,38] Some investigators have reported that the size of the transition zone correlates with an increased risk of acute urinary retention.[39] Using an MRI-guiding technique, Thomas and colleagues reported that the transition zone volume was the only significant predictor of acute urinary retention in a multivariate analysis ($p < .01$).[39] Merrick and colleagues evaluated the relationship between transition zone index (TZI = transition zone volume/prostate gland volume) and urinary dysfunction using IPSSs in 170 consecutive patients undergoing PPI.[40] The TZI correlated with the time for IPSS normalization and the maximum increase in IPSS after brachytherapy. These authors concluded that the preimplant TZI correlated with the need for a subsequent transurethral resection. They also reported that TZI did not correlate with prolonged catheterization or α-blocker dependency. Thus, large prostates may be problematic not just because of their predilection for pubic arch interference but also because there may be physiologic issues that can complicate urinary function after implantation.

The temporary implant is usually used as a boost in conjunction with EBRT. Typically, this involves 4 to 5 weeks of EBRT treatment with one or multiple implants at the beginning, sandwiched between or at the end of the EBRT. As a result, patients selected for temporary implant are generally those with greater risk of extracapsular extension or patients who already need external beam treatment. Because of the flexible nature of the after-loading technology, the treatment is not as limited by the patient's anatomy. Based on cost considerations resulting from shorter hospital stays, as well as the accuracy and flexibility of the HDR after-loading technology, most centers in the United States that use temporary prostate implants have switched from LDR to delivering HDR treatment.

RESULTS OF PERMANENT SEED IMPLANT ALONE

Fifteen-year data are available from two institutions with a long track record of prostate brachytherapy.[41,42] The largest series was reported by Zelefsky and colleagues and included 1,078 patients treated between March 1970 and December 1987 via a retropubic approach.[41] All patients underwent bilateral pelvic lymphadenectomy before implantation. The patients included in this series were very different from patients included in contemporary series, with 20% of these patients having T3 disease and 32% having positive lymph nodes. With a median follow-up of 11 years, multivariate analysis identified nodal involvement, high-grade disease, clinical stage, and implant dose less than 140 Gy as independent predictors of local relapse. The local recurrence-free survival rates for patients with negative nodes at 5, 10, and 15 years were 69, 44, and 24%, respectively. The authors concluded that iodine 125 implantation via the retropubic approach was associated with a greater than expected incidence of local relapse at 15 years. Unfortunately, pretreatment PSA was not available for these patients, and it is likely that they had very unfavorable disease by today's standards.

The series reported by Schellhammer and colleagues is unique because of the long follow-up and excellent PSA data.[42] The records of 126 patients who underwent open PPI more than 15 years previously were reviewed and compared with the first 126 patients treated by TRUS-guided PPI. Of the 13 patients with a confirmed diagnosis who were clinically free of disease, 4 had a PSA level of 0.2 ng/mL or less, 4 had a PSA level between 0.21 and 0.9 ng/mL, and 5 had a PSA level between 1 and 2.5 ng/mL. These authors concluded that patients who were alive and clinically free of disease longer than 15 years after therapy achieved low PSA levels. Of note, their findings do not support the assertion that PSA levels need to be less than 0.2 ng/mL to support "cure," as suggested by Critz and colleagues.[43]

Using the modern TRUS-based approach, Blasko and colleagues reported their experience using radioactive iodine 125 seed implant as the sole treatment for prostate cancer at the Northwest Tumor Institute (NWTI) in 1995.[44] A total of 197 patients with clinically staged T1b–T2b disease (AJCC, 1992 staging system), Gleason score 2 to 6, and median pretreatment PSA of 7.0 ng/mL were treated between 1988 and 1992. In 97% of patients with an abnormal pretreatment PSA, the post-treatment PSA value decreased to less than 1.0 ng/mL at 48 months postimplant. The actuarial freedom from biochemical failure was 93% at 5 years. Ragde and colleagues subsequently updated their experience.[45] A total of 126 patients treated between 1988 and 1990 with a median follow-up of 5.8 years were evaluated. The 7-year actuarial freedom from biochemical failure was 89%. More recently, the NWTI's experience was updated at 10 years.[46,47] This analysis included 125 consecutive patients who were treated with iodine 125 brachytherapy. The biochemical disease–free rate was 87% for low-risk (PSA < 10, Gleason sum 2 to 6, T1–2b) patients. The NWTI also reported their experience using palladium 103.[48] Ninety-seven patients with clinical stage T1b–T2c disease were treated between 1987 and 1992 with palladium 103 alone. With a median follow-up of 37 months, 86% remained disease free with a PSA < 1.0 ng/mL. The NWTI has reported the longest and the most favorable results using permanent seed implantation. This group is credited with training many radiation oncologists and urologists to perform permanent seed implantation (Table 17–1).

Beyer and Priestley reported their experience at Boswell Memorial Hospital using iodine 125 seed implant.[49] Their experience with 133 patients was first presented by Priestley and Beyer and subsequently updated by Beyer et al.[50] A total of 489 patients with clinical stage T1a–T2c, Gleason score 2 to 10, and median pretreatment PSA of 7.3 ng/mL were treated between 1988 and 1993. The 5-year actuarial biochemical disease–free survival was 79%.

Wallner and colleagues reported their experience with iodine 125 implant at Memorial Sloan-Kettering Cancer Center (MSKCC) using a CT-based implant technique.[51,52] Between 1988 and 1994, 92 patients with clinical stage T1b-T2c disease, Gleason score 2 to 7 (very few Gleason scores equal 7), and median pretreatment PSA of 9 ng/mL were treated using iodine 125 seed implant alone. With a median follow-up of 36 months, the 4-year actuarial biochemical progression–free rate was 63%.

The technique and experience with seed implant at Mount Sinai Hospital in New York was reported by Stone and Stock and their colleagues,[53,54] who examined 97 patients with stage T1b–T2c disease treated between 1990 and 1994 using radioactive iodine 125 or palladium 103. Eighty-one% of the patients had laparoscopic pelvic lymph node dissection, and 14% of the patients had hormonal therapy. With a median follow-up of 18 months, 76% remained disease free at 2 years.

Sharkey and colleagues reported their experience with palladium 103 implantation. Between 1991 and 1996, 434 patients with clinical stage T1–2 disease were treated with palladium 103 implants.[55] Forty-eight percent of the patients received hormonal ther-

Table 17–1. SELECTED SERIES USING PERMANENT RADIOACTIVE SEED IMPLANTATION ALONE

Institution	Patient Characteristics	Treatment	No. and Follow-up (mo)	Results (Definition)	Complications
NWTI,[46] 1998	T1a–T3a, GS 2–10, PSA 0.4–138, mean = 11.0 ng/mL	Iodine 125 (N = 98), 45 Gy + Iodine 125 (N = 54)	N = 152, 119 median	60% 10-yr PFS (iodine 125 only PSA > 0.5)	NS
NWTI,[47] 2000	T1a–T2c, GS 2–6	Iodine 125	N = 126, 69.3 median	87% biochemical DFS	NS
NWTI,[48] 1995	T1b–T2c, GS 2–7, PSA 0.8–32.4, 7.0 median	Palladium 103	N = 97, 37 median	86% 4-yr PFS (PSA 1)	Superficial urethral necrosis in patient with TURP
Boswell Memorial Hospital, AZ[49,50]	T1a–T2c, GS 2–10, PSA 0.1–89, 7.3 median	Iodine 125	N = 489, 35 median	79% 5-yr BDFS (PSA > 4)	4.2% obstruction, 1% incontinence, 3/489 proctitis, pelvic pain (1/489)
MSKCC[51,52]	T1b–T2c, GS 2–7, PSA 1–90, 9 median	Iodine 125	N = 92, 36 median	63% 4-yr BPFS (plateaued PSA > 1)	14% Foley catheter, 9% TURP, 3% incontinence, 5% rectal ulceration, 3 required colostomy for prostatic-rectal fistula, 14% at 3 yrs impotence
Mount Sinai, NY[53,54]	T1b–T2c, GS 2–7, PSA 0– > 20, pN0	Iodine 125 (71), Palladium 103 (12), HT + Palladium 103 (14)	N = 97, 18 median	76% 2-yr FFBF (2 PSA increases)	4% Foley catheter 1–2 days, 1/97 suprapubic catheter 3 month, 1/97 G2 proctitis, 21% at 2 yrs impotence
Urology Health Center, FL[55]	T1–T2, GS 2–10, PSA 0.1–48, 7.4 mean, pN0	Palladium 103 (224), HT + palladium 103 (210)	N = 434, 27.6 mean	80% 4-yr DFS (PSA = 1.5)	< 5% incontinence, < 15% impotence
Southeast Alabama Medical Center[56]	T1b–T2c, GS = 7, PSA 0.7–67.1, 10.6 mean	Iodine 125	N = 142, 30 median	76% 5-yr DFS (abnormal exam; 2 increases in PSA)	1.4% G3 urinary retention, (1/142) G3 hematuria, 5% incontinence, 1/142 colostomy, 1/142 pulmonary embolus

NWTI = Northwest Tumor Institute; GS = Gleason score; PSA = prostate-specific antigen; PFS = progression-free survival; NS = not stated; DFS = disease-free survival; TURP = transurethral resecton of the prostate; BDFS = boichemical disease-free survival; MSKCC = Memorial Sloan-Kettering Cancer Center; BPFS = biochemical progression–free survival; HT = hormonal therapy; FFBF = freedom from biochemical failure.

apy because of gland size larger than 50 cc. With a mean follow-up of 27.6 months, it was estimated that 80% would remain biochemical disease free at 4 years. Stokes and colleagues reported their experience with iodine 125 implant. A total of 142 patients with stage T1b–T2c disease, Gleason score ≤ 7, and a mean pretreatment PSA of 10.6 ng/mL were treated between 1988 and 1992.[56] With a median follow-up of 30 months, 76% of the patients remained disease free at 5 years.

Other than the results reported by the NWTI, most of the published series on permanent seed implantation have a limited number of patients with short follow-up. Although the reported results are fairly comparable to EBRT, it is unclear if the patient populations are comparable. It is also unclear at this time if the published results can be reproduced for the general population because of the "learning curve" associated with any new technique.

Results of Permanent Seed Implant Boost in Combination with External Beam Radiotherapy

The results of permanent seed implant boost in combination with external beam radiotherapy are summarized in Table 17–2. Ragde and colleagues reported the NWTI experience using combined 45 Gy of external beam and iodine 125 implant boost.[46] Fifty-four patients with stages T1b–T3a disease were treated between 1987 and 1988. They reported a 10-year progression-free survival of 76% with a PSA of 0.5 ng/mL.

Most patients receiving a combined approach are treated by EBRT followed by PPI. Some physicians have chosen the opposite sequence. Critz and colleagues reported their experience using iodine 125 implant followed by 45 Gy of EBRT.[57] Their analysis included patients with clinical stage T1–T2 disease and a Gleason score of 2 to 10 treated between 1984 and 1994. Thirty-five percent of the patients were treated using ultrasonography guidance; the rest were treated using the retropubic implant technique. Eighty-eight percent of the patients had pretreatment PSA. With a median follow-up of 40 months, 5-year progression-free survival was between 81 and 97% depending on pretreatment PSA. Zeitlin and colleagues reported their experience using iodine 125 and palladium 103 implantation followed by 45 Gy of EBRT.[58] A total of 212 patients with stage T1b–T3 disease and a Gleason score of 2 to 10 were treated between 1991 and 1996. Patients with stage T2b or greater, pretreatment PSA of 20 ng/mL or greater, or Gleason score of 7 or greater were surgically staged to be N0. With a mean follow-up of 33 months, the 5-year disease-free survival rate was 91%.

Dattoli and colleagues reported their experiences using 41 Gy of EBRT followed by palladium 103 implantation.[59] Seventy-three patients with clinical stage T2a–T3 disease, Gleason score 4 to 9, and a median pretreatment PSA of 12 ng/mL were treated between 1991 and 1994. Thirteen percent of the patients received a short course of hormonal therapy prior to treatment, and one patient underwent staging lymphadenectomy. At a median follow-up of 24 months, 79% of the patients remained biochemically free of disease with a PSA ≤ 1.0 ng/mL. It is unclear from the review of literature which patients should be selected for the combined treatment.

Result of Temporary Brachytherapy Boost in Combination with External Beam Radiotherapy

Most of the reported experiences with temporary LDR boost in combination with EBRT include patients treated prior to the PSA era. None of the groups used TRUS guidance. With these limitations in mind, a majority of the groups reported reasonably good results, with a low to moderate risk of gastrointestinal toxicity. A summary of the results is presented in Table 17–3.[60–65]

Table 17–4 summarizes the results of HDR brachytherapy boost in combination with EBRT. Kovacs and colleagues reported one of the earliest experiences using HDR brachytherapy boost at the University of Kiel. Most patients treated had clinical stage T2b–T3 disease and poorly differentiated tumors. They used a combination of split-course EBRT and two 15-Gy HDR treatments. They reported an 18% positive biopsy rate at 18 months post-treatment.[66] The results were updated at 10 years; 78% of 171 patients remained free of disease at a median follow-up of 55 months.[67]

Mate and Gottesman at Swedish Medical Center reported their experience with HDR brachytherapy. They used a more moderate hypofractionated schema with four treatments of 3- to 4-Gy fractions of HDR treatments combined with 45 to 50 Gy of EBRT. Routine cystoscopy at the end of the implant procedure was done to ensure that the catheters were placed at the proper depth and to avoid injuring the urethra. Pretreatment characteristics included clinical stage T1b to T3c disease, mean initial PSA of 12.9 ng/mL, and Gleason score ranging from 3 to 9. They reported an 84% 5-year PSA disease-free survival.[68,69]

Martinez and colleagues at the William Beaumont Hospital reported an ongoing prospective dose escalation trial using HDR brachytherapy as a boost. There have been multiple updates of their results.[70–73] They have continued to dose escalate using increasingly larger fractions of HDR treatment ranging from 5.5 to 6.5 Gy × 3 to 8.25 to 9.5 Gy × 2 combined with 46 Gy of EBRT. In a recent update, they have showed acceptable toxicity using 9.5 Gy × 2 treatments. Patients with a PSA of 10 ng/mL, tumor stage T2b, and Gleason score 7 were selected for the trial. Despite the high frequency of poor prognostic factors, the actuarial biochemical control rate was 89% at 2 years and 63% at 5 years. The 5-year actuarial rates of local failure and distant metastasis were 16% and 14%, respectively.

Borghede and colleagues at Göteborg University in Sweden reported their experience using 50 Gy of EBRT combined with two fractions of a 10-Gy HDR boost.[74,75] They used ultrasonography to target tumor nodules inside the prostate and give an additional 5-Gy boost to these areas. They reported a 4% positive biopsy rate at 18 months post-treatment. No hormonal therapy was used. After a median follow-up of 45 months, a post-treatment PSA level of 1.0 ng/mL was achieved in 84% of the patients. Dinges and colleagues at the University of Berlin reported their experience combining 40 to 45 Gy of EBRT with a 9- to 10-Gy HDR boost. With a median follow-up of 24 months, the local control rate was 79.5%.[76]

COMPLICATIONS AND LIMITATIONS OF THE AVAILABLE DATA

Perhaps the most important and controversial issue related to brachytherapy is the risk of morbidity. Unfortunately, most of the available published data are based on physician-reported complications and

Table 17–2. SELECTED SERIES USING PERMANENT RADIOACTIVE SEED IMPLANTATION IN COMBINATION WITH EXTERNAL BEAM RADIOTHERAPY

Institution	Patients	Treatment	No. and Follow-up (mo)	Results	Complications
NWTI[46]	T1a–T3a, GS 2–10, PSA 0.4–138, 11.0 mean	45 Gy + iodine 125 (54), iodine 125 (98)	152, 119 median	76% 10-yr PFS (PSA > 0.5)	NS
Radiotherapy Clinic of Georgia[57]	T1–T2, GS 2–10, PSA 0.3–188, 8.4 median	RP iodine 125 80 Gy + 45 Gy (346), US iodine 125 80 Gy + 45 Gy (190)	536, 40 median	81–97% 5-yr PFS (2–3 PSA increases)	NS
Staten Island University Hospital,[58]	T1b–T3, GS 2–10, PSA < 4–> 20, pN0 (T2b, GS = 7, PSA = 20)	Iodine 125 120 Gy + 45 Gy, palladium 103 90 Gy + 45 Gy	212, 33 mean	91% DFS (PSA > 0.5 increase to = 1; increase to 2 if < 0.5)	1.5% urinary retention, 3.8% incontinence, 0.5% urethral stricture, 21.4% proctitis, 2.8% colostomy, 2.4% recto-prostate fistula, 0.5% rectal wall breakdown, 38% impotence
University Community Hospital[59]	T2a–T3, GS 4–9, PSA 4–147, 12 median pN0(1)	41 Gy, palladium 103 80 Gy, HT + 41 Gy + implant (10)	73, 24	79% 3-yr BPFS (PSA > 1)	2/73 TURP, 1/73 incontinence, 23% impotence

NWTI = Northwest Tumor Institute; GS = Gleason score; PSA = prostate-specific antigen; RP = retropubic approach (not TRUS based); PFS = progression-free survival; NS = not stated; DFS = disease-free survival; BPFS = biochemical progression–free survival.

Table 17–3. SELECTED SERIES USING TEMPORARY LDR BRACHYTHERAPY BOOST IN COMBINATION WITH EXTERNAL BEAM RADIOTHERAPY

Author	Patients	Treatment	No. and Follow-up	Results	Complications
Prestidge[60]	T2b–T3	EB 45–50 Gy, iodine 125, irradium 192 30–35 Gy	34	NS	NS
Khan[61]	T1b–T3	EB 34 Gy, irradium 192 31 Gy	321	NS	NS
Syed [62]	A2–C, pN0, GS 2–10	EB 40 Gy, irradium 192 30–35 Gy	200, 7 yr	85% 5-yr actuarial survival	6 colostomies, 15/200 moderate to severe complication
Stromberg,[63] Brindle[64]	B2–C, pN0–1	EB 30.6 Gy, irradium 192 30–35 Gy	57, 72 mo	85% 5-yr actuarial survival, 63% 5-yr DFS	4.5% G4 rectal ulceration, 3/57 G4 urinary incontinence, 3/57 G3 or 4 chronic perineal pain
Donnelly[65]	A2–D1	EB 45 Gy, irradium 192 35 Gy	170	NS	NS

LDR = low-dose rate; EB = external beam; NS = not stated; DFS = disease-free survival.

not on the use of validated instruments. Significant discrepancies have been noted between patient reports and physician-reported rates of complications. For example, in one study, patients reported urinary incontinence and pelvic pain more often than physicians.[77] In contrast, nocturia was reported more often by physicians than by patients. Highly significant statistical differences were also observed for interest in sex, sexual activity, urinary incontinence, and cystitis. Thus, physicians treating prostate cancer should follow their patients using validated instruments. This will allow us to share our rates of complications with patients considering this procedure and compare it to other approaches (Table 17–5).

TREATMENT COMPLICATIONS WITH PERMANENT PROSTATE SEED IMPLANTATION ALONE

Complications from permanent seed implant alone are summarized in Table 17–1. Ragde and colleagues reported the experience at the NWTI.[46] Most patients experienced some degree of urinary urgency, frequency, and varying degrees of outlet obstruction that usually subsided within 5 to 10

Table 17–4. SELECTED SERIES USING TEMPORARY HDR BRACHYTHERAPY BOOST IN COMBINATION WITH EXTERNAL BEAM RADIOTHERAPY

Institution	Patients	Treatment	No. and Follow-up (mo)	Results	Complications
University of Kiel[67]	T1–T3, G1–G3	EB (30) 50 Gy, IS 15 Gy × 2	171, 55 mo	78% clinical disease free	5/171 G3 proctitis, 3/171 G3 dysuria cystitis, 9/171 incontinence
Swedish Tumor Institute[69]	T1–T3, PSA 12.9, GS 3–9	EB 50.4 Gy, IS 3–4 Gy × 4	104, 46 mo	84% at 5-yr actuarial (3 increases)	6.7% stricture, 1% necrosis
William Beaumont Hospital[72]	T2b–T3, PSA, GS 7	EB 46, IS 5.5–6.5 Gy × 3, 8.25–9.5 Gy × 2	142, 2.1 yr	89% DFS at 5 yr, 95% OS at 5 yr	5% G3 acute toxicity, 9% 5-yr actuarial, G3 late toxicity
Goteborg University[74,75]	T1–T3pN0, G1–3	EB 50 Gy, IS 10–15 Gy × 2	50, 45 mo	84% PSA 1.0, 4% positive Bx at 18 mo	4% dysuria, 6% frequency, 8% diarrhea, 2% proctitis, 12% impotence
University of Berlin[76]	T2–T3pN0, G1–3, PSA 14.0	EB 40–45 Gy, IS 9–10 Gy × 2	82, 24 mo	52.9% PSA < 1.0, 26.9% positive Bx at 24 mo	7/82 G3 stricture, 6/82 G3 incontinence, 3/82 G4 proctitis

HDR = high-dose rate; EB = external beam; PSA = prostate-specific antigen; DFS = disease-free survival; OS = overall survival; Bx = biopsy.

Table 17–5. SELECTED SERIES COMPARING PERMANENT SEED IMPLANTS TO CONVENTIONAL RADIOTHERAPY AND/OR SURGERY

Lead Author (year)	No. of Patients	Details	Conclusions
Seung (1998)[97]	EBRT = 187	Patients treated with EBRT from UCSF who were thought to have been candidates for BT compared to literature	Wide range of results overlapping with EBRT results
D'Amico (1998)[99]	BT = 66, EBRT = 766, RP = 888	EBRT at Harvard versus radical retropubic prostatectomy and BT at University of Penn	The outcome was similar for low-risk patients regardless of treatment type; however high- and intermediate-risk patients did worse with BT
King (1998)[100]	BT = 63, EBRT = 85, RP = 73	Comparison of results from patients with T1/2 disease treated at Yale University	EBRT patients did the worse than RP or BT; mean EBRT only dose 66 Gy and had higher Gleason scores and PSAs than BT patients; RP patients were N0
Beyer (2000)[98]	BT = 695, EBRT = 1,527	Retrospective study of large multiphysician practice	Patients with GS ≥ 7 or PSA > 10 ng/mL did significantly better with EBRT than BT
Krupski (2000)[101]	BT = 70, EBRT+ BT = 4, RP = 27	Retrospective quality of life survey	Quality of life score was significantly lower in EBRT + BT; BT and RP had similar scores, but urinary symptoms score was lowest with RP
Brandeis (2000)[96]	RP = 74, BT = 48	Compares general and disease-specific health-related quality of life in men undergoing BT to those undergoing radical RP and age-matched healthy controls	Urinary leakage was better in the BT than in the RP group; BT patients had more irritative urinary symptoms and worse bowel function than controls; patients with BT and EBRT performed worse in general and disease-specific health-related quality of life domains than with BT alone
Davis (2001)[102]	BT = 122, EBRT = 188, RP = 220	Retrospective quality of life survey	General health-related quality of life mostly unaffected by the treatment modality; EBRT had worse bowel "bothersomeness"; RP had worse urinary function; RP worse sexual function; urinary symptoms score initially worse with BT but equal to other modalities after 12 mo
Lee (2001)[103]	BT = 44, EBRT = 23, RP = 23	Prospective quality of life survey	Health-related quality of life decreases significantly in the first month after BT or RP but not after EBRT; differences in the score were not significant 12 mo post-treatment

EBRT = external beam radiation therapy; UCSF = University of California at San Francisco; BT = permanent prostate brachytherapy; RP = radical prostatectomy; PSA = prostate-specific antigen.

months. Rectal symptoms, such as diarrhea, tenesmus, urgency, and bleeding, were rarely encountered. Among 118 patients, 5.1% developed urinary incontinence, 2.5% developed severe urinary stricture and required urinary diversion, and 12% developed short urinary strictures and required dilatation. All patients who developed urinary incontinence had a history of TURP.

Beyer and Priestley also reported that obstructive and irritative voiding symptoms were common after implantation.[49] Prolonged symptoms developed in 4.2% of 489 patients. Sixty-seven percent of these patients required intervention postimplant. One percent of the patients developed urinary incontinence. Three patients developed proctitis, and one patient developed chronic pelvic pain. Wallner and colleagues reported that most patients developed urinary symptoms within several weeks of implantation, with 46% requiring medication.[51,52,78] For persistent urinary obstructive symptoms, 9% of the patients required TURP. Three percent of the patients reported urinary incontinence. Five percent (5/92) of the patients developed rectal ulceration within 11 to 22 months. Three percent (3/92) ultimately required colostomy for prostatic-rectal fistula. Of 56 patients who were sexually potent prior to treatment, 86% remained potent at 3 years.

Stone and Stock and their colleagues reported that irritative symptoms were common in most patients 6 months following implantation.[53,54] Four percent (4/97) developed obstructive symptoms that required placement of a Foley catheter for 24 to 48 hours immediately postimplant. Two percent (2/97) required TURP, and one required suprapubic catheter for 3 months. One patient experienced proctitis. They also assessed erectile function in 64 patients who were potent prior to implant. Seventy-nine percent remained potent at 2 years. Sharkey and colleagues reported short-term bladder and bowel irritation in most patients but no readmission for urinary retention.[55] Less than 5% of the patients developed incontinence. Impotence was reported in less than 15%. Stokes and colleagues reported transient urethritis in most patients.[56] Significant morbidity occurred in 8.4% (12/142), which included urinary incontinence in 5%, urinary retention in two patients, hematuria in one patient, colostomy in one patient, and fatal pulmonary embolus in one patient. They also reported a decrease in the incidence of urethral morbidity by decreasing the central prostate dose.

Han and colleagues used a patient questionnaire-based assessment of complications on 160 consecutive patients treated with prostate brachytherapy. They reported that 5% of patients required hospital admission for an average of 2 days and 38% required nonroutine visits with a physician as a result of the procedure.[79] Furthermore, 32% of the patients required urinary catheterization at some point after the implant. The authors concluded that there is generally an underreporting of the short-term complications by physicians, and patient survey provided a more realistic assessment.

A review of the brachytherapy literature suggests that treatment-related side effects occur in a significant proportion of patients and may be prolonged and irritative in nature. Although these symptoms may not always be classified as "complications," they can have deleterious effects on patient quality of life.[80] In recent years, much attention has been directed toward assessing quality of life after treatment. Various validated quality of life instruments have been developed and are currently being used to evaluate this issue.[81–88]

Rectal complications appear to be less common but can be severe and more bothersome than urinary complications, which tend to be common but mild. Rectal bleeding, ulcers, and rectourethral fistulae are additional complications of note.[89–94] Rectal bleeding can be bothersome but usually is not associated with pain. Bleeding can be very cautiously treated with argon lasers; however, whenever possible conservative management is preferred.[95]

TREATMENT COMPLICATIONS FOLLOWING EXTERNAL BEAM RADIATION THERAPY AND BRACHYTHERAPY

Treatment complications following combination radiotherapy are generally similar to that of PPI monotherapy. Some authors are of the opinion that the addition of EBRT increases treatment-related complications for patients undergoing brachytherapy.[96] Brandeis and colleagues reported on a cohort of 48 men treated with brachytherapy with and without pretreatment EBRT who completed the Rand 36-item general health survey. Patients who underwent brachytherapy after EBRT performed worse in all general and disease-specific health-related quality of life domains compared with those who did not undergo pretreatment radiation therapy.

Physicians routinely using a combined approach have reported rates of complications not dissimilar to those expected with PPI monotherapy. For example, Zeitlin and colleagues reported their experience using iodine 125 implant followed by 45 Gy of EBRT.[58] Although they reported irritative voiding symptoms in most patients, they were controlled with medication, and these symptoms persisted for more than 1 year in only 5% of the patients. Urinary incontinence developed in 3.8% of the patients, and urethral stricture in 0.5%. Proctitis occurred in 21.4% of the patients. Overall, 2.8% required colostomy. These patients included five with rectoprostatic fistula and one patient with rectal wall breakdown. Of 100 patients who were potent prior to treatment, 62% retained potency. Dattoli and colleagues reported their experience using 41 Gy of EBRT followed by a palladium 103 implant boost.[59] They reported Radiation Therapy Oncology Group (RTOG) grade 1 to 2 urinary symptoms in most patients postimplant. Table 17–6 is the RTOG toxicity grading system. Six patients underwent transurethral incision of the prostate (TUIP) during implantation owing to substantial pretreatment prostatic obstructive symptoms, two required TURP for persistent urinary obstructive symptoms, and one developed urinary incontinence. None developed

Table 17–6. RTOG TOXICITY SCALES*

	0	1	2	3	4	5
Acute grade (day 1–90)						
Diarrhea	None	Increase of 2 to 3 stools per day over pre-Rx	Increase of 4 to 6 stools per day; nocturnal stools; moderate cramping	Increase of 7 to 9 stools per day or incontinence, severe cramping	Increase of ≥ 10 stools per day; grossly bloody diarrhea or need for parenteral support	Death
Lower GI including pelvis	None	Increased frequency; change in quality of bowel habits not requiring medication; rectal discomfort not requiring analgesics	Diarrhea requiring parasympatholytic drugs/mucus discharge not necessitating sanitary pads; rectal or abdominal pain requiring analgesics	Diarrhea requiring parasympatholytic drugs/mucus discharge not necessitating sanitary pads; rectal or abdominal pain requiring analgesics	Acute or subacute obstruction, fistula or perforation, GI bleeding requiring transfusion; abdominal pain or tenesmus requiring tube decompression or bowel diversion	Death
GU (hematuria)	None	Microscopic	Gross/no clots	Gross + clots	Requires transfusion	Death
Late grade (> 90 days)						
GU	None	Frequency of urination or nocturia twice pretreatment habit/ dysuria, urgency not requiring medication	Frequency of urination or nocturia that is less frequent than every hour; dysuria, urgency, bladder spasm requiring local anesthetic (eg, pyridium)	Frequency with urgency and nocturia hourly or more frequently/dysuria, pelvis pain or bladder spasm requiring regular, frequent narcotic/gross hematuria with/ without clot passage	Hematuria requiring transfusion/acute bladder obstruction not secondary to clot passage, ulceration or necrosis	Death
Small/large intestine	None	Mild diarrhea, mild cramping, bowel movement 5 times daily, slight rectal discharge or bleeding	Moderate diarrhea and colic; bowel movement > 5 times daily; excessive rectal mucus or intermittent bleeding	Obstruction or bleeding requiring surgery	Necrosis/perforation; fistula	Death
Bladder	None	Slight epithelial atrophy, minor telangiectasia (microscopic hematuria)	Moderate frequency; generalized telangiectasia; intermittent macroscopic hematuria	Severe frequency; severe generalized telangiectasia; intermittent frequent hematuria; reduction in bladder capacity (< 150 cc)	Necrosis/contracted bladder (< 100 cc); severe hemorrhagic cystitis	Death

GU = genitourinary; GI = gastrointestinal; Rx = therapy.
* Modified from the Radiation Therapy Oncology (RTOG) Group Web site.

rectal ulceration. Seventy-seven percent of 46 patients who were sexually potent prior to treatment were potent at 3 years.

TREATMENT COMPLICATIONS WITH HIGH DOSE RATE BRACHYTHERAPY

A summary of treatment complications from HDR brachytherapy boost in combination with EBRT is listed in Table 17–4. Kovács and colleagues reported 3% RTOG-European Organization for the Research and Treatment of Cancer (EORTC) G3 proctitis, 2% G3 dysuria/cystitis, and 5% urinary incontinence (all in patients who had previous TURP). One patient developed osteoradionecrosis of the pubic ramus.[67] Mate and colleagues had a slightly different experience, with 6% urethral stricture and 1% urethral necrosis. There were no significant gastrointestinal complications.[69] Martinez and colleagues reported a similar result with 5% RTOG acute G3 toxicity. Five-year actuarial G3 late toxicity was 9%. All of the G3 toxicities were urethral strictures, and the median time to late complication was 2.4 years. There were no G4 or G5 complications.[72]

6. Bagshaw MA, Kaplan HS, Sagerman RH. Linear accelerator supervoltage radiotherapy. VII carcinoma of the prostate. Radiology 1965;85:121–9.
7. Del Regato JA. Radiotherapy in the conservative treatment of operable and locally inoperable carcinoma of the prostate. Radiology 1967;88:761–6.
8. George FW, Carlson CE, Dykehuizen RF. Cobalt-60 telecurie-therapy in the definitive treatment of carcinoma of the prostate: a preliminary report. J Urol 1965;92:102–9.
9. Ragde H, Grado GL, Nadir B, Elgamal A-A. Modern prostate brachytherapy. CA Cancer J Clin 2000;50:380–93.
10. Holm H, Juul N, Pedersen J, et al. Transperineal iodine-125 seed implanatation in prostate cancer guided by transrectal ultrasonography. J Urol 1983;130:283–6.
11. Benoit RM, Naslund MJ, Cohen JK. A comparison of complications between ultrasound-guided prostate brachytherapy and open prostate brachytherapy. Int J Radiat Oncol Biol Phys 2000;47:909–13.
12. Roach M 3rd. The role of PSA in the radiotherapy of prostate cancer. Oncology (Huntingt) 1996;10:1143–53; discussion 1154–61.
13. Hall E. Radiobiology for the radiologist. Philadelphia: JB Lippincott; 1994. p. 211–29.
14. Dale RG. The application of the linear-quadratic dose-effect equation to fractionated and protracted radiotherapy. Br J Radiol 1985;58:515–28.
15. Dale RG. Radiobiological assessment of permanent implants using tumor repopulation factors in the linear-quadratic model. Br J Radiol 1989;62:241–4.
16. Stock RG, Stone NN, DeWyngaert JK. PSA findings and biopsy results following interactive ultrasound guided transperineal brachytherapy for early stage prostate cancer. Presented at the 78th Annual Meeting of the American Radium Society, Paris, France, 1995.
17. Beyer DC, Puente F, Rogers KL, Gurgoze EM. Prostate brachytherapy: comparison of dose distribution with different. Radiology 2001;221:623–7.
18. Ling CC, Li WX, Anderson LL. The relative biological effectiveness of I-125 and Pd-103. Int J Radiat Oncol Biol Phys 1995;32:373–8.
19. Cha CM, Potters L, Ashley R, et al. Isotope selection for patients undergoing prostate brachytherapy. Int J Radiat Oncol Biol Phys 1999;45:391–5.
20. Waterman F, Yue N, Corn B, Dicker A. Edema associated with I-125 or Pd-103 prostate brachytherapy and its impact on post-implant dosimetry: an analysis based on serial CT acquisition. Int J Radiat Oncol Biol Phys 1998;41:1069–77.
21. Prestige BR, Bice WS, Kiefer EJ, et al. Timing of computed tomography-based postimplant assessment following permanent transperineal prostate brachytherapy. Int J Radiat Oncol Biol Phys 1998;40:1111–5.
22. Speight JL, Shinohara K, Pickett B, et al. Prostate volume change after radioactive seed implantation: possible benefit of improved dose volume histogram with perioperative steroid. Int J Radiat Oncol Biol Phys 2000;48:1461–7.
23. Stock R, Stone N, Tabert A, et al. A dose-response study for I-125 prostate implants. Int J Radiat Oncol Biol Phys 1998;41:101–8.
24. Potters L, Cao Y, Calugaru E, et al. A comprehensive review of CT-based dosimetry parameters and biochemical control in patients treated with permanent prostate brachytherapy. Int J Radiat Oncol Biol Phys 2001;50:605–14.
25. Lessard E, Pouliot J. Inverse planning anatomy-based dose optimization for HDR-brachytherapy of the prostate using fast simulated annealing algorithm and dedicated objective function. Med Phys 2001;28:773–9.
26. Kolkman-Deurloo IKK, Visser AG, Niël CGJH, et al. Optimization of interstitial volume implants. Radiother Oncol 1994;31:229–39.
27. Brenner DJ, Hall EJ. Fractionation and protraction for radiotherapy of prostate carcinoma. Int J Radiat Oncol Biol Phys 1999;43:1095–101.
28. King CR, Fowler JF. A simple analytic derivation suggests that prostate cancer alpha/beta ratio is low. Int J Radiat Oncol Biol Phys 2001;51:213–4.
29. Fowler J, Chappell R, Ritter M. Is alpha/beta for prostate tumors really low? Int J Radiat Oncol Biol Phys 2001; 50:1021–31.
30. Duchesne GM, Peters LJ. What is the alpha/beta ratio for prostate cancer? Rationale for hypofractionated high-dose-rate brachytherapy [editorial]. Int J Radiat Oncol Biol Phys 1999;44:747–8.
31. Hsu I-C, Pickett B, Shinohara K, et al. Normal tissue dosimetric comparison between HDR prostate implant boost and conformal external beam radiotherapy boost: potential for dose escalation. Int J Radiat Oncol Biol Phys 2000;46:851–8.
32. D'Souza WD, Thames HD. Is the alpha/beta ratio for prostate cancer low? Int J Radiat Oncol Biol Phys 2001;51:1–3.
33. Yoshioka Y, Nose T, Yoshida K, et al. High-dose-rate interstitial brachytherapy as a monotherapy for localized prostate cancer: treatment description and preliminary results of a phase I/II clinical trial. Int J Radiat Oncol Biol Phys 2000; 48:675–81.
34. Martinez AA, Pataki I, Edmundson G, et al. Phase II prospective study of the use of conformal high-dose-rate brachytherapy as monotherapy for the treatment of favorable stage prostate cancer: a feasibility report. Int J Radiat Oncol Biol Phys 2001;49:61–9.
35. Critz FA, Tarlton RS, Holladay DA. Prostate specific antigen-monitored combination radiotherapy for patients with prostate cancer. I-125 implant followed by external-beam radiation. Cancer 1995;75:2383–91.
36. Critz FA, Levinson AK, Williams WH, et al. Simultaneous radiotherapy for prostate cancer: 125I prostate implant followed by external-beam radiation. Cancer J Sci Am 1998;4:359–63.
37. Wang H, Wallner K, Sutlief S, et al. Transperineal brachytherapy in patients with large prostate glands. Int J Cancer 2000;90:199–205.
38. Stone NN, Stock RG. Prostate brachytherapy in patients with prostate volumes >/= 50 cm(3): dosimetic analysis of implant quality. Int J Radiat Oncol Biol Phys 2000;46: 1199–204.
39. Thomas MD, Cormack R, Tempany CM, et al. Identifying the predictors of acute urinary retention following magnetic-resonance-guided prostate brachytherapy. Int J Radiat Oncol Biol Phys 2000;47:905–8.
40. Merrick GS, Butler WM, Galbreath RW, et al. Relationship between the transition zone index of the prostate gland

and urinary morbidity after brachytherapy. Urology 2001; 57:524–9.

41. Zelefsky MJ, Whitmore WF Jr. Long-term results of retropubic permanent 125 iodine implantation of the prostate for clinically localized prostatic cancer. J Urol 1997;158: 23–9; discussion 29–30.
42. Schellhammer PF, Moriarty R, Bostwick D, Kuban D. Fifteen-year minimum follow-up of a prostate brachytherapy series: comparing the past with the present. Urology 2000;56:436–9.
43. Critz FA, Williams WH, Holladay CT, et al. Post-treatment PSA < or = 0.2 ng/mL defines disease freedom after radiotherapy for prostate cancer using modern techniques. Urology 1999;54:968–71.
44. Blasko JC, Wallner K, Grimm PD, Ragde H. Prostate specific antigen based disease control following ultrasound guided 125 iodine implantation for stage T1/T2 prostatic carcinoma. J Urol 1995;154:1096–9.
45. Ragde H, Blasko JC, Grimm PD, et al. Interstitial iodine-125 radiation without adjuvant therapy in the treatment of clinically localized prostate carcinoma. Cancer 1997;80: 442–53.
46. Ragde H, Elgamal AA, Snow PB, et al. Ten-year disease free survival after transperineal sonography-guided iodine-125 brachytherapy with or without 45-gray external beam irradiation in the treatment of patients with clinically localized, low to high Gleason grade prostate carcinoma. Cancer 1998;83:989–1001.
47. Grimm P, Blasko J, Sylvester J, et al. 10-year biochemical (prostate-specific antigen) control of prostate cancer with I-125 brachytherapy. Int J Radiat Oncol Biol Phys 2000; 51:31–40.
48. Blasko JC, Ragde H, Grimm PD. Transperineal ultrasound guided palladium-103 brachytherapy for prostate carcinoma. J Urol 1995;153:385.
49. Beyer DC, Priestley JB Jr. Biochemical disease-free survival following 125I prostate implantation. Int J Radiat Oncol Biol Phys 1997;37:559–63.
50. Priestly JB, Beyer DC. Guided brachytherapy for treatment of confined prostate cancer. Urology 1992;40:27–32.
51. Wallner K, Roy J, Zelefsky M. Short-term freedom from disease progression after I-125 prostate implantation. Int J Radiat Oncol Biol Phys 1994;30:405.
52. Wallner K, Roy J, Harrison L. Tumor control and morbidity following transperineal iodine 125 implantation for stage T1/T2 prostatic carcinoma. J Clin Oncol 1996;14:449–53.
53. Stone NN, Ramin SA, Wesson MF, et al. Laparoscopic pelvic lymph node dissection combined with real-time interactive transrectal ultrasound guided transperineal radioactive seed implantation of the prostate. J Urol 1995;153:1555–60.
54. Stock RG, Stone NN, DeWyngaert JK, et al. Prostate specific antigen findings and biopsy results following interactive ultrasound guided transperineal brachytherapy for early stage prostate carcinoma. Cancer 1996;77:2386–92.
55. Sharkey J, Chovnick SD, Behar RJ, et al. Outpatient ultrasound-guided palladium 103 brachytherapy for localized adenocarcinoma of the prostate: a preliminary report of 434 patients. Urology 1998;51:796–803.
56. Stokes SH, Real JD, Adams PW, et al. Transperineal ultrasound-guided radioactive seed implantation for organ-confined carcinoma of the prostate. Int J Radiat Oncol Biol Phys 1997;37:337–41.
57. Critz FA, Levinson AK, Williams WH, Holladay DA. Prostate-specific antigen nadir: the optimum level after irradiation for prostate cancer. J Clin Oncol 1996;14:2893–900.
58. Zeitlin SI, Sherman J, Raboy A, et al. High dose combination radiotherapy for the treatment of localized prostate cancer. J Urol 1998;160:91–6.
59. Dattoli M, Wallner K, Sorace R, et al. 103Pd brachytherapy and external beam irradiation for clinically localized, high-risk prostatic carcinoma. Int J Radiat Oncol Biol Phys 1996;35:875–9.
60. Prestidge B, Butler B, Shaw D, McComas V. Ultrasound guided placement of transperineal prostatic afterloading catheters. Int J Radiat Oncol Biol Phys 1993;28:263–6.
61. Khan K, Thompson W, Bush S, Stidley C. Transperineal percutaneous iridium-192 intersititial template implant of the prostate: results and complications in 321 patients. Int J Radiat Oncol Biol Phys 1992;22:935–9.
62. Syed AMN, Puthawala A, Austin P, et al. Temporary iridium-192 implant in the management of carcinoma of the prostate. Cancer 1992;69:2515–24.
63. Stromberg J, Martinez A, Benson R, et al. Improved local control and survival for surgically staged patients with locally advanced prostate cancer treated with up-front low dose rate iridium-192 prostate implantation and external beam irradiation. Int J Radiat Oncol Biol Phys 1994;28:67–75.
64. Brindle J, Martinez A, Schray M, et al. Pelvic lymphadenectomy and transperineal interstitial implantation of Ir-192 combined with external beam radiotherapy for bulky stage C prostate carcinoma. Int J Radiat Oncol Biol Phys 1989;17:1063–6.
65. Donnelly BJ, Pedersen JE, Porter AT, McPhee MS. Iridium 192 brachytherapy in the treatment of cancer of the prostate. Urol Clin North Am 1991;18:481–3.
66. Kovacs G, Wirth B, Bertermann H, et al. Prostate preservation by combined external beam and HDR brachytherapy at nodal negative prostate cancer patients—an intermediate analysis after ten years experience. Int J Radiat Oncol Biol Phys 1996;36:198.
67. Kovács G, Galalae R, Loch T, et al. Prostate preservation by combined external beam and HDR brachytherapy in nodal negative prostate cancer. Strahlenther Onkol 1999;175 Suppl 2:87–8.
68. Mate T, Gottesman J. Fractionated HDR conformal prostate brachytherapy. Presented at the 8th International Brachytherapy Conference, 1995.
69. Mate TP, Gottesman JE, Hatton J, et al. High dose-rate afterloading 192 Iridium prostate brachytherapy: feasibility report. Int J Radiat Oncol Biol Phys 1998;41:525–33.
70. Martinez A, Orton C, Mould R. Brachytherapy HDR and LDR. In: Bertermann H, Brix F, editors. Ultrasound guided interstitial high dose brachytherapy with iridium-192: technique and preliminary results in locally confined prostate cancer. Columbia (MD): Nucletron; 1990. p. 281–303.
71. Martinez A, Gonzalez J, Stromberg J, et al. Conformal prostate brachytherapy: initial experience of a phase I/II dose-escalating trial. Int J Radiat Oncol Biol Phys 1995; 33:1019–27.
72. Martinez AA, Kestin LL, Stromberg JS, et al. Interim report of image-guided conformal high-dose-rate brachytherapy for patients with unfavorable prostate cancer: The William Beaumont Phase II dose-escalating trial. Int J Radiat Oncol Biol Phys 2000;47:343–52.

73. Stromberg JS, Martinez AA, Horwitz EM, et al. Conformal high dose rate iridium-192 boost brachytherapy in locally advanced prostate cancer: superior prostate-specific antigen response compared with external beam treatment. Cancer J Sci Am 1997;3:346–52.
74. Borghede G, Hedelin H, Holmäng S, et al. Irradiation of localized prostatic carcinoma with a combination of high dose rate iridium-192 brachytherapy and external beam radiotherapy with three target definitions and dose levels inside the prostate gland. Radiother Oncol 1997;44:245–50.
75. Borghede G, Hedelin H, Holmäng S, et al. Combined treatment with temporary short-term high dose rate iridium-192 brachytherapy and external beam radiotherapy for irradiation of localized prostatic carcinoma. Radiother Oncol 1997;44:237–44.
76. Dinges S, Deger S, Koswig S, et al. High-dose rate interstitial with external beam irradiation for localized prostate cancer—results of a prospective trial. Radiother Oncol 1998;48:197–202.
77. Joly F, Brune D, Couette JE, et al. Health-related quality of life and sequelae in patients treated with brachytherapy and external beam irradiation for localized prostate cancer. Ann Oncol 1998;9:751–7.
78. Wallner K, Lee H, Wasserman S, Dattoli M. Low risk of urinary incontinence following prostate brachytherapy in patients with a prior transurethreal prostate resection. Int J Radiat Oncol Biol Phys 1997;37:565–9.
79. Han BH, Demel KC, Wallner K, et al. Patient reported complications after prostate brachytherapy. J Urol 2001;166: 953–7.
80. Lee WR, McQuellon RP, McCullough DL. A prospective analysis of patient-reported quality of life after prostate brachytherapy. Sem Urol Oncol 2000;18:147–51.
81. Borghede G, Sullivan M. Measurement of quality of life in localized prostatic cancer patients treated with radiotherapy — development of a prostate cancer-specific module supplementing the EORTC Qlq-C30. Qual Life Res 1996; 5:212–22.
82. Cella DF, Tulsky DS, Gray G, et al. The Functional Assessment of Cancer Therapy scale: development and validation of the general measure. J Clin Oncol 1993;11:570–9.
83. Dale W, Campbell T, Ignacio L, et al. Self-assessed health-related quality of life in men being treated for prostate cancer with radiotherapy: instrument validation and its relation to patient-assessed bother of symptoms. Urology 1999;53:359–66.
84. Esper P, Mo F, Chodak G, et al. Measuring quality of life in men with prostate cancer using the functional assessment of cancer therapy-prostate instrument. Urology 1997;50: 920–8.
85. Barry MJ, Fowler FJ Jr, O'Leary MP, et al. The American Urological Association symptom index for benign prostatic hyperplasia. The Measurement Committee of the American Urological Association. J Urol 1992;148: 1549–57; discussion 1564.
86. Litwin MS, Hays RD, Fink A, et al. The UCLA Prostate Cancer Index—development, reliability, and validity of a health-related quality of life measure. Med Care 1998; 36:1002–12.
87. Wei JT, Dunn RL, Litwin MS, et al. Development and validation of the expanded prostate cancer index composite (EPIC) for comprehensive assessment of health-related quality of life in men with prostate cancer. Urology 2000; 56:899–905.
88. Stockler MR, Osoba D, Corey P, et al. Convergent discriminitive, and predictive validity of the Prostate Cancer Specific Quality of Life Instrument (PROSQOLI) assessment and comparison with analogous scales from the EORTC QLQ-C30 and a trial-specific module. J Clin Epidemiol 1999;52:653–66.
89. Gelblum DY, Potters L. Rectal complications associated with transperineal interstitial brachytherapy for prostate cancer. Int J Radiat Oncol Biol Phys 2000;48:119–24.
90. Davis JW, Schellhammer PF. Prostatorectal fistula 14 years following brachytherapy for prostate cancer. J Urol 2001; 165:189.
91. Davis BJ, Pfeifer EA, Wilson TM, et al. Prostate brachytherapy seed migration to the right ventricle found at autopsy following acute cardiac dysrhythmia. J Urol 2000;164: 1661.
92. Cherr GS, Hall C, Pineau BC, Waters GS. Rectourethral fistula and massive rectal bleeding from iodine-125 prostate brachytherapy: a case report. Am Surg 2001;67:131–4.
93. Merrick GS, Butler WM, Dorsey AT, et al. Rectal function following prostate brachytherapy. Int J Radiat Oncol Biol Phys 2000;48:667–74.
94. Merrick GS, Butler WM, Dorsey AT, Dorsey JT 3rd. The effect of constipation on rectal dosimetry following prostate brachytherapy. Med Dosim 2000;25:237–41.
95. Smith S, Wallner K, Dominitz JA, et al. Argon plasma coagulation for rectal bleeding after prostate brachytherapy. Int J Radiat Oncol Biol Phys 2001;51:636–42.
96. Brandeis JM, Litwin MS, Burnison CM, Reiter RE. Quality of life outcomes after brachytherapy for early stage prostate cancer. J Urol 2000;163:851–7.
97. Seung SK, Kroll S, Wilder RB, et al. Candidates for prostate radioactive seed implantation treated by external beam radiotherapy Cancer J Sci Am 1998;4:168–74.
98. Beyer DC, Brachman DG. Failure free survival following brachytherapy alone for prostate cancer: comparison with external beam radiotherapy. Radiother Oncol 2000;57: 263–7.
99. D'Amico AV, Whittington R, Malkowicz SB, et al. Biochemical outcome after radical prostatectomy, external beam radiation therapy, or interstitial radiation therapy for clinically localized prostate cancer. JAMA 1998;280:969–74.
100. King CR, Sanzone J, Anderson KR. Definitive therapy for stage T1/T2 prostate carcinoma: PSA-based comparison between surgery, external beam, and implant radiotherapy. Int J Brachyther 1998;14:169–77.
101. Krupski T, Petroni GR, Bissonette EA, Theodorescu D. Quality-of-life comparison of radical prostatectomy and interstitial brachytherapy in the treatment of clinically localized prostate cancer. Urology 2000;55:736–42.
102. Davis JW, Kuban DA, Lynch DF, Schellhammer PF. Quality of life after treatment for localized prostate cancer: differences based on treatment modality. J Urol 2001;166:947–52.
103. Lee WR, Hall MC, McQuellon RP, et al. A prospective quality-of-life study in men with clinically localized prostate carcinoma treated with radical prostatectomy, external beam radiotherapy, or interstitial brachytherapy. Int J Radiat Oncol Biol Phys 2001;51:614–23.

18

New Forms of Focal Therapy

KATSUTO SHINOHARA, MD

The treatment of prostate cancer remains controversial. Radical prostatectomy, radiation therapy, and watchful waiting are options for clinically localized prostate cancer, and their risks and benefits are frequently discussed. Radical prostatectomy has been perceived as morbid, with decreased quality of life after treatment, whereas radiation therapy has been criticized for its uncertain efficacy.[1–3] Although surveillance may be an early option for some patients, such patients frequently receive more conventional treatment in follow-up.[4] Such concerns regarding conventional treatment have stimulated a search by both patients and physicians for alternative treatments, which may be effective and associated with limited morbidity.

In experienced hands, and when carried out for the appropriate indication, radical surgery is associated with minimal mortality and acceptably low morbidity rates and remains the treatment of choice among many for localized prostate cancer in healthy, younger (<60 years) patients.[5–7] The optimal therapy for older patients or patients with locally advanced disease (T3) is more controversial.[6] The need for treatment of older (>70 years) patients is uncertain, and treatment may be associated with high complication rates in this population.[1] Patients with stage T3 disease have a higher risk of local recurrence (compared with patients with T1 and T2 disease) when treated with conventional therapies.[8] In addition, treatment options for local failure after primary treatment are limited. Such salvage treatment has been associated with significant morbidity and limited efficacy.[9,10] Attention has recently focused on alternative minimally invasive therapy as a potential treatment that may be applicable to the older patient, any patient with T3 disease, or the patient who develops local recurrence after primary therapy.[11]

Many different energy sources have been under investigation for ablation of benign prostate hyperplasia and prostate cancer. These energy sources include electric or water-induced heat conduction,[12] microwave,[13] radiofrequency,[14] laser,[15] high-intensity focused ultrasonography (HIFU),[16] photodynamic therapy,[17] and cryoablation[18] (Table 18–1). This chapter describes the current status of minimally invasive treatment modalities for prostate cancer using such energy sources.

BIOLOGIC BASIS OF THERMAL AND CRYOABLATION

Thermal Effect

Heat applied to tissue results in various changes in cellular composition. Cytoplasmic and nuclear protein denaturation, deoxyribonucleic acid (DNA) and ribonucleic acid (RNA) changes, and cellular membrane function change are observed. Of those, it is assumed that proteins are the molecules at risk for cell inactivation by heat.[19] Treatments using heat to destroy tissue are generally divided into three categories (Table 18–2). Hyperthermia is a treatment with tissue temperature below 46°C. This does not create tissue necrosis, but it changes tissue compositions that can be repared completely. Cellular membrane permeability and cell metabolism are increased. Also, increased tissue blood perfusion and subsequent tissue oxygen partial pressure are observed. During the period of tissue change, cells are more susceptible to other insults, such as radiation or chemotherapy.

Table 18–1. ENERGY SOURCES APPLICABLE TO PROSTATE ABLATION

- Cryogenic
  - Liquid nitrogen
  - Liquid argon
- Thermal ablation
  - External
    - High-intensity focused ultrasound (HIFU)
    - Microwave
    - Radiofrequency
    - Water-induced heat conduction
  - Interstitial
    - Radiofrequency (RITA)
    - Ferromagnetic thermal ablation
    - Microwave
    - Interstitial LASER
    - Resistance wire heater
    - Water-induced heat conduction
    - Tubular ultrasound radiators
- Others
  - Interstitial photon radiation
  - Photodynamic therapy
  - Chemical ablation (absolute ethanol)
  - Biologic ablation (adenovirus)

Thermotherapy is defined as a treatment temperature between 46°C and 70°C. With this tissue temperature, nonreversible cellular protein denaturation takes place, resulting in coagulative tissue necrosis in the treatment area. However, tissue temperature has to be sustained for a long period of time (30 minutes or longer) to produce a large area of tissue necrosis. Thermoablation requires tissue temperature of more than 70°C. Cell death is almost immediately achieved with this temperature, and an extensive coagulative necrosis is created. Therefore, the tissue destruction is a product of tissue temperature and treatment time. A low tissue temperature requires a longer treatment time, whereas a high-temperature treatment produces the same tissue effect in a short period of time. This relation is expressed as a thermal isoeffect dose (Figure 18–1).

Table 18–2. CLASSIFICATION OF HEAT THERAPY

	Temperature	Tissue Effect
Hyperthermia	41–45°C	Reversible Increased cellular metabolism, cell wall permeability, and blood flow
Thermotherapy	46–70°C	Irreversible Cellular death with sustained time
Thermoablation	> 70°C	Cellular death immediately

Cryogenic Effect

The mechanism of cell death after freezing has been carefully analyzed in the past. There are multiple factors that result in tissue necrosis. The two parameters that correlate with the likelihood of cell destruction are the cooling rate during freezing and the lowest temperature achieved. Cell death may occur owing to chemical damage or intracellular ice formation.[20] Zippe summarized this destructive process as follows: Freezing of the extracellular compartment and withdrawal of water from the cells occurs at –15°C, creating dehydration. Intracellular ice crystal formation occurs at –20°C to –40°C, leading to mechanical cellular wall damage and denaturation of the proteins. Thawing results in fluid shift into the cells and cellular wall disruption. Cell death may be mediated by ischemia owing to vascular thrombosis precipitated by the freezing of the vessels.[21]

Tatsutani and colleagues described the effect of tissue temperature and rate of freezing in an in vivo prostate cancer cell experiment.[22] These investigators showed that complete cell death is unlikely to occur at temperatures higher than –20°C, and temperatures lower than –40°C are required to completely destroy cells. Larson and colleagues reported that cryoablation results in two tissue zones: a central zone of complete cellular necrosis surrounded by a more

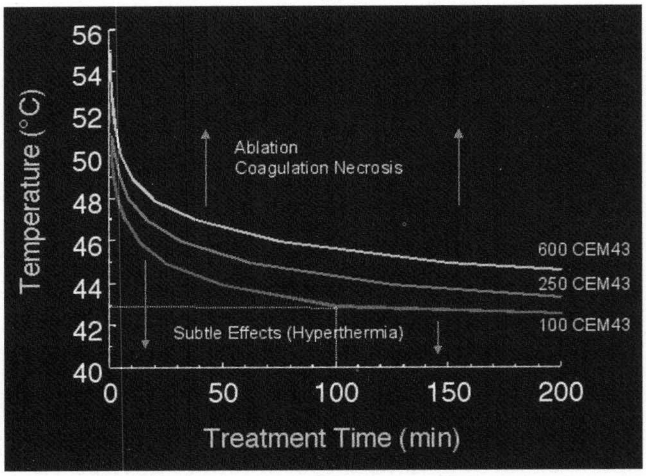

Figure 18–1. Tissue temperature and length of treatment define thermal isoeffect dose. CEM43 stands for cumulative equivalent minutes at 43°C. 100 CEM 43 is the thermal effect equivalent to 100 minutes of 43°C treatment. More than 600 CEM 43 causes coagulative necrosis (thermotherapy), whereas less than 100 CEM 43 causes a subtle tissue effect (hyperthermia). Adapted from Chris Diederich, PhD, personal communication.

peripheral zone of cell damage but not necrosis.[23] The central zone of complete cellular necrosis can be significantly enlarged by a second freezing cycle (Figure 18–2). In a historical study by Gage, it was described that a double-freezing process created a larger area of tissue necrosis than single freezing, even though the achieved temperatures were no different in both groups.[24] The experiment by Tatsutani and colleagues previously described showed that the rate of temperature change and number of freezing cycles significantly influenced the required temperature for cell death.[22]

Compared with thermoablation, which requires a temperature change less than 10°C from body temperature to create cell death, cryoablation requires more than 70°C of temperature change. Because the temperature gradation is so wide, cryoablation creates a rather unclear boundary of necrosis with a tissue mixed with vital and nonvital cells at the edge. Thermal ablation can create more clearly demarcated areas of tissue necrosis; however, on the other hand, it can be affected more easily by the existence of heat sinks, such as vessels.

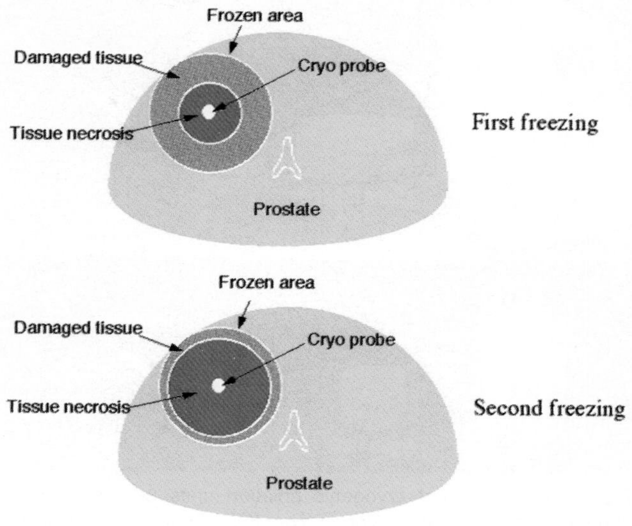

Figure 18–2. With cryoablation, first freezing causes tissue necrosis surrounded by damaged tissue that is not necessarily nonviable tissue. On second freezing, the area of tissue necrosis significantly enlarges, and the amount of damaged tissue area reduces.

CRYOABLATION OF PROSTATE

History

The first report describing cryoablation of benign prostate hyperplasia using circulating liquid nitrogen in a closed system appeared in 1966.[25] An attempt to destroy prostate cancer by using a transperineally introduced probe was reported by Reuter in 1972.[26] That same year, urologists at the University of Iowa reported their experience with the open transperineal approach of cryoablation to treat patients with various stages of prostate cancer.[27] These initial attempts to effectively treat prostate cancer failed for a variety of reasons, including an inability to effectively monitor the freezing process. In 1984, Onik and colleagues demonstrated that the frozen area could be seen as a well-marginated hyperechoic rim with acoustic shadowing monitored by ultrasonography.[28] As transrectal ultrasound technology was in widespread use in the 1990s for the early detection of prostate cancer, a transperineal, percutaneously introduced, multiple-cryoprobe system for prostate cancer treatment was developed.[29] The first clinical application of such a system was reported in 1993.[18]

Equipment and Procedure

Currently, three cryosurgical devices for prostate cancer treatment are available in the United States. The CMS AccuProbe system (Cryo Medical Sciences, Inc, Ewing, New Jersey) uses ultra-cooled liquid nitrogen in which the nitrogen is compressed and cooled to –206°C. At this temperature, the liquid nitrogen becomes partly frozen (slush). This will cool tissue to approximately –185°C. The Cryocare system (Endocare, Inc, Irvine, California) uses liquid argon as the source of freezing and can freeze up to eight probes simultaneously. More recently, a system developed by Galil (Galil Medical USA, Woburn, Massachusetts) uses liquid argon as a cryogen, and up to 30 needle-shaped probes can be used to create a more conformal freezing pattern.

Liquid nitrogen or argon is delivered through a thin lumen in the center to the tip of the probe. Partially evaporated gas returns through the outer chamber just underneath the surface of the probe. The Joule-Thompson principle of an expanding gas draws heat into the circulating gas (Figure 18–3).

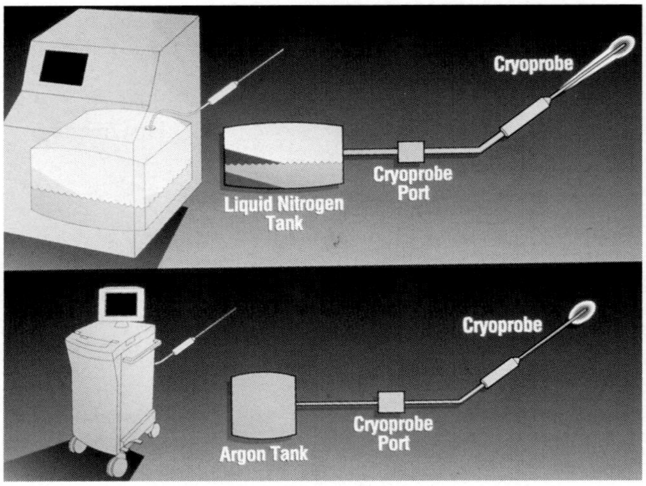

Figure 18–3. Current cryogenic ablation units use either liquid nitrogen or argon as the cryogen. The Joule-Thompson principle of an expanding gas draws heat into the gas circulating through the probe tip.

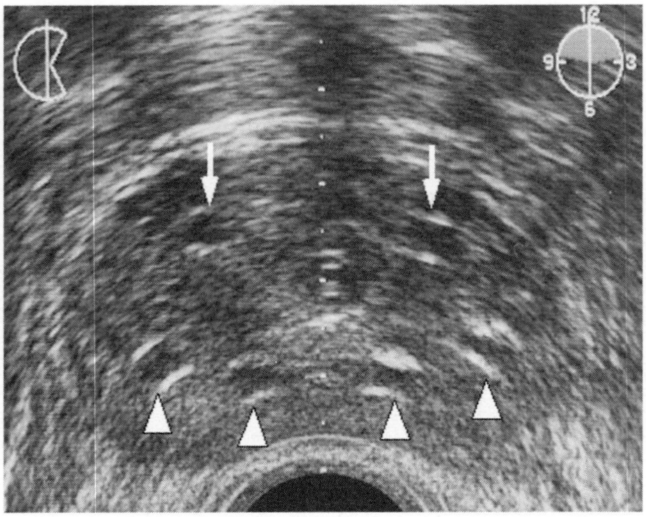

Figure 18–4. A transrectal ultrasonographic image after dilation of tracts just before insertion of cryoprobes. Generally, two anterior tracts (*arrows*) and four posterior tracts (*arrowheads*) are dilated for the preparation of probe insertion.

Procedure

Patients undergo light bowel preparation consisting of oral magnesium citrate the day before the procedure and have a Fleet enema the morning of the procedure. After induction of regional or general anesthesia, the patient is placed in the lithotomy position. A transrectal ultrasound probe is inserted in the rectum, and the prostate gland is carefully examined for size and tumor location. The exact positioning of each needle and probe is determined at this point. An 18-gauge, diamond-tipped, hollow-core needle is inserted into the prostate gland under ultrasound guidance. The needle locations are seen as bright dots on ultrasound imaging. Each needle is advanced up to the desired location (usually up to the base of the prostate). Generally, six needles are inserted: two anteromedially, two posterolaterally, and two posteromedially (Figure 18–4). To avoid urethral freezing, needles are placed at least 8 mm from the urethra. Once the needle is in position, a guidewire is advanced through, and dilators followed by 12F cannulas are inserted into the prostate over the guidewires.

Prior to the placement of the cryoprobes, the urethral warmer must be in position, and irrigation with warm saline must be started. The cryoprobes are placed, and the cannulas are retracted to expose the tip of each probe. The probes are secured in position by freezing each probe to –50 to 70°C ("stick" temperature). This will create a small ice ball around the tip of each probe. The cryogen (liquid argon or nitrogen) is circulated through the anterior probes first, and the resulting freezing zones or "ice balls" are monitored by ultrasonography. The ice ball is allowed to extend posteriorly and laterally. The posterior ice balls are allowed to extend to the muscularis propria of the rectal wall (Figure 18–5). Freez-

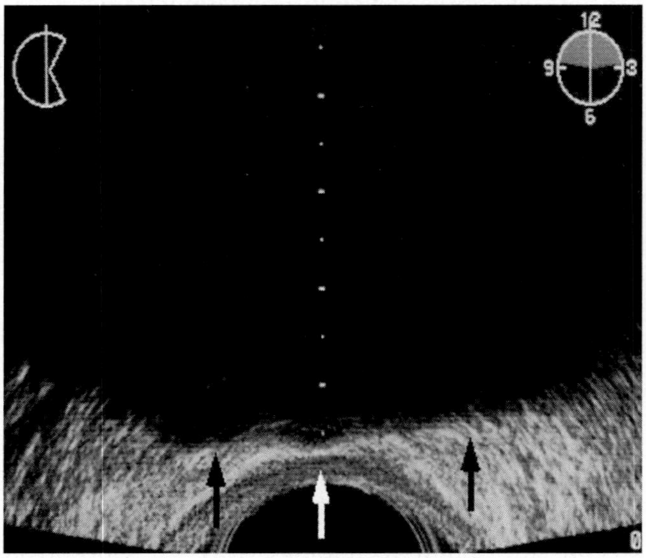

Figure 18–5. Frozen edge is clearly visible by transrectal ultrasonography (*black arrows*). The ice ball is allowed to extend to touch the propria muscularis of the rectum (*white arrow*).

ing beyond this may result in damage to the rectum and formation of a rectourethral fistula. Most surgeons routinely perform two freeze/thaw cycles in all patients. If the ice ball does not adequately extend to the apex of the prostate, the cryoprobes are pulled backward into the apex, and additional freezing is performed. Patients who undergo cryosurgery alone rarely require hospitalization, and the procedure is usually performed on an ambulatory basis. A urethral or suprapubic catheter is left in place for 3 weeks as such a period of catheterization appears to be associated with a lower likelihood of postoperative tissue sloughing and urinary retention.

Results of Primary Therapy

Local Control

Commonly, patients who have been treated with cryotherapy have undergone repeat prostatic biopsy 6 to 12 months after the procedure. The positive biopsy rate after cryoablation ranges between 7.7 and 25 percent (Table 18–3). There is a relationship, not surprisingly, between clinical stage and the likelihood of a positive post-treatment biopsy following cryotherapy. The likelihood of a positive biopsy is approximately 9% for those with clinical stages T1 and T2 disease and at least 21 percent for those with T3 disease.[30] Shinohara and colleagues reported a 64 percent positive biopsy rate in 15 patients treated with a single freeze/thaw cycle. The local recurrence rate was significantly lowered to 11 percent in 63 patients treated with two freeze/thaw cycles.[31] A similar result was reported by Pisters and colleagues in radiation-recurrent prostate cancer cases. A 29 percent positive biopsy rate was observed in cases treated with a single freeze/thaw cycle, whereas only 9 percent were positive for residual cancer in the group treated with two freeze/thaw cycles.[31] Lee and colleagues reported significantly less residual glandular tissue in cases treated by a six- to eight-probe system compared with cases treated by a conventional five-probe system.[32]

Recurrence was more common in cancers located at the apex and seminal vesicles in contrast to those located in the midgland and base.[33,34]

Biochemical Failure

The serum prostate-specific antigen (PSA) level after a definitive form of treatment such as radical prostatectomy or radiation therapy has been shown to be an important determinant of eventual outcome. Serum PSA levels after cryosurgery reported from several series are summarized in Table 18–3. What constitutes an acceptable PSA following cryotherapy has not been well evaluated. Radiation or cryotherapy does not result in complete destruction of all prostate tissue. Detectable levels of PSA may be attributable to either malignant or benign epithelial elements. Therefore, a low but stable PSA after cryotherapy may not be associated with disease progression as seen in radiation therapy.[35] Biochemical failure (subsequent rise in PSA > 0.2 ng/mL) appears to be lowest in those who achieve PSA nadirs < 0.1 ng/mL (21%) and is more common in those with higher nadir values. Moreover, biopsy failure also appears to be lowest

Table 18–3. RESULTS OF PROSTATE CRYOSURGERY

Study	Number of Patients	Residual Cancer, %	Post-treatment Prostate-Specific Antigen
Onik et al, 1993[18]	23	17.4	2.8 ng/mL (mean 3 mo)
Miller et al, 1994[87]	62	21.0	0.59 ± 1.66 ng/mL (mean 3 mo)
Bahn et al, 1995[34]	130	7.7	0.35 ± 0.75 ng/mL
Coogan and McKiel, 1995[42]	87	17.0	≤ 0.2 ng/mL in 33.3% (1 yr)
Weider et al, 1995[45]	61	13.1	< 0.5 ng/mL in 57.4% (3 mo)
Bales et al, 1995[88]*	23	14.0	< 0.3 ng/mL in 14% (1 yr)
Shinohara et al, 1996[31]	102	23.0	< 0.1 ng/mL in 48% (3 mo)
Wake et al, 1996[89]	63	25.0	< 0.1 ng/mL in 25% (3 mo)
Cohen et al, 1996[43]	383	18.0	< 0.4 ng/mL in 55% (2 yr)
Pisters et al, 1997[39]*	150	18.0	No increase > 0.2 ng/mL in 46%
Lee et al, 1999[32]	81	2.5	0.12 and 0.07 ng/mL (mean and median)
Long et al, 2001[90]	975	18	< 0.5 in 60%, 45% and 36% for low-, intermediate-, and high-risk group (5 yr)
Chin et al, 2001[91]*	118	6	< 0.5 ng/mL in 34% (50 mo)

*Radiation failure cases only.

in those with PSA nadirs < 0.1 ng/mL (1.5%) and those with nadirs < 0.4 ng/mL (10%). In contrast, 55% of patients with PSA nadir values > 0.5 ng/mL had a positive prostate biopsy in follow-up.[33] Greene and colleagues similarly showed that a serum PSA > 0.5 ng/mL was highly predictive of biopsy and biochemical failure after cryotherapy.[36] Long and colleagues analyzed a very well-characterized series of 145 patients.[37] The crude rates of maintaining either a negative biopsy or a serum PSA < 0.3 ng/mL at 6 and 24 months after the procedure were 87 and 73 percent, respectively. However, the overall actuarial rate at 42 months of maintaining a serum PSA < 0.3 ng/mL was 59 percent. Gould described 27 cases of "total cryosurgery" in which concomitant transurethral resection was performed to remove any transition or central zone tissue not ablated by the freezing process.[38] A post-treatment PSA level of < 0.2 ng/mL was achieved in 96 percent of these patients.

Recent advancement in technique has improved the results significantly. Double freezing, the use of thermosensors, increasing the number of probes, and removal of remaining urethral tissue with transurethral resection of the prostate (TURP) all appeared to improve the outcomes of the procedure.

Results of Salvage Therapy After Radiation

Treatment options for those who fail locally after radiation therapy are limited. Salvage cryosurgery has been offered to patients with residual/recurrent cancer in the absence of metastatic disease. Pisters and colleague reported a PSA relapse-free rate of 66 percent and a biopsy-negative rate of 93 percent in those who were treated with two consecutive freeze/thaw cycles.[39] However, the complication rate was significant, with urinary incontinence and urinary obstruction occurring in 73 and 67 percent of their patients, respectively. Those with preoperative PSA levels of more than 10 ng/mL and a Gleason score of ≥ 8 were more likely to develop recurrence of disease during follow-up.[40] More recently, de la Taille and colleagues reported the results of 43 cases of salvage cryosurgery. They noted a biochemical failure-free rate of 66 percent at 12 months. Incontinence and urinary obstruction were seen in only 9 percent and 5 percent of the patients, respectively. A PSA nadir level of > 0.1 ng/mL was an independent predictor of eventual biochemical failure.[41]

Complications

Impotence

Impotence after cryosurgery is common. Bahn and colleagues[34] and Coogan and McKiel[42] reported the incidence of impotence after cryosurgery to be 40 and 47 percent, respectively. However, more contemporary series report higher rates of 80 percent or more.[31,37] This is probably because of the use of multiple freeze/thaw cycles and extension of the ice ball beyond the prostate into the area of the neurovascular bundles (Table 18–4).

Incontinence

The incidence of incontinence following cryosurgery varies among series, probably owing to varying definitions of incontinence. In a large series by Cohen and colleagues,[43] incontinence was reported to occur in 4 percent of patients, whereas Cox and Crawford reported that incontinence was found in 27 percent.[44] Shinohara and colleagues noted that patients who underwent TURP after cryosurgery were more likely to suffer incontinence.[31] Incontinence to some degree was observed in more than 70 percent of the patients who underwent cryosurgery for management of recurrent cancer following radiation (see Table 18–4).

Tissue Sloughing

After cryosurgery, prostate tissue becomes necrotic. The necrotic tissue is gradually absorbed and replaced with fibrous tissue. The urethra-warming device protects the urethral tissue from complete freezing. If urethral freezing occurs, necrotic prostate tissue is exposed to the urinary tract and may become infected. Such infection does not respond well to systemic antibiotics because of poor regional blood flow. Tissue may then slough into the urethra. This condition is manifested by irritative and obstructive voiding symptoms. Pyuria is noted as well. Urinary retention is not uncommon. This

Table 18–4. COMPLICATIONS ASSOCIATED WITH PROSTATE CRYOSURGERY

Study	Number of Patients	Tissue Sloughing, %	Impotence, %	Incontinence, %	Rectourethal Fistula, %
Previously untreated prostate cancer					
Bahn et al, 1995[34]	210	NR	40	9	2.4
Cox and Crawford, 1995[44]	63	19	NR	27	3
Wieder et al, 1995[45]	83	3.8	80	2.5	0
Coogan and McKiel, 1995[42]	95	10	47	3.5	1
Cohen et al, 1996[43]	239	9.8	NR	4	0.4
Sosa et al, 1996[92]	1467	9.9	100	11	1.4
Shinohara et al, 1996[31]	102	23	86	15	1
Long et al, 1998[37]	145	8.9	88	2.0	0
Radiation-recurrent cancer					
Miller et al, 1994[87]	33	15.4	NR	10.3	0
Bales et al, 1995[88]	23	40.9	100	95.5	0
Pisters et al, 1997[39]	150	44	72	73	1.5
Long et al, 1998[37]	18	8.9	88	83	11
de la Taille et al, 2000[41]	43	5	NR	9	0
Chin et al, 2001[91]	118	5.1	NR	33.3	3.3

NR = not reported.

condition typically occurs 3 to 8 weeks after the procedure. Tissue sloughing is reported to occur in 3.8 to 23% of cases after cryoablation.[31,37,42,43,45]

Occasionally, patients complain of pelvic or rectal pain after the procedure. This complication occurs in 0.4 to 11 percent of the patients who undergo cryosurgery.[31,37,42,43,45]

Penile Numbness

Shinohara and colleagues reported that 10 percent of patients treated with cryosurgery developed transient penile numbness.[31]

Rectourethral Fistula

Rectourethral fistula formation is reported to occur in 0 to 3 percent of the patients who undergo cryosurgery of the prostate.[37,44] This complication is most commonly seen in those previously treated with radiation (see Table 18–4).

Urethral Stricture

A urethral stricture rarely forms after cryoablation if an effective urethra-warming device is used at the time of the procedure. However, if extensive tissue sloughing occurs, stricture at the bladder neck or even in the middle of the prostatic urethra can occur. Transurethral incision or balloon dilation is usually successful. Calcification of the stricture may occur, necessitating transurethral resection.

THERMAL ABLATION

The use of heat for the treatment of cancer is not new and predates the use of radiation. Heat has also been used in combination with radiation; however, this clinical application has not become widely accepted.[46] Therapeutic hyperthermia involves inducing a temperature between 41°C and 45°C, within an organism or a part of it, such that the physiologic temperature regulation of the body is partially and temporarily overcome. More recently, higher-temperature therapies known as thermotherapy, thermal therapy, or thermal ablation have been employed for the treatment of cancerous and benign conditions. Thermotherapy uses temperatures greater than 45°C and as high as 100°C in destroying cells. Significant improvement has been noted in using thermotherapy compared to hyperthermia in the treatment of prostate disease.[47] Many methods have been used for the delivery of heat.

Ferromagnetic Thermoablation

Metals with ferrous property are known to produce heat under magnetic field. This occurs through oscillation of the magnetic field, which induces electric current flow (Eddy current) in the metal and produces resistive heat.[48] Based on the composition of ferrous and nonferrous metal in the alloy, it loses its magnetic property at a certain temperature (Curie point transition). This phenomenon results in automatically shutting off the Eddy current. The ThermoRod is an interstitially implantable, small, 14-mm-long, 1-mm-diameter, biocompatible palladium/cobalt alloy rod (Figure 18–6). ThermoRods are placed into the prostate using a minimally invasive technique similar to radioactive seed implantation (brachytherapy), through a transperineal approach using transrectal ultrasonography, and fluoroscopic guidance, with appropriate anesthesia (Figure 18–7). The patient is then treated for an hour with the thermotherapy system which consists of a coil system creating a magnetic field around the patient's pelvis (Figure 18–8). This extracorporeal coil causes heat induction in the percutaneously implanted palladium-cobalt rods. Depending on the cobalt and palladium ratio, the Curie point can be set at various temperatures, such as 55°C, 65°C, and 70°C. This results in an autoregulation of temperature in the treatment area. Each rod heats about 1 to 2 cm^3 of tissue.

Animal Study

A series of studies in dogs were performed using temperature self-regulating interstitial rods.[49] The canine studies demonstrated that interstitial rods with a self-regulating temperature of 55°C achieved adequate tissue ablation. Moderately uniform treatment temperatures were observed with the 55°C rods. This temperature produced necrosis and resulting fibrosis in the dog prostate. Thermal monitoring demonstrated that ablative temperatures were confined

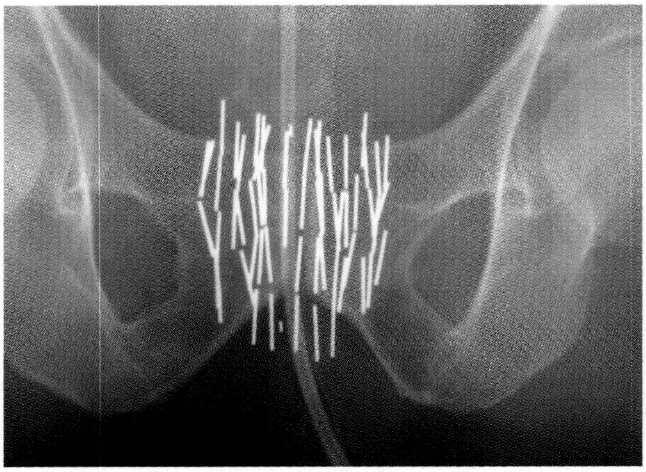

Figure 18–7. Plain radiograph of the pelvis after insertion of ThermoRods in the prostate. ThermoRods are inserted in the prostate transperineally under transrectal ultrasound guidance.

within the prostatic capsule. All dogs tolerated 1 hour of treatment, with no visible side effects or complications. Additional canine studies demonstrated that repeated thermal ablation treatments would be tolerated and effective when separated by 24 hours.

Clinical Study

The initial safety study in humans was performed in prostate cancer patients who had local tumor recurrence following primary radiation therapy. Nine patients had between 14 and 38 self-regulating 55°C rods implanted. Each patient had six 1-hour treatments, during which heat was induced by the application of a magnetic field around the patient's pelvis. The therapy was well tolerated, with no thermal injury and no serious side effects observed with up to 12 months of follow-up. One patient who

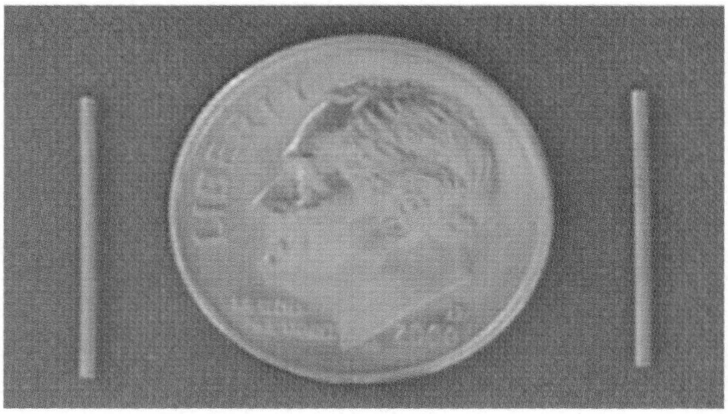

Figure 18–6. The ThermoRod is a biocompatible 14-mm-long, 1-mm-diameter palladium and cobalt alloy rod.

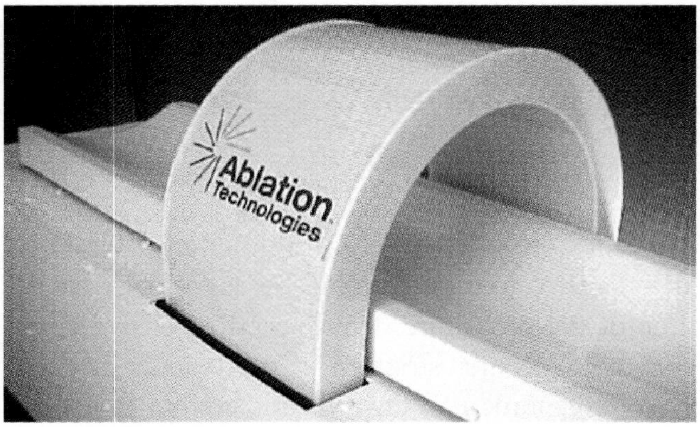

Figure 18–8. Magnetic coil table for ThermoRod treatment.

experienced urinary retention following a treatment session required catheterization, with normal micturition returning within 24 hours.[50]

ThermoRod ablation was carried out in prostate cancer patients who were scheduled to have radical prostatectomy. ThermoRods with Curie points of 55°C, 60°C, and 70°C were used. Radical prostatectomy specimens showed that 70°C ThermoRods implanted at 1-cm intervals created homogeneous tissue necrosis between rods. However, temperature at the edge of array dropped off quickly.[51]

Once the rods are placed, they can provide hyperthermia repeatedly by placing the patient in the treatment coil. ThermoRods with a low Curie point at 55°C are ideal for hyperthermia combined with radiation therapy. Deger and colleagues treated 41 prostate cancer patients with radiation therapy combined with hyperthermia using ThermoRods. No major side effects were observed during the hyperthermia session. The median PSA level decreased from 11.25 ng/mL to 0.88 ng/mL 3 months after treatment and to 0.38 ng/mL 12 months after treatment, with a median follow-up of 10 months.[52]

Salvage Therapy at the University of California at San Francisco

ThermoRod ablation therapy was carried out in 11 patients as a salvage therapy for local recurrence of prostate cancer after radiation therapy.[53] Eleven men enrolled in the study with an average age of 71 years (61–83). All had biopsy-proven cancer in the prostate, with a rising PSA (1.0 to 10.3). The patients had 70°C ThermoRods placed under transrectal ultrasound guidance similar to that of brachytherapy. The urethra was protected by a urethra-cooling catheter during the treatment. All men had preradiation Gleason scores between 3 and 7. The average length of time since radiation was 5.0 years (range 1.1 to 11.4 years). Prostate-specific antien nadir values after radiation ranged between 0.3 and 2.2 ng/mL. Prostatic tissue temperature was homogeneously elevated to > 50°C, whereas rectum and urethra temperature did not exceed 44°C at any point. Data from 10 men were available beyond 6 months of follow-up for review. At 6 months, 6 of 10 (60%) men had a PSA value < 0.1 ng/mL. Two subjects had a continued elevation of PSA after treatment. Two subjects whose PSA dropped below 1 ng/mL by 1-month post-treatment now have a rising PSA (Figure 18–9). Prostate biopsy at 6 months revealed no evidence of disease in nine patients and residual cancer in the seminal vesicle in one patient. The most common side effects were seen in the early subjects with urinary tract infection, obstruction, and urinary incontinence.

Radiofrequency

Radiofrequency energy has been clinically used to treat benign prostatic hyperplasia tissue. Transurethral needle ablation of the prostate has been

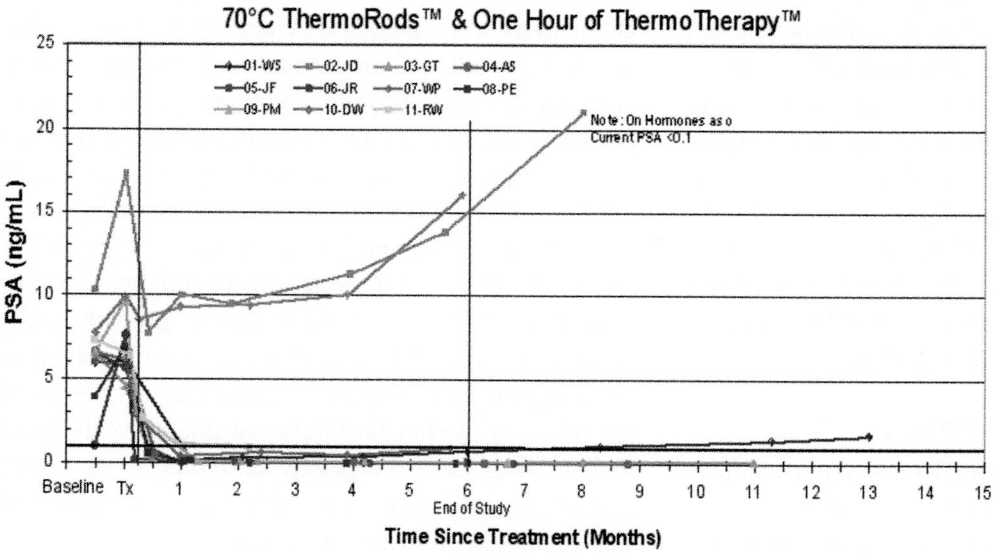

Figure 18–9. Prostate-specific antigen (PSA) changes after ThermoRod treatment in 11 patients with local recurrence of prostate cancer after radiation therapy.

shown to be an effective treatment method for bladder outlet obstruction caused by benign prostatic hyperplasia.[54] However, the transurethral approach is not ideal to treat the periphery of prostate, where most prostate cancers arise. A radiofrequency interstitial tumor ablation (RITA) system (RITA Medical Systems, Inc, Mountain View, California) has been applied to various tumors, such as hepatoma and renal cell carcinoma.[55–57] This system consists of a small needle with multiple antennas that extend from the tip of the needle once the needle is inserted in the tissue (Figure 18–10). The 490-Hz low-power radiowave energy heats the tissues surrounding the multihook antenna to 100°C, resulting in thermal damage and subsequent necrosis of spherical shape tissue, 2 cm in diameter. Multiple needles can be inserted in the tissue to achieve larger areas of necrosis.

The major advantage of this treatment is that it can be performed under local anesthesia. Tissue ablation is achieved rather quickly compared with cryoablation or HIFU (see below). The procedure can be done in the office setting. The antenna is 15 gauge, which is significantly smaller than a cryoprobe and less traumatic to the gland. The major disadvantage is that tissue ablation is not monitorable by ultrasonography. Temperature monitoring and size of possible tissue ablation have to be predetermined to design needle localization.

Technique

The procedure can be performed under general, spinal, or local anesthesia. The patient is placed in the lithotomy position and a TRUS probe is inserted in the rectum. Using ultrasound guidance, a RITA probe is inserted in the prostate transperineally into the area of interest determined by ultrasonographic image. The antennas are extended after insertion of the probes in the designated area, and radiofrequency is applied. The area of treatment is not monitorable by ultrasonography. Treatment control has to be based on the needle position and the theoretical size of the lesion created by RITA.

Clinical Study

Zlotta and colleagues performed 15 RITA procedures using a transperineally placed antenna prior to radical prostatectomy. This study showed a clearly delineated necrotic lesion created in the prostate. The size of the lesions created by RITA on a pathologic specimen correlated well with the predicted size. One patient was treated with multiple RITA procedures only. This patient achieved an undetectable PSA 3 months after the treatment. There was no adverse effect of the treatment observed during or after radical prostatectomy.[58] Radiofrequency interstitial tumor ablation was also performed in 10 prostate cancer patients by Djavan and colleagues. Magnetic resonance imaging (MRI) after the treatment followed by radical prostatectomy was performed in 9 patients. They concluded that the procedure was safe and the lesion was predictable in size and location based on MRI and histologic correlation.[59]

Shariat and colleagues performed RITA on 11 patients with radiation-recurrent adenocarcinoma as a salvage treatment. These treatments were performed under local anesthesia in the clinic setting. Only areas of biopsy-proven cancer were focally ablated. In 90 percent of patients, a PSA decline of more than 50 percent was observed. Follow-up biopsies from the site of ablation were negative in 67 percent of patients. They concluded that this minimally invasive office procedure might delay or prevent progression of tumor. Moreover, repeat RITA may lead to complete eradication of disease.[60]

High-Intensity Focused Ultrasonography (HIFU)

The energy from an ultrasound wave is gradually attenuated and is converted to heat as it travels, achieving thermal ablation in a small area instantaneously. High-intensity focused ultrasonography is an extracorporeal treatment modality that can produce designated areas of tissue necrosis. The technique has been used for treatment of benign prostate hyperplasia in the past.[16,61] The treatment, however, requires general or spinal anesthesia, and the treatment time can be very long. These facts have discouraged the procedure as a minimally invasive treatment modality for benign prostatic hyperplasia. Because tissue ablation produced by HIFU is predictable and controllable with direct vision using ultrasonography and precise computer control, recent interest has shifted the application of this technology to cancer treatment.

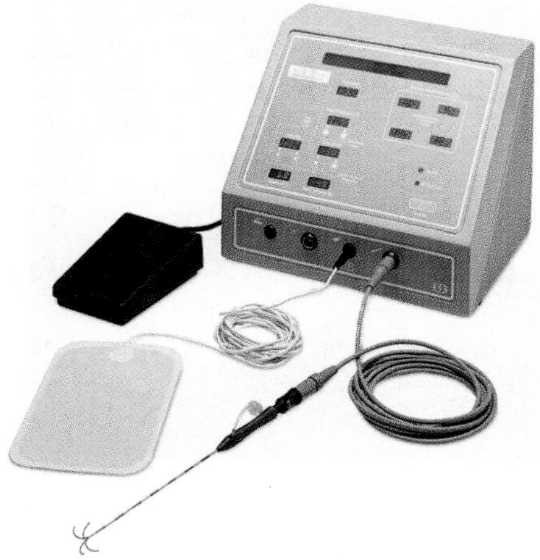

Figure 18–10. A radiofrequency interstitial tumor ablation (RITA) system consists of a generator and a needle with multiple antennas extending from the tip.

Equipment and Technique

Currently, two HIFU systems (Ablatherm, EDAP-Technomed, Lyon, France, and Sonablate, Focus Surgery, Indianapolis, Indiana) are clinically available. Both systems use the transrectal approach, and their probes have both an imaging and a treatment transducer. The treatment transducer is a large single pyezoelectric crystal that has a tightly focused area about 2 to 3 cm from the probe (Figure 18–11). When the transducer is activated, ultrasound energy is converted to heat at the focus, producing 100°C of tissue temperature in seconds. The lesion created by HIFU is a small 1 to 2 mm in diameter and 1- to 1.5-cm-long cylindrical shape. A computer control system gradually moves the focus according to the preprogrammed plan.

The procedure is performed under spinal anesthesia. The patient is placed in the left lateral decubitus position with hips and knees flexed to 90 degrees, and the body is immobilized with multiple belts and pads. A treatment probe is inserted in the rectum, and the prostate gland is visualized by transrectal ultrasonography. The probe position is fixed, and the treatment plan is performed. After activating the treatment crystal, the probe moves step by step, creating a small lesion at each site to create a designed area of tissue necrosis. The rectal cavity is continuously cooled with cold fluid to prevent heat conduction to the rectum. Either a suprapubic tube or a Foley catheter is required after treatment for urine drainage since, temporally, urinary retention is quite common after this procedure.

Animal Study

High-intensity focused ultrasonography has been applied as an experimental cancer treatment study since the 1970s.[62–64] Chapelon and colleagues reported a tumor destruction experiment using the Ablatherm system in a rat prostate cancer model in 1992.[65] Foster and colleagues reported tissue destruction in the canine prostate using the Sonablate system in 1993.[66]

Clinical Study

Gelet and colleagues attempted partial ablation of organ-confined prostate cancer using HIFU in 14 patients. Average PSA decreased significantly, and repeat biopsy showed 50 percent of patients with no evidence of cancer.[67] Beerlage and colleagues reported a histopathologic correlation study of HIFU prior to radical prostatectomy. The HIFU lesions correlated well with the location and size of the treatment plan.[68] Recently, clinical applications of HIFU alone for prostate cancer treatment have been extensively performed in Europe. A recent clinical report by Chaussy and Thüroff included 3-year follow-up on 184 prostate cancer patients treated with HIFU. Their results demonstrated a negative biopsy rate of 80 percent. A PSA nadir < 0.5 ng/mL was achieved in 61 percent of the patients treated. Not surprisingly, there was a significant learning curve for this treatment. Complications were relatively frequent in the initial 96 patients, with stress incontinence in 24 per-

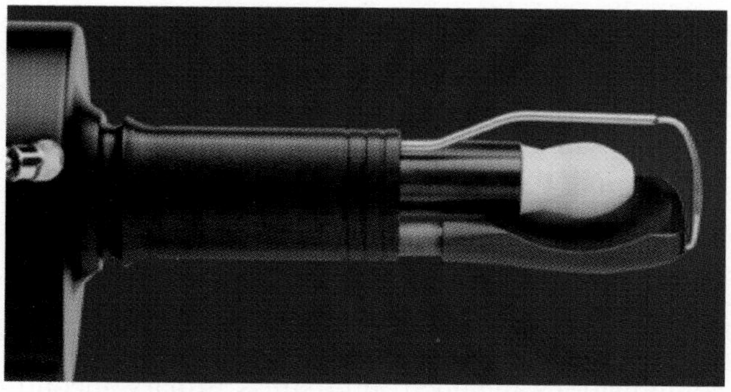

Figure 18–11. A high-intensity focused ultrasound (HIFU) probe consists of an imaging transducer in the middle and a large treatment transducer behind it.

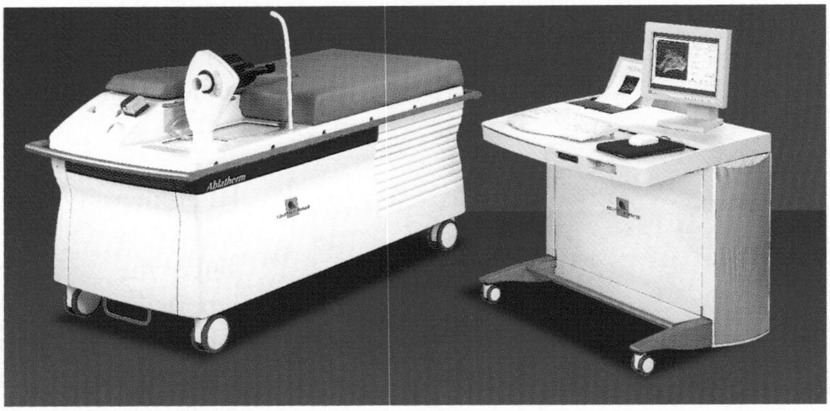

Figure 18–12. A high-intensity focused ultrasound (HIFU) unit (Ablatherm) consists of a treatment table, a probe, a rectal cooling pump, and a control panel.

cent and rectourethral fistula in 3.1 percent. These complications were reduced to 1 and 0 percent, respectively, in the last 100 patients. On average, 29 days of bladder drainage using a suprapubic tube was required, and 33 percent of the patients underwent TURP to resect necrotic debris from the urethra.[69] Gelet and colleagues treated 102 patients with T1–2 prostate cancer with HIFU. With a mean follow-up of 19 months, 34 percent of patients showed either local failure by biopsy or three consecutive rises in PSA after reaching a nadir level.[70] Current equipment cannot treat a large prostate gland since the lesion size is limited to 18 mm in length. An MRI study after HIFU therapy revealed that approximately 8 cc of the anterior prostate remained untreated in a 44-cc prostate gland.[71] Future development of more widely adjustable equipment may popularize this treatment.

Salvage Therapy in US

Twenty-six patients with recurrent carcinoma of the prostate after radiation have been treated at three academic centers. Twenty-four patients have at least 3 months follow-up, and 17 patients had the PSA level decrease to < 1 ng/mL (71%). Fifteen patients have at least 12 months follow-up, and 10 have a sustained reduction of PSA to < 1 ng/mL (67%). Sextant biopsies at 6 months were negative in 16 of 21 patients (76%) and at 12 months were negative in 11 of 14 patients (79%). The most common complication was urinary tract infection in 40 percent of patients. Other complications included mild stress urinary incontinence (one to two pads/day or less) in 38 percent and significant lower urinary tract obstructive symptoms requiring transurethral resection of necrotic tissue in 29 percent. There were no rectal or bladder injuries and no rectourethral fistulae (BJ Miles and colleagues, personal communication, 2000).

Microwave Therapy

Current microwave therapy uses a catheter-associated antenna that is positioned similar to a Foley catheter. This treatment is known as transurethral microwave therapy. Treatment is given using a 915- or 1,296-MHz microwave transducer that produces a zone of hyperthermia surrounding the antenna.[72,73] Temperatures greater than 46°C are achieved, which results in coagulative necrosis after just 30 minutes of therapy. Because of its current antenna configuration, the hyperthermia occurs in the transition zone of the prostate surrounding the urethra. Although this may be effective for benign hyperplasia, cancer that is mostly located in the peripheral zone is not likely to be adequately treated using this modality.

Transurethral microwave therapy, in its current form, includes no real-time imaging to guide the antenna position or to direct the therapy. However, transperineally insertable interstitial microwave fibers similar to RITA have been developed for prostate cancer treatment.[74] Sherar and colleagues recently reported their experience using interstitial microwave thermal ablation (Precision Hyperthermia System, BSD Medical Corp., Salt Lake City, Utah) for radiation-recurrent prostate cancer. Twenty-five patients were treated with five microwave antennae inserted transperineally. Peripheral prostatic temperature reached 55°C, whereas urethral and rectal temperatures were kept below 42°C. The PSA nadir was 0.5 ng/mL in 52 percent of cases. The negative biopsy rate at 24 weeks was 64 percent. No major complications were noted, and stress incontinence was seen in only 5 percent of patients.[75]

Photodynamic Therapy

Photodynamic therapy is currently under early evaluation for use in prostate cancer. In this technique, a photosensitizing chemical is given intravenously. Owing to the abnormal, leaky neovascularity associated with tumors, these sensitizing agents accumulate around tumors. The tissue is then exposed to a red light of an appropriate wavelength. The light converts the chemical to a cytotoxic metabolite. By exposing the sensitized and diseased tissue to the appropriate wavelength of light, targeted tissue destruction can be achieved.[17,76,77] Early feasibility studies demonstrated adequate chemical uptake by prostatic tissues, and its localization allowed for both transurethral and transrectal access for the light source.[78] In addition, the light absorption characteristic of the prostate seemed to allow for more scattering of light rather than absorption.[79] This allows for larger areas of the prostate to be treated with each light fiber. Nathan and colleagues reported photodynamic therapy applied to 12 patients with local recurrence of prostate cancer after radiation therapy.[80] The patients received 0.15 mg/kg meso-tetrahydroxyphenyl chrolin intravenously for photosensitization. Three days later, up to eight catheters were inserted in the prostate transperineally, and the prostate was treated with a diode laser light source. The PSA fell in 7 patients, including 2 with PSA levels less than 0.5 ng/mL. Incontinence occurred in 2 patients and impotence in 50 percent of patients. Total ablation of the prostate may prove difficult and unnecessary if cancer location can be predicted. It may be possible in cases of focally limited cancer to concentrate treatment to the diseased areas. Side effects to the sensitizer agents do occur. For the agents with a longer half-life, cutaneous photosensitivity can be a problem. Like all focal therapies, treatment can be repeated relatively easily in cases of persistent or recurrent disease.

ALCOHOL INJECTION

Absolute ethanol is known to destroy tissue by causing dehydration and protein degeneration and has been used in a variety of medical applications. Recently, some clinical studies using transurethrally or transperineally injected absolute ethanol into benign prostatic hyperplasia tissue to treat bladder outlet obstruction have been reported.[81–83] This material can be injected into an area of cancer under TRUS guidance to achieve tumor destruction. Levy and colleagues described a canine prostate model study using absolute ethanol with or without carmustine injected under ultrasound guidance. They concluded that ethanol injection was readily controllable and resulted in hemorrhagic and coagulative necrosis of prostatic tissue with minimal morbidity.[84] However, feasibility studies in humans using absolute ethanol as a cancer treatment have not yet been performed.

PROSTATE-SPECIFIC ANTIGEN–DEPENDENT ONCOLYTIC ADENOVIRUS THERAPY

An adenovirus that specifically infects cell lines that produce PSA was created by inserting minimal enhancer/promoter constructs derived from the 5' flank of the human PSA gene into adenovirus type 5. This virus, CN706 (Calydon, Sunnyvale, California), destroyed large PSA-producing LNCaP tumors (1×10^9 cells) and abolished PSA production in mouse xenograft models with a single intratumoral injection.[85] A number of small aliquots of virus suspension can be injected transperineally into the prostate using a technique similar to that of permanent radioactive seed implantation. The virus selectively infects PSA-producing cancer cells in the prostate, destroying them by replicating within the cell. The virus may then re-infect surrounding prostate cells. This, theoretically, results in selective tumor ablation within the prostate gland. DeWeese and colleagues reported the results of a phase I trial using the CN706 virus injected into the prostate gland as a treatment of localized radiation-recurrent adenocarcinoma.[86] This dose-response study showed that there was no severe toxicity associated with the treatment using up to 1×10^{13} virus particles. Fifty percent of patients treated with the highest dose of virus achieved a decrease in PSA of ≥ 50 percent. These authors demonstrated the feasibility of this virus-induced prostate cancer ablation therapy, suggesting that further investigation using a higher dose is warranted.

CONCLUSION

Conventional prostate cancer treatments, such as radical prostatectomy and external beam radiation, continue to evolve. With more knowledge and experience, radical prostatectomy has been shown to be a very efficacious and low morbid procedure with minimum incontinence risk and good potency preservation; remember that this is with more knowledge and experience, and does not apply to inexperienced surgeons. With advancement of technology, such as three-dimensional conformal and intensity-modulation techniques, external beam radiation has also become safer and more effective. Recent advancements in brachytherapy have made this modality a minimally invasive and effective treatment option for well-selected patients with prostate cancer. The newer forms of treatment discussed in this chapter are still under investigation. Even cryoablation, which has been recognized as an established treatment option for prostate cancer, requires further improvements to achieve comparable efficacy and morbidity with current radical prostatectomy or radiation therapy as a primary treatment. All of the ablation therapies discussed require more precise control of energy to prevent urethral, sphincteric, and neurovasular bundle injury and to completely ablate all local tumors. Advancements in imaging modalities in the future may precisely delineate tumor location within the gland. If this technology is established, and these energy sources can be properly designed to increase efficacy while decreasing morbidity, (side effects, such as urinary obstruction, incontinence, and sexual dysfunction), a new concept of intraprostatic focal ablation therapy using the technologies discussed here may be feasible.

In addition to use as primary therapy for patients with clinically localized disease, ablation modalities may prove to be useful in patients with local disease recurrence after surgery or radiation and in those with locally advanced prostate cancer. In this latter group of patients, prostate ablation may achieve effective tumor debulking with limited morbidity. Such treatments could potentially be combined with radiation therapy to offer more effective treatment for patients with a high risk of disease recurrence.

REFERENCES

1. Fowler FJ, Barry MJ, Lu-Yao G, et al. Patient-reported complications and follow-up treatment after radical prostatectomy. The National Medicare Experience: 1988–1990 (updated June 1993). Urology 1993;42:622–9.
2. Benoit RM, Naslund MJ, Cohen JK. Complications after radical retropubic prostatectomy in the medicare population. Urology 2000;56:116–20.
3. Kabalin JN, Hodge KK, McNeal JE, et al. Identification of residual cancer in the prostate following radiation therapy: role of transrectal ultrasound guided biopsy and prostate specific antigen. J Urol 1989;142(2 Pt 1):326–31.
4. Koppie TM, Grossfeld GD, Miller D, et al. Patterns of treatment of patients with prostate cancer initially managed with surveillance: results from The CaPSURE database. Cancer of the Prostate Strategic Urological Research Endeavor. J Urol 2000;164:81–8.
5. Zincke H, Oesterling JE, Blute ML, et al. Long-term (15 years) results after radical prostatectomy for clinically localized (stage T2c or lower) prostate cancer. J Urol 1994; 152(5 Pt 2):1850–7.
6. Murphy GP, Mettlin C, Menck H, et al. National patterns of prostate cancer treatment by radical prostatectomy: results of a survey by the American College of Surgeons Commission on Cancer. J Urol 1994;152(5 Pt 2):1817–9.
7. Walsh PC, Partin AW, Epstein JI. Cancer control and quality of life following anatomical radical retropubic prostatectomy: results at 10 years. J Urol 1994;152(5 Pt 2):1831–6.
8. Epstein JI, Pizov G, Walsh PC. Correlation of pathologic findings with progression after radical retropubic prostatectomy. Cancer 1993;71:3582–93.
9. Brenner PC, Russo P, Wood DP, et al. Salvage radical prostatectomy in the management of locally recurrent prostate cancer after 125I implantation. Br J Urol 1995;75:44–7.
10. Rogers E, Ohori M, Kassabian VS, et al. Salvage radical prostatectomy: outcome measured by serum prostate specific antigen levels. J Urol 1995;153:104–10.
11. Benoit RM, Cohen JK, Miller RJ Jr. Counseling patients about cryotherapy for prostate cancer in the information age. Semin Urol Oncol 2000;18:226–32.
12. Cioanta I, Muschter R. Water-induced thermotherapy for benign prostatic hyperplasia. Tech Urol 2000;6:294–9.
13. Laduc R, Bloem FA, Debruyne FM. Transurethral microwave thermotherapy in symptomatic benign prostatic hyperplasia. Eur Urol 1993;23:275–81.
14. Ramon J, Goldwasser B, Shenfeld O, et al. Needle ablation using radio frequency current as a treatment for benign prostatic hyperplasia: experimental results in ex vivo human prostate. Eur Urol 1993;24:406–10.
15. Muschter R, de la Rosette JJ, Whitfield H, et al. Initial human clinical experience with diode laser interstitial treatment of benign prostatic hyperplasia. Urology 1996;48:223–8.
16. Madersbacher S, Kratzik C, Szabo N, et al. Tissue ablation in benign prostatic hyperplasia with high-intensity focused ultrasound. Eur Urol 1993;23 Suppl 1:39–43.
17. Chang SC, Buonaccorsi G, MacRobert A, Bown SG. Interstitial and transurethral photodynamic therapy of the canine prostate using meso-tetra-(m-hydroxyphenyl) chlorin. Int J Cancer 1996;67:555–62.
18. Onik GM, Cohen JK, Reyes GD, et al. Transrectal ultrasound-guided percutaneous radical cryosurgical ablation of the prostate. Cancer 1993;72:1291–9.

19. Streffer C. Biological basis of thermotherapy. In: Gautherie M, editor. Biological basis of oncologic thermotherapy. Berlin: Springer-Verlag; 1990. p. 39–43.
20. Mazur P. Cryobiology: the freezing of biological systems. Science 1970;168:939–49.
21. Zippe CD. Cryosurgical ablation for prostate cancer: a current review. Semin Urol 1995;13:148–56.
22. Tatsutani K, Rubinsky B, Onik G, Dahiya R. Effect of thermal variables on frozen human primary prostatic adenocarcinoma cells. Urology 1996;48:441–7.
23. Larson TR, Rrobertson DW, Corica A, Bostwick DG. In vivo interstitial temperature mapping of the human prostate during cryosurgery with correlation to histopathologic outcomes. Urology 2000;55:547–52.
24. Gage AA. Experimental cryogenic injury of the palate: observations pertinent to cryosurgical destruction of tumors. Cryobiology 1978;15:415–25.
25. Soanes WA, Gonder MJ, Shulman S. Apparatus and technique for cryosurgery of the prostate. J Urol 1966;96:508–11.
26. Reuter HJ. Endoscopic cryosurgery of prostate and bladder tumors. J Urol 1972;107:389–93.
27. Flocks RH, Nelson CM, Boatman DL. Perineal cryosurgery for prostatic carcinoma. J Urol 1972;108:933–5.
28. Onik G, Cooper C, Goldberg HI, et al. Ultrasonic characteristics of frozen liver. Cryobiology 1984;21:321–8.
29. Chang Z, Finkelstein JJ, Ma H, Baust J. Development of a high-performance multiprobe cryosurgical device. Biomed Instrum Technol 1994;28:383–90.
30. Connolly JA, Shinohara K, Presti JC, Carroll PR. Prostate-specific antigen after cryosurgical ablation of the prostate. Defining the appropriate response. Urol Clin North Am 1997;24:415–20.
31. Shinohara K, Connolly JA, Presti JC, Carroll PR. Cryosurgical treatment of localized prostate cancer (stages T1 to T4): preliminary results. J Urol 1996;156:115–20; discussion 120–1.
32. Lee F, Bahn DK, Badalament RA, et al. Cryosurgery for prostate cancer: improved glandular ablation by use of 6 to 8 cryoprobes. Urology 1999;54:135–40.
33. Shinohara K, Rhee B, Presti JC, Carroll PR. Cryosurgical ablation of prostate cancer: patterns of cancer recurrence. J Urol 1997;158:2206–9; discussion 2209–10.
34. Bahn DK, Lee F, Solomon MH, et al. Prostate cancer: US-guided percutaneous cryoablation. Work in progress. Radiology 1995;194:551–6.
35. Consensus statement: guidelines for PSA following radiation therapy. American Society for Therapeutic Radiology and Oncology Consensus Panel. Int J Radiat Oncol Biol Phys 1997;37:1035–41.
36. Greene G, Pisters L, Scott S, Eschenbach AV. Predicitive value of prostate specific antigen nadir following salvage cryotherapy [abstract]. J Urol 1997;157:419A.
37. Long JP, Fallick ML, LaRock DR, Rand W. Preliminary outcomes following cryosurgical ablation of the prostate in patients with clinically localized prostate carcinoma. J Urol 1998;159:477–84.
38. Gould RS. Total cryosurgery of the prostate versus standard cryosurgery versus radical prostatectomy: comparison of early results and the role of transurethral resection in cryosurgery. J Urol 1999;162:1653–7.
39. Pisters LL, von Eschenbach AC, Scott SM, et al. The efficacy and complications of salvage cryotherapy of the prostate. J Urol 1997;157:921–5.
40. Pisters LL, Perrotte P, Scott SM, et al. Patient selection for salvage cryotherapy for locally recurrent prostate cancer after radiation therapy. J Clin Oncol 1999;17:2514–20.
41. de la Taille A, Hayek O, Benson MC, et al. Salvage cryotherapy for recurrent prostate cancer after radiation therapy: the Columbia experience. Urology 2000;55:79–84.
42. Coogan CL, McKiel CF. Percutaneous cryoablation of the prostate: preliminary results after 95 procedures. J Urol 1995;154:1813–7.
43. Cohen JK, Miller RJ, Rooker GM, Shuman BA. Cryosurgical ablation of the prostate: two-year prostate-specific antigen and biopsy results. Urology 1996;47:395–401.
44. Cox RC, Crawford ED. Complications of cryosurgical ablation of the prostate to treat localized adenocarcinoma of the prostate. Urology 1995;45:932–5.
45. Wieder J, Schmidt JD, Casola G, et al. Transrectal ultrasound-guided transperineal cryoablation in the treatment of prostate carcinoma: preliminary results. J Urol 1995;154 (2 Pt 1):435–41.
46. Hall E. Radiobiology for the radiologist. Hagestown: Harper and Row; 1978.
47. Cavaliere R, Ciocatto EC, Giovanella BC, et al. Selective heat sensitivity of cancer cells. Biochemical and clinical studies. Cancer 1967;20:1351–81.
48. Lilly MB, Brezovich IA, Atkinson WJ. Hyperthermia induction with thermally self-regulated ferromagnetic implants. Radiology 1985;154:243–4.
49. Paulus JA, Tucker RD, Loening SA, Flanagan SW. Thermal ablation of canine prostate using interstitial temperature self-regulating seeds: new treatment for prostate cancer. J Endourol 1997;11:295–300.
50. Friedrichs R, Loening SA, Rudolf B, et al. Local recurrence of prostate cancer: treatment by thermal ablation using interstitial temperature self-regulating seeds. Presented at the European Urological Association Annual Meeting, 1998.
51. Tucker RD, Huidobro C, Larson T, Platz CE. Use of permanent interstitial temperature self-regulating rods for ablation of prostate cancer. J Endourol 2000;14:511–7.
52. Deger S, Bohmer D, Turk I, et al. [Thermoradiotherapy with interstitial thermoseeds in treatment of local prostatic carcinoma. Initial results of a phase II study]. Urologe A 2001;40:195–8.
53. Shinohara K, Master V, Carroll PR. Preliminary report of thermal ablation therapy using ferromagnetic rods (ThermoRod) in locally recurrent prostate cancer following external beam radiation therapy. J Urol 2001;165(5 Suppl): 388.
54. Roehrborn CG, Issa MM, Bruskewitz RC, et al. Transurethral needle ablation for benign prostatic hyperplasia: 12-month results of a prospective, multicenter U.S. study. Urology 1998;51:415–21.
55. Siperstein A, Garland A, Engle K, et al. Laparoscopic radiofrequency ablation of primary and metastatic liver tumors. Technical considerations. Surg Endosc 2000;14:400–5.
56. Lewin JS, Connell CF, Duerk JL, et al. Interactive MRI-guided radiofrequency interstitial thermal ablation of abdominal tumors: clinical trial for evaluation of safety and feasibility. J Magn Reson Imaging 1998;8(1):40–7.
57. Wood BJ, Bates S. Radiofrequency thermal ablation of a splenic metastasis. J Vasc Interv Radiol 2001;12:261–3.
58. Zlotta AR, Djavan B, Matos C, et al. Percutaneous transperineal radiofrequency ablation of prostate tumour: safety,

feasibility and pathological effects on human prostate cancer. Br J Urol 1998;81:265–75.
59. Djavan B, Susani M, Shariat S, et al. Transperineal radiofrequency interstitial tumor ablation (RITA) of the prostate. Tech Urol 1998;4:103–9.
60. Shariat S, LA, Bergamaschi F, Slawin K. Initial experience with radiofrequency interstitial tumor ablation (RITA) for the treatment of prostate cancer. J Urol 2001;165 Suppl: 288. #1186.
61. Sanghvi NT, Foster RS, Bihrle R, et al. Noninvasive surgery of prostate tissue by high intensity focused ultrasound: an updated report. Eur J Ultrasound 1999;9(1):19–29.
62. Fry FJ, Johnson LK. Tumor irradiation with intense ultrasound. Ultrasound Med Biol 1978;4:337–41.
63. Moore WE, Lopez RM, Matthews DE, et al. Evaluation of high-intensity therapeutic ultrasound irradiation in the treatment of experimental hepatoma. J Pediatr Surg 1989;24(1):30–3; discussion 33.
64. Yang R, Reilly CR, Rescorla FJ, et al. High-intensity focused ultrasound in the treatment of experimental liver cancer. Arch Surg 1991;126:1002–9; discussion 1009–10.
65. Chapelon JY, Margonari J, Vernier F, et al. In vivo effects of high-intensity ultrasound on prostatic adenocarcinoma Dunning R3327. Cancer Res 1992;52:6353–7.
66. Foster RS, Bihrle R, Sanghvi NT, et al. High-intensity focused ultrasound in the treatment of prostatic disease. Eur Urol 1993;23 Suppl 1:29–33.
67. Gelet A, Chapelon JY, Bouvier R, et al. Treatment of prostate cancer with transrectal focused ultrasound: early clinical experience. Eur Urol 1996;29:174–83.
68. Beerlage HP, van Leenders GJ, Oosterhof GO, et al. High-intensity focused ultrasound (HIFU) followed after one to two weeks by radical retropubic prostatectomy: results of a prospective study. Prostate 1999;39:41–6.
69. Chaussy C, Thuroff S. Results and side effects of high-intensity focused ultrasound in localized prostate cancer. J Endourol 2001;15:437–40; discussion 447–8.
70. Gelet A, Chapelon JY, Bouvier R, et al. Transrectal high intensity focused ultrasound for the treatment of localized prostate cancer: factors influencing the outcome. Eur Urol 2001;40:124–9.
71. Rouviere O, Lyonnet D, Raudrant A, et al. MRI appearance of prostate following transrectal HIFU ablation of localized cancer. Eur Urol 2001;40:265–74.
72. Blute ML, Tomera KM, Hellerstein DK, et al. Transurethral microwave thermotherapy for management of benign prostatic hyperplasia: results of the United States Prostatron Cooperative Study. J Urol 1993;150(5 Pt 2):1591–6.
73. Larson TR, Blute ML, Bruskewitz RC, et al. A high-efficiency microwave thermoablation system for the treatment of benign prostatic hyperplasia: results of a randomized, sham-controlled, prospective, double-blind, multicenter clinical trial. Urology 1998;51:731–42.
74. Trachtenberg J, Chen J, Kucharczyk W, et al. Microwave thermoablation for localized prostate cancer after failed radiation therapy: role of neoadjuvant hormonal therapy. Mol Urol 1999;3:247–50.
75. Sherar MD, Gertner MR, Yue CK, et al. Interstitial microwave thermal therapy for prostate cancer: method of treatment and results of a phase I/II trial. J Urol 2001;166:1707–14.
76. Whitehurst C, Pantelides ML, Moore JV, et al. In vivo laser light distribution in human prostatic carcinoma. J Urol 1994;151:1411–5.
77. Lee LK, Whitehurst C, Pantelides ML, Moore JV. An interstitial light assembly for photodynamic therapy in prostatic carcinoma. BJU Int 1999;84:821–6.
78. Selman SH, Keck RW. The effect of transurethral light on the canine prostate after sensitization with the photosensitizer tin (II) etiopurpurin dichloride: a pilot study. J Urol 1994;152(6 Pt 1):2129–32.
79. Pantelides ML, Whitehurst C, Moore JV, et al. Photodynamic therapy for localised prostatic cancer: light penetration in the human prostate gland. J Urol 1990;143:398–401.
80. Nathan TR, Whitelaw DE, Lees WR, et al. Photodynamic therapy (PDT) for prostate cancer: a phase I study in locally recurrent disease after radiotherapy. J Urol 1999; 161 Suppl:340.
81. Sharma GD, Goel PP. Transperineal intraprostatic injection treatment of benign prostatic enlargement. Aust N Z J Surg 1977;47:220–2.
82. Goya N, Ishikawa N, Ito F, et al. Ethanol injection therapy of the prostate for benign prostatic hyperplasia: preliminary report on application of a new technique. J Urol 1999;162: 383–6.
83. Savoca G, De Stefani S, Gattuccio I, et al. Percutaneous ethanol injection of the prostate as minimally invasive treatment for benign prostatic hyperplasia: preliminary report. Eur Urol 2001;40:504–8.
84. Levy DA, Cromeens DM, Evans R, et al. Transrectal ultrasound-guided intraprostatic injection of absolute ethanol with and without carmustine: a feasibility study in the canine model. Urology 1999;53:1245–51.
85. Rodriguez R, Schuur ER, Lim HY, et al. Prostate attenuated replication competent adenovirus (ARCA) CN706: a selective cytotoxic for prostate-specific antigen-positive prostate cancer cells. Cancer Res 1997;57:2559–63.
86. DeWeese TL, van der Poel H, Li S, et al. A phase I trial of CV706, a replication-competent, PSA selective oncolytic adenovirus, for the treatment of locally recurrent prostate cancer following radiation therapy. Cancer Res 2001;61: 7464–72.
87. Miller RJ Jr, Cohen JK, Merlotti LA. Percutaneous transperineal cryosurgical ablation of the prostate for the primary treatment of clinical stage C adenocarcinoma of the prostate. Urology 1994;44:170–4.
88. Bales GT, Williams MJ, Sinner M, et al. Short-term outcomes after cryosurgical ablation of the prostate in men with recurrent prostate carcinoma following radiation therapy. Urology 1995;46:676–80.
89. Wake RW, Hollabaugh RS, Bond KH. Cryosurgical ablation of the prostate for localized adenocarcinoma: a preliminary experience. J Urol 1996;155:1663–6.
90. Long JP, Bahn D, Lee F, et al. Five-year retrospective, multi-institutional pooled analysis of cancer-related outcomes after cryosurgical ablation of the prostate. Urology 2001;57:518–23.
91. Chin JL, Pautler SE, Mouraviev V, et al. Results of salvage cryoablation of the prostate after radiation: identifying predictors of treatment failure and complications. J Urol 2001;165(6 Pt 1):1937–41; discussion 1941–2.
92. Sosa RE, Martin T, Lynn K. Cryosurgical treatment of prostate cancer: a multicenter review of complications. J Urol 1996;155 Suppl:401A.

19

Local Therapy for Prostate-Specific Antigen Recurrence after Definitive Treatment

MAXWELL V. MENG, MD
GARY D. GROSSFELD, MD, FACS
PETER R. CARROLL, MD, FACS

The use of prostate-specific antigen (PSA) screening in conjunction with digital rectal examination and transrectal ultrasonography (TRUS) has resulted in earlier cancer diagnosis and increased opportunities for cure. Nevertheless, disease recurrence after local therapy for prostate cancer is increasingly common. In part this is attributable to clinical understaging of the cancer, which occurs in up to 50% of patients undergoing radical prostatectomy.[1] An analysis of patients enrolled in a disease registry of patients with prostate cancer demonstrated that 22% of patients who received initial treatment with radical prostatectomy, radiation therapy, or cryotherapy required a second form of prostate cancer treatment within 3 years of initial therapy.[2] Most of these treatments were administered in a nonadjuvant (therapeutic) fashion for apparent evidence of disease recurrence. Patients managed with radical prostatectomy had the lowest rate of second cancer treatment. Similar results have been reported by others, with at least 16 to 35% of radical prostatectomy patients and 24% of radiotherapy patients receiving second cancer treatments within 5 years of primary treatment.[3–5] Currently, failure of therapy is most often manifest solely by a rising PSA level. Moul estimated that up to 50,000 men per year may have PSA-only recurrence after definitive treatment.[6] However, there are no adequate studies comparing the outcomes of these secondary treatments, and the specific indications and optimal timing for additional therapy are equally undefined. Herein, we discuss the various treatment options with definitive, curative intent in patients whose cancers recur locally after radical prostatectomy, radiation therapy, or cryotherapy.

RISK FACTORS FOR RECURRENCE

Multiple studies have examined predictors of recurrence after definitive treatment for prostate cancer. Most of these data are derived from analysis of outcomes of patients treated by radical prostatectomy (Table 19–1).[7–21] Pre-treatment clinical features that correlate with prognosis include T stage, biopsy Gleason score, and serum PSA level.[22] As one would expect, higher stage, the presence of Gleason pattern 4 or greater or a Gleason sum greater than 7, and PSA levels exceeding 10 ng/mL are associated with an increased risk of progression after surgery. These elements have been combined to more accurately predict tumor extent or pathologic stage and therefore prognosis; such probability tables and multivariate models have been based on a larger number of men who have undergone radical prostatectomy.[23–25] Pathologic criteria that are independent factors include tumor grade, surgical margin status, and the presence of extracapsular disease, seminal vesicle invasion, or involvement of pelvic lymph

Table 19–1. RISK FACTORS FOR RECURRENCE AFTER RADICAL PROSTATECTOMY

Pretreatment features
Higher stage[7–13]
Biopsy Gleason grade (any pattern 4, sum > 7)[7–13]
Preoperative PSA (> 10 ng/mL)[7–13]
Greater number of positive biopsies[14]
Pathologic features
Higher stage (seminal vesicle, lymph node involvement)[7,10,12,15,16]
Higher tumor Gleason grade[7,8,15,17]
Positive surgical margin[7,15,18,19]
DNA ploidy[20]
Vascular invasion[21]

PSA = prostate-specific antigen.

nodes (ie, pathologic stage greater than T2N0M0).[26] A recent analysis of clinicopathologic factors confirmed that pathologic category, based on tumor extent and margin status, was the variable most strongly associated with biochemical failure.[21] Interestingly, vascular invasion was the only other variable significantly associated with failure after radical prostatectomy. Similarly, in patients receiving radiation therapy and cryotherapy, risks of recurrence are associated with pretreatment serum PSA, tumor grade, and clinical stage. In addition, PSA nadir following treatment predicts risk for treatment failure.[27] Thus, multiple predictors are available to help identify patients receiving definitive therapy for localized prostate cancer who are at increased risk for disease recurrence.

IDENTIFYING RECURRENCE AND ITS SITE

Prostate-Specific Antigen

Prostate-specific antigen is a powerful tool in the monitoring of patients after definitive treatment of clinically localized prostate cancer. Typically, biochemical failure precedes clinical disease recurrence by 6 to 48 months.[28] Pound and colleagues characterized disease progression after PSA elevation in patients undergoing radical prostatectomy. Actuarial time to metastases was 8 years from the time of PSA failure and was predicted by time from surgery to biochemical failure, Gleason score, and PSA doubling time.[29] The serum PSA of patients after radical prostatectomy should fall to undetectable levels, and initial testing should begin at 2 to 3 months. Serial PSA measurements provide the most reliable method in detecting recurrence as tumor progression rarely occurs in the absence of PSA elevation. Likewise, PSA is used as an end point in monitoring outcomes after radiotherapy. In these cases, however, PSA declines to low but often detectable levels, and the PSA response to treatment is unpredictable.[30] As a result, definitions of treatment success and failure are variable and no consensus exists. Recent recommendations from the American Society of Therapeutic Radiology and Oncology (ASTRO) define recurrence after radiotherapy as three consecutive rises in serum PSA independent of PSA nadir.[31] Only a single study has validated this definition by correlation with clinical outcomes.[32] Critz and colleagues proposed a PSA nadir of 0.5 ng/mL or more to define brachytherapy treatment failure, demonstrating a significant likelihood of disease-free survival at 5 and 10 years in those with nadir PSA values less than 0.5 ng/mL.[33,34] However, the prognostic value of this nadir depends on most men achieving a nadir of 0.2 ng/mL or less.[35] Time to reach PSA nadir varies with treatment modality. Prostate-specific antigen nadir is typically achieved within 6 weeks after radical prostatectomy. Following radiation therapy, time to PSA nadir ranges from 8 to 18 months and even longer with brachytherapy. Ragde and colleagues reported an average of 42 months to PSA nadir in a series of 152 patients receiving brachytherapy.[36] Patterns of PSA failure, such as time to failure, nadir PSA reached, time to nadir PSA level, and PSA velocity, are the current methods to further evaluate for treatment failure.[33,34,37,38] Another confounding factor in patients treated with radiation therapy is the concomitant use of androgen deprivation. No standard regimens or recommendations exist to address the optimal timing and duration of neoadjuvant or adjuvant hormonal therapy, resulting in difficulty assessing treatment success, degree of recurrence, and efficacy (ie, disease-specific survival) of initial or salvage therapy. Thus, despite the widespread use of PSA to monitor disease activity after radiotherapy, controversy exists regarding exact definitions of treatment failure. In addition, it is important to keep in mind that most studies use PSA failure as a surrogate end point for cancer-specific survival. Although PSA may be a sensitive indicator of recurrent or residual disease, it may not accurately reflect the more relevant outcome of survival.[39] The development of alternative intermediate end point biomarkers is needed. Recent studies demonstrate serum acid phosphatase and quantitative nuclear grade as independent predictors of postprostatectomy biochemical progression and suggest their potential use as novel biomarkers of treatment outcome.[40,41]

Distinguishing between local recurrence and distant failure is important in making subsequent treatment decisions (Figure 19–1). Physical examination of the prostate or surgical bed by digital rectal examination is neither sensitive nor specific in detection or localization of low-volume disease recurrence because of irradiated and postsurgical changes in the prostatic fossa.[42,43] Changes in serial examinations over time, however, may help to detect local disease.[44] More recently, the need for anastomotic biopsy has been questioned. Data from our patients receiving radiotherapy after prostatectomy show no differences in outcomes between those treated for biochemical failure alone and those treated for biopsy-proven recurrence, suggesting that biopsy may not be necessary to define patients most appropriate for salvage local therapy.[45]

In conjunction with pathologic stage and Gleason grade, PSA kinetics may provide the best means of identifying the location of tumor failure. Patients with low-grade disease generally have local recurrence, whereas those with seminal vesicle invasion or positive lymph nodes are more likely to fail distantly. Prostate-specific antigen velocity less than 0.75 ng/mL/year was observed in 94% of patients with local recurrence.[46] Conversely, over 50% of men with metastatic disease had a PSA velocity greater than 0.75 ng/mL/year. In the same study, earlier postoperative elevations in PSA, within 2 years, were associated with distant disease. Clearly, a PSA doubling time less than 6 months suggests distant disease. Trapasso and colleagues described a median PSA doubling time of 4.3 months in patients ultimately progressing with distant failure, whereas those patients with clinically

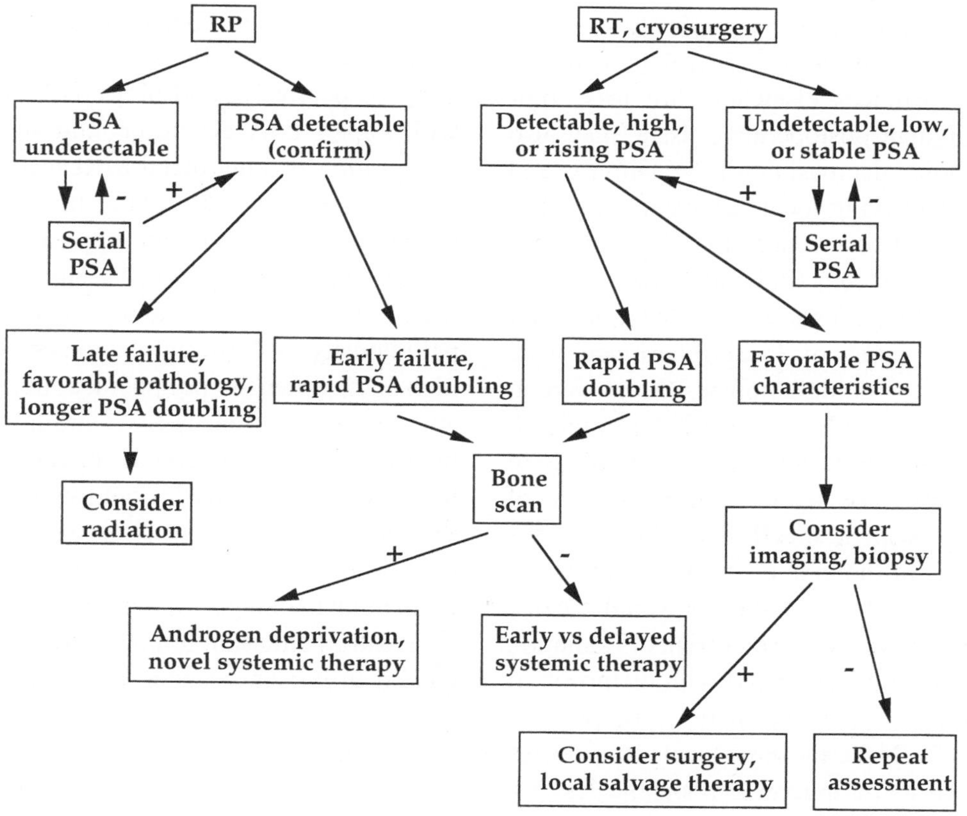

Figure 19–1. Algorithm for evaluation, diagnosis, and treatment of recurrent prostate cancer. RP = radical prostatectomy; RT = radiotherapy; PSA = prostate-specific antigen.

detected local failure or biochemical failure had a PSA doubling time of only 11.7 months.[47] Shorter PSA doubling times also predict increased risk for and shorter time to the appearance of clinical disease.[48,49]

IMAGING

Imaging studies complement clinical and pathologic information in localizing primary treatment failure (Figure 19–2). These modalities include TRUS, bone scan, pelvic computed tomography (CT) and magnetic resonance imaging (MRI), positron emission tomography (PET), and single-photon emission computed tomography (SPECT; ie, ProstaScint).

The probability of a positive anastomotic biopsy performed for an elevated PSA is between 40% and 50% and is not dependent on rectal examination findings.[50–52] Transrectal ultrasonography alone does not increase detection of local recurrence but guides needle placement to the vesicourethral anastomosis. Pelvic anatomy after radical prostatectomy is well described.[52–54] Bladder neck tissue can be seen as a homogeneous, hyperechoic ring at the level of the anastomosis. Recurrent disease is typically seen as a hypoechoic mass posterior or posterolateral to the anastomosis; recurrences elsewhere are less common.[52] Nonmalignant postoperative tissue may also appear hypoechoic, decreasing the sensitivity and specificity for identifying local recurrence. In addition, up to a third of recurrences may have an isoechoic appearance. A recent study addressed some of these issues.[55] Of 99 patients with PSA failure after prostatectomy, 41 cases of local recurrence were detected using TRUS-guided biopsies. Most were at the anastomosis and bladder neck (82%), although lesions noted in the retrovesical space were likely to represent recurrent disease. Overall sensitivity of TRUS was 76%, with a specificity of 67%. Post-treatment changes of the in situ organ after radiation or cryotherapy make the use of TRUS even more difficult in the detection of local recurrence. Radiation creates a small, hyperechoic gland with distortion of normal tissue planes; after cryotherapy, the prostate appears "fuzzy."[50] Nevertheless, local recurrences can be visualized as peripheral hypoechoic lesions. As mentioned earlier, TRUS-guided biopsies may not be necessary after radical prostatectomy to confirm local recurrence. In a cohort of 67 patients receiving radiation therapy after radical prostatectomy, outcomes were equivalent in those undergoing treatment for PSA-only recurrence and those with biopsy-proven disease.[45] Indications for TRUS-guided biopsy after radiation and cryotherapy are also not clear. Most would agree that biopsies should be considered in patients who show serial elevations in serum PSA after reaching a PSA nadir. Nadir levels of PSA are usually reached within 8 to 18 months after radiation and within 3 months after cryotherapy.

Most patients with evidence of disease recurrence undergo both bone scan and CT; however, the utility of these tests is unclear in patients with PSA-only progression. Oesterling suggested that radionucleotide bone scintigraphy is not cost effective in those with minimal PSA elevation after prostatectomy.[56] Cher and colleagues reported that bone scans are rarely positive (5%) until PSA reaches 30 to 40 ng/mL; most patients who fail are detected at significantly lower PSA levels.[57] Bone scans are most useful in patients with rapidly rising PSA (5 ng/mL/month) or new skeletal symptoms. Likewise, cross-sectional imaging to detect local recurrence or lymphadenopathy is fairly insensitive (60% and 30 to 80%, respectively) and plays a greater role in men with higher PSA elevations and shorter PSA doubling time.[58,59] Endorectal MRI increases resolution to 3 mm, appreciably greater than TRUS.[60,61] Most recurrences after surgery appear on T1-weighted images as isointense lesions relative to the surrounding levator ani muscles and as areas of reduced signal intensity on T2-weighted images in the normally high signal intensity peripheral zone. After radiotherapy, tumor recurrences have similar characteristics: hyperintense on T2-weighted images when compared to the levator ani muscles but hypointense relative to the peripheral zone. As technology in high-resolution CT and MRI/spectroscopy evolves, so too will their roles in visualizing local and distant recurrence.

Positron emission tomography is not well characterized in prostate cancer. Imaging takes advantage of differential cellular uptake and metabolism of a radiolabeled compound, such as the glucose analogue 18-fluoro-2-deoxyglucose.[62] Theoretically, the increased positron emission by tumor cells is detected and allows localization. Early studies report sensitivity and specificity of 75% and 67%, respectively, in detecting lymph node metastases, although the utility of PET in recurrent prostate cancer, especially after radiotherapy and cryotherapy, is unclear.[63]

The ProstaScint scan is based on a murine monoclonal antibody, recognizing prostate-specific membrane antigen, conjugated to a linker-chelator and the radioisotope indium 111.[64] Early data do not indicate a clear role for the capromab pendetide immunoscintography, but it appears to detect prostatic fossa recurrence with reasonable accuracy.[65] Kahn and colleagues reported on SPECT findings and the ability to predict response to salvage radiotherapy in 32 patients.[66] Seventy percent of those patients with a normal scan or evidence of only local disease had a durable, complete response to radiotherapy, whereas only 22% with capromab pendetide findings outside the prostatic fossa responded.

RECURRENCE AFTER RADICAL PROSTATECTOMY

Despite earlier diagnosis, improved patient selection, and evolution in surgical technique, as many as 35 to 50% of patients undergoing radical prostatectomy develop biochemical recurrence after treatment. Up to half of these men have local recurrence, with the remainder having distant disease alone or combined local and distant failure.[67] Therefore, it is important to define the role of regional therapy in patients after radical prostatectomy who may potentially benefit from further treatment.

Treatment of biochemical disease recurrence with radiation can often result in an undetectable PSA. In general, freedom from biochemical recurrence has been reported in 30 to 65% of men following therapeutic, or salvage, radiotherapy (Table 19–2).[68–77] Schild and colleagues reported an overall 50% disease-free survival at 3 years; however, 78% of those patients with a preradiation PSA less than 1.0 ng/mL were disease free, whereas only 18% of men with PSA greater than 1.0 ng/mL remained disease free.[68] Forman and colleagues also reported improved disease-free survival in patients with lower preradiation PSA (< 2.0 ng/mL).[73] More recently, in a cohort of 166 patients treated with radiotherapy after prostatectomy, 46% were free of biochemical relapse at 5 years of follow-up.[74] Multivariate analysis identified pathologic stage, tumor grade, and preradiation PSA as independent factors associated with PSA relapse. Leventis and colleagues studied the response to salvage radiation in a group of 49 men with biopsy-proven recurrence after prostatectomy.[78] Preradiation PSA and postrecurrence PSA doubling time before radiation were the only predictors of response to secondary therapy. In our series of 34 men with biopsy-proven recurrence after radical prostatectomy, 47% achieved favorable PSA response (< 0.1 ng/mL or stable PSA < 0.5 ng/mL) at a mean of 38.3 months after salvage external beam radiotherapy.[79] Predictors of secondary treatment success included prostatectomy Gleason sum less than 7 and preradiation PSA ≤ 4.0 ng/mL. Other investigators have reported no differences between adjuvant and therapeutic radiotherapy in patients with initially undetectable PSA after surgery.[80] Similarly, Coetzee and colleagues noted a more durable response to radiation in men who failed after an initial undetectable PSA when compared with men with a persistently detectable PSA (66% at 40 months versus 20% at 12 months, respectively).[71] We recently evaluated our experience with radiation following radical prostatectomy in 105 patients at the University of California at San Francisco (UCSF).[81] The overall 5-year disease-free survival rate was 43%, with failure after radiation defined as PSA greater than 0.2 ng/mL. Outcomes were equivalent in those men receiving adjuvant and salvage radiotherapy when therapeutic radiation was initiated with a low serum PSA (< 1.0 ng/mL)

Table 19–2. RESULTS OF THERAPEUTIC RADIOTHERAPY AFTER PROSTATECTOMY

Study	Number of Patients	Percentage with Undetectable PSA	Length of Follow-up
Hudson and Catalona[69]	21	29	12.6 mo
Schild et al[68]	46	50	5 yr
Wu et al[72]	53	23	2 yr
McCarthy et al[75]	37	54	27.5–36 mo
Morris et al[76]	48	47	3 yr
Forman et al[73]	47	73	36 mo
Cadeddu et al[82]	30	37	At least 2 yr
vander Kooy et al[70]	30	56	8 yr
Coetzee et al[71]	45	51	33 mo
Nudell et al[81]	47	41	3 yr
Pisansky et al[74]	166	46	5 yr

(Figure 19–3). There were no differences between the adjuvant and salvage radiotherapy groups with respect to preprostatectomy PSA, tumor grade, or pathologic stage. In univariate analyses, low stage prior to prostatectomy and low Gleason sum predicted a response to radiotherapy, whereas in multivariate analysis, preprostatectomy PSA under 20 ng/mL predicted radiotherapy success. Our data, as well as those from Vicini and colleagues, also demonstrate that the indication for radiotherapy (adjuvant versus therapeutic) was an independent prognostic factor associated with biochemical control.[77] However, no other clinical, pathologic, or treatment-related factors were associated with 5-year outcome in their patients. Cadeddu and colleagues presented more pessimistic data.[82] Only 21% of men had an undetectable PSA for over 2 years after therapeutic radiation following prostatectomy. No patients with Gleason score 9 or greater, positive seminal vesicles, or positive lymph nodes had undetectable PSA levels greater than 2 years. Finally, early treatment at lower PSA or isolated PSA elevation without documented local recurrence did not predict a favorable response to therapy. Thus, although it appears that adjuvant radiotherapy is a viable option in patients at higher risk for local recurrence, radiation may be used with efficacy in a therapeutic fashion when tumor volume, as reflected by serum PSA, is low. Patients most likely to benefit from salvage radiation after prostatectomy include those with low- to moderate-grade tumors with an undetectable postoperative PSA that rises more than 1 year after surgery. The exact timing of radiation has yet to be determined, although a PSA cutpoint of 2.0 ng/mL currently appears reasonable. The recent ASTRO Consensus Panel recommendations regarding salvage radiotherapy include a dose of at least 6,400 cGy given when PSA is less than 1.5 ng/mL.[83]

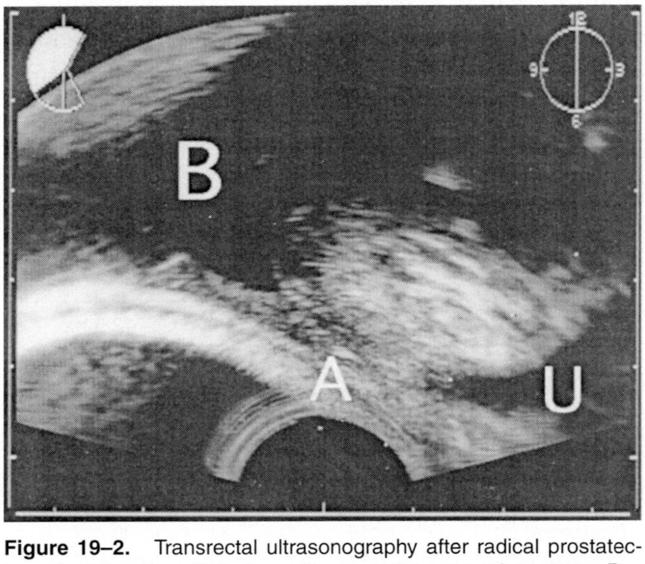

Figure 19–2. Transrectal ultrasonography after radical prostatectomy in the midsagittal plane demonstrating normal anatomy. B = bladder; A = vesicourethral anastomosis; U = bulbar urethra.

Other forms of treatment for locally recurrent disease after radical prostatectomy have been reported but are not well characterized. These include brachytherapy and cryosurgical ablation. Kotrouvelis and colleagues treated five patients with salvage brachytherapy after prostatectomy with acceptable morbidity and results.[84] At UCSF, we have treated three cases of local recurrence after prostatectomy with cryoablation; one of the three patients has maintained an undetectable PSA for 3 years. We have treated one patient with salvage brachytherapy after prostatectomy, and 18 months after the procedure, his PSA was 0.03 ng/mL. Further studies are required before the routine use of either cryotherapy or brachytherapy after radical prostatectomy can be recommended.

A caveat has been raised regarding residual benign prostate glands as a potential source for post-prostatectomy elevations in PSA. Djavan and colleagues found benign prostatic glands in the surgical margins of 95 of 351 prostatectomy specimens (27%).[85] These were found most commonly in the posterior and lateral areas. A large fraction (79%) of patients with pT2 disease and benign glands at the surgical margin had detectable postoperative PSA, ranging from 0.6 to 2.0 ng/mL. They concluded that the remaining benign prostate glands may be a cause of apparent biochemical failure after surgery. More recently, Shah and colleagues reported a significantly lower incidence of benign prostatic glands at the surgical margins.[86] A prospective analysis of 119 consecutive prostatectomy specimens was performed with whole-mount sectioning at 3-mm intervals. Only 13 cases (11%) demonstrated benign glands, with most focally involving the apex. Higher Gleason score and larger prostate gland volume were significantly associated with the finding of benign glands on the surgical margins. No patients with benign glands on the inked margins had PSA recurrences; however, follow-up was relatively short, with a median of 2 months. Thus, one may consider benign prostate glands as a source for detectable PSA after surgery, but recurrent or persistent cancer must be sought and presumed to be present in those with high-risk disease characteristics.

RECURRENCE AFTER RADIATION THERAPY

Radiation therapy, both external beam and brachytherapy, is increasingly used for patients with organ-confined cancers.[87] A certain percentage of patients receiving radiation will fail locally owing to either inadequate localization of the target, inadequate dose, or radiation resistance. Therefore, issues of detection and localization of recurrence after radiation and subsequent treatment options are important to elucidate.

As discussed, various definitions of PSA failure after radiation have been used. Nevertheless, any rising PSA level after radiation therapy may signal active, residual disease. An exception may be those who have been treated with neoadjuvant hormonal therapy, in whom androgen levels and PSA may rise after androgen deprivation is ceased. In addition, an interesting phenomenon has been noted in about one-third of patients who receive brachytherapy but not other forms of radiation. A self-limited, temporary rise in serum PSA often occurs 12 to 18 months after the procedure ("PSA bounce"); this benign PSA flare is unrelated to tumor progression.[36] In a report of 591 men treated with brachytherapy, a significant fraction exhibited a temporary increase in post-treatment PSA (between 0.3 and 3.4 ng/mL) at a mean of 24.8 months after implant.[88] Importantly, this spiking of PSA was not associated with a higher risk of subsequent clinical failure or risk factors for recurrent disease.

As many as one-third of patients may demonstrate rising PSA at 3 years and as many as half may fail clinically within 5 to 7 years after radiotherapy.[89–91] Recurrence rates may have decreased with the use of techniques that target the prostate better and allow for delivery of higher doses. In those patients with recurrent or persistent localized disease, the curative options traditionally included salvage prostatectomy or cryoablation. Most commonly, however, androgen ablation is instituted with postirradiation recurrence. We found that androgen deprivation is the most common form (88%) of secondary treatment after radiotherapy, suggesting limited curative options for those patients currently failing initial radiation.[2]

Salvage prostatectomy after radiotherapy has been approached with caution in the past. It is often technically difficult but has been demonstrated to be feasible, with acceptable morbidity and cure rates. Overall, cancer-specific survival and disease-free rates have ranged from 70 to 90% and 30 to 50% at 8 to 10 years, respectively.[92–94] Pathologically organ-confined disease is found in 20 to 50% of cases and is an important prognostic factor. Tefilli and colleagues reported that all patients with organ-confined disease were disease free at 34 months.[95] Amling and colleagues reported a 10-year disease-free survival of 43% in 108 patients, similar to results from Rogers and colleagues and Moul and Paulson.[94,96,97] Both DNA ploidy and preoperative serum PSA were significant predictors of outcome following surgery. Another study also reported radical prostatectomy Gleason score as an independent predictor of cancer-specific survival.[98] Other factors influencing outcomes of salvage prostatectomy include preradiation clinical stage and preoperative PSA.[99] Data suggest that PSA levels less than 10 ng/mL prior to surgery may predict pathologically localized disease and reduced recurrence. In general, salvage prostatectomy after radiation should be reserved for men with few comorbidities and a 10-year life expectancy in whom recurrence is not locally advanced. Parameters guiding the decision include Gleason sum less than 7, PSA less than 10 ng/mL, and clinical stage T2 or less at the time of both radiation and surgery. However, accurate presurgical staging is often difficult after radiation and may make appropriate patient selection difficult.

Interest in both primary and salvage cryosurgical ablation of the prostate has re-emerged with technical innovations and the desire for minimally invasive procedures. High-resolution TRUS allows precise placement of the probes and real-time visualization of the freezing process. In addition, freezing may cause greater tumor destruction of a heterogeneous, radioresistant cell population, even outside the

MORBIDITY FROM SECONDARY TREATMENT

In evaluating additional treatments for prostate cancer recurrence, both local and distant, factors other than PSA-free or overall survival must be considered. All modalities, including salvage surgery, radiation, cryotherapy, and traditional hormonal therapy, have significant side effects and morbidity. Nevertheless, few studies carefully address these points. Tefilli and colleagues examined quality of life in 68 men undergoing salvage procedures.[118] They reported significantly worse outcomes in urinary continence and physical well-being after salvage prostatectomy; however, similar satisfaction with respect to overall quality of life and potency was found after salvage prostatectomy and salvage radiotherapy.

Morbidity of therapeutic external beam radiation after radical prostatectomy has not been carefully reported. Typically, 45 to 65 Gy are delivered to the prostatic bed and are generally well tolerated. Short-term complications, including bowel and bladder irritability, are seen in approximately 10% of patients, whereas long-term and significant complications are less well defined but approach 20% of the population.[119,120] A retrospective study of 294 men analyzed the effects of adjuvant external beam radiation on urinary continence and potency after nerve-sparing prostatectomy.[121] With a median follow-up of 2.6 years, no significant impact of postoperative radiation was seen on urinary continence or erectile dysfunction. However, a more recent study suggested that primary external beam radiation therapy may lead to hypogonadism, with lower testosterone, free testosterone, and dihydrotestosterone levels, as well as increased luteinizing and follicle-stimulating hormone levels.[122] Although lower doses of radiation may be administered as secondary therapy, this report suggests that salvage radiotherapy may potentially cause testicular damage and resultant hypogonadism.

Complications of salvage prostatectomy are more common when compared with primary prostatectomy. Urinary incontinence is seen in 20 to 60% of patients and bladder neck contracture in approximately 20%, and impotence is virtually universal. Rectal injury may occur in fewer than 10% of patients but rarely necessitates fecal diversion.[92,94,123,124] Contemporary series report better outcomes owing to improved patient selection, earlier identification of failure, and improved surgical techniques. Vaidya and Soloway performed salvage prostatectomy in six patients with isolated local recurrence after radiotherapy.[125] Although all were rendered impotent, five were continent and operative morbidity was excellent, with mean operative time, blood loss, and hospitalization of 195 minutes, 680 mL, and 3.2 days, respectively. Nevertheless, patients must be informed of all potential outcomes, including cystoprostatectomy and urinary diversion, temporary diverting colostomy, and inoperability owing to pelvic desmoplasia. Some have proposed planned cystoprostatectomy with urinary diversion at the time of salvage surgery to maximize subsequent lower urinary tract function.[126–128] Careful preoperative evaluation is necessary to identify manifestations of radiation injury, such as intractable hematuria, low-volume bladder, and irritative lower urinary tract symptoms, which may alter treatment decisions.

A study of salvage cryotherapy has recently been published.[129] The data support the importance of urethral warming with respect to several aspects of quality of life, and the authors concluded that salvage cryotherapy is not superior to salvage prostatectomy when considering morbidity. Patients should be made aware of these issues, and the decision-making process should weigh these factors against potential benefits in prognosis. Moreover, additional studies are necessary to clarify questions of morbidity and quality of life in secondary treatments for recurrent prostate cancer.

CONCLUSIONS

Recurrence after definitive treatment for prostate cancer is a significant problem. Few studies exist examining the optimal diagnostic and therapeutic strategies following either radical prostatectomy or radiation therapy where there is evidence of local disease. Limited curative options are available in many situations. We await the development of more efficacious and less morbid treatment options.

Promising areas of research include molecular characterization and earlier detection of prostate cancer relapse. Pathologic and immunohistochemical markers may add information to determine prognosis. It remains to be determined if genetic markers can predict disease recurrence or metastatic potential. If found, this information could direct the type and timing of additional treatments. Moreover, it may be recognized that not all patients who fail initial therapy as evidenced by biochemical relapse will suffer disease-specific morbidity or mortality. Identification of such patients would spare them the inconvenience, cost, and morbidity of complex testing and/or treatment. Earlier determination of PSA failure and prompt institution of salvage therapy may be possible with the ultrasensitive PSA assay. The lead time may increase the efficacy of second treatments such as radiotherapy after prostatectomy by minimizing tumor burden. Finally, patients may fail both primary and salvage therapy because of undetected metastatic, or micrometastatic, disease. Development of better diagnostic techniques and systemic treatments may address this issue by affecting both local and distant prostate cancer cells. New approaches currently undergoing evaluation, such as antiangiogenesis agents or gene therapy, may revolutionize therapy of prostate cancer.

REFERENCES

1. Johansson JE, Holmberg L, Johansson S, et al. Fifteen-year survival in prostate cancer. A prospective, population-based study in Sweden. JAMA 1997;277:467–71.
2. Grossfeld GD, Stier DM, Flanders SC, et al. Use of second treatment following definitive local therapy for prostate cancer: data from the CaPSURE database. J Urol 1998;160:1398–404.
3. Lu-Yao GL, Potosky AL, Albertsen PC, et al. Follow-up prostate cancer treatments after radical prostatectomy: a population-based study. J Natl Cancer Inst 1996;88:166–73.
4. Fowler FJ Jr, Barry MJ, Lu-Yao G, et al. Patient-reported complications and follow-up treatment after radical prostatectomy. The National Medicare Experience: 1988-1990 (updated June 1993). Urology 1993;42:622–9.
5. Fowler FJ Jr, Barry MJ, Lu-Yao G, et al. Outcomes of external-beam radiation therapy for prostate cancer: a study of Medicare beneficiaries in three surveillance, epidemiology, and end results areas. J Clin Oncol 1996;14:2258–65.
6. Moul JW. Prostate specific antigen only progression of prostate cancer. J Urol 2000;163:1632–42.
7. Eastham JA, Scardino PT. Radical prostatectomy. In: Walsh PC, Retik AB, Vaughan ED Jr, Wein AJ, editors. Campbell's urology. 7th ed. Philadelphia: WB Saunders, 1998. p. 2547–64.
8. Partin AW, Pound CR, Clemens JQ, et al. Prostate-specific antigen after anatomic radical prostatectomy: The Johns Hopkins experience after ten years. Urol Clin North Am 1993;20:713–25.
9. Zincke OH, Oesterling JE, Blute ML, et al. Long-term (15 years) results after radical prostatectomy for clinically localized (stage T2c or lower) prostate cancer. J Urol 1994;152:1850–7.
10. D'Amico AV, Whittington R, Malkowicz SB, et al. A multivariate analysis of clinical and pathological factors that predict for prostate specific antigen failure after radical prostatectomy for prostate cancer. J Urol 1995;154:131–8.
11. Zietman Al, Edelstein RA, Coen JJ, et al. Radical prostatectomy for adenocarcinoma of the prostate: the influence of preoperative and pathologic findings on biochemical disease-free outcome. Urology 1994;43:828–33.
12. Catalona WJ, Smith DJ. Five-year tumor recurrence rates after anatomic radical retropubic prostatectomy for prostate cancer. J Urol 1994;152:1837–42.
13. Ohori M, Goad JR, Wheeler TM, et al. Can radical prostatectomy alter the progression of poorly differentiated prostate cancer? J Urol 1994;152:1843–9.
14. Presti JC Jr, Shinohara K, Bacchetti P, et al. Positive fraction of systematic biopsies predicts risk of relapse after radical prostatectomy. Urology 1998;52:1079–84.
15. Epstein JI, Pizov G, Walsh PC. Correlation of pathologic findings with progression after radical retropubic prostatectomy. Cancer 1993;71:3582–43.
16. Epstein JI, Partin AAW. Sauvageot J, Walsh PC. Prediction of progression following radical prostatectomy: a multivariate analysis of 721 men with long-term follow-up. Am J Surg Pathol 1996;20:286–92.
17. Epstein JI, CarMichael MJ, Pizov G, Walsh PC. Influence of capsular penetration on progression following radical prostatectomy: a study of 196 cases with long-term follow-up. J Urol 1993;150:135–41.
18. Ohori M, Wheeler TM, Kattan MW, et al. Prognostic significance of positive surgical margins in radical prostatectomy specimens. J Urol 1995;154:1818–24.
19. Montie JE. Significant and treatment of positive margins or seminal vesicle invasion after radical prostatectomy. Urol Clin North AM 1990;17:803–12.
20. CarMichael MJ, Veltri RW, Partin AW, et al. Deoxyribonucleic acid ploidy analysis as a predictor of recurrence following radical prostatectomy for stage T2 disease. J Urol 1995;153:1015–9.
21. Babaian RJ, Troncoso P, Bhadkamkar VA, Johnston DA. Analysis of clinicopathologic factors predicting outcome after radical prostatectomy. Cancer 2001;91:1414–22.
22. Nasseri KK, Austenfeld MS. PSA recurrence after definitive treatment of clinically localized prostate cancer. AUA Update Series 1997;16:82–7.
23. Partin AW, Subong ENP, Walsh PC, et al. Combination of prostate-specific antigen, clinical stage, and Gleason score to predict pathological stage of localized prostate cancer: a multi-institutional update. JAMA 1997;277:1445–51.
24. Kattan MW, Wheeler TM, Scardino PT. Postoperative nomogram for disease recurrence after radical prostatectomy for prostate cancer. J Clin Oncol 1999;17:1499–507.
25. D'Amico AV, Chang H, Holoupka E. Calculated prostate cancer volume: the optimal predictor of the actual prostate cancer volume. Urology 1997;49:385–91.
26. Epstein JI. Pathology of adenocarcinoma of the prostate. In: Walsh PC, Retik AB, Vaughan ED Jr, Wein AJ, editors. Campbell's urology. 7th ed. Philadelphia: WB Saunders; 1998. p. 2497–505.

94. Rogers E, Ohori M, Kasabian VS, et al. Salvage radical prostatectomy: outcome measure by serum prostate specific antigen levels. J Urol 1995;153:104–10.
95. Tefilli MV, Gheiler EL, Tiguert R, et al. Salvage surgery or salvage radiotherapy for locally recurrent prostate cancer. Urology 1998;52:224–9.
96. Moul JW, Paulson DF. The role of radical surgery in the management of radiation recurrent and large volume prostate cancer. Cancer 1991;68:1265–71.
97. Amling CL, Lerner SE, Martin SK, et al. Deoxyribonucleic acid ploidy and serum prostate specific antigen predict outcome following salvage prostatectomy for radiation refractory prostate cancer. J Urol 1999;161:857–62.
98. Cheng L, Sebo TJ, Slezak J, et al. Predictors of survival for prostate carcinoma patients treated with salvage radical prostatectomy after radiation therapy. Cancer 1998;83:2164–71.
99. Gheiler El, Tefilli MV, Tiguert R, et al. Predictors for maximal outcome in patients undergoing salvage surgery for radio-recurrent prostate cancer. Urology 1998;51:789–95.
100. Pister LL, Von Eschenbach AC, Scott SM, et al. The efficacy and complications of salvage cryotherapy of the prostate. J Urol 1997;157:921–5.
101. Izawa JI, Perrotte P, Greene GF, et al. Local tumor control with salvage cryotherapy for locally recurrent prostate cancer after external beam radiotherapy. J Urol 2001;165:867–70.
102. Bales GT, Wiliams MJ, Sinner M, et al. Short-term outcomes after cryosurgical ablation of the prostate in men with recurrent prostate carcinoma following radiation therapy. Urology 1995;46:676–80.
103. de la Taille A, Hayek O, Benson MC, et al. Salvage cryotherapy for recurrent prostate cancer after radiation therapy: the Columbia experience. Urology 2000;55:79–84.
104. Chin JL, Pautler SE, Mouraviev V, et al. Results of salvage cryoablation of the prostate after radiation: identifying predictors of treatment failure and complications. J Urol 2001;165:1937–41.
105. Greene GF, Pisters LL, Scott SM, et al. Predictive value of prostate specific antigen nadir after salvage cryotherapy. J Urol 1998;160:86–90.
106. Grado GL, Collins JM, Kriegshauser JS, et al. Salvage brachytherapy for localized prostated cancer after radiotherapy failure. Urology 1999;53:2–10.
107. Beyer DC. Permanent brachytherapy as salvage treatment for recurrent prostate cancer. Urology 1999;54:880–3.
108. Madersbacher S, Pedevilla M, Vingers L, et al. Effect of high-intensity focused ultrasound on human prostate cancer in vivo. Cancer Res 1995;55:3346–51.
109. Beerlage HP, van Leenders GJ, Oosterhof GO, et al. High-intensity focused ultrasound (HIFU) followed after one to two weeks by radical retropubic prostatectomy: results of a prospective study. Prostate 1999;39:41–6.
110. Zlotta AR, Djavan B, Matos C, et al. Percutaneous transperineal radiofrequency ablatin of prostate tumour: safety, feasibility and pathological effects of human prostate cancer. Br J Urol 1998;81:265–75.
111. Gelet A, Chapelon JY, Bouvier R, et al. Local control of prostate cancer by transrectal high intensity focused ultrasound therapy: preliminary results. J Urol 1999;161:156–61.
112. Shinohara K, Master VA, Carroll PR. Preliminary report of thermal ablation therapy using ferromagnetic rods (ThermoRod™) in locally recurrent prostate cancer following external beam radiation therapy. J Urol 2001;165:388A.
113. Koppie TM, Shinohara K, Grossfeld GD, et al. The efficacy of cryosurgical ablation of prostate cancer: the University of California, San Francisco experience. J Urol 1999;162:427–32.
114. Long JP, Fallick ML, LaRock DR, Rand W. Preliminary outcomes following cryosurgical ablation of the prostate in patients with clinically localized prostate carcinoma. J Urol 1998;159:477–84.
115. Grampsas SA, Miller GJ, Crawford ED. Salvage radical prostatectomy after failed transperineal cryotherapy: histologic findings from prostate whole-mount specimens correlated with intraoperative transrectal ultrasound images. Urology 1995;45:936–41.
116. Pisters LL, Dinney CP, Pettaway CA, et al. A feasibility study of cryotherapy followed by radical prostatectomy for locally advanced prostate cancer. J Urol 1999;161:509–14.
117. Burton S, Brown DM, Colonias A. Salvage radiotherapy for prostate cancer recurrence after cryosurgical ablation. Urology 2000;56:833–8.
118. Tefilli MV, Gheiler El, Tiguert R, et al. Quality of life in patients undergoing salvage procedures for locally recurrent prostate cancer. J Surg Oncol 1998;69:156–61.
119. Ornstein DK, Oh J, Herschman JD, Andriole GL. Evaluation and management of the man who has failed primary curative therapy for prostate cancer. Urol Clin North Am 1998;25:591–601.
120. Grossfeld GD, Tigrani VS, Nudell D, et al. Management of a positive surgical margin after radical prostatectomy: decision analysis. J Urol 2000;164:93–9.
121. Formenti SC, Lieskovsky G, Simoneau AR, et al. Impact of moderate dose of postoperative radiation on urinary continence and potency in patients with prostate cancer treated with nerve sparing prostatectomy. J Urol 1996;155:616–9.
122. Daniell HW, Clark JC, Pereira SE. Hypogonadism following prostate-bed radiation therapy for prostate carcinoma. Cancer 2001;91:1889–95.
123. Pontes JE, Montie J, Klein E, Huben R. Salvage surgery for radiation failure in prostate cancer. Cancer 1993;71:976–80.
124. Zincke H. Radical prostatectomy and exenterative procedures for local failure after radiotherapy with curative intent: comparison of outcomes. J Urol 1992;147:894–9.
125. Vaidya A, Soloway MS. Salvage radical prostatectomy for radiorecurrent prostate cancer: morbidity revisited. J Urol 2000;164:1998–2001.
126. Bochner BH, Figueroa AJ, Skinner EC, et al. Salvage radical cystoprostatectomy and orthotopic urinary diversion following radiation failure. J Urol 1998;160:29–33.
127. Gheiler El, Wood DP Jr, Montie JE, Pontes JE. Orthotopic urinary diversion is a viable option in patients undergoing salvage cystoprostatectomy for recurrent prostate cancer after definitive radiation therapy. Urology 1997;50:580–4.
128. Pisters LL, English SF, Dinney CPN, McGuire EJ. Salvage prostatectomy with continent catheterizable urinary reconstruction: a novel approach to recurrent prostate cancer following radiation therapy. J Urol 1999;161:335A.
129. Perrotte P, Litwin MS, McGuire EJ, et al. Quality of life after salvage cryotherapy: the impact of treatment parameters. J Urol 1999;162:398–402.

20

Androgen Deprivation Therapy: Timing and Type

KATHERINE A. HARRIS, MD, PhD
ERIC J. SMALL, MD

Prostate cancer is the most common malignancy in men, and in 1999 accounted for more than 37,000 deaths in the United States.[1] Over half of patients will have metastases at some time during the course of their disease.[2] A relationship between testicular factors and prostate growth was postulated as early as the late 18th century, and castration was used as treatment for patients with enlarged prostate glands in the 19th century.[3,4] However, it was the pioneering work of Huggins and colleagues in the early 1940s that truly ushered in the modern era of hormonal therapy for advanced prostate cancer.[5,6] Huggins's group demonstrated that castration with orchiectomy or with estrogen therapy in men with metastatic prostate cancer resulted in declines in serum acid phosphatase and amelioration of symptoms in a large proportion of patients. Administration of testosterone after castration reversed these beneficial effects, establishing that androgen deprivation was responsible for disease improvement. Subsequently, it has been found that more than 85% of patients with metastatic disease will have an objective response to hormonal therapy.[7] In the era of prostate-specific antigen (PSA) testing, it has been found that hormonal therapy reduces the PSA by over 95% in 90 to 99% of patients.[8]

Knowledge of androgen physiology has been greatly advanced since the time of Huggins. The testes are the major source of androgens, secreting approximately 5 to 10 mg of testosterone each day.[9] Testicular Leydig's cells synthesize and release testosterone in response to stimulation by luteinizing hormone (LH) from the pituitary. Luteinizing hormone secretion is, in turn, dependent on LH–releasing hormone (LH-RH) from the hypothalamus. The adrenal glands, under the influence of pituitary adrenocorticotropic hormone, are an alternate source of androgens. More than 95% of the circulating testosterone in plasma is bound to sex hormone–binding globulin and, to a lesser extent, albumin. The unbound moiety is the biologically active form. On entrance into the cell, testosterone is converted into a number of metabolites that mediate the intracellular processes under androgenic control. The most active of these metabolites, dihydrotestosterone (DHT), is produced by the action of 5α-reductase. In the cytoplasm, DHT binds with high affinity to the androgen receptor, which also binds testosterone with a 4 to 5 times lower affinity. The hormone-receptor complex is then translocated to the nucleus, where it influences the transcriptional activity of androgen-responsive genes. In the prostate, androgens function primarily as growth and survival factors. After androgen deprivation, the gland rapidly involutes, and the glandular cells undergo apoptosis.[10] However, a population of cells remains viable and is capable of regenerating the gland if androgens are provided.

ORCHIECTOMY

Since the observations of Huggins and colleagues, surgical castration has been a mainstay in achieving androgen deprivation. Bilateral total or subcapsular orchiectomy is a relatively simple, safe, and inexpensive procedure. The main side effects are those of androgen withdrawal: loss of libido, impotence, and, in up to 60% of men, development of hot flashes. Orchiectomy rapidly reduces circulating testosterone by around 95% to levels of < 20 ng/mL; castrate levels of testosterone are reached within 24 hours.[11] The intraprostatic concentration of DHT is less affected and may remain at 30 to 40% of normal levels.[12,13] Despite its advantages, the psychological consequences make this option unacceptable to many patients.[14,15] In addition, the procedure is irreversible, which precludes the option of intermittent hormonal therapy (discussed below).

ESTROGEN THERAPY

For many years, estrogens, particularly diethylstilbestrol (DES), were the only hormonal alternative to orchiectomy. Estrogens are believed to exert their effect centrally by suppressing hypothalamic secretion of LH-RH.[16] The first Veterans Administration Cooperative Urological Research Group study (VACURG I), demonstrated that DES administered at 5 mg daily produced outcomes that were not significantly different from those achieved with orchiectomy.[17] The combination did not appear to be superior to either treatment alone. Of note, an excess of cardiovascular mortality was associated with this dose of DES. Other side effects included thromboembolism, fluid retention, gynecomastia, impotence, and loss of libido. The second study, VACURG II, showed that administration of DES at a dose of 1 mg daily was as effective as the higher dose, with fewer cardiovascular side effects, although castrate levels of testosterone were not consistently obtained and levels tended to rise after 6 to 12 months of treatment.[18] Because of concerns of inadequate suppression of androgens, many clinicians have administered a dose of 3 mg daily, which provides castrate levels of testosterone in 7 to 21 days.[19] A large prospective trial demonstrated that this intermediate dose was effective in up to 46% of men, although cardiovascular complications, including thromboembolism, were not insignificant.[7] Estrogens are currently only rarely used in the treatment of advanced prostate cancer. This is in large part owing to concerns about thromboembolic disease, a problem that is not seen with LH-RH agonists. In addition, production of DES was recently discontinued.

GONADOTROPIN-RELEASING HORMONE AGONISTS

Luteinizing hormone–releasing hormone was isolated in the early 1970s.[20] Subsequently, long-acting agonists were designed. Administering a bolus of an LH-RH analogue initially causes a release of LH and an increase in testosterone production, called the "flare" phenomenon. However, continuous administration of LH-RH agonists renders the pituitary refractory to hypothalamic stimulation with a consequent loss of normal pituitary follicle-stimulating hormone and LH secretion. As a result, after a short period of 4 to 5 days during which testosterone levels rise above baseline, castrate levels of serum androgens are achieved by 4 weeks in 90% of men and remain suppressed for the duration of treatment.[21] In effect, the administration of LH-RH agonists achieves medical castration.

Several studies have examined the efficacy of LH-RH analogues versus DES or orchiectomy. The Leuprolide Study Group randomized almost 200 patients with newly diagnosed advanced prostate cancer to receive either leuprolide acetate 1 mg subcutaneously each day or DES 3 mg each day.[7] Median survival was similar in both arms. The results of overall complete response, partial response, and stable disease were equivalent in the two arms. The side-effect profile, however, showed a greater incidence of gynecomastia and cardiovascular complications in the DES arm. The leuprolide arm had a higher incidence of hot flushes. Similar results have been seen comparing goserelin with DES 3 mg daily.[22] Another randomized trial compared the use of the LH-RH agonist buserelin with that of DES or orchiectomy in 160 patients with advanced disease. There was no difference between treatment groups in terms of best response, progression-free survival, or overall survival.[23] The LH-RH agonist goserelin has also been shown to be equivalent to surgical castration on the basis of degree of serum testosterone suppression, objective response rates, duration of response, and survival.[24,25]

Luteinizing hormone–releasing hormone analogues are generally well tolerated. The main side effects are similar to those with surgical castration: loss of libido, impotence, and hot flashes. The reversible nature of the androgen suppression makes intermittent therapy an option, as discussed below. The disadvantages to these medications are twofold. First, the flare phenomenon previously described may account for worsening of symptoms, particularly bone pain, in up to 5% of patients.[26–28] This phenomenon can have potentially serious side effects in patients with impending ureteral or spinal cord compression. Treatment with an antiandrogen 7 to 10 days before, or concomitantly with, the first injection of the LH-RH analogue can prevent this surge of serum testosterone and control the exacerbation of symptoms.[29–31] Luteinizing hormone–releasing hormone antagonists, which do not cause an initial flare,[32,33] are currently under investigation. The second disadvantage of LH-RH agonists is their relatively high cost. The issue of cost is of more concern in patients treated at earlier stages of disease who are likely to be treated for a prolonged period of time. However, costs may be offset by the use of intermittent androgen deprivation in these patients.

NONSTEROIDAL ANTIANDROGENS: MONOTHERAPY

Antiandrogens act at the cellular level to competitively block the binding of testosterone or its metabolite DHT to the androgen receptor. Nonsteroidal antiandrogens available in the United States include flutamide, bicalutamide, and nilutamide. Side effects common to all these agents include gynecomastia (25 to 35%) and flushing (15 to 30%). Loss of libido and potency is reported in 20 to 30% of men treated with antiandrogen monotherapy.[34,35] Additional side effects of flutamide include diarrhea (10 to 15%) and liver function abnormalities (30%).[36] Severe, sometimes fatal hepatotoxicity occurs but appears to be rare.[37,38] Bicalutamide appears to be better tolerated than flutamide, largely owing to a smaller incidence of diarrhea and also possibly owing to less hepatotoxicity.[39–41] Additional side effects observed with nilutamide include the impairment of visual adaptation to dark (20%), alcohol intolerance (20%), and interstitial pneumonitis (1 to 3%).[42,43]

Although these antiandrogens are approved for use in combination with gonadal androgen deprivation, several studies have examined their use as monotherapy in metastatic disease (Table 20–1).[34,44–54] This approach is attractive since monotherapy with an antiandrogen does not result in LH suppression, and testosterone levels increase with long-term treatment. The benefit is that potency and libido are sometimes maintained. A theoretical concern exists that elevated testosterone levels may overcome the antiandrogen action and ultimately stimulate the growth of prostate cancer cells. The majority of reported series are small noncomparative studies, and response criteria vary substantially, making it difficult to draw firm conclusions. Although the results do indicate that monotherapy with an antiandrogen is usually better tolerated than gonadal androgen deprivation, there is a suggestion that the response rate and duration may be inferior with this approach. Two early randomized European trials

Table 20–1. SELECTED TRIALS USING ANTIANDROGEN MONOTHERAPY

Lead Author	Drug/Dose	N	Clinical Response (%)*
Jacobo[44]	Flutamide		
	750 mg/d	4	0
	1,500 mg/d	4	50
Sogani[45]	Flutamide 750 mg/d	21	90
Sogani[46]	Flutamide 750 mg/d	74	87.5
MacFarlane[47]	Flutamide 750 mg/d	3	67
Lundgren[48]	Flutamide 750 mg/d	10	20
Lund[49]	Flutamide 750 mg/d	21	65
Prout[50]	Flutamide 750 mg/d	52	50
Decensi[34]	Nilutamide 300 mg/d	26	38
Delaere[51]	Flutamide 750 mg/d	35	86
Iversen[52]	Bicalutamide 50 mg/d	267	55
Chodak[53]	Bicalutamide 50 mg/d	243	58
Soloway[54]	Bicalutamide 50 mg/d	151	50

*Defined as improvement in imaging studies or symptoms, including pain.

found flutamide to have equivalent response rates to 1 to 3mg of DES daily.[45,55] However, a more recent Eastern Cooperative Oncology Group study demonstrated that survival was inferior in patients treated with flutamide when compared with DES 3 mg daily.[56] Another recent trial found that 50 mg of bicalutamide daily resulted in fewer PSA declines and a higher likelihood of treatment failure compared to medical or surgical castration. As of the last report, median survival had not yet been reached in this study.[53] A combined analysis of more than 1,000 patients showed that bicalutamide at 50 mg daily was inferior to castration. Treatment failure rate (53% versus 41%), objective progression (46% versus 35%), and survival (25 versus 28 months) were all inferior in those patients receiving bicalutamide monotherapy.[57]

High-dose bicalutamide (150 mg daily) has also been studied. A combined analysis of two multicenter randomized trials comparing this to gonadal androgen ablation achieved by either LH-RH agonists or orchiectomy showed a survival benefit of 6 weeks for patients with metastatic disease treated with gonadal androgen ablation.[58] In patients with nonmetastatic disease, however, high dose may prove equivalent in terms of survival, although mature data on this point are lacking.[58,59] In a separate series of 53 men treated with 200 mg of bicalutamide daily, 88% had PSA reductions of > 80%, 48% had bone scan improvements, and median time to progression was 14 months,[60] although a comparison to medical or surgical castration was not undertaken. A recent randomized trial compared bicalutamide 150 mg daily to continuous therapy with goserelin and flutamide.[61] Although the primary end point of overall survival was not different between the groups, methodologic flaws such as potential imbalances in the treatment arms and relatively short follow-up combined with inadequate power make it difficult to interpret the results.

Taken in aggregate, these data suggest that antiandrogen monotherapy can produce PSA reductions and objective improvement in some patients with advanced prostate cancer. The side-effect profile appears to be favorable, and preservation of sexual function occurs in a majority of men who are potent at the time treatment is initiated with standard doses of antiandrogens. However, some evidence suggests that the duration of response, and perhaps survival, may be compromised with this approach, particularly in patients with metastatic disease. For these reasons, this form of treatment is not recommended outside the setting of a clinical trial.

STEROIDAL ANTIANDROGENS

Prior to the development of the nonsteroidal antiandrogens, the steroidal antiandrogens cyproterone acetate and megestrol acetate were used to inhibit androgen action. Both have progestational properties. These drugs act both to block androgen action at the cellular level and to suppress LH release from the pituitary. Cyproterone acetate has been extensively studied in Europe; it is not available in the United States. Overall, it appears to be as effective as estrogen but with a somewhat lower incidence of cardiovascular side effects (10 to 15%).[62,63] Treatment with megestrol acetate at doses of 80 to 100 mg daily achieves castrate levels of testosterone after approximately 1 month. Subsequently, an escape phenomenon occurs, and testosterone levels return toward normal.[64] The addition of low doses of estrogen can prevent this rise in testosterone levels.[65] Megestrol acetate, given alone or with low doses of estrogen, appears to have significant activity, with objective response rates of up to 70% reported.[66–68] Cardiovascular side effects, including thromboembolic events, are similar to those seen with DES. Because of the side-effect profile, megestrol acetate is generally not used in first-line therapy of prostate cancer.

COMBINED ANDROGEN BLOCKADE

The concept of combined androgen blockade (CAB) is based on the premise that adrenal androgens contribute to the progression of prostate cancer. Theoretically, simultaneous blockade of gonadal and adrenal androgens would provide a clinical advantage. Although generally viewed as a modern therapeutic approach, this concept was first explored in 1945, when Huggins and Scott performed bilateral adrenalectomy in four patients in whom initial hormonal therapy for prostate cancer failed.[69] Owing to a lack of glucocorticoid replacement, survival was limited. More than 20 years later, Bracci revisited the idea by combining cyproterone with bilateral orchiectomy.[70] The development of LH-RH agonists and nonsteroidal antiandrogens rekindled interest in CAB. Labrie and coworkers were the first to report on the use of leuprolide and flutamide as primary therapy.[71] The dramatic results in this study—a 95% objective response rate and an 89% 2-year survival—led to multiple trials comparing CAB to monotherapy with an LH-RH agonist (Table 20–2).[72–81] Three large randomized trials demonstrated a statistically significant improvement for CAB in time to progression and length of survival.[72,77,80] The largest of these, the National Cancer Institute (NCI) Intergroup study, enrolled over 600 patients with previously untreated metastatic disease.[72] Patients were assigned to receive either leuprolide plus placebo or leuprolide plus flutamide. Median time to progression and median survival were both superior in the combined treatment arm. In a retrospective subset analysis, these differences were particularly striking in men with minimal disease and good performance status. In this subset of patients, median survival was 61 months in the combined therapy group versus only 41 months in the monotherapy group. A European Organization for Research and Treatment of Cancer (EORTC) trial comparing orchiectomy to the combination of goserelin plus flutamide confirmed these results.[77] Median time to progression and median survival were superior in men receiving CAB. As in the NCI Intergroup study, men with minimal metastatic disease appeared to gain the most benefit. A third large study supporting these results demonstrated an improvement in median and progression-free survival in men receiving orchiectomy plus nilutamide as opposed to orchiectomy alone.[80]

However, several other published studies have failed to demonstrate a significant advantage for CAB over monotherapy. The largest and most recent study was a randomized, controlled trial of bilateral orchiectomy with placebo or flutamide in 1,387 patients with metastatic prostate cancer.[81] Although

Table 20–2. SELECTED RANDOMIZED TRIALS OF COMBINED ANDROGEN BLOCKADE

Series	Treatment	TTP	Survival
Crawford[72]	Leuprolide + flutamide vs leuprolide + placebo	13.8 mo vs 16.9 mo $p = .039$	29.3 mo vs 35.1 mo $p = .035$
Beland[73]	Orchiectomy + nilutamide vs orchiectomy + placebo	12.9 mo vs 11.9 mo p = NS	24.7 mo vs 19.2 mo p = NS
Tyrrell[74]	Goserelin + flutamide vs goserelin	760 d vs 965 d p = NS	29 mo vs 26.9 mo p = NS
Marshall[75]	Orchiectomy + flutamide vs orchiectomy + placebo	NR	23 mo vs 31 mo p = NS
Boccardo[76]	Goserelin + flutamide vs goserelin	12 mo vs 12 mo p = NS	34 mo vs 32 mo p = NS
Denis[77]	Buserelin + flutamide vs orchiectomy	71 wk vs 46 wk $p = .002$	34.4 mo vs 27.1 mo $p = .02$
Iversen[78,79]	Goserelin + flutamide vs orchiectomy	16.5 mo vs 16.8 mo p = NS	22.7 mo vs 27.6 mo p = NS
Janknegt[80]	Orchiectomy + nilutamide vs orchiectomy + placebo	20.8 mo vs 14.9 mo $p = .005$	27.3 mo vs 24.2 mo p = NS
Eisenberger[81]	Orchiectomy + flutamide vs orchiectomy + placebo	20.4 mo vs 18.6 mo p = NS	33.5 mo vs 29.9 mo p = NS

TTP = time to progression; NS = not significant; NR = not reported.

the percentage of patients achieving a PSA of $\leq$ 4 ng/mL was significantly higher in those receiving flutamide, neither overall nor progression-free survival was statistically different in the two arms. Subgroup analysis of survival in patients with minimal versus extensive disease showed no benefit in either group. It should be pointed out that in many of these studies, patients on the placebo or control arm were treated at the time of disease progression with the addition of an antiandrogen. Thus, many of these trials really address the question of early versus late CAB. The utility of late CAB was further delineated by Fowler and colleagues, who reported on the impact of deferred flutamide treatment after gonadal androgen ablation in 45 patients with localized disease and 50 patients with metastatic disease.[82] Prostate-specific antigen declined by more than 50% in 32 (80%) of those with localized cancer and in 27 (54%) of those with metastatic cancer. In general, however, the PSA responses were brief (median duration 5 months for patients with metastatic disease) and were followed by progressive PSA elevation.

In an attempt to reconcile these conflicting data, two meta-analyses have been performed. An initial meta-analysis included seven randomized trials enrolling a total of 1,191 patients treated with orchiectomy versus orchiectomy plus nilutamide.[83] The addition of nilutamide resulted in a statistically significant reduction of 16% in the risk of progression and a statistically nonsignificant 10% reduction in the risk of death. In an update of the analysis, including 2 more years of follow-up, this reduction in risk of progression remained significant.[84] The Prostate Cancer Trialist's Collaborative Group pooled data from 22 randomized trials involving 5,710 patients treated with either castration (medical or surgical) or CAB (various regimens).[85] There was no advantage to CAB over monotherapy detected. Methodologic flaws in the conduct of this study have raised questions about the validity of its conclusions, however.[86–88]

In summary, the overall findings of a large number of studies suggest that CAB is at least equivalent to monotherapy with gonadal androgen ablation followed by deferred treatment with an antiandrogen at progression. Whether CAB is superior remains controversial. Evidence suggests that, particularly in men with minimal metastatic disease and good performance status, it may offer a survival advantage. This is particularly relevant today, with increasing numbers of patients being diagnosed at earlier stages of disease. It should be pointed out that there are no data on the utility of CAB versus monotherapy with gonadal androgen ablation in patients other than men with metastatic prostate cancer, so the extrapolation of these data to patients with nonmetastatic disease is probably not appropriate. Issues of tolerability and cost may also come into play when considering CAB versus gonadal androgen ablation alone.

EARLY VERSUS DELAYED THERAPY

There is general agreement that symptomatic patients with metastatic disease should be offered hormone therapy. The timing of androgen suppression in the asymptomatic patient, however, remains somewhat controversial. In the 1950s, instituting hormonal therapy immediately was thought to be fundamental to improved survival based on three studies showing improved survival of patients treated with orchiectomy or DES compared to controls from the 1930s.[88–91] In the mid-1960s, however, the Veterans Administration Cooperative Urological Research Group's trials allowed for an indirect comparison of early versus delayed hormonal therapy since most patients in the placebo groups whose disease progressed were subsequently begun on hormonal therapy.[17,18] The first study showed no difference in survival between groups. However, an update of the second study suggested a survival benefit to 1 mg of DES daily compared with either placebo, 0.2 mg DES, or 5 mg of DES. This benefit was noted in patients younger than 74 years who had higher Gleason scores (sum of $\geq$ 7). A recent large randomized trial conducted by the Medical Research Council directly compared immediate treatment with orchiectomy or an LH-RH agonist to the same treatment deferred until an indication for therapy occurred.[92] Disease progression occurred more rapidly, and the development of serious complications such as spinal cord compression was increased in patients who receive delayed hormonal treatment compared with those who received immediate treatment. A survival advantage to early therapy was also observed. Although these data are provocative, this study has been criticized for methodologic flaws. Further direct evidence favoring early hormonal therapy comes from a recently completed Intergroup study that randomized 98 patients with node-positive prostate cancer after radical prostatectomy to receive either orchiectomy or goserelin versus the same hormonal therapy administered at the time of objective progression. Early hormonal therapy significantly prolonged survival compared with observation and delayed hormonal therapy. In the early hormonal therapy arm, 6 of 46 patients have expired (13%), 2 from prostate cancer (4.3%); in the delayed therapy arm, 18 of 52 men have expired (34.6%), 16 from prostate cancer (30.8%).[93]

Indirect support of the early use of hormonal therapy also comes from the NCI Intergroup study comparing LH-RH and flutamide to LH-RH and placebo in men with metastatic prostate cancer.[72] A marked difference in survival was noted in patients with minimal disease treated with the combination of hormone therapy compared with those treated with monotherapy. In those patients with minimal disease, a 20-month survival benefit was noted with early institution of CAB, compared with only 4 months benefit in patients with extensive disease, suggesting that the use of CAB at earlier stages of the disease was of clinical benefit. Further indirect evidence supporting earlier use of hormones comes from a randomized trial comparing external irradiation with or without 3 years of goserelin therapy in patients with locally advanced disease.[94] Because patients in the radiation-only arm frequently received hormonal therapy at the time of progression, this trial indirectly compares early versus late androgen deprivation. Overall and disease-free survival at 5 years were statistically superior in the combined treatment group (79% versus 62% and 85% versus 48%, respectively). Although these results could be attributed to synergy between radiation and androgen deprivation, they could just as easily be attributed to the earlier use of hormones in the experimental treatment arm. In aggregate, these data support the use of earlier androgen deprivation, although there are insufficient data to reach conclusions about whether hormonal therapy is appropriate in patients with very early disease (eg, serologic progression after local therapy).

INTERMITTENT ANDROGEN DEPRIVATION

Unfortunately, no hormonal therapy is capable of producing durable responses in any but a small minority of patients with advanced disease, and the median duration of response to androgen deprivation is approximately 18 months.[2] Essentially all patients treated with androgen blockade will eventually develop progressive hormone-insensitive disease manifested by increasing PSA levels, new lesions on radiographic studies, or worsening symptoms. This has led to the search for ways in which to increase the duration of efficacy of hormonal therapy. In the 1970s, Noble reported that intermittent hormonal therapy delayed the progression to hormonal independence in an androgen-dependent rat breast tumor model.[95] In 1990, Bruchovsky and colleagues demonstrated that androgen withdrawal led to a dramatic increase in the proportion of androgen-independent stem cells in an androgen-dependent mouse mammary carcinoma (the Shionogi mouse model).[96] This group postulated that intermittent stimulation of the stem cells with androgens would prompt them to differentiate into androgen-dependent tumors, which would then be susceptible to further androgen withdrawal. Thus, intermittent androgen deprivation (IAD) may increase the period during which the tumor remains sensitive to hormonal manipulation. Subsequently, it was shown that IAD did, in fact, prolong the time to development of androgen independence in the Shionogi mouse model.[97]

This information, coupled with a desire to minimize the side effects and costs of androgen deprivation therapy, spurred a number of single-institution phase II clinical trials of IAD. Two large, randomized Intergroup trials are ongoing. Nevertheless, the data so far have provided valuable information. The first clinical trial to evaluate IAD was reported in the 1980s.[98] Twenty patients were treated with DES until a clinical response was achieved, and then the drug was discontinued until progressive disease occurred. All patients responded to at least two cycles of therapy. The median time off treatment was 8 months; during this time, many patients reported return of sexual function and improved quality of life.

Several subsequent trials have been reported in the era of LH-RH agonists and nonsteroidal antiandrogens (Table 20–3).[99–106] Although there is hetero-

Table 20–3. SELECTED TRIALS USING INTERMITTENT ANDROGEN DEPRIVATION

Series	N	Treatment Regimen	Median Time off Hormones (mo) (% of total cycle length)
Goldenberg[99]	47	LH-RH + antiandrogen	7.6 (41–45)
Higano[100]	22	LH-RH + antiandrogen	6.0 (38–51)
Oliver[101]	20	LH-RH + antiandrogen (12) LH-RH (6) DES (2)	24.0 (NR)
Gleave[102]	70	LH-RH + antiandrogen	9.0 (NR)
Grossfeld[103]	47	LH-RH + antiandrogen (33) LH-RH (14)	7.5 (47)
Theyer[104]	52	LH-RH + antiandrogen	16.0 (NR)
Crook[105]	54	LH-RH + antiandrogen	8.0 (52)
Kurek[106]	44	LH-RH + antiandrogen	11.6 (44–58)

LH-RH = luteinizing hormone–releasing hormone agonist; DES = diethylstilbestrol.

geneity in various aspects of the studies, some generalizations can be made. The most common treatment scheme is to treat until serum PSA becomes undetectable, at which time, androgen deprivation is stopped. This initial cycle generally lasts 6 to 9 months. Serum PSA is then monitored, and treatment is resumed once a predetermined value is reached; progression of disease also warrants resumption of hormonal therapy. The threshold PSA level at which androgen ablation is resumed is usually 50% of the pretreatment value or an absolute value of greater than 5 to 10 ng/mL. Most patients initially have 6 to 9 months off therapy during the initial cycle; this may decrease somewhat during subsequent cycles. Notably, some patients with minimal disease may enjoy off periods lasting 3 or more years. The vast majority of patients will respond to androgen deprivation when it is resumed after the first cycle. It is not known if this approach results in a longer time to development of hormone independence compared to continuous androgen deprivation or if such an approach has an impact on survival.

Quality of life may also be improved with IAD. Serum testosterone levels often recover to normal levels after 3 to 4 months, and some patients report a coincident reduction in symptoms associated with androgen deprivation.[98,100] Weight gain and hot flashes have been reported to improve in over half of patients, as do energy and a sense of well-being.[107] Younger patients who are potent prior to initiation of therapy may recover sexual function, and libido may return.[98,100,107] The influence of IAD on the long-term side effects of androgen deprivation—such as osteoporosis and anemia—needs to be further studied. Initial reports from one study suggest that although bone mineral density declined during the initial cycle of hormonal therapy, stabilization or partial recovery was seen during the first off-treatment period.[108] Controversy exists as to whether factors such as initial extent of disease, Gleason grade, PSA doubling time, and time to relapse after primary therapy influence the efficacy of IAD.[103,109] Furthermore, if testosterone remains low during the periods off therapy, short- and long-term side effects may not be affected significantly and quality of life also may not be influenced. In this regard, age may be an important factor to consider as patients older than 70 may be less likely to recover testicular function after 6 to 12 months of androgen deprivation.[106] In sum, it appears that IAD is feasible and, at least in some patients, achieves the goal of successful long-term treatment with periods of decreased side effects. Whether this approach prolongs survival awaits completion of randomized trials.

REFERENCES

1. Landis S, Murray T, Bolden S, Wingo P. Cancer statistics, 1999. CA Cancer J Clin 1999;49:8–31.
2. Gittes R. Carcinoma of the prostate. N Engl J Med 1991;324:236–45.
3. Cabot A. The question of castration for enlarged prostate. Ann Surg 1896;24:265.
4. White J. The present position of the surgery of the hypertrophied prostate. Ann Surg 1893;18:152.
5. Huggins C, Hodges C. Studies on prostatic cancer: I. The effect of castration, of estrogen, and of androgen injection on serum phosphatases in metastatic carcinoma of the prostate. Cancer Res 1941;1:293–7.

6. Huggins C, Stevens R, Hodges C. Studies on prostatic carcinoma: II. The effect of castration on advanced carcinoma of the prostate gland. Arch Surg 1941;43:209–33.
7. The Leuprolide Study Group. Leuprolide versus diethylstilbestrol for metastatic prostate cancer. N Engl J Med 1984;311:1281–6.
8. Schellhammer P. Combined androgen blockade for the treatment of metastatic carcinoma of the prostate. Urology 1996;47:622–8.
9. Vermeulen A. The androgens. In: Grey C, James V, editors. Hormones in blood. Vol 3. London: Academic Press; 1979.
10. Kyprianou N, Isaacs J. Activation of programmed cell death in the rat ventral prostate after castration. Endocrinology 1988;122:552–62.
11. Labrie F, Dupont A, Belanger A. A complete androgen blockade for the treatment of prostate cancer. In: DeVita V, Hellman S, Rosenberg S, editors. Important advances in oncology. Philadelphia: JB Lippincott; 1985.
12. Labrie F, Luthy I, Veilleuz R, et al. New concepts on the androgen sensitivity of prostate cancer. Prog Clin Biol Res 1987;243A:145–72.
13. Geller J, Albert J, Vik A. Advantages of total androgen blockade in the treatment of advanced prostate cancer. Semin Oncol 1988;15:53–61.
14. Cassileth B, Soloway M, Vogelzang N, et al. Patient's choice of treatment in stage D prostate cancer. Urology 1989; 33:57–62.
15. Fossa S, Aass N, Opjordsmoen S. Assessment of quality of life in patients with prostate cancer. Semin Oncol 1994; 21:657–61.
16. Byar D, Corle D. Hormone therapy for prostate cancer: results of the Veterans Administration Cooperative Urological Research Group studies. Natl Cancer Inst Monogr 1988;7:165–70.
17. Veterans Administration Cooperative Urological Research Group. Treatment and survival of patients with cancer of the prostate. Surg Gynecol Obstet 1967;124:1011–7.
18. Byar D. The Veterans Administration Cooperative Urological Research Group's studies of cancer of the prostate. Cancer 1973;32:1126–30.
19. Citrin D, Kies M, Wallemark C, et al. A phase II study of high-dose estrogens (diethylstilbestrol diphosphate) in prostate cancer. Cancer 1985;56:457–60.
20. Shally A, Arimura A, Baba Y, et al. Isolation and properties of the FSH and LH-releasing hormone. Biochem Biophys Res Commun 1971;43:393–9.
21. Linde R, Doelle G, Alexander N, et al. Reversible inhibition of testicular steroidogenesis and spermatogenesis by a potent gonadotropin-releasing hormone agonist in normal men: an approach toward the development of a male contraceptive. N Engl J Med 1981;305:663–7.
22. Emtage L, Trethowan C, Hilton C, et al. Interim report of a randomized trial comparing Zoladex 3.6 mg depot with diethylstilbestrol 3 mg/day in advanced prostate cancer. Am J Clin Oncol 1988;11:173–5.
23. Klioze S, Miller M, Spiro T. A randomized, comparative study of buserelin with DES/orchiectomy in the treatment of stage D2 prostatic cancer patients. Am J Clin Oncol 1988;2:S5176–82.
24. Debruyne F, Denis L, Lunglmayr G, et al. Long-term therapy with a depot luteinizing hormone-releasing hormone analogue (Zoladex) in patients with advanced prostatic carcinoma. J Urol 1988;140:775–7.
25. Kaisary A, Tyrrell C, Peeling W, Griffiths K. Comparison of LH-RH analogue (Zoladex) with orchiectomy in patients with metastatic prostatic carcinoma. Br J Urol 1991; 67:502–8.
26. Brewster S, Gillatt D. Advanced prostate cancer: what's new in hormonal manipulation? Br J Hosp Med 1993;49:710–5.
27. Bruchovsky N, Goldenberg S, Akakura K, Rennie P. Luteinizing hormone-releasing hormone agonists in prostate cancer. Cancer 1993;72:1685–91.
28. Dijkman G, Debruyne F, Fernandez del Moral P, et al. A randomized trial comparing the safety and efficacy of the Zoladex 10.8 mg depot, administered every 12 weeks to that of the Zoladex 3.6 mg depot, administered every 4 weeks, in patients with advanced prostate cancer. Eur Urol 1995;27:43–6.
29. Boccon-Gibod L, Laudat M, Dugue M, Steg A. Cyproterone acetate lead-in prevents initial rise of serum testosterone induced by luteinizing hormone-releasing hormone analogues in the treatment of metastatic carcinoma of the prostate. Eur Urol 1986;12:400–2.
30. Labrie F, Dupont A, Belanger A, Lachance R. Flutamide eliminates the risk of disease flare in prostatic cancer patients treated with a luteinizing hormone-releasing hormone agonist. J Urol 1987;138:804–6.
31. Kuhn J-M, Billebaud T, Navratil H, et al. Prevention of the transient adverse effects of a gonadotropin-releasing hormone analogue (buserelin) in metastatic prostate carcinoma by administration of an antiandrogen (nilutamide). N Engl J Med 1989;321:413–8.
32. Campion M, Kuca B, Garnick M. The magnitude of Lupron (L) or Zoladex (Z) testosterone (T) and luteinizing hormone (LH) surge is dependent on formulation: comparative results of L and Z vs abarelix-depot (A-D), a GnRH antagonist devoid of androgen surge [abstract]. Proc Am Soc Clin Oncol 1999;18:320a.
33. Garnick M, Tomera K, Campion M, et al. Abarelix-depot (A-D), a sustained-release (SR) formulation of a potent GnRH pure antagonist in patients (pts) with prostate cancer (PrCA): phase II clinical results and endocrine comparison with superagonists Lupron (L) and Zoladex (Z) [abstract]. Proc Am Soc Clin Oncol 1999;18:321a.
34. Decensi A, Boccardo F, Guarneri D, et al. Monotherapy with nilutamide, a pure nonsteroidal antiandrogen in untreated patients with metastatic carcinoma of the prostate. The Italian Prostatic Cancer Project. J Urol 1991;146:377–81.
35. Kaisary A. Current clinical studies with a new nonsteroidal antiandrogen, Casodex. Prostate 1994;5:27–33.
36. Burton S, Trachtenberg J. Effectiveness of antiandrogens in the rat. J Urol 1986;136:932–5.
37. Wysowski D, Freiman J, Tourtelot J, Horton M. Fatal and nonfatal hepatotoxicity associated with flutamide. Ann Intern Med 1993;118:860–4.
38. Wysowski D, Fourcroy D. Flutamide hepatotoxicity. J Urol 1996;155:209–12.
39. Tyrrell C. Casodex: a pure non-steroidal antiandrogen used as monotherapy in advanced prostate cancer. Prostate 1992;4:97–104.

21

Second-Line Hormonal Therapy

SANDY SRINIVAS, MD

Prostate cancer is exquisitely sensitive to hormonal therapy. Any treatment aimed at depriving or depleting testosterone results in a fall in serum prostate-specific antigen (PSA) and objective responses in more than 80% of patients. Eventually, however, resistant disease develops in almost all individuals, as manifested by a rising serum PSA, progression on radiographic studies, and, ultimately, worsening of symptoms. This clinical state is generally defined as hormone-refractory prostate cancer (HRPC) and is associated with a dismal prognosis, with a median survival of 6 to 12 months after relapse.

The use of the term HRPC is a misnomer, however. There are clearly subsets of patients who will respond to additional hormonal maneuvers after the failure of medical or surgical castration. To account for these observations, various schemes have been devised to categorize patients with advanced prostate cancer. One of the more useful systems was developed by Scher and colleagues, who proposed that tumors be categorized as hormone naive, androgen independent but hormone sensitive, and hormone independent (Table 21–1).[1]

The focus of this chapter is on the various therapeutic options for patients with androgen-independent but hormone-sensitive tumors. These patients have a climbing serum PSA or objective progression despite adequate androgen ablation and castrate levels of testosterone, but they may still respond to alternative hormonal maneuvers.

ASSESSING RESPONSE

One of the principal difficulties in evaluating new drugs in advanced prostate cancer is measuring response. Since more than 75% of patients have bone metastases only, serum PSA has been used as an end point to assess response. Significant data now exist that suggest that, at least for cytotoxic agents, declines in PSA correlate with improved survival. Declines in serum PSA from a pretreatment level of greater than 50%, 75%, or 80% have been used to define responders.[2] Myers and coworkers demonstrated that patients who had a greater than 75% fall in serum PSA had a longer survival after treatment with suramin sodium.[3] Kelly and colleagues reported that those patients treated on various chemotherapy trials who had a greater than 50% fall in serum PSA by 2 months of treatment had a longer survival.[4] Smith and colleagues confirmed that a declining serum PSA value after 8 weeks of chemotherapy was most predictive of survival and response.[5]

Although these data strongly suggest that serum PSA is a valid surrogate end point in patients treated with cytotoxic agents, the use of PSA to assess response to secondary hormonal manipulations may be more problematic. Some agents may, at least in theory, affect PSA secretion without retarding tumor cell proliferation.[2] However, in the absence of reliable alternatives for assessing response, the use of PSA can be considered an appropriate screen for the activity of secondary hormonal agents.

Clearly, there is a need for consensus in defining response criteria in HRPC. Dawson, in her report of a survey of 35 investigators, found consensus on eligibility criteria for clinical trials but less consensus in reporting outcomes.[6] To introduce some uniformity into reporting practices, a standardized set of eligibility and response criteria for the use of serum PSA in androgen-independent prostate cancer was recently proposed by the Prostate-Specific Antigen

Table 21–1. CLASSIFICATION OF PATIENTS WITH ADVANCED PROSTATE CANCER

1. Hormone naive: patients without prior hormonal therapy
2. Androgen independent but hormone sensitive: patients with castrate levels of testosterone who respond to second-line hormonal therapy
3. Hormone independent: patients who no longer respond to any hormonal manipulation

Working Group.[7] These guidelines advocate simply reporting actual PSA trends in each patient on an investigational protocol without defining response as a specified decline (eg, greater than 50%) in PSA. The definitions as proposed will need to be validated; nonetheless, they are useful guidelines that allow clinical investigators who are evaluating new regimens in androgen-independent prostate cancer to use standard response criteria.

MAINTAINING ANDROGEN DEPRIVATION

There are some data to suggest that patients with HRPC who are being treated with secondary hormonal agents or chemotherapy derive benefit from continued androgen suppression. Taylor and colleagues reported that continuation of androgen suppression was an independent predictor of survival among patients with HRPC.[8] A Southwest Oncology Group study, in contrast, failed to demonstrate a survival advantage to continuing testicular suppression.[9] It should be noted, however, that in the latter trial, median survival for all patients was very short (6 months), so any effect of continued androgen suppression would likely be negligible.

Further support for the importance of continued androgen deprivation comes from trials in which androgens were used to stimulate tumor growth prior to chemotherapy or radiopharmaceuticals. Fowler and Whitmore, for example, reported that 87% of 52 men who were treated with exogenous testosterone at the time of systemic chemotherapy had progressive disease and increased morbidity, including rapidly escalating pain and serious complications such as spinal cord compression.[10] Thus, in the absence of prospective data, it seems appropriate to view the modest potential benefits against the minimal risk of treatment and to continue androgen suppression indefinitely in patients with HRPC.

SECONDARY HORMONAL MANIPULATIONS

The following will serve as a brief overview of available secondary hormonal manipulations. In general, secondary hormonal maneuvers can be divided broadly into three categories: use of second antiandrogens (or withdrawal of antiandrogen in patients receiving it), adrenal suppression, and use of alternative steroid hormones (Table 21–2).

Addition of Antiandrogens

Most patients in the United States are treated with a combination of castration (medical or surgical) and an oral antiandrogen when hormonal therapy is initiated. For those patients treated with castration alone, the addition of an antiandrogen at the time of progression may cause PSA declines in approximately 50% of patients.[11] However, the duration of response tends to be brief (2 to 4 months), and these patients should be monitored closely for evidence of disease progression. Because of their modest efficacy, the use of antiandrogens in this situation is most appropriate for patients unable to tolerate other therapies.

Of the antiandrogens, high-dose bicalutamide has been studied most extensively in patients with androgen-independent prostate cancer. The rationale for the use of high-dose bicalutamide is that the level of blockade that can be achieved is dependent on the relative number of molecules of the agonist and the competitive antagonist around the receptor. Increasing the dose of the competitive inhibitor may therefore increase the level of blockade. Joyce and colleagues demonstrated a greater than 50% fall in serum PSA in 7 of 31 patients with androgen-independent prostate cancer treated with 150 mg of bicalutamide daily.[12] Interestingly, responses were more commonly observed in patients previously treated with long-term flutamide as part of a complete

Table 21–2. THERAPEUTIC OPTIONS FOR PATIENTS WITH ANDROGEN INDEPENDENT PROSTATE CANCER

Use of second antiandrogens
Antiandrogen withdrawal
Aminoglutethimide
Ketoconazole
Glucocorticoids
Estrogens
PC-SPES

PC-SPES = an eight herb mixture.

prostate cancer. In one early study focusing on symptomatic end points, prednisone produced improved quality of life in 40% of patients.[44] In a randomized trial comparing mitoxantrone and prednisone with prednisone alone, Tannock and colleagues demonstrated that 21% of patients on the prednisone arm had an improvement in quality of life, with a decrease in pain intensity.[45] Other steroid preparations such as hydrocortisone and dexamethasone have also shown subjective responses with minimal toxicity. Thus, glucocorticoids should be considered for all patients with advanced HRPC as a palliative maneuver.

In addition to conventional therapy, alternative treatments may have hormonal activity in advanced prostate cancer. PC-SPES, an herbal mixture composed of eight different herbs (chrysanthemum, Isatis indigotica, licorice, Ganoderma Lucidum, *Panax pseudo ginseng*, Rabdosia Rubescens, saw palmetto, and Scutellaria), has been widely used in the last several years, and emerging data suggest that this compound has activity in both hormone-naive and androgen-independent disease. DiPaolo and colleagues reported results in eight patients with androgen-dependent prostate cancer treated with PC-SPES and noted PSA declines in all patients.[46] Estrogenic side effects were seen in all patients, with a decline of serum testosterone to castrate levels. Despite its estrogenic activity, high-performance liquid chromatography, gas chromatography, and mass spectrometry have failed to identify estradiol, estrone, or DES in PC-SPES, indicating that its estrogenic activity resides in some other compound. Pfeifer and colleagues reported on 16 patients with androgen-independent prostate cancer treated with PC-SPES and noted that 13 patients (81%) had a greater than 50% fall in PSA.[47] Significant improvements in quality-of-life measures and reductions in patient's pain rating were also noted. Small and his colleagues treated 70 patients with PC-SPES, 37 of whom were androgen independent.[48] Fifty-four percent of patients had a PSA decline of greater than 50%. The median duration of PSA decline was 18 weeks. Two patients had improvement in bone scans. The side-effect profile was similar to estrogens and resulted in gynecomastia in 93% and hot flashes in 62% of patients. Interestingly, those patients who had hot flashes at baseline had a complete or near complete resolution of hot flashes on therapy with PC-SPES. Thromboembolic events were reported in 4.3%. It is yet to be determined how PC-SPES would compare to single-agent DES, but these data suggest that this herbal preparation may have a role in the treatment of advanced prostate cancer.

CONCLUSIONS

The use of secondary hormonal manipulations is a viable option for the majority of patients with HRPC. These agents produce PSA responses in approximately 50% of patients and are particularly well suited for the patient with asymptomatic disease with a rising PSA. Additional trials will be required to determine if one agent is superior and whether combinations of these drugs have added efficacy.

REFERENCES

1. Scher HI, Steineck G, Kelly WK. Hormone refractory (D3) prostate cancer: refining the concept. Urology 1995;46: 142–8.
2. Eisenberger MA, Nelson WG. How much can we rely on the level of prostate specific antigen as an endpoint for evaluation of clinical trails? A word of caution. J Natl Cance Inst 1996;88:779–81.
3. Myers C, Cooper M, Stein C, et al. Suramin: a novel growth factor antagonist with activity in hormone refractory metastatic prostate cancer. J Clin Oncol 1992;10:881–9.
4. Kelly WK, Scher HL, Mazumdhar M, et al. Prostate specific antigen as a measure of disease outcome in metastatic hormone refractory prostate cancer. J Clin Oncol 1993; 11:607–15.
5. Smith DC, Dunn RL, Sttrawderman MS, Pienta K. Change in serum prostate specific antigen as a marker of response to cytotoxic therapy for hormone refractory prostate cancer. J Clin Oncol 1998;16:1835–43.
6. Dawson NA. Apples and oranges: building a consensus for standardized eligibility criteria and endpoints in prostate cancer clinical trials. J Clin Oncol 1995;16:3398–405.
7. Bubley GJ, Carducci M, Dahut W, et al. Eligibility and response guidelines for phase II clinical trials in androgen-independent prostate cancer: recommendations from the Prostate-Specific Antigen Working Group. J Clin Oncol 1999;17:3461–7.
8. Taylor CD, Elson P, Trump DL. Importance of continued testicular suppression in hormone refractory prostate cancer. J Clin Oncol 1993;11:2167–72.
9. Hussain M, Wolf M, Marshall E, et al. Effects of continued androgen deprived therapy and other prognostic factors on response and survival in phase II chemotherapy trials for hormone refractory prostate cancer: a Southwest Oncology Group report. J Clin Oncol 1994;12:1868–75.
10. Fowler JE, Whitmore WF. Consideration for the use of testosterone with systemic chemotherapy for prostate cancer. Cancer 1982;49:1373–7.
11. Fowler JE Jr, Pandey P, Seaver LE, Feliz TP. Prostate specific

antigen after gonadal withdrawal and deferred flutamide treatment. J Urol 1995;154:448–53.
12. Joyce R, Fenton MA, Rode P, et al. High dose bicalutamide for androgen independent prostate cancer: effect of prior hormonal therapy. J Urol 1998;159:149–53.
13. Kacuk O, Blumenstein B, Moinpour C, et al. Phase II trial of Casodex in advanced prostate cancer patients who fail conventional hormonal manipulations: a SWOG study. Proc Am Soc Oncol 1996;15:245A.
14. Blackledge GR. High dose bicalutamide monotherapy for the treatment of prostate cancer. Urology 1996;47:44–7.
15. Kelly WK, Scher HI. Prostate specific antigen decline after antiandrogen withdrawal: the flutamide withdrawal syndrome. J Urol 1993;149:607–9.
16. Small EJ, Srinivas S. The antiandrogen withdrawal syndrome. Experience in a large cohort of unselected advanced prostate cancer patients. Cancer 1995;76:1428–34.
17. Scher HI, Kelly WK. Flutamide withdrawal syndrome: its impact on clinical trials in hormone refractory prostate cancer. J clin Oncol 1993;11:1566–72.
18. Figg WD, Sartor O, Cooper MR, et al. Prostate specific antigen decline following the discontinuation of flutamide in patients with stage D2 prostate cancer. Am J Med 1995; 98:412–4.
19. Kelly WK. Endocrine withdrawal syndrome and its relevance to the management of hormone refractory prostate cancer. Eur Urol 1998;34:18–23.
20. Longmore L, Foley JP, Rozanski TA, et al. Prolonged serum prostate specific antigen response in flutamide withdrawal despite disease progression. South Med J 1998;91:573–5.
21. Taplin ME, Bubley GJ, Shuster TD, et al. Mutation of the androgen receptor gene in metastatic androgen independent prostate cancer. N Engl J Med 1995;332:1393–8.
22. Akakura K, Bruchovsky N, Goldberg SL, et al. Effects of intermittent androgen suppression on androgen dependent tumors. Cancer 1993;71:2782–90.
23. Visakorpi T, Hyytinen E, Koivisto P, et al. In vivo amplification of the androgen receptor gene and progression of human prostate cancer. Nat Genet 1995;9:401–5.
24. Berrevoets CA, Veldscholte J, Mulder E. Effects of antiandrogens on transformation activation of wild type and mutated LNCaP androgen receptors. J Steroid Biochem Mol Biol 1993;46:731–6.
25. Nieh PT. Withdrawal phenomena with antiandrogen Casodex. J Urol 1995;153:1070–2.
26. Sella A, Flex D, Sulkes A, Baniel J. Antiandrogen withdrawal syndrome with cyproterone actetate. Urology 1998;52: 1091–3.
27. Huan SD, Gerridzar RG, Yau JC, Stewart DJ. Antiandrogen withdrawal syndrome with nilutamide. Urology 1997;49: 632–4.
28. Akakura K, Akimoto S, Furuya Y, Ito H. Incidence and characteristics of antiandrogen withdrawal syndrome in prostate cancer after treatment with chlormadinone acteate. Eur Urol 1998;33:567–71.
29. Dawson NA, McLeod DG. Dramatic prostate specific antigen decrease in response to discontinuation of megestrol acetate in advanced prostate cancer: expansion of the antiandrogen withdrawal syndrome. J Urol 1995;15:1946–7.
30. Sartor O, Cooper M, Weinberfer M, et al. Surprising activity of flutamide withdrawal, when combined with aminoglutethimide, in treatment of "hormone refractory" prostate cancer. Natl Cancer Inst 1994;86:222–7.
31. Dupont A, Gomez JL, Cusan L, et al. Response to flutamide withdrawal in advanced prostate cancer in progression under combination therapy. J Urol 1993;150:908–13.
32. Figg WD, Kroog G, Duray P, et al. Flutamide withdrawal plus hydrocortisone resulted in clinical complete response in a patient with prostate carcinoma. Cancer 1997;79:1964–8.
33. Small EJ, Baron A, Bok R. Simultaneous antiandrogen withdrawal and treatment with ketoconazole and hydrocortisone in patients with advanced prostate carcinoma. Cancer 1997;80:1755–9.
34. Trump DL, Havlin KH, Messing EM, et al. High dose ketoconazole in advanced hormone refractory prostate cancer. Endocrinologic and clinical effects. J Clin Oncol 1989; 7:1093–8.
35. Verhelst J, Denis L. Ketoconazole and liarozole in the treatment of advanced prostate cancer. Cancer 1993;71;1068–73.
36. Small EJ, Baron AD, Fippin LD, Apodaca D. Ketoconazole retains activity in advanced prostate cancer patients with progression despite flutamide withdrawal. J Urol 1997; 157:1204–7.
37. Crombie C, Raghavan D, Page J, et al. Phase II study of megestrol acetate for metastatic carcinoma of the prostate. Br J Urol 1987;59:443–6.
38. Patel SR, Kvols LK, Hahn RG, et al. A phase II randomized trial of megestrol acetate or dexamethasone in the treatment of hormonally refractory advanced carcinoma of the prostate. Cancer 1990;66:655–8.
39. Dawson NA, Conaway M, Halabi S, et al. A randomized study comparing standard versus moderately high dose megestrol acetate for patients with advanced prostatic carcinoma: Cancer and Leukemia Group B. Cancer 2000;88:825–34.
40. Klotz L, McNeil I, Fleshner N. A phase 1-2 trial of diethylstilbestrol plus low dose warfarin in advanced prostate carcinoma. J Urol 1999;16:169–72.
41. Smith DC, Redman BG, Flaherty LE, et al. A phase II trial of oral diethylstilbestrol as a second-line hormonal agent in advanced prostate cancer. Urology 1998;52:257–60.
42. Orlando M, Chacon M, Salum G, Chacon DR. Low-dose continuous oral fosfestrol is highly active in "hormone refractory" prostate cancer. Ann Oncol 2000;11:177–81.
43. Droz JP, Kattan J, Bonnay M, et al. High-dose continuous infusion fosfestrol in hormone resistant prostate cancer. Cancer 1993;71:1123–30.
44. Tannock I, Gospodarowicz M, Meakin W, et al. Treatment of metastatic prostate cancer with low dose prednisone: evaluation of pain and quality of life as pragmatic indices of response. J Clin Oncol 1989;7:590–7.
45. Tannock IF, Osoba D, Stockler M, et al. Chemotherapy with mitoxantrone plus prednisone or prednisone alone for symptomatic hormone resistant prostate cancer: a Canadian randomized study with palliative end points. J Clin Oncol 1996;14:1756–64.
46. DiPaola RS, Zhang H, Lambert GH, et al. Clinical and biologic activity of an estrogenic herbal combination (PC-SPES) in prostate cancer. N Engl J Med 1998;339:785–91.
47. Pfeifer BL, Pirani JF, Hamann SR, Klippel KF. PC-SPES, a dietary supplement for the treatment of hormone refractory prostate cancer. BJU Int 2000;85:481–5.
48. Small EJ, Frolich MW, Bok R, et al. Prospective trial of the herbal supplement PC-SPES in patients with progressive prostate cancer. J Clin Oncol 2000;18:3595–603.

22

Role of Chemotherapy in the Treatment of Hormone-Refractory Prostate Cancer

DAVID M. REESE, MD

The initial treatment of metastatic prostate cancer involves the suppression of testicular androgen production by medical or surgical castration, a therapy that has not changed significantly since the reports of Huggins and Hodges more than 50 years ago.[1,2] Although the large majority of patients will experience tumor regression after androgen ablation, most will eventually develop disease progression despite the maintenance of castrate levels of testosterone. The development of hormone-refractory prostate cancer (HRPC) is often an ominous clinical finding since median survival remains approximately 1 year.[3]

A variety of treatment approaches have been used in HRPC, including antiandrogen withdrawal, secondary hormonal manipulation, and palliative measures alone. Until recently, cytotoxic chemotherapy was believed to be largely ineffective in the management of HRPC, based primarily on the low objective response rates (< 20%) observed with most single agents.[4] Two influential reviews in the mid-1980s concluded that chemotherapy had little role to play in the treatment of HRPC and that for comparison studies, a palliative care arm was appropriate.[5,6] However, many early chemotherapy trials were performed before the advent of prostate-specific antigen (PSA) as a tumor marker and relied on traditional assessments of measurable disease, which is present in only 10 to 30% of patients. More modern trials of combination regimens have demonstrated PSA response rates of 40 to 60%, and there is renewed interest in the use of cytotoxics to treat HRPC.

EVALUATING RESPONSE TO CHEMOTHERAPY

One of the major barriers in the development of new chemotherapy regimens for HRPC has been the difficulty in quantifying disease response to treatment. The majority of patients (> 70%) with metastatic HRPC have disease limited to bone, a site in which lesions are not easily quantifiable or measurable with standard technetium bone scans. To surmount this problem, many trials performed in the 1970s and 1980s incorporated response criteria that included clinical stabilization of disease as a favorable outcome. However, this approach was flawed because it appeared to inflate the percentage of true responders to various chemotherapy treatment regimens.[7] Other clinical trials were therefore often limited to the 20 to 30% of patients with bidimensionally measurable (soft tissue) disease, but this population may have a worse prognosis.[8] Thus, in the past, the evaluation of new chemotherapeutic programs was hampered by the lack of reliable ways in which to assess disease response.

In the 1990s, the use of serum PSA declines as a surrogate for tumor response has emerged as an alternative method of assessing treatment outcome. There is a growing body of evidence that suggests that declines in PSA of 50% or more identify a subset of patients with HRPC who have improved survival after treatment with cytotoxic chemotherapy. In a retrospective analysis of patients treated with a variety of systemic agents, Kelly and colleagues found that a 50% decline in PSA level 2 months after therapy was associated with improved survival (8.6 months versus > 25 months, respectively).[9] Investigators at the University of Michigan have also recently reported that PSA decreases of more than 50% were associated with enhanced survival among patients treated with estramustine and etoposide on sequential clinical trials.[10] More recently, Scher and colleagues analyzed a large number of patients on phase II trials for HRPC and found that a post-therapy decline of 50% or more at 8 and 12 weeks was an independent factor associated with improved survival.[11]

There is thus an emerging consensus that PSA response to chemotherapy is a useful marker of treatment efficacy. However, there is no general agreement about the magnitude or duration of PSA decline necessary to translate into clinical benefit. To resolve some of the issues surrounding use of PSA as a marker for response in HRPC, an expert panel was recently convened under the auspices of the National Cancer Institute.[12] This panel has recommended a standardization of reporting criteria for PSA response, including a 50% PSA decline as a possible measure of treatment efficacy. In the future, all trials investigating new therapeutics for HRPC should adhere to these reporting guidelines. For the purposes of this review, a PSA response is defined as a 50% decline in PSA values from an initial level that is maintained for a defined period of time, usually at least 4 to 8 weeks.

The remainder of this chapter is devoted to a discussion of currently used chemotherapy programs for HRPC.

MITOXANTRONE COMBINATIONS

Mitoxantrone is a synthetic aminoanthraquinone with a spectrum of antineoplastic activity similar to that of members of the anthracycline family. Mitoxantrone, delivered by continuous infusion, was originally investigated as a single agent in HRPC, with modest response rates.[13] More recently, however, mitoxantrone has been combined with low-dose prednisone in patients with metastatic HRPC.

Based on a preliminary study indicating clinical benefit in some patients,[14] Tannock and colleagues conducted a randomized trial comparing the mitoxantrone-prednisone combination with prednisone alone in 161 patients with HRPC.[15] Mitoxantrone (12 mg/m^2) was administered intravenously every 3 weeks, and all patients received 10 mg of prednisone daily. Importantly, the primary end points of this trial were measures of clinical benefit and included reduction of pain as assessed by a standardized pain scale and analgesic use. Changes in quality of life were also compared between treatment arms. Twenty-nine percent of those treated with the combination experienced decreased pain, compared with 12% treated with prednisone alone, a difference that was statistically significant. Patients receiving mitoxantrone and prednisone also had a significantly greater improvement in some quality of life measures such as relief of constipation and improved mood. In terms of objective response, 33% of those in the mitoxantrone-prednisone arm had a greater than 50% reduction in PSA level, whereas 50% PSA declines were seen in 22% of those receiving prednisone. This difference was not statistically significant. Toxicity of the combination regimen was generally mild, and febrile neutropenia occurred in less than 2% of treatment courses. Median survival for both groups was about 12 months, although the crossover design of the study makes survival comparisons problematic.

In light of the above data, the US Food and Drug Administration (FDA) approved mitoxantrone and prednisone for use in HRPC. This approval was significant in that it indicated that the FDA might now consider palliative end points as well as survival in the evaluation of new drugs for the treatment of HRPC.

Mitoxantrone has also been evaluated in combination with hydrocortisone. The Cancer and Leukemia Group B conducted a randomized study comparing mitoxantrone and hydrocortisone with hydrocortisone alone in 242 patients with HRPC.[16] The results of this trial in general mirror those reported in the Tannock et al study. There was a delay in time to treatment failure and disease progression in favor of the mitoxantrone arm, and quality of life appeared to be better in those receiving mitoxantrone. There was, however, no difference in overall survival (12.3 versus 12.6 months), a significant observation since this trial had no crossover design.

The above studies suggest that mitoxantrone in combination with a steroid may provide palliative benefit for up to 40% of patients with HRPC, although there is no convincing evidence for a survival benefit. The favorable toxicity profile makes these regimens an acceptable choice for patients unable to tolerate more aggressive therapy. In addition, mitoxantrone-based regimens may serve as an appropriate control arm for future randomized studies evaluating new agents.

ESTRAMUSTINE-BASED REGIMENS

Estramustine, an oral drug consisting of estradiol linked to a nornitrogen mustard, was developed three decades ago to target hormonally responsive cancers.[17] It was initially assumed that the steroid component induced uptake by hormone-sensitive tumor cells, followed by alkylation by the nitrogen mustard. However, it is now clear that estramustine's principal mechanism of action is probably unrelated to being a vehicle for delivery of an alkylating agent. The dephosphorylated form of the drug binds to microtubule proteins, structural nuclear proteins, and the nuclear matrix.[18,19] In addition, estramustine may modulate the function of the P-glycoprotein efflux pump in target tumor cells.[20]

Estramustine was originally used in high doses as a single agent for the treatment of HRPC. When given at a dose of 14 mg/kg daily, estramustine has reported objective response rates ranging from 14 to 69%.[21,22] However, in the experience of most investigators, estramustine has low response rates when used alone. In addition, when used continuously at the above doses, there may be substantial toxicity, including gastrointestinal upset, thromboembolic sequelae such as deep venous thrombosis or pulmonary embolism, and fluid retention.

Because estramustine has profound effects on microtubules and the nuclear matrix, its efficacy in combination with other antimicrotubule agents has been investigated both in the laboratory and the clinic. In vitro studies have suggested a potent synergistic antiproliferative effect when estramustine is used in conjunction with vinblastine, etoposide, paclitaxel, or docetaxel.[23–26] Based on these data, a number of phase II studies using these agents with estramustine have been performed (Table 22–1).[27–37] Most of these studies have reported PSA response rates of 50% or greater, although no definitive improvement in median survival has yet been demonstrated. Several ongoing estramustine combination studies are also using clinical benefit end points to investigate the palliative benefit of treatment.

Estramustine combinations typically produce mild to moderate toxicity, primarily leukopenia, nausea and vomiting, edema, and occasional thromboembolic events. With the exception of leukopenia, most side effects can be attributed to estramustine itself, and many investigators now use lower doses (eg, 140 to 280 mg three times daily for a brief period each

Table 22–1. ESTRAMUSTINE-BASED REGIMENS FOR HORMONE-REFRACTORY PROSTATE CANCER

Lead Author	Year	Agent(s)	N	PSA Response (%)	Median Survival (mo)
Hudes[27]	1992	Vinblastine	36	61	10
Pienta[28]	1994	Etoposide	42	58	NR
Reese[29]	1996	Vinorelbine	14	50	NR
Pienta[30]	1997	Etoposide	62	39	13
Hudes[31]	1997	Paclitaxel	34	53	16
Dimopoulos[32]	1997	Etoposide	56	58	13
Colleoni[33]	1997	Etoposide			
		Vinorelbine	25	56	NR
Kelly[34]	1998	Paclitaxel			
		Carboplatin	25	56	NR
Petrylak[35]	1999	Docetaxel	33	63	NR
Smith[36]	1999	Etoposide			
		Paclitaxel	37	65	13
Kreis[37]	1999	Docetaxel	17	82	NR

NR= not reported.

treatment cycle) in an attempt to limit toxicity. We have noted excellent tolerability when using low-dose, limited-duration estramustine in conjunction with the taxanes and, based on the results of the above phase II clinical trials, consider the use of estramustine-based regimens an appropriate treatment strategy for patients with HRPC in whom off-protocol cytotoxic chemotherapy is planned. Whether one of these regimens is superior is unknown, but ongoing or planned phase III clinical trials should establish whether one of these regimens is preferred in terms of response rate and survival.

OTHER REGIMENS

In addition to mitoxantrone and estramustine combinations, several other regimens may have activity in HRPC. Most of the combinations with reported efficacy incorporate doxorubicin or cyclophosphamide into the treatment program.

Cyclophosphomide has been relatively extensively investigated for the treatment of HRPC. When given intravenously, cyclophosphamide alone or in combination with other standard agents such as methotrexate has demonstrated minor antitumor acitvity.[38] However, prolonged administration of oral cyclophosphamide may have significant palliative benefit. For example, in an early trial, oral cyclophosphamide was given for 14 days of a 28-day cycle; 60% of patients experienced a symptomatic response, with minimal toxicity.[39] Oral cyclophosphamide has also been combined with oral etoposide in one study, with more than 70% of patients experiencing relief of bone pain and 35% having PSA responses.[40]

Other trials have examined dose intensity for traditional agents. Small et al investigated dose-escalated cyclophosphamide with doxorubicin and granulocyte colony-stimulating factor support and noted a 46% PSA response rate, although hematologic toxicity was common, with grade 4 neutropenia encountered in 33% of cycles.[41] Weekly doxorubicin has also been combined with ketoconazole, an oral antifungal agent with activity as a secondary hormonal therapy and possible direct cytotoxic effects on prostate tumor cells.[42] In that study, a 55% PSA response rate was observed and a median survival of 15 months was reported. Toxicity was significant, however, with 45% of patients requiring hospitalization for complications such as severe mucositis, stomatitis, acral erythema, or infection. These regimens require further investigation before they can be routinely recommended outside the setting of a clinical trial.

Camptothecin and its analogues have also been investigated for the treatment of HRPC. These drugs inhibit DNA topoisomerase type I and in preclinical models have shown efficacy against a wide variety of solid tumors. Unfortunately, they do not appear to be effective in HRPC. Hudes and colleagues treated 34 patients with topotecan in standard doses and noted PSA responses in only 6 (18%).[43] Four patients had relief of pain, leading the authors to conclude that topotecan has minimal activity in HRPC. Likewise, a phase II study of single-agent irinotecan in 15 patients with HRPC demonstrated no PSA responses.[44] Thus, camptothecins are unlikely to play a significant role in the treatment of HRPC when used alone, although combining them with other agents such as the topoisomerase type II inhibitor etoposide is currently being investigated.

FUTURE DIRECTIONS

It is now clear that cytotoxic chemotherapy may provide palliative benefit for many patients with HRPC. In particular, the estramustine-based regimens appear to have significant activity and acceptable toxicity profiles and are suitable for use in most patients. However, a number of unresolved questions need to be addressed to determine the optimal use of chemotherapy in this patient population.

One important issue is the relative importance of estramustine in the combination antimicrotubule regimens. Preliminary results from one randomized trial comparing vinblastine alone versus vinblastine plus estramustine suggest that the combination is superior in terms of progression-free survival, although no survival benefit has yet been reported.[45] These data, coupled with the preclinical evidence of synergistic interactions, suggest that estramustine is necessary in these regimens. However, other studies of newer drugs indicate significant single-agent activity. For example, there is preliminary evidence

23

Novel Systemic Therapy

LAWRENCE FONG, MD
ERIC J. SMALL, MD

Although androgen deprivation has remained the cornerstone of therapy for advanced prostate cancer over the last 60 years,[1] novel therapies are evolving that almost certainly will expand the current treatment armamentarium. New therapies are evolving in the treatment of hormone-resistant prostate cancer that may improve on current limited options. Over the last 5 years, several new agents have been approved for advanced prostate cancer, and there are also many novel agents at various stages of development.

The diagnosis of advanced prostate cancer spans a broad spectrum of disease, from hormonally responsive to hormone-refractory disease. Disease progression during each of these phases typically has a different tempo. Moreover, the pace of disease progression can vary significantly between different patients. This heterogeneity in tumor biology can make defining therapeutic end points a challenge in developing novel therapies.

ASSESSMENT OF RESPONSE IN ADVANCED PROSTATE CANCER

Advanced prostate cancer encompasses clinical entities ranging from patients with asymptomatic elevations in their serum prostate-specific antigen (PSA) levels following local primary therapy to patients with overt metastatic disease. Recurrences following primary treatment can manifest as a detectable and rising PSA level either with or, more commonly, without objective local or distant sites of disease. In addition to its use as a primary screening test, serum PSA has emerged as a sensitive method to detect recurrences and monitor responses to therapy.[2] Patients who relapse biochemically after primary therapy remain a therapeutic challenge in that no standard treatment option exists for these patients. These patients are ideal candidates for clinical trials, particularly with novel agents with minimal side effects such as immunotherapy.

In addition to its routine use for cancer surveillance, the serum PSA level is routinely used to follow patients with advanced disease and more recently as a surrogate marker of tumor response. Given the long natural history of prostate cancer, defining therapeutic efficacy on the basis of survival alone generally precludes the development of therapies in a timely fashion. Retrospective studies suggest that PSA declines of ≥ 50% correlate with improved survival in patients with second-line hormonal therapy and chemotherapy.[3] However, the use of PSA decline as a surrogate remains problematic because confounding factors such as the effects of ancillary treatments on PSA synthesis or secretion can affect serum levels. For example, concurrent administration of corticosteroids can decrease PSA.[4,5] The availability of in vitro assays, which test the effect of novel agents on PSA production in tissue culture, add a level of complexity to interpreting post-therapy PSA declines. Some agents, such as suramin sodium, may decrease PSA production of prostate cancer cell lines in vitro, with little effect on cancer cell viability.[6] Other agents, such as phenylbutyrate[7] and TNP-470,[8] can actually increase PSA secretion from prostate cancer cell lines. Although these observations mandate caution in interpreting

PSA as an end point, it should be pointed out that the utility of these in vitro assays, and their correlation with in vivo effects, has not been demonstrated to date. Finally, PSA declines associated with withdrawal of different agents, antiandrogens in particular, can confound results, particularly if inadequate time has elapsed before initiating new treatment.[9] Despite these caveats, PSA decline remains a reasonable surrogate end point for evaluating novel therapies in phase II trials, with the understanding that the efficacy of promising therapies identified with this surrogate must ultimately be confirmed with other end points such as survival or improvements in quality of life.

Radiologic modalities can also be used to assess response to treatment. Bone scans, although useful, visualize lesions that, in general, cannot be measured. As a result, 70 to 80% of patients with prostate cancer lack bidimensionally measurable disease. Moreover, bone scintigraphy is insensitive in detecting responses in bony disease. Computed tomographic scanning can be effective in assessing soft tissue responses, although these metastases occur less frequently. Radioimmunodetection with labeled monoclonal antibodies directed at proteins expressed on prostate cells represents another modality used to identify metastatic disease. One system (ProstaScint®) relies on indium 111–labeled antibody directed against prostate-specific membrane antigen (PSMA) to detect cell deposits of prostate cancer. Although such technology seems theoretically powerful, problems with nonspecific binding and limits of detection have limited its usefulness. In the setting of evaluating patients for residual or recurrent disease, ProstaScint scanning yielded a sensitivity of 49% and a specificity of 71% when compared with prostatic fossa biopsy.[10] Moreover, because antibodies used in this study are derived from mice, patients undergoing this study can develop human antimouse antibodies that may preclude the readministration of murine antibodies in the future as well as potentially affecting laboratory assays (eg, PSA, digoxin) that rely on mouse antibodies as reagents.

More recently, quality of life has been used as an end point in developing therapies for hormone-refractory prostate cancer. Standardized questionnaire and pain scoring has transformed what was previously considered to be subjective assessments into quantitative measures. Commonly used instruments include the European Organization for Research and Treatment of Cancer Quality-of-Life Questionnaire, Functional Assessment of Cancer Therapy—Prostate, and Quality-of-Life Index. In fact, treatment-associated improvements in quality of life led to the approval of mitoxantrone for patients with hormone-refractory disease.[11]

Alternative intermediate end points used in prostate cancer include time to progression as measured by PSA or radiologic studies (eg, bone scan). Specific therapeutic approaches may require unique end points relevant to that intervention. For example, in the development of bisphosphonates, reduction of skeleton-related events, such as pathologic fractures and cord compression, has been used as an end point. Cancer vaccine trials should assess immune responses as an investigational end point.

EMERGING THERAPIES

Chemotherapy

Although no chemotherapy used as a single agent has an objective response rate of > 30%, new drug combinations have led to considerable progress in developing active regimens in prostate cancer. Estramustine, an oral drug consisting of estradiol linked to nitrogen mustard that inhibits nuclear matrix microtubules, has limited activity as a single agent but shows significant promise when used in combinations: in phase II studies, 40 to 60% of patients had PSA responses (≥ 50% decline) to estramustine combined with etoposide, vinorelbine, paclitaxel, or docetaxel.[12–15] Other novel combinations and new drugs are currently being tested and are described by Reese elsewhere in this publication. Moreover, as discussed below, chemotherapy is increasingly being combined with other treatment approaches, including antiangiogenesis and differentiating agents (Table 23–1).

Bisphosphonates

Bisphosphonates, in combination with chemotherapy, have clearly demonstrated efficacy in decreasing skeletal events in multiple myeloma and breast cancer.[16,17] Because of prostate cancer's tropism for

Table 23–1. EMERGING THERAPIES IN PROSTATE CANCER

Class of Agent	Target	Agent
Chemotherapy	Nuclear matrix microtubules	Estramustine
Bisphosphonates	Bone turnover	Zoledronate
Matrix metalloproteinase inhibitors		Marimastat
		Prinomastat
Antiangiogenesis		Angiostatin
		Endostatin
Growth factor inhibitors		Suramin
Differentiation agents	Retinoid receptors	Retinoids
	Induction of AR expression	Vitamin D analogues
Gene therapy	Selective viral replication	Caledon
Immunotherapy		
Antibodies	*HER2/NEU*	Herceptin
	TAG-72	CC-49
Vaccines	PSA	Dendritic cells
		Liposomes
	PSMA	Dendritic cells
		DNA vaccination
		Adenovirus
	PAP	Dendritic cells
	Globo H hexasaccharide	KLH conjugates
	Unspecified antigens	GM-CSF–transduced tumor cells

AR = androgen receptor; PSA = prostate-specific antigen; PSMA = prostate-specific membrane antigen; PAP = prostatic acid phosphatase; KLH = keyhole-limpet hemocyanin; GM-CSF = granulocyte-macrophage colony–stimulating factor; TAG = tumor-associated glycoprotein.

bone, bisphosphonates have also been evaluated in metastatic prostate cancer, with varying success.[18,19] Trials with third-generation bisphosphonates such as zoledronate, which is 100 to 1,000 times more potent than prior agents,[20] are currently under way to assess the ability of these drugs to prevent skeletal events.

Matrix Metalloproteinase Inhibitors

Tumors must break down the extracellular matrix with proteases and establish new blood vessels to grow or spread. Matrix metalloproteinases represent a family of at least 16 proteins that can digest the extracellular matrix and basement membrane.[21] These enzymes are regulated by specific (eg, tissue inhibitors of metalloproteinases) and nonspecific proteinase inhibitors. Plasma levels of matrix metalloproteinases were found to be elevated in patients with metastatic prostate cancer when compared with patients with prostatic hypertrophy or nonmetastatic cancer.[22] Several matrix metalloproteinase inhibitors, including marimastat and AG3340 (prinomastat), are at various stages of clinical trials.[23] Moreover, trials using these agents in combination with chemotherapy are also under way.

Antiangiogenesis

The formation of new blood vessels is critical in tumor growth and in the development of metastases. As with matrix metalloproteinases, angiogenesis is controlled by a balance in positive and negative regulatory factors.[24] Examples of the former include vascular endothelial growth factor (VEGF), fibroblast growth factor, transforming growth factor α and β, and tumor necrosis factor α (TNF-α). Examples of the latter include angiostatin, endostatin, thrombospondin, retinoic acid, and interferons α, β, and γ. Curiously, PSA itself has recently been described to possess antiangiogenic activity in vitro and in vivo.[25]

It has been established that prostate cancer cells can elaborate proangiogenic factors, such as VEGF and platelet-derived growth factor (PDGF).[26] Moreover, increased angiogenesis in prostatectomy specimens, as determined by microvessel density, has been correlated with metastatic disease.[27] Plasma levels of VEGF are increased in patients with metastatic prostate cancer.[28] Antibodies targeting VEGF and small molecules blocking PDGF signaling and the VEGF receptor have also entered clinical trials in prostate cancer. Thalidomide, another drug with antiangiogenic activity,[29] is also being studied in prostate cancer. Because these approaches may be cytostatic rather than cytocidal, many of these therapies are being investigated in combination with conventional chemotherapy.

Growth Factor Inhibitors

Several new agents that act by blocking growth factor receptor signaling are being investigated in prostate cancer. Suramin sodium, a polysulfonated naphthylurea, represents one of the earliest agents in this class to be investigated. Although complex dosing schedules and serum monitoring were required to minimize toxicities during this drug's development, suramin and hydrocortisone have been demonstrated to produce a 33% PSA response rate compared with 16% for hydrocortisone plus placebo in a randomized trial.[30] Furthermore, there was a significant improvement in the likelihood of obtaining a pain response with suramin (43% versus 28%), and duration of pain control was significantly improved (240 days versus 69 days). Suramin also had a modest impact on prolonging time to progression (relative risk = 1.5; 95% CI = 1.2 to 1.9).[31] Regardless of the ultimate role of suramin in the care of patients with prostate cancer, it represents the first biologic agent to have been shown to have antiprostate cancer activity. Specific targets for inhibition that are currently under development include the PDGF and endothelial growth factor receptor pathways.

Differentiation and Cell Cycle Inhibition

Inducing cellular differentiation and/or blocking cell cycle progression are two approaches that are being explored in prostate cancer. This approach uses agents such as retinoids, vitamin D analogues, phenylacetate, and phenylbutyrate to affect gene expression within cancer cells that should result in growth arrest. Retinoids, one of the principal family of endogenous compounds that control epithelial cell growth and differentiation, have been demonstrated to induce the expression of androgen receptors.[32] Retinoids and inhibitors of retinoid metabolism such as liarazole have been evaluated. Although liarazole appears to demonstrate some anticancer activity, its commercial development has been halted.[33] Phenylacetate affects cell cycle regulation by inducing up-regulation of P21,[34] which results in retinoblastoma protein dephosphorylation, and has also entered clinical trials.

The antitumor effects of vitamin D may act through a similar mechanism[35] or through the induction of androgen receptor expression.[32] Preclinical studies have demonstrated antiproliferative effects on prostate cancer cell lines.[36] In early trials, 1,25-dihydroxyvitamin D has been shown to have some slowing on the rate of PSA rise.[37] Analogues have been developed to reduce the hypercalcemic effects of the parent compound and are undergoing clinical trials. The vitamin D receptor acts as a heterodimer with the retinoid X receptor, so functional interactions between 1,25-dihydroxyvitamin D_3 and retinoids may exist. In fact, synergism with vitamin D and retinoids has been demonstrated in vitro and could serve as the basis for combination of these agents.[38,39] As with antiangiogenesis agents, these agents may cause growth arrest rather than cell death, which would affect response assessment. Moreover, toxicities associated with treatment will be extremely important given the long-term treatment that may be necessary with these cytostatic agents.

Gene Therapy

Gene therapy approaches include developing replacement vectors for tumor suppressor genes commonly mutated in prostate cancer such as *P53* and *BRCA1*.[40] As new generations of vectors are developed that improve transfection efficiency and reduce their immunogenicity, gene replacement strategies will continue to improve. An alternate approach focuses on delivery of suicide genes to prostate cancer cells. One such approach employs a modified adenovirus in which the expression of certain viral products (E1A, E1B) is controlled by prostate-specific enhancer/promoter elements such as those for PSA. As a result, lytic replication of this engineered virus occurs preferentially in prostate-derived tissues.[41] Clinical trials are under way exploring the feasibility and efficacy of these approaches. For now, the utility of therapy mediated by viral vectors is limited by the need for direct injection into tumor sites (eg, patients with local recurrence after local therapy).

Immunotherapy

Immunotherapy focuses on exploiting the various effector arms of the immune system to kill tumor cells. Immune effectors can be classified as antibody, cytokine, and vaccine based. Antibody-based therapies rely on targeting proteins specifically expressed on tumor cells. Unlike antibodies against CD20 for non-Hodgkin's lymphoma and against *HER2/NEU* for breast cancer, specific antibodies that trigger cell death in prostate cancer have yet to be identified, although a preclinical study has demonstrated some activity of *anti-HER2/NEU* antibodies against prostate cancer xenografts.[42] Unfortunately, *HER2/NEU* does not appear to be frequently overexpressed in prostate cancer specimens. Nevertheless, clinical trials using Herceptin®, a monoclonal antibody against *HER2/NEU*, are under way. With most antibody trials currently under way, antibodies are coupled to cytotoxic agents, such as radioisotopes and toxins, and are used to target the complexes to sites of tumor. CC49, an antibody that recognizes the pancarcinoma antigen TAG-72, has been shown to generate disease responses in ovarian cancer.[43] This antigen is expressed on prostate cancer cells,[44] and is being studied in clinical trials for prostate cancer. As with ProstaScint scans, problems with specificity and adequate delivery of antibodies into tumor tissues must be addressed as this treatment approach is developed clinically.[45]

The goal of tumor vaccine development is to induce antibody and/or T-lymphocyte immune responses targeted at cancer cells. The majority of antigens identified in the prostate, including PSA, PSMA, and prostatic acid phosphatase (PAP), represent "self proteins." As a result, these proteins are not inherently immunogenic. By delivering antigens in a manner that stimulates an immune response, cancer vaccines attempt to generate cytotoxic T cells and/or antibodies from B lymphocytes, overcoming the preexisting immune tolerance to these antigens. The ability to generate immunity against PSA,[46] PSMA,[47] and PAP[48,49] through various immunization approaches has been demonstrated in clinical trials.

The most straightforward vaccines involve admixing tumor-associated proteins with nonspecific immunostimulatory adjuvants. One such trial used recombinant PSA encapsulated in liposomes and mixed with bacille Calmette-Guérin as the vaccination and has generated both antibody and T-cell responses.[46] Another trial used the prostate antigen globo H hexasaccharide conjugated to keyhole-limpet hemocyanin and was administered with the immunologic adjuvant QS-21 as another vaccine approach.[50]

Recombinant viruses that express prostate antigens have also been developed as a vaccination. One trial employs a vaccinia vector expressing PSA.[51] Despite preexisting immunity to the underlying viral construct, antibodies against PSA could be generated in vivo with the vaccine.

Prostate tumor cells have also been used as cancer vaccines. Preclinical models have demonstrated that tumor cells, when transduced with cytokine genes[52] or costimulatory molecules,[53] can be used to immunize animals and protect them from developing tumors. Clinical trials have been performed using either autologous prostate cancer cells or, more recently, allogeneic prostate cancer cell lines transduced with cytokine genes such as granulocyte-macrophage colony–stimulating factor (GM-CSF) as a vaccine.[54]

An alternative approach uses the patient's own dendritic cells (DCs) as a cellular vaccine. Dendritic cells are rare, bone marrow–derived antigen-presenting cells that are uniquely capable of sensitizing naive T cells to new antigens. Presumably, many of the vaccine approaches rely on targeting antigen to DCs to generate immunity. By loading the DCs themselves with tumor antigens, this approach hopes to accentuate immune responses to the targeted antigens. The first described clinical trial with DC-based vaccination demonstrated the generation of immunity and antitumor activity in non-Hodgkin's lymphoma.[55] Trials on the prostate have since been performed. One such trial has focused on immunizing patients with PSMA-derived peptides loaded onto DCs.[47] Trials ongoing at our institutions have focused on PAP as the target antigen.[48,49]

Finally, cytokines have been used as an immunotherapeutic approach for prostate cancer. Whereas some cytokines can be cytotoxic to tumor cells, most of the cytokines studied in prostate cancer are directed at enhancing the presentation of antigens from the prostate. For example, GM-CSF administered to patients with androgen-insensitive prostate cancer led to a PSA response rate of 22%, including one patient who had a sustained dramatic decline.[56] Presumably, such a therapy may work by stimulating the function and/or number of antigen-presenting cells, including DCs, in situ. Studies with other cytokines including interleukin-1β (IL-1β), IL-2, GM-CSF, interferon-γ, TNF-α, and Flt3L are ongoing.

FUTURE DIRECTIONS

Some of the emerging treatments discussed may eventually demonstrate efficacy in advanced prostate cancer. However, many of these approaches (eg, immunotherapy) may be more effective in settings of lower disease burdens, so exploring these treatments in patients with minimal residual disease will be important. Combinations of different modalities are just beginning to be explored and may also hold significant promise.

With the ongoing developments in genomics and the advent of microarrays, the genetic and molecular defects involved in prostate carcinogenesis will most certainly be more thoroughly dissected in the coming years. This knowledge will lead the way for targeted, more effective therapies for patients with prostate cancer.

REFERENCES

1. Huggins C, Hodges CV. Studies on prostatic cancer. I. The effect of castration, of estrogen and androgen injection on serum phosphatases in metastatic carcinoma of the prostate. CA Cancer J Clin 1972;22:232–40.
2. Hudson MA, Bahnson RR, Catalona WJ. Clinical use of prostate specific antigen in patients with prostate cancer. J Urol 1989;142:1011–7.
3. Smith DC, Pienta KJ. The use of prostate-specific antigen as a surrogate end point in the treatment of patients with hormone refractory prostate cancer. Urol Clin North Am 1997;24:433–7.
4. Plowman PN, Perry LA, Chard T. Androgen suppression by hydrocortisone without aminoglutethimide in orchiectomised men with prostatic cancer. Br J Urol 1987; 59:255–7.
5. Storlie JA, Buckner JC, Wiseman GA, et al. Prostate specific antigen levels and clinical response to low dose dexamethasone for hormone-refractory metastatic prostate carcinoma. Cancer 1995;76:96–100.
6. Thalmann GN, Sikes RA, Chang SM, et al. Suramin-induced decrease in prostate-specific antigen expression with no effect on tumor growth in the LNCaP model of human prostate cancer. J Natl Cancer Inst 1996;88:794–801.
7. Walls R, Thibault A, Liu L, et al. The differentiating agent phenylacetate increases prostate-specific antigen production by prostate cancer cells. Prostate 1996;29:177–82.
8. Horti J, Dixon SC, Logothetis CJ, et al. Increased transcriptional activity of prostate-specific antigen in the presence of TNP-470, an angiogenesis inhibitor. Br J Cancer 1999;79:1588–93.
9. Small EJ, Srinivas S. The antiandrogen withdrawal syndrome. Experience in a large cohort of unselected patients with advanced prostate cancer. Cancer 1995;76:1428–34.
10. Kahn D, Williams RD, Manyak MJ, et al. 111Indium-capromab pendetide in the evaluation of patients with residual or recurrent prostate cancer after radical prostatectomy. The ProstaScint Study Group. J Urol 1998;159:2041–6; discussion 2046–7.
11. Tannock IF, Osoba D, Stockler MR, et al. Chemotherapy with mitoxantrone plus prednisone or prednisone alone for symptomatic hormone-resistant prostate cancer: a Canadian randomized trial with palliative end points. J Clin Oncol 1996;14:1756–64.
12. Pienta KJ, Redman BG, Bandekar R, et al. A phase II trial of oral estramustine and oral etoposide in hormone refractory prostate cancer. Urology 1997;50:401–6; discussion 406–7.
13. Colleoni M, Graiff C, Vicario G, et al. Phase II study of estramustine, oral etoposide, and vinorelbine in hormone-refractory prostate cancer. Am J Clin Oncol 1997;20:383–6.
14. Smith DC, Pienta KJ. Paclitaxel in the treatment of hormone-refractory prostate cancer. Semin Oncol 1999;26:109–11.
15. Petrylak DP, Macarthur RB, O'Connor J, et al. Phase I trial of docetaxel with estramustine in androgen-independent prostate cancer. J Clin Oncol 1999;17:958–67.
16. Berenson JR, Lichtenstein A, Porter L, et al. Long-term pamidronate treatment of advanced multiple myeloma patients reduces skeletal events. Myeloma Aredia Study Group. J Clin Oncol 1998;16:593–602.
17. Hortobagyi GN, Theriault RL, Lipton A, et al. Long-term prevention of skeletal complications of metastatic breast cancer with pamidronate. Protocol 19 Aredia Breast Cancer Study Group. J Clin Oncol 1998;16:2038–44.
18. Bloomfield DJ. Should bisphosphonates be part of the standard therapy of patients with multiple myeloma or bone metastases from other cancers? An evidence- based review. J Clin Oncol 1998;16:1218–25.
19. Pelger RC, Hamdy NA, Zwinderman AH, et al. Effects of the bisphosphonate olpadronate in patients with carcinoma of the prostate metastatic to the skeleton. Bone 1998;22: 403–8.
20. Green JR, Muller K, Jaeggi KA. Preclinical pharmacology of CGP 42'446, a new, potent, heterocyclic bisphosphonate compound. J Bone Miner Res 1994;9:745–51.
21. Chambers AF, Matrisian LM. Changing views of the role of matrix metalloproteinases in metastasis. J Natl Cancer Inst 1997;89:1260–70.
22. Lein M, Nowak L, Jung K, et al. Metalloproteinases and tissue inhibitors of matrix-metalloproteinases in plasma of patients with prostate cancer and in prostate cancer tissue. Ann N Y Acad Sci 1999;878:544–6.
23. Shalinsky DR, Brekken J, Zou H, et al. Broad antitumor and antiangiogenic activities of AG3340, a potent and selective MMP inhibitor undergoing advanced oncology clinical trials. Ann N Y Acad Sci 1999;878:236–70.
24. Folkman J. Angiogenesis in cancer, vascular, rheumatoid and other disease. Nat Med 1995;1:27–31.
25. Fortier AH, Nelson BJ, Grella DK, Holaday JW. Antiangiogenic activity of prostate-specific antigen. J Natl Cancer Inst 1999;91:1635–40.

improved understanding of the cellular and molecular processes involved in the colonization of bone by prostate cancer cells is a prerequisite to the development of new, biologically based treatment approaches to bone metastasis. Because the skeleton is the most common site of metastasis, therapies specifically targeting prostate cancer–bone interactions have the potential to reduce morbidity and may even contribute to improved survival. This chapter reviews some of the aspects of the relationship between prostate cancer and the bone microenvironment.

MECHANISMS OF METASTASIS

According to the multistep model of metastasis, a clinically significant metastatic deposit will develop only after the cancer cell completes a number of biologically discrete steps. Beginning in the prostate, the epithelial carcinoma cells are initially limited by a basement membrane that surrounds the prostate glands, including glands containing prostatic intraepithelial neoplasia. A carcinoma cell or gland destined to metastasize must possess the biologic capability to invade through the basement membrane surrounding the gland and enter into the extracellular matrix or stroma of the prostate. Then, as a prerequisite to systemic dissemination, the cell or gland must invade either the vasculature or lymphatic spaces. To reach the bone, cells must first survive in the bloodstream and then attach and invade at the distant site. The carcinoma cells may attach to bone marrow endothelial cells; alternatively, they may pass unimpeded through fenestrations in the bone marrow endothelium and attach directly to extracellular bone surfaces via receptors for moieties such as collagens, laminin, and/or other bone matrix proteins. Finally, cells must establish a metastatic colony by cellular proliferation and angiogenesis.[6] As described below, metastatic colonies often induce an intense reaction in the bone, and this reaction likely contributes to the establishment and survival of the metastatic deposit. Because of the number of steps involved and the nature of the barriers that must be overcome by the metastasizing cell, the entire process has been characterized as inefficient, with only specific subpopulations of cells able to complete the process.[7] It is presumed that only a tiny fraction of tumor cells escape the primary tumor, and only a fraction of circulating cells end up forming a macroscopic metastatic deposit.

The early steps of metastasis are common to all carcinomas: invasion through the basement membrane and entrance into the stroma of the primary organ, vascular/lymphatic invasion, systemic dissemination, and survival in the circulation. The final steps of metastasis may be unique to prostate cancer. Why does prostate cancer prefer bone? Although the specific answer to this question remains to be determined, on a general level, the preference of prostate cancer for bone may be explained by either enhanced targeting of cells to bone and/or enhanced proliferation of cells in bone once they have arrived in the bone marrow.

IS THERE TARGETING OF THE BONE BY CIRCULATING PROSTATE CANCER CELLS?

As mentioned, the predilection for prostate cancer to metastasize to bone may be explained, at least in part, by preferential targeting of bone. Some investigators have used the term "homing" to describe this phenomenon. Enhanced homing might be explained by either preferential delivery of tumor cells or preferential attachment of tumor cells at the distant site. In spontaneous metastasis assays, in which human prostate cancer cells are implanted into the mouse prostate, circulating cells reach virtually all organs.[8] A simplistic conclusion from these studies is that homing or targeting cannot be attributable to enhanced delivery of circulating tumor cells. Nonetheless, a popular and traditional hypothesis regarding the pattern of prostate cancer metastasis does indeed invoke blood flow patterns. According to this hypothesis, the lower axial skeleton is a prime landing spot for circulating prostate cancer cells because of a portal system of veins between the prostate and the lower lumbar vertebrae termed Batson's plexus.[9,10] In anatomic studies on human cadavers, Batson injected dye into the dorsal venous complex of the penis (which communicates with the periprostatic venous complex) and then found the dye in the paravertebral venous complex.

Experimental evidence supporting this hypothesis comes from Shevrin and colleagues.[11] These investigators injected human prostate cancer cells into the tail vein of immunodeficient mice with simultaneous compression of the vena cava through the abdominal wall. The incidence of experimental metastasis to the lower lumbar spine could be increased by abdominal compression. The authors suggested that these data lend support to the hypothesis that entry of cells into the vertebral venous circulation is an important step in the development of lumbar spine metastases.

There are other anatomic factors in the architecture of the bone marrow cavity that may give the bone an advantage with regard to "delivery" of circulating tumor cells. In this protected space, blood flows at a slow rate, which may give circulating cancer cells increased time and opportunity to adhere to the bone marrow endothelium. Furthermore, the bone marrow endothelium is known to contain small openings or "fenestrations" through which hematopoietic cells are known to pass.[12] These fenestrations in the bone marrow endothelium and the sinusoidal structure of the marrow vasculature may facilitate tumor cell extravasation into the bone marrow extracellular space, thereby bypassing the steps of attachment to and invasion through the endothelium.

Is there an advantage to the bone with respect to the adhesion of circulating tumor cells? The colonization of bone marrow by prostate cancer cells is likely to involve adhesion to specific ligands found either on endothelial or bone marrow parenchymal cells or within the extracellular matrix of the bone marrow environment. In an in vitro study, Lehr and Pienta found that prostate cancer cells adhered preferentially to bone marrow endothelial cells as opposed to endothelial cells derived from other organs.[13] With regard to extracellular matrix proteins such as laminin, collagen, fibronectin, and vitronectin, tumor cell adhesion is mediated, at least in part, by transmembrane proteins termed integrins. An integrin receptor is a noncovalently linked heterodimer consisting of an α and a β subunit, each with large extracellular and intracellular domains.[14,15] Cell-surface integrins adhere specifically to matrix proteins through interaction with Arg-Gly-Asp (R-G-D) amino-acid motifs in the matrix molecules. It has been demonstrated that various bone components can stimulate tumor cell adhesion and chemotaxis,[16] and Kostenuik et al[17] found that prostate cancer cells adhere to type I collagen in osteoblast extracellular matrix via the $\alpha_2\beta_1$ integrin. These types of interactions may lead to preferential adhesion of circulating cells to elements of the bone microenvironment.

As described above, physical considerations and cellular adhesion mechanisms may explain the preferential targeting of prostate cancer cells to the bone marrow. However, clinical studies of micrometastatic disease suggest that seeding is not sufficient to account for the preferential growth of prostate cancer cells in the bone marrow microenvironment. A number of studies have documented microscopic seeding of bone marrow in clinically localized colorectal and gastric carcinomas, two tumor types that rarely produce clinically significant, macroscopic bone metastases. In these types of cancers, the finding of low numbers of carcinoma cells in the bone marrow indicates a worse prognosis,[18,19] just as in prostate cancer.[20] However, unlike with prostate cancer, patients with colorectal and gastric cancers usually succumb to large soft tissue metastases without developing grossly evident metastatic bone deposits. These observations emphasize the special relationship between prostate cancer cells and bone and suggest that alternative mechanisms play a role in the preference of prostate cancer cells for bone.

IS THERE ENHANCED PROLIFERATION OF PROSTATE CANCER CELLS ONCE THEY REACH THE BONE?

The alternative explanation is that enhanced proliferation, rather than enhanced targeting, explains the phenomenon of prostate cancer bone metastases. This theory was initially articulated by Paget[21] in 1889 and has become known as the "seed and soil hypothesis." According to this hypothesis, specific types of tumor cells (seed) have a special biologic affinity for the microenvironment (soil) of certain target organs of metastasis. Paget's epidemiologic data came from a large autopsy study of patients who died of various types of metastatic disease.

Presently, many laboratories are devoting significant efforts to try to gain a molecular understanding of the seed and soil hypothesis.

Direct experimental evidence supporting Paget's theory comes from the severe combined immunodeficient-human model of prostate cancer bone metastasis developed in our laboratory.[22] We implanted macroscopic human fetal bone fragments and other human organ fragments into the subcutaneous space of immunodeficient mice (Figure 24–1). Several weeks later, we injected human prostate cancer cells into the mice either intravenously or directly into the implanted human organs. We found that circulating human prostate cancer cells formed tumors in the implanted human bones but not in the in situ mouse bones or other implanted human organs. Furthermore, the directly injected cells preferred to proliferate in the human bone microenvironment as compared with other human or murine organ microenvironments. These data support the hypothesis that there is a special and unique interaction between prostate cancer cells and the bone microenvironment.

A variety of experimental approaches have been used to demonstrate the inductive capacity of bone and bone-derived factors on the growth of prostate cancer cells. Using coculture techniques, Lang and colleagues found that close contact with bone marrow stromal cells in culture can stimulate the growth of cells derived from primary prostate tumors.[23] Close physical interaction with bone cells has also been shown to enhance tumorigenicity of normally nontumorigenic LNCaP prostate cancer cells.[24] Subcutaneous tumors formed in nude mice following co-injection of LNCaP cells with either bone or prostate fibroblasts but not with kidney or lung fibroblasts. Manipulation of this system through multiple rounds of co-injection, subculturing, and androgen withdrawal has resulted in sublines of LNCaP that are tumorigenic, androgen independent,[25] and able to metastasize to lymph nodes and bone.[26] Gleave and colleagues also noted that soluble factors produced by bone fibroblasts could induce tumor formation by LNCaP in nude mice, suggesting that paracrine interactions might be involved.[24] Tissue culture studies have also shown that soluble factors derived from bone marrow[27] or osteoblast-like cells[28] could stimulate growth of various prostate cancer cell lines, although

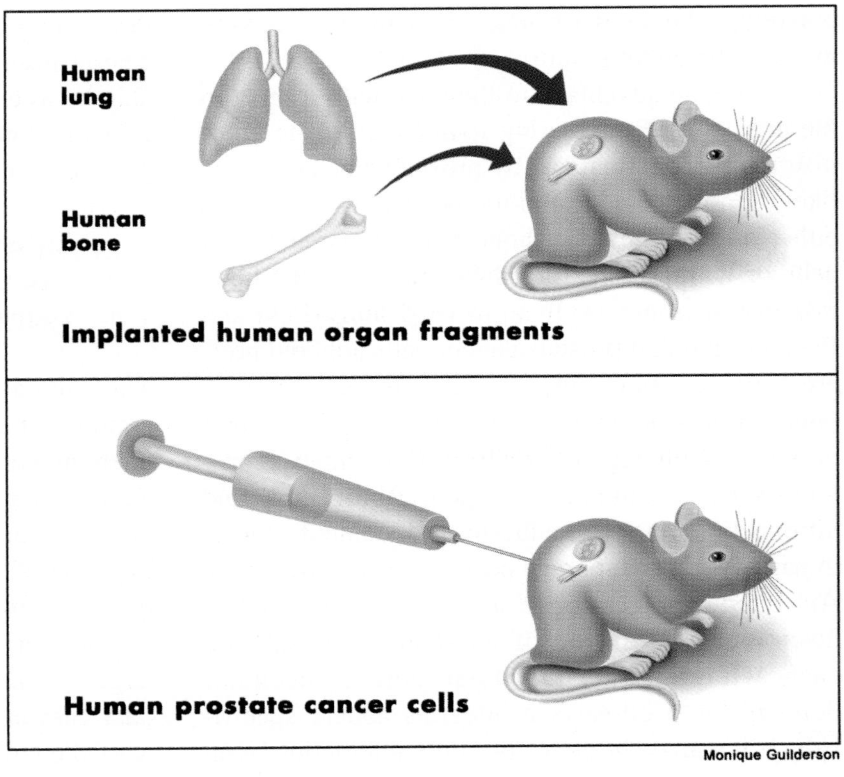

Figure 24–1. Severe combined immunodeficient-human model of prostate cancer bone metastasis. Severe combined immunodeficient-human mice are created by subcutaneous implantation of human organ fragments into immunodeficient mice. A few weeks later, human prostate cancer cells are injected either intravenously or directly into the implanted fragment.

the factors responsible for this stimulation remain incompletely described.

A number of in vitro studies have focused on possible growth factor interactions that may promote prostate cancer cell growth in the bone marrow. Bone and bone marrow are rich sources of growth factors and cytokines, which normally regulate bone growth and hematopoiesis, and a number of these factors could enhance the formation of metastatic deposits by prostate cells. As noted above, soluble factors derived from bone or bone marrow can stimulate prostate cancer cell growth in culture, but attempts to replicate this effect by adding purified growth factors known to be present in bone marrow have met with limited success.[27,29] The following discussion addresses some of the growth factor systems present in bone that may contribute to the specific growth of prostate cancer metastases.

The insulin-like growth factor (IGF) system consists of IGF-I and IGF-II, the type I and type II receptors, and IGF-binding proteins 2 through 6, which are known to modulate the activity of the IGFs (reviewed in Jones Clemmons[30]). Cohen and colleagues demonstrated the ability of IGFs to stimulate the growth of normal prostatic epithelial cells in culture and suggested that mechanisms involving IGFs and the binding proteins may participate in prostate growth control in vivo.[31] Insulin-like growth factors may also be involved in prostate tumorigenesis, since the DU145, LNCaP, and PC3 prostate cancer cell lines all respond to IGF in culture,[32] and all three cell lines secrete IGFs, suggesting a possible autocrine loop.[33] Insulin-like growth factor-I and -II have also been detected in bone,[34] and it has been suggested that the presence of IGFs may promote the formation of prostate cancer bone metastases through increased proliferation and chemotaxis.[29]

Transforming growth factor-β (TGF-β) is a multifunctional growth factor that acts as a potent growth inhibitor of epithelial cells in culture, including prostate cancer cells.[35] Transforming growth factor-β has different effects in vivo. Steiner and Barrack found that overexpression of TGF-β by a rodent prostate cancer cell line enhanced tumor formation and growth rate.[36] In addition, levels of TGF-β are typically higher in prostate cancer tissues than in normal prostate tissue[37,38] and appear to correlate with histologic grade of cancer. Furthermore, bone is known to be a rich source of TGF-β, where it is produced by osteoblasts[39] and stored in the bone matrix.[40] Much study has been done to reconcile the growth-suppressive effects of TGF-β with its ability to promote tumor formation. Among the mechanisms by which TGF-β may enhance tumor growth are stimulation of angiogenesis[41] through induction of vascular endothelial growth factor secretion,[42] induction of cell motility and extracellular matrix deposition,[43] and suppression of the immune system.[44] Certain properties of the tumor cells themselves or their environment may also help them escape the growth-suppressive effects of TGF-β in vivo. For example, interaction with other growth factors such as epidermal growth factor (EGF) can alleviate the negative effects of TGF-β on primary prostate cells.[45] Growth of prostate cancer cells on purified matrix proteins can also blunt the growth-inhibitory effects of TGF-β, although the cells can still respond with increased motility.[46] Tumor cells may also alter their response to TGF-β. At low concentrations and certain culture conditions, TGF-β is mildly stimulatory for PC3 and DU145 cancer cell lines,[28] and the TSU-Pr1 cell line is highly stimulated by TGF-β.[47] Finally, loss of expression of the type I or type II TGF-β receptor has been detected in prostate cancer specimens and was linked to increased tumor grade.[48–50] Therefore, the presence of high levels of TGF-β in the bone marrow environment could contribute to the formation of prostate cancer metastases through several mechanisms.

Epidermal growth factor is a potent stimulator of prostate epithelial cell growth. Most of the well-characterized human prostate cancer cell lines express the EGF receptor and respond to EGF from either autocrine or exogenous sources (reviewed in Ware[51]). Epidermal growth factor protein has been found in the bone marrow stroma. Furthermore, EGF can stimulate the migration of prostate cancer cells in culture, and it has been suggested that this chemotactic property might be involved in the seeding of lymph nodes and bone by prostate cancer cells.[52] It is possible that a combination of EGF-related effects (migration/chemotaxis, growth stimulation, relief of growth inhibition by TGF-β) plays an important role in the formation and growth of prostate cancer bone metastases.

Basic fibroblast growth factor (bFGF) can be found in bone, where it is produced by osteoblasts and sequestered in the bone matrix.[53] The potential role for bFGF in prostate tumorigenesis was demonstrated by Gleave and colleagues.[24] In this study, subcutaneous injection of LNCaP cells into nude mice did not result in tumors; however, tumors did form when the cells were co-injected with bFGF. Basic FGF has also been found to be expressed by prostate tumors[54, 55] and thus may act in both a paracrine and an autocrine fashion. In addition to its direct growth-stimulatory effects, production of bFGF by tumor cells may also enhance tumor formation through induction of angiogenesis.[56]

The cytokine interleukin-6 (IL-6) is present at high levels in the bone marrow environment and functions primarily in the induction of B-cell maturation and immunoglobulin production.[57] Recently, its potential role in a number of cancers has become apparent, including renal cell carcinoma,[58] cervical carcinoma,[59] and prostate carcinoma. Message for the IL-6 receptor has been detected in a high proportion of prostate cancer specimens and some benign hyperplastic prostate tissues, suggesting a possible role in the progression of prostate disease.[60] The three human prostate cancer cell lines, LNCaP, DU145, and PC3, also express both the IL-6 receptor and IL-6,[61] and it appears to act as an autocrine growth factor for these cells as well.[62,63] In the bone, IL-6 is produced by osteoblasts and induces the formation and activity of osteoclasts. It is also negatively regulated by androgen and is involved in the clinical loss of bone mass that accompanies androgen withdrawal.[64] This raises questions regarding the use of androgen withdrawal as a therapy for advanced prostate cancer since increased IL-6 production by bone cells following androgen withdrawal therapy may actually stimulate growth of prostate cancer cells in the bone marrow. Theoretically, this mechanism could reduce the effectiveness of this therapy. Furthermore, autocrine production of IL-6 by prostate cancer cells can confer resistance to cytotoxic agents such as tumor necrosis factor-α, etoposide, and *cis*-platinum.[65] These observations could be important when designing treatment strategies involving chemotherapy and androgen withdrawal.

Urokinase-type plasminogen activator (uPA, urokinase) is a protein that may play a very important role in prostate cancer growth and metastasis. The primary function of urokinase is the conversion of plasminogen to its active form, plasmin[66]; however, this enzyme has also been found at high levels in cancer systems, where it is thought to be involved in tissue remodeling and cell migration.[67] In a study on prostate cancer bone metastases, Kirchheimer and colleagues found much higher levels of urokinase activity in extracts from bone metastases versus their primary tumor counterparts.[68] In experimental systems, overexpression of urokinase was able to enhance bone metastasis by the rat prostate cancer cell line MatLyLu[69]; conversely, inhibition of urokinase activity through overexpression of its natural inhibitor PAI-1 slowed the growth and decreased the incidence of metastasis by PC3 cells in nude mice.[70] The mechanism by which urokinase enhances prostate cancer growth is unclear but may involve its ability to modulate the activity of a number of growth factors. Koutsilieris and colleagues found that urokinase can cleave various IGF binding proteins, thus altering the availability and activity of IGF.[71] In fact, proteolysis of the IGF binding protein 3 by urokinase appears to be involved in autocrine stimulation of PC3 cells.[72] Urokinase also can release matrix-bound bFGF,[73] and this mechanism is thought to play a role in angiogenesis. Generation of the osteoblastic reaction to metastatic prostate cells may also involve urokinase. A short amino-terminal fragment of uPA has been identified that can stimulate proliferation of osteoblasts directly.[74] Production of urokinase by prostate cancer cells and generation of this stimulatory fragment could lead to a "vicious cycle" of tumor growth, whereby prostate cell–derived urokinase induces osteoblast proliferation, and, in turn, increased numbers of osteoblasts produce more stimulatory factors for prostate cancer cells.

In addition to growth factors and cytokines, prostate cancer cells may interact specifically with extracellular matrix proteins. These interactions may play a part in supporting growth of metastatic prostate cancer colonies, although there is very little information in the literature specifically addressing bone extracellular matrix. Experimentally, growth of prostate cells on reconstituted basement membrane and purified matrix proteins has striking effects on cellular behavior. Growth on basement membrane proteins was found to enhance production of PSA, slow proliferation, and increase the sensitivity to androgen in normal prostate epithelial cells[75] and in LNCaP carcinoma cells.[76] However, growth of a rat prostate cell line, NbMC-2, in a basement membrane gel resulted in enhancement of malignant properties.[77] Therefore, the response to matrix proteins appears to be cell type specific.

As mentioned earlier, prostate cancer cells may interact with the extracellular matrix via integrins on their cell surface. In addition to their role in adhesion, integrins are involved in intracellular signaling and greatly influence cell behavior and phenotype. For example, binding of cells to a substrate via the $\alpha v\beta 3$ integrin can potentiate the stimulatory effects of insulin and IGF (reviewed in Ruoslahti[78]). However, activation of certain integrin subunits can also result in growth arrest.[79] Interaction with extracellular matrix through the $\alpha_5\beta_1$ integrin has also been shown to protect cells from apoptosis in serum-free culture conditions through a mechanism involving BCL2.[78] As mentioned above, growth of rodent prostate cancer cells on matrix components can relieve the growth-inhibitory effects of TGF-β, although the cells can still respond with enhanced motility and matrix production.[46] Therefore, integrin signaling may contribute to the specificity of prostate cancer metastasis to bone through interaction with the specific subset of extracellular matrix proteins present in the bone environment.

REACTION OF THE BONE TO THE PRESENCE OF PROSTATE CANCER CELLS: A VICIOUS CYCLE

As mentioned, prostate cancer bone metastases cause a relatively unique reaction in bone. This reaction usually results in osteoblastic findings on radiographic imaging studies. Examination of plain film radiographs or computed tomographic scans shows expansion of the bone with areas of increased radiographic density corresponding to areas of formation of dense, new, mineralized bone matrix. The appearance of these lesions is characteristic of prostate cancer metastasis (Figure 24–2). However, indiscriminate application of the term osteoblastic to describe prostate cancer metastasis can lead to an incomplete understanding of the biology of prostate cancer's interaction with bone. As mentioned, from a clinical standpoint, the term osteoblastic simply describes increased radiographic density obvious on casual examination of imaging studies. Using such a radiologic definition, a series of untreated prostate cancer metastases were classified into five types: osteoblastic (15%), mainly osteoblastic (31%), mainly osteolytic (17%), osteolytic (10%), and undetermined (27%).[80] Also, computed tomographic imaging often identifies lytic areas within predominantly osteoblastic lesions,[81] and quantitative x-ray absorptiometry shows reduced bone mass in the bony pelvis of patients with metastatic prostate cancer, mainly owing to the predominance of bone resorption within radiologically defined osteoblastic metastases.[82,83] Thus, even by radiographic criteria, prostate cancer bone metastases demonstrate both lytic and blastic activity. In addition, several studies have demonstrated lytic and blastic activity on a cellular and a biochemical level. Histomorphometric studies of prostate cancer metastases have demonstrated increased bone resorption at the tumor site.[84] Serum and/or urine biochemical markers of bone resorption and formation are elevated specifically in

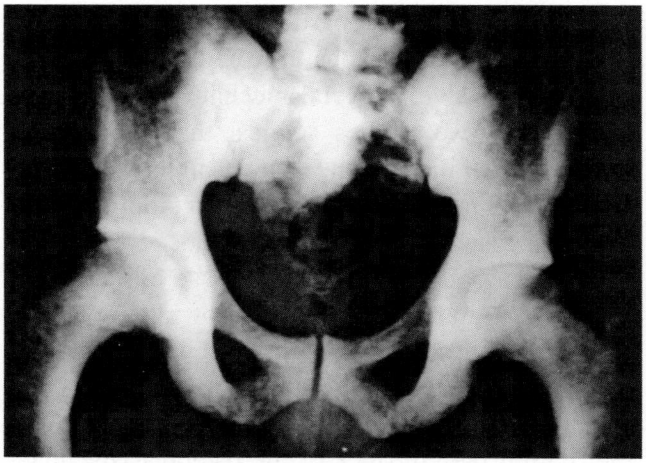

Figure 24–2. Plain film radiograph of a patient with prostate cancer. This patient has widespread bone metastasis throughout his pelvis and vertebral column.

patients with prostate cancer bone metastasis, and the levels correlate with metastatic load and response to treatment.[83,85–93] In some studies, markers of bone resorption correlate better with metastatic load than markers of bone formation.[89,90,93] Thus, prostate cancer bone metastasis is associated with increased metabolic bone turnover, including both bone loss and new bone formation. In any case, bone exhibits a tremendous response to the presence of prostate cancer; this response is part of a bidirectional communication between prostate cancer cells and bone, as described below.

In both normal and pathologic states, bone remodeling is a sequential process by which there is resorption and subsequent formation of bone extracellular matrix. This process has long been described as a series of steps[94] and has recently been reviewed.[95] In the current model, bone matrix degradation involves osteoclast recruitment (differentiation and migration), digestion of a superficial layer of nonmineralized collagen by osteoblasts (in preparation for osteoclast attachment), and mineralized matrix degradation by osteoclasts. Mineralized matrix resorption occurs via the action of cysteine proteases and matrix metalloproteinases (MMPs), both of which are produced by osteoclasts and secreted into the osteoclast resorption lacuna.[96] Osteoblasts are responsible for synthesis of new bone matrix.

In metastatic disease, turnover of bone matrix is stimulated by paracrine communication between tumor cells and bone cells. This phenomenon has been a topic of interest, particularly in breast cancer, in which the bone lesions are predominantly osteolytic (destructive). Several mechanisms have been described.[97] Two studies suggest that cancer cells degrade mineralized bone matrix directly, possibly via the secretion of MMPs.[98,99] In addition, one study suggested that MMP-2, produced by cancer cells, was associated with the release of collagen I fragments from bone.[100] However, owing to pH considerations, most investigators feel that metastatic cells cannot directly degrade the mineralized compartment of bone matrix; a low pH can be attained only within the confines of the osteoclast lacuna.[97] There is ample experimental evidence of a local, bidirectional communication between prostate cancer cells and bone cells including both osteoblasts and osteoclasts,[101] and the predominance of the literature suggests that cancer cells in bone stimulate osteoblasts and osteoclasts in a paracrine fashion to digest and synthesize new mineralized matrix.[102,103] Candidates for the stimulation and/or recruitment of osteoclasts include TGF-α, EGF, IL-1, IL-6, IL-11, TNF-α, prostaglandins, and parathyroid hormone–related peptide.[6,104] Leading molecular candidates for the paracrine stimulation of bone formation include the IGFs,[105] TGF-β,[36] FGF,[24] bone morphogenetic proteins[106] and the amino-terminal fragment of urokinase.[107] It is likely that bone matrix turnover actually contributes to the establishment and growth of metastatic prostate cancer colonies by the release of factors into the microenvironment during the degradative stages. Such a vicious cycle involving prostate cancer cells, bone cells, bone matrix turnover, and the release of stimulatory factors can easily be understood to form the basis of the propensity of prostate cancer to proliferate within the bone microenvironment (Figure 24–3).

CONCLUSIONS

Although many of the structural factors and molecular and cellular interactions described above exhibit tumor- and metastasis-promoting activity, it is unlikely that any one of these factors alone explains the preferential growth of prostate cancer in bone. It is also clear that individual factors influence the response of prostate cancer cells to other factors in a complex and interactive fashion. Within the context of the bone environment, the relative contribution of each of these factors, and perhaps many others, remains to be determined. Further studies directed toward understanding the interactions of various growth factor signaling pathways, cell–extracellular matrix interactions, and direct cell-cell communication may provide more clues to the bone specificity of prostate cancer metastasis. These studies may eventually lead to the development of treatment strategies designed specifically to inhibit the growth of metastatic prostate cancer cells in the bone microenvironment, and such strategies may ultimately prove to be beneficial to our patients.

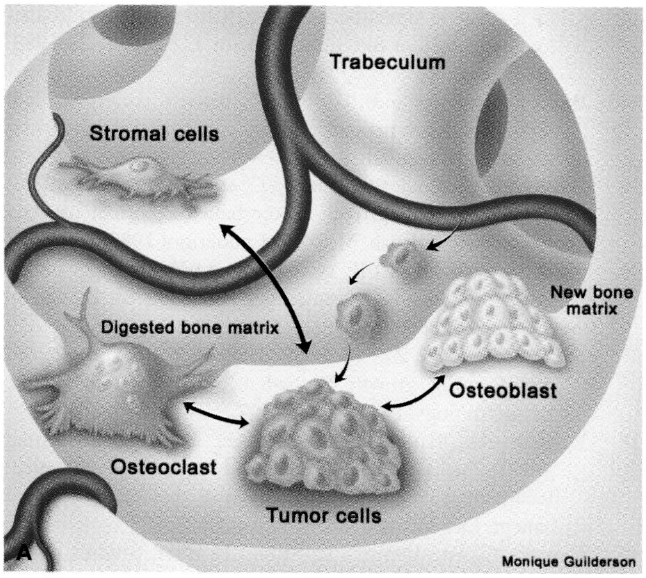

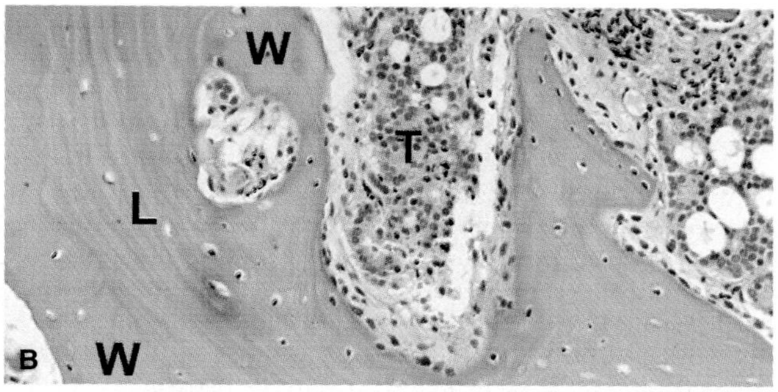

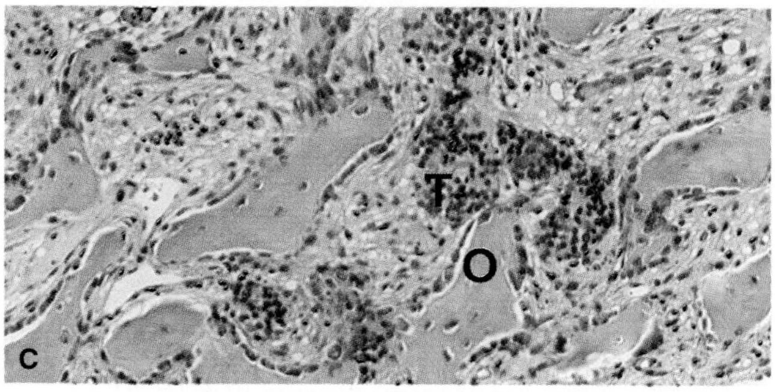

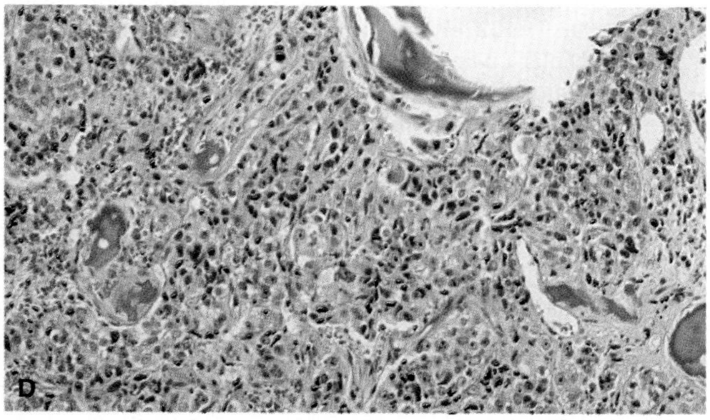

Figure 24–3. Vicious cycle of tumor cell proliferation and bone matrix turnover. Tumor cells enter the bone marrow microenvironment via the sinusoidal endothelium. The cells enter by attachment and invasion or through fenestrations in the endothelium. Tumor cells adhere to the extracellular matrix of bone trabeculae and secrete cytokines and growth factors that stimulate bone cells, including osteoclasts, osteoblasts, and bone marrow stromal cells. Osteoclastic degradation of the organic bone matrix releases other factors and matrix protein fragments that are stimulatory to the cancer cells. Osteoblasts and tumor cells also communicate in a bidirectional fashion. Osteoblasts form new organic bone matrix, resulting in the typical osteoblastic appearance on imaging studies.

REFERENCES

1. Schwartz KL, Grignon DJ, Sakr WA, Wood DP Jr. Prostate cancer histologic trends in the metropolitan Detroit area, 1982 to 1996. Urology 1999;53:769–74.
2. Sakr WA, Grignon DJ, Crissman JD, et al. High grade prostatic intraepithelial neoplasia (HGPIN) and prostatic adenocarcinoma between the ages of 20–69: an autopsy study of 249 cases. In Vivo 1994;8:439–43.
3. Saitoh H, Hida M, Shimbo T, et al. Metastatic patterns of prostatic cancer. Correlation between sites and number of organs involved. Cancer 1984;54:3078–84.
4. Glaves D. Mechanisms of metastasis: prostate cancer. Prog Clin Biol Res 1987;239:329–45.
5. Eisenberger MA. Chemotherapy for hormone resistant prostate cancer. In: Walsh PC, Retik AC, Vaughan ED, Wein AJ, editors. Campbell's urology. Vol 3. Philadelphia: WB Saunders; 1998. p. 2645–58.
6. Goltzman D. Mechanisms of the development of osteoblastic metastases. Cancer 1997;80:1581–7.
7. Fidler IJ. Modulation of the organ microenvironment for treatment of cancer metastasis. J Natl Cancer Inst 1995; 87:1588–92.
8. Yang M, Jiang P, Sun FX, et al. A fluorescent orthotopic bone metastasis model of human prostate cancer. Cancer Res 1999;59:781–6.
9. Batson OV. The role of the vertebral veins in metastatic processes. Ann Intern Med 1942;16:38–45.
10. Batson OV. Function of vertebral veins and their role in spread of metastases. Ann Surg 1940;112:138–49.
11. Shevrin DH, Kukreja SC, Ghosh L, Lad TE. Development of skeletal metastasis by human prostate cancer in athymic nude mice. Clin Exp Metastasis 1988;6:401–9.
12. Weiss L. Bone marrow. In: Mitchell CW, editor. Histology, cell and tissue biology. Baltimore: Urban & Schwarzenberg; 1983.
13. Lehr JE, Pienta KJ. Preferential adhesion of prostate cancer cells to a human bone marrow endothelial cell line. J Natl Cancer Inst 1998;90:118–23.
14. Albelda SM, Buck CA. Integrins and other cell adhesion molecules. FASEB J 1990;4:2868–80.
15. Hynes RO. Integrins: versatility, modulation, and signaling in cell adhesion. Cell 1992;69:11–25.
16. Magro C, Orr FW, Manishen WJ, et al. Adhesion, chemotaxis, and aggregation of Walker carcinosarcoma cells in

response to products of resorbing bone. J Natl Cancer Inst 1985;74:829–38.

17. Kostenuik PJ, Sanchez-Sweatman O, Orr FW, Singh G. Bone cell matrix promotes the adhesion of human prostatic carcinoma cells via the alpha 2 beta 1 integrin. Clin Exp Metastasis 1996;14:19–26.
18. Lindemann F, Schlimok G, Dirschedl P, et al. Prognostic significance of micrometastatic tumour cells in bone marrow of colorectal cancer patients. Lancet 1992;340:685–9.
19. Jauch KW, Heiss MM, Gruetzner U, et al. Prognostic significance of bone marrow micrometastases in patients with gastric cancer. J Clin Oncol 1996;14:1810–7.
20. Wood DP Jr, Banerjee M. Presence of circulating prostate cells in the bone marrow of patients undergoing radical prostatectomy is predictive of disease-free survival. J Clin Oncol 1997;15:3451–7.
21. Paget S. The distribution of secondary growths in cancer of the breast. Lancet 1889;1:571–73.
22. Nemeth JA, Harb JF, Barroso U Jr, et al. Severe combined immunodeficient-human model of human prostate cancer metastasis to human bone. Cancer Res 1999;59:1987–93.
23. Lang SH, Clarke NW, George NJ, et al. Interaction of prostate epithelial cells from benign and malignant tumor tissue with bone-marrow stroma. Prostate 1998;34:203–13.
24. Gleave M, Hsieh JT, Gao CA, et al. Acceleration of human prostate cancer growth in vivo by factors produced by prostate and bone fibroblasts. Cancer Res 1991;51: 3753–61.
25. Wu HC, Hsieh JT, Gleave ME, et al. Derivation of androgen-independent human LNCaP prostatic cancer cell sublines: role of bone stromal cells. Int J Cancer 1994;57:406–12.
26. Thalmann GN, Anezinis PE, Chang SM, et al. Androgen-independent cancer progression and bone metastasis in the LNCaP model of human prostate cancer [published erratum appears in Cancer Res 1994;54:3953]. Cancer Res 1994;54:2577–81.
27. Chackal-Roy M, Niemeyer C, Moore M, Zetter BR. Stimulation of human prostatic carcinoma cell growth by factors present in human bone marrow. J Clin Invest 1989; 84:43–50.
28. Lang SH, Miller WR, Habib FK. Stimulation of human prostate cancer cell lines by factors present in human osteoblast-like cells but not in bone marrow. Prostate 1995;27:287–93.
29. Ritchie CK, Andrews LR, Thomas KG, et al. The effects of growth factors associated with osteoblasts on prostate carcinoma proliferation and chemotaxis: implications for the development of metastatic disease. Endocrinology 1997;138:1145–50.
30. Jones JI, Clemmons DR. Insulin-like growth factors and their binding proteins: biological actions. Endocr Rev 1995;16:3–34.
31. Cohen P, Peehl DM, Lamson G, Rosenfeld RG. Insulin-like growth factors (IGFs), IGF receptors, and IGF-binding proteins in primary cultures of prostate epithelial cells. J Clin Endocrinol Metab 1991;73:401–7.
32. Iwamura M, Sluss PM, Casamento JB, Cockett AT. Insulin-like growth factor I: action and receptor characterization in human prostate cancer cell lines. Prostate 1993;22:243–52.
33. Pietrzkowski Z, Mulholland G, Gomella L, et al. Inhibition of growth of prostatic cancer cell lines by peptide analogues of insulin-like growth factor 1. Cancer Res 1993; 53:1102–6.
34. Bautista CM, Mohan S, Baylink DJ. Insulin-like growth factors I and II are present in the skeletal tissues of ten vertebrates. Metabolism 1990;39:96–100.
35. Wilding G, Zugmeier G, Knabbe C, et al. Differential effects of transforming growth factor beta on human prostate cancer cells in vitro. Mol Cell Endocrinol 1989;62:79–87.
36. Steiner MS, Barrack ER. Transforming growth factor-beta 1 overproduction in prostate cancer: effects on growth in vivo and in vitro. Mol Endocrinol 1992;6:15–25.
37. Steiner MS, Zhou ZZ, Tonb DC, Barrack ER. Expression of transforming growth factor-beta 1 in prostate cancer. Endocrinology 1994;135:2240–7.
38. Eastham JA, Truong LD, Rogers E, et al. Transforming growth factor-beta 1: comparative immunohistochemical localization in human primary and metastatic prostate cancer. Lab Invest 1995;73:628–35.
39. Kasperk C, Fitzsimmons R, Strong D, et al. Studies of the mechanism by which androgens enhance mitogenesis and differentiation in bone cells. J Clin Endocrinol Metab 1990;71:1322–9.
40. Pfeilschifter J, Mundy GR. Modulation of type beta transforming growth factor activity in bone cultures by osteotropic hormones. Proc Natl Acad Sci U S A 1987;84:2024–8.
41. Roberts AB, Sporn MB, Assoian RK, et al. Transforming growth factor type beta: rapid induction of fibrosis and angiogenesis in vivo and stimulation of collagen formation in vitro. Proc Natl Acad Sci U S A 1986;83:4167–71.
42. Pertovaara L, Kaipainen A, Mustonen T, et al. Vascular endothelial growth factor is induced in response to transforming growth factor-beta in fibroblastic and epithelial cells. J Biol Chem 1994;269:6271–4.
43. Massague J. The transforming growth factor-beta family. Annu Rev Cell Biol 1990;6:597–641.
44. Torre-Amione G, Beauchamp RD, Koeppen H, et al. A highly immunogenic tumor transfected with a murine transforming growth factor type beta 1 cDNA escapes immune surveillance. Proc Natl Acad Sci U S A 1990;87:1486–90.
45. Sutkowski DM, Fong CJ, Sensibar JA, et al. Interaction of epidermal growth factor and transforming growth factor beta in human prostatic epithelial cells in culture. Prostate 1992;21:133–43.
46. Morton DM, Barrack ER. Modulation of transforming growth factor beta 1 effects on prostate cancer cell proliferation by growth factors and extracellular matrix. Cancer Res 1995;55:2596–602.
47. Lamm ML, Sintich SM, Lee C. A proliferative effect of transforming growth factor-beta1 on a human prostate cancer cell line, TSU-Pr1. Endocrinology 1998;139:787–90.
48. Guo Y, Jacobs SC, Kyprianou N. Down-regulation of protein and mRNA expression for transforming growth factor-beta (TGF-beta1) type I and type II receptors in human prostate cancer. Int J Cancer 1997;71:573–9.
49. Kim IY, Ahn HJ, Zelner DJ, et al. Loss of expression of transforming growth factor beta type I and type II receptors correlates with tumor grade in human prostate cancer tissues. Clin Cancer Res 1996;2:1255–61.
50. Williams RH, Stapleton AM, Yang G, et al. Reduced levels of

transforming growth factor beta receptor type II in human prostate cancer: an immunohistochemical study. Clin Cancer Res 1996;2:635–40.

51. Ware JL. Growth factors and their receptors as determinants in the proliferation and metastasis of human prostate cancer. Cancer Metastasis Rev 1993;12:287–301.
52. Rajan R, Vanderslice R, Kapur S, et al. Epidermal growth factor (EGF) promotes chemomigration of a human prostate tumor cell line, and EGF immunoreactive proteins are present at sites of metastasis in the stroma of lymph nodes and medullary bone. Prostate 1996;28:1–9.
53. Globus RK, Plouet J, Gospodarowicz D. Cultured bovine bone cells synthesize basic fibroblast growth factor and store it in their extracellular matrix. Endocrinology 1989;124:1539–47.
54. Mydlo JH, Michaeli J, Heston WD, Fair WR. Expression of basic fibroblast growth factor mRNA in benign prostatic hyperplasia and prostatic carcinoma. Prostate 1988;13: 241–7.
55. Story MT, Sasse J, Jacobs SC, Lawson RK. Prostatic growth factor: purification and structural relationship to basic fibroblast growth factor. Biochemistry 1987;26:3843–9.
56. Shing Y, Folkman J, Haudenschild C, et al. Angiogenesis is stimulated by a tumor-derived endothelial cell growth factor. J Cell Biochem 1985;29:275–87.
57. Gauldie J, Richards C, Harnish D, et al. Interferon beta 2/B-cell stimulatory factor type 2 shares identity with monocyte-derived hepatocyte-stimulating factor and regulates the major acute phase protein response in liver cells. Proc Natl Acad Sci U S A 1987;84:7251–5.
58. Takenawa J, Kaneko Y, Fukumoto M, et al. Enhanced expression of interleukin-6 in primary human renal cell carcinomas. J Natl Cancer Inst 1991;83:1668–72.
59. Eustace D, Han X, Gooding R, et al. Interleukin-6 (IL-6) functions as an autocrine growth factor in cervical carcinomas in vitro. Gynecol Oncol 1993;50:15–9.
60. Siegsmund MJ, Yamazaki H, Pastan I. Interleukin 6 receptor mRNA in prostate carcinomas and benign prostate hyperplasia. J Urol 1994;151:1396–9.
61. Siegall CB, Schwab G, Nordan RP, et al. Expression of the interleukin 6 receptor and interleukin 6 in prostate carcinoma cells. Cancer Res 1990;50:7786–8.
62. Okamoto M, Lee C, Oyasu R. Interleukin-6 as a paracrine and autocrine growth factor in human prostatic carcinoma cells in vitro. Cancer Res 1997;57:141–6.
63. Okamoto M, Lee C, Oyasu R. Autocrine effect of androgen on proliferation of an androgen responsive prostatic carcinoma cell line, LNCAP: role of interleukin-6. Endocrinology 1997;138:5071–4.
64. Bellido T, Jilka RL, Boyce BF, et al. Regulation of interleukin-6, osteoclastogenesis, and bone mass by androgens. The role of the androgen receptor. J Clin Invest 1995;95: 2886–95.
65. Borsellino N, Belldegrun A, Bonavida B. Endogenous interleukin 6 is a resistance factor for *cis*-diamminedichloroplatinum and etoposide-mediated cytotoxicity of human prostate carcinoma cell lines. Cancer Res 1995;55:4633–9.
66. Saksela O. Plasminogen activation and regulation of pericellular proteolysis. Biochim Biophys Acta 1985;823:35–65.
67. Dano K, Andreasen PA, Grondahl-Hansen J, et al. Plasminogen activators, tissue degradation, and cancer. Adv Cancer Res 1985;44:139–266.
68. Kirchheimer JC, Pfluger H, Ritschl P, et al. Plasminogen activator activity in bone metastases of prostatic carcinomas as compared to primary tumors. Invasion Metastasis 1985;5:344–55.
69. Achbarou A, Kaiser S, Tremblay G, et al. Urokinase overproduction results in increased skeletal metastasis by prostate cancer cells in vivo. Cancer Res 1994;54:2372–7.
70. Soff GA, Sanderowitz J, Gately S, et al. Expression of plasminogen activator inhibitor type 1 by human prostate carcinoma cells inhibits primary tumor growth, tumor-associated angiogenesis, and metastasis to lung and liver in an athymic mouse model. J Clin Invest 1995;96:2593–600.
71. Koutsilieris M, Frenette G, Lazure C, et al. Urokinase-type plasminogen activator: a paracrine factor regulating the bioavailability of IGFs in PA-III cell-induced osteoblastic metastases. Anticancer Res 1993;13:481–6.
72. Angelloz-Nicoud P, Binoux M. Autocrine regulation of cell proliferation by the insulin-like growth factor (IGF) and IGF binding protein-3 protease system in a human prostate carcinoma cell line (PC-3). Endocrinology 1995;136:5485–92.
73. Saksela O, Rifkin DB. Release of basic fibroblast growth factor-heparan sulfate complexes from endothelial cells by plasminogen activator-mediated proteolytic activity. J Cell Biol 1990;110:767–75.
74. Rabbani SA, Desjardins J, Bell AW, et al. An amino-terminal fragment of urokinase isolated from a prostate cancer cell line (PC-3) is mitogenic for osteoblast-like cells. Biochem Biophys Res Commun 1990;173:1058–64.
75. Fong CJ, Sherwood ER, Sutkowski DM, et al. Reconstituted basement membrane promotes morphological and functional differentiation of primary human prostatic epithelial cells. Prostate 1991;19:221–35.
76. Fong CJ, Sherwood ER, Braun EJ, et al. Regulation of prostatic carcinoma cell proliferation and secretory activity by extracellular matrix and stromal secretions. Prostate 1992;21:121–31.
77. Freeman MR, Bagli DJ, Lamb CC, et al. Culture of a prostatic cell line in basement membrane gels results in an enhancement of malignant properties and constitutive alterations in gene expression. J Cell Physiol 1994;158:325–36.
78. Ruoslahti E. Integrins as signaling molecules and targets for tumor therapy. Kidney Int 1997;51:1413–7.
79. Zheng DQ, Fornaro M, Bofetiado CJ, et al. Modulation of cell proliferation by the integrin cytoplasmic domain. Kidney Int 1997;51:1434–40.
80. Shimazaki J, Higa T, Akimoto S, et al. Clinical course of bone metastasis from prostatic cancer following endocrine therapy: examination with bone x-ray. Adv Exp Med Biol 1992;324:269–75.
81. Rubens RD. The nature of metastatic bone disease. In: Rubens RD, Fogelman I, editors. Bone metastases: diagnosis and treatment. London: Springer-Verlag; 1991. p. 1–8.
82. Rico H, Chapado MS, Revilla M, et al. Total and regional bone mass in metastatic cancer of the prostate. Eur Urol 1996;30:73–6.
83. Revilla M, Arribas I, Sanchez CM, et al. Total and regional bone mass and biochemical markers of bone remodeling in metastatic prostate cancer. Prostate 1998;35:243–7.

84. Urwin GH, Percival RC, Harris S, et al. Generalised increase in bone resorption in carcinoma of the prostate. Br J Urol 1985;57:721–3.
85. Akimoto S, Furuya Y, Akakura K, Ito H. Comparison of markers of bone formation and resorption in prostate cancer patients to predict bone metastasis. Endocr J 1998;45:97–104.
86. Buchs N, Bonjour JP, Rizzoli R. Renal tubular reabsorption of phosphate is positively related to the extent of bone metastatic load in patients with prostate cancer. J Clin Endocrinol Metab 1998;83:1535–41.
87. Yoshida K, Sumi S, Arai K, et al. Serum concentration of type I collagen metabolites as a quantitative marker of bone metastases in patients with prostate carcinoma. Cancer 1997;80:1760–7.
88. Samma S, Kagebayashi Y, Yasukawa M, et al. Sequential changes of urinary pyridinoline and deoxypyridinoline as markers of metastatic bone tumor in patients with prostate cancer: a preliminary study. Jpn J Clin Oncol 1997;27:26–30.
89. Westerhuis LW, Delaere KP. Diagnostic value of some biochemical bone markers for the detection of bone metastases in prostate cancer. Eur J Clin Chem Clin Biochem 1997;35:89–94.
90. Maeda H, Koizumi M, Yoshimura K, et al. Correlation between bone metabolic markers and bone scan in prostatic cancer. J Urol 1997;157:539–43.
91. Papatheofanis FJ. Quantitation of biochemical markers of bone resorption following strontium-89-chloride therapy for metastatic prostatic carcinoma. J Nucl Med 1997;38:1175–9.
92. Takeuchi S, Arai K, Saitoh H, et al. Urinary pyridinoline and deoxypyridinoline as potential markers of bone metastasis in patients with prostate cancer. J Urol 1996;156:1691–5.
93. Kylmala T, Tammela TL, Risteli L, et al. Type I collagen degradation product (ICTP) gives information about the nature of bone metastases and has prognostic value in prostate cancer. B J Cancer 1995;71:1061–4.
94. Hattner R, Epker BN, Frost HM. Suggested sequential mode of control of changes in cell behaviour in adult bone remodelling. Nature 1965;206:489–90.
95. Chenu C, Delmas PD. Physiology of bone remodeling. In: Zaidi M, editor. Molecular and cellular biology of bone. Vol 5A. Stamford (CT): JAI Press; 1998. p. 45–64.
96. Kokubo T, Ishibashi O, Kumegawa M. Role of proteases in osteoclastic resorption. In: Zaidi M, editor. Molecular and cellular biology of bone. Vol 5B. Stamford (CT): JAI Press; 1998. p. 359–70.
97. Mundy GR. Mechanisms of bone metastasis [review]. Cancer 1997;
98. Eilon G, Mundy GR. Direct resorption of bone by human breast cancer cells in vitro. Nature 1978;276:726–8.
99. Sanchez SO, Lee J, Orr FW, Singh G. Direct osteolysis induced by metastatic murine melanoma cells: role of matrix metalloproteinases. Eur J Cancer 1997;33:918–25.
100. Stearns ME. Alendronate blocks TGF-beta1 stimulated collagen 1 degradation by human prostate PC-3 ML cells. Clin Exp Metastasis 1998;16:332–9.
101. Gleave ME, Hsieh JT, von Eschenbach AC, Chung LW. Prostate and bone fibroblasts induce human prostate cancer growth in vivo: implications for bidirectional tumor-stromal cell interaction in prostate carcinoma growth and metastasis. J Urol 1992;147:1151–9.
102. Morinaga Y, Fujita N, Ohishi K, Tsuruo T. Stimulation of interleukin-11 production from osteoblast-like cells by transforming growth factor-beta and tumor cell factors. Int J Cancer 1997;71:422–8.
103. Zhang Y, Fujita N, Oh HT, et al. Production of interleukin-11 in bone-derived endothelial cells and its role in the formation of osteolytic bone metastasis. Oncogene 1998;16:693–703.
104. de la Mata J, Uy HL, Guise TA, et al. Interleukin-6 enhances hypercalcemia and bone resorption mediated by parathyroid hormone-related protein in vivo. J Clin Invest 1995;95:2846–52.
105. Polychronakos C, Janthly U, Lehoux JG, Koutsilieris M. Mitogenic effects of insulin and insulin-like growth factors on PA-III rat prostate adenocarcinoma cells: characterization of the receptors involved. Prostate 1991;19:313–21.
106. Harris SE, Harris MA, Mahy P, et al. Expression of bone morphogenetic protein messenger RNAs by normal rat and human prostate and prostate cancer cells. Prostate 1994;24:204–11.
107. Rabbani SA, Gladu J, Mazar AP, et al. Induction in human osteoblastic cells (SaOS2) of the early response genes fos, jun, and myc by the amino terminal fragment (ATF) of urokinase. J Cell Physiol 1997;172:137–45.

25

Complementary and Alternative Medicine

DAVID S. WU, MD
DEBORAH P. LUBECK, PhD
GARY D. GROSSFELD, MD, FACS
PETER R. CARROLL, MD, FACS

Complementary and alternative medicine (CAM) is a term that encompasses a variety of unconventional therapies and beliefs that include acupuncture, diet therapy, supplements, megavitamins, mind-body techniques, energy healing, and herbal remedies, among others. The National Institutes of Health's Office of Alternative Medicine (OAM) defines alternative medicine as therapies outside of conventional medical practice, the efficacy of which has yet to be proven. In a 1995 OAM panel discussion, CAM was defined as

> a broad domain of healing resources that encompass all health systems, modalities, and practices and their accompanying theories and beliefs, other than those intrinsic to the politically dominant health system of a particular society or culture in a given historical period. It includes all such practices and ideas self-defined by their users as preventing or treating illness or promoting health and well-being.[1]

Despite its unproven nature, CAM is frequently used as an adjunct to contemporary medical care for chronic ailments and diseases such as arthritis,[2,3] back pain,[4,5] neuropathies,[6,7] gastrointestinal problems,[8,9] benign prostatic hyperplasia,[10] and cancer.[11–14] Its advocates point to improvements in quality-of-life outcomes and stress reduction, as well as chemopreventive benefits with certain types of CAM. Today, CAM use has gained wide acceptance as adjunctive therapy both in the general public and for patients with cancer. It is estimated that more than one-third of adults in the United States use some form of CAM.[11,15,16] Furthermore, Americans made more visits to complementary medicine providers than to allopathic primary care physicians during the 1990s.[17–20] In 1997, there were 629 million visits to alternative medicine practitioners, up 47% from 1993. That was 243 million more patient visits to CAM practitioners than to all primary care physicians combined. These patients spent between $27.0 to $34.4 billion dollars in out-of-pocket physician services in the United States for that same year.[16,19] Furthermore, acceptance of CAM is growing. Most major health plans now have or are considering CAM coverage, and funding from the National Institutes of Health continues to increase.[16,21] Paralleling this interest, medical investigators have sought to better characterize CAM use and their impact on patient outcomes. This interest is reflected by the increasing number of scientific publications of CAM use in the treatment of cancer patients. Although the primary goal of complementary therapy may not necessarily be to cure the patient of cancer or to replace conventional treatments, CAM may have a role in improving patient well-being and quality of life.[22–24] This chapter reviews the prevalence of CAM use in prostate cancer, the rationale of their use, and their impact on prostate cancer control.

PREVALENCE OF COMPLEMENTARY AND ALTERNATIVE MEDICINE USE FOR PROSTATE CANCER

Determination of the prevalence of the use of alternative medicine in the treatment of prostate cancer is problematic because the definition of what constitutes an alternative treatment modality is often not clear. A treatment modality that one physician considers alternative medicine another believes to be conventional care. Further yet, some may not view it as treatment at all. Studies of the prevalence of CAM use by patients with prostate cancer vary. An 8.8% rate was reported by a study that combined patients with prostate cancer and those with testicular carcinomas.[25] In another study of 234 men with localized prostate cancer, Lippert and colleagues reported a CAM prevalence of 43%.[13] However, this rate may be artificially high as the definition of CAM was less stringent and included spiritual "therapies" such as prayer or religious practices. Nam and colleagues reported CAM use in 32.8% of their patients with prostate cancer.[14]

From CaPSURE (Cancer of the Prostate Strategic Urologic Research Endeavor), a longitudinal observational database of over 4,000 patients with prostate cancer recruited from 35 urology practice sites throughout the country, we measured the prevalence of CAM use. We identified 1,055 patients (22.6%) newly diagnosed with prostate cancer who completed at least two questionnaires detailing their use of complementary and alternative treatments. A total of 191 patients (18.2%) reported the use of complementary therapies such as acupuncture, herbal medicine, diet/lifestyle modification, vitamins/mineral supplements, homeopathic remedies, chiropractor visits, and meditation/biofeedback. A total of 864 patients (81.9%) reported never using CAM treatments. The most common types of complementary therapies used by the patients with prostate cancer are reported in Table 25–1 along with common CAM used by the American public. In decreasing order of reported frequency, the most common therapies used in the current study were chiropractor visits (11.4%), herbal medicine (7.2%), supplements (3.3%), diet/lifestyle modifications (2.4%), homeopathic remedies (0.6%), meditation/biofeedback (0.5%), and acupuncture (< 0.5%). The mean ages at diagnosis of users and nonusers were similar at 66.1 years and 66.9 years, respectively ($p = .796$). There were no significant differences in the disease stage, biopsy Gleason grade, or prostate-specific antigen (PSA) at diagnosis between users and nonusers of CAM (Table 25–2).

Patients' home living arrangements, ethnicity, education level, and household income data were also analyzed (see Table 25–2). There was no difference in home living arrangements, but the two groups differed in ethnicity, education, and income. Complementary therapy users consisted of 91.6% Whites, 6.8% Blacks, and 1.0% from other ethnicities. The ethnic distribution of nonusers was significantly different at 81.6% Whites, 14.1% Blacks, and 3.9% other ($p = .002$). Furthermore, CAM users had more formal education than nonusers. Forty-three percent of users were college graduates, and 20.9% went on to graduate or professional schools. In the nonuser group, only 27.8% graduated from college, and 14.7% went on to pursue further formal education ($p < .001$). Higher household income was also associated with the use of nontraditional therapies. In the complementary therapy users group, 20.9% reported an annual income of over $75,000, compared with 11.9% in the nonusers groups. When analyzing patients with annual incomes of less than $30,000, the proportions of users and nonusers were 23.5% and 35.3%, respectively ($p < .001$).

It is essential that physicians caring for patients with prostate cancer possess some knowledge of these treatments. Patients frequently ask questions about possible alternative treatments that may serve as an adjunct to the conventional therapy that they are already receiving. It is equally important to note

Table 25–1. COMPLEMENTARY THERAPIES USED BY 1,055 PATIENTS WITH PROSTATE CANCER AND BY ADULTS IN THE UNITED STATES

	Patients Reporting Use (%)	
Type of Treatment	CaPSURE Patients	General Public[16]
Chiropractor	11.4	11.0
Herbal medicine	7.2	12.1
Vitamins/minerals/supplements	3.3	5.5
Diet/nutrition/lifestyle modifications	2.4	8.4
Homeopathic remedies	0.6	3.4
Biofeedback	0.5	1.0
Acupuncture	< 0.5	1.0

that a significant proportion of patients receive alternative treatments or ingest vitamins, herbs, etc without notifying their physician. Although the efficacy of these alternative forms of treatment remains to be proven, numerous laboratory studies and epidemiologic surveys support their use. Here, we highlight some of the various forms of CAM used by patients with prostate cancer (Tables 25–3 to 25–5).

VITAMIN D

Vitamin D is a secosteroid that is involved in calcium homeostasis. Although vitamin D forms a number of metabolites, calcitriol (1,25-dihydroxycholecalciferol) is the principal active form of vitamin D. Studies have shown that calcitriol can inhibit the growth and differentiation of normal and malignant cells; however, it was Schwartz and Hulka who first suggested a role for calcitriol in the development of prostate cancer.[26] They noted that the major risk factors for prostate cancer (age, African-American ethnicity, living in a northern latitude) were all associated with low vitamin D levels.[26] The incidence of prostate cancer significantly increases with age. Interestingly, calcitriol production decreases with age. Furthermore, Blacks have higher levels of melanin in their skin, which corresponds to lower production of calcitriol. That Asians have lower rates of prostate cancer is interesting because vitamin D is more abundant in Asian diets and may therefore confer protection against the development of prostate cancer. Finally, those who reside in more northern latitudes tend to live in a colder climate and have less exposure to sunlight. Consequently, endogenous production of vitamin D is less in these individuals. An epidemiologic study in various counties across the United States revealed such an inverse relationship between ultraviolet light exposure and mortality rates from prostate cancer.[27]

In a prospective study, Corder and colleagues measured vitamin D levels in the stored sera of 181 men who subsequently developed prostate cancer.[28] This was compared to age-matched controls who did not develop prostate cancer. Men with prostate cancer were found to have vitamin D levels that were 1.8 pg/mL lower than those in the control group ($p < .002$). Schwartz reported results that support

Table 25–2. CLINICAL AND DEMOGRAPHIC CHARACTERISTICS OF 1,055 PATIENTS WITH PROSTATE CANCER AND THE USE OF COMPLEMENTARY THERAPIES

	User (n = 191)	Nonuser (n = 864)	*p* Value
Age	66	67	0.796
PSA at diagnosis	14 ng/mL	16 ng/mL	NS
TNM stage			
T1	25	26	NS
T2	67	63	
T3/4N0M0	3	6	
TanyN+M+	6	5	
Biopsy Gleason sum			
2–4	12	8	NS
5–6	52	53	
7	22	21	
8–10	14	12	
Ethnicity			
White	92	82	.002
Black	7	14	
Hispanic, Asian, other	1	4	
Education level			
Some high school or less	10	22	< .001
High school	26	26	
Some college	18	19	
College graduate	23	13	
Graduate or professional school	21	15	
Annual household income			
< 20,000	10	21	< .001
20,000–30,000	14	15	
30,000–50,000	25	20	
50,000–75,000	12	12	
> 75,000	21	12	
Missing	19	20	

NS = not significant.

these findings.[29] However, Braun and colleagues and Gann and Hennekens saw no correlation between low vitamin D levels and the development of prostate cancer.[30,31]

Miller and colleagues have reported the presence of vitamin D receptors in LNCaP cells, a hormone-responsive human prostate cancer cell line.[32] They noted that calcitriol at high doses was effective in inhibiting LNCaP growth and PSA production.[33] Vitamin D receptors have also been found in other prostate cancer cell lines, notably PC-3 and DU-145. Calcitriol appears to have antiproliferative effects on these cell lines as well.[34] Through in vitro gel invasion assay, calcitriol has also been noted to inhibit the invasive properties of prostate cancer cells.[35] The mechanism of action of calcitriol on prostate cancer cells is believed to be mediated through ligand-receptor binding of vitamin D receptors; however,

At the present time, there is no reason to recommend daily soy consumption for patients with localized prostate cancer. However, it may be used as an adjunct to conventional treatment because it appears that a moderate increase in soy intake is not harmful.[74] In fact, soy has been shown to prevent osteoporosis and to decrease cholesterol levels. Yet whether soy will play an important role in the treatment or prevention of prostate cancer remains to be seen.

LYCOPENE

Lycopene is a type of carotenoid abundantly found in tomatoes. It is of special interest because it has been suggested that lycopene consumption may reduce the risk of developing breast and prostate cancer.[75–77] An epidemiologic analysis of mortality data from 41 countries revealed that there was a high association between tomato consumption and reduced prostate cancer mortality rates.[78] A prospective study of 578 men who subsequently developed prostate cancer with 1,294 age- and smoking-matched controls demonstrated that lycopene levels were significantly lower in men with prostate cancer than in the matched controls.[79] Of the five different types of carotenoids measured, only lycopene was found to have an association with decreased risk of prostate cancer. In vitro studies have also shown that lycopene can inhibit growth of particular prostate cancer cell lines such as DU-145.[80]

PC-SPES

PC-SPES is a supplement composed of a mixture of herbs that has become popular among patients with prostate cancer.[81,82] Studies have shown that PC-SPES has strong estrogenic properties.[83,84] Thus, patients with prostate cancer have been using PC-SPES as an alternative to conventional androgen deprivation therapy.

PC-SPES has exhibited antitumor activity in vitro.[85] It has been shown to inhibit proliferation of LNCaP human prostate cancer cells. It can induce cell cycle arrest in prostate cancer cell lines such as LNCaP, PC-3, and DU-145.[86] Clinical studies have also demonstrated PSA decline in patients receiving PC-SPES. A recent phase 2 trial reported a significant decline in serum PSA in all 33 patients with androgen-dependent prostate cancer receiving PC-SPES.[87] The average PSA decline was greater than 80%. Approximately half of 35 patients with androgen-independent prostate cancer also experienced a PSA decline of greater than 50%. Of note, 3 patients in this study experienced thromboembolic events. Other side effects of PC-SPES include gynecosmastia, gynecodynia, leg cramps, and diarrhea. These findings suggest that the clinical efficacy of PC-SPES may be mediated through its estrogenic activity. However, high-performance gas chromatography, liquid chromatography, and mass spectrometry have failed to identify estradiol, estrone, or diethylstilbestrol in PC-SPES.[84] This suggests that PC-SPES's putative estrogenic properties may not be attributable to previously characterized estrogenic compounds.

PC-SPES supplementation can also be quite expensive. A patient receiving three capsules a day incurs a cost of over $150 per month. In light of the fact that this herbal remedy may produce potentially serious side effects, future studies are needed to elucidate the mechanism of action and efficacy of this compound before PC-SPES can be accepted as a safe, valid, complementary treatment for prostate cancer.

SAW PALMETTO

Saw palmetto is a herbal blend used by patients with prostate cancer. This herb is better known for its use in the treatment of men with benign prostatic hyperplasia and lower urinary tract symptoms.[88,89] In vitro studies have shown that saw palmetto exhibits α_1-adrenoreceptor-inhibitory properties.[90] However, clinical studies comparing saw palmetto with placebo have failed to demonstrate significant improvements in objective measures of bladder outlet obstruction.[91] This herbal remedy is well tolerated and has minimal side effects. Consequently, many men use saw palmetto for benign prostatic hyperplasia. However, there is no evidence of the efficacy of saw palmetto in prostate cancer. Much work is still needed to determine whether saw palmetto will have a role in the treatment of prostate cancer.

ST. JOHN'S WORT

Currently, there is more clinical research regarding St. John's wort (*Hypericum perforatum*) than any other herbal remedy.[92] Its components of hypericin and pseudohypericin are well studied, but the precise mechanism of their actions remains unknown.[93] As an over-the-counter supplement, St. John's wort has been shown to be an effective alternative therapy in the treatment of depression.[92] Twenty-five percent of patients with advanced prostate cancer will experience significant clinical depression.[94] Thus, it may be used to treat depression in patients with prostate cancer.

The safest way to obtain St. John's wort is to purchase a formulation with at least 0.3% hypericin. Suggested dosage is 300 to 900 mg per day (divided dosages). Results can be anticipated in 4 to 6 weeks.[92] Side effects are less than those of conventional antidepressants.[95] However, patients should still be warned of possible side effects such as photosensitivity, gastrointestinal upset, dizziness, restlessness, sedation, and constipation.[96]

GINKGO

Ginkgo biloba has been used by patients with prostate cancer for treatment of erectile dysfunction.[96] There is good evidence that ginkgo extracts may improve tissue perfusion; however, many of these studies focused on its use in dementia and chronic cerebral insufficiency.[97,98] In fact, it is approved for the treatment of dementia in Germany. However, its use in erectile dysfunction is not yet supported by clinical evidence. A placebo-controlled, double-blind study found no significant difference in the erectile function between patients receiving ginkgo extracts versus those receiving placebo.[99] More studies are needed to address this issue because of its widespread use in the general public.

KAVA

Kava (*Piper methysticum*) is an herbal supplement with reported anticonvulsant, anxiolytic, and muscle-relaxant properties.[100,101] A number of clinical trials have shown that kavalactone can be used to manage anxiety and tension. Thus, kava is used by patients with prostate cancer to control anxiety and tension after the diagnosis of cancer. Preparations of kava are available that contain 100 to 200 mg of kavalactones per day.[100]

MEDITATION

A diagnosis of prostate cancer produces considerable stress in any man's life. Therefore, it is not surprising that patients with prostate cancer are increasingly turning to alternative therapies such as meditation and yoga to reduce anxiety and stress and to provide themselves with a greater sense of control. It is, however, quite difficult to objectively assess the benefits of meditation. There is also a paucity of evidence examining the association between meditation and treatment of prostate cancer. In a 1994 study, mindful meditation was shown to be associated with an increase in melatonin levels.[102] A later study of 14 patients with hormone-refractory prostate cancer revealed that 57% of the patients receiving oral melatonin had a 50% decrease in serum PSA. The study also showed that 64% of these patients had survival of at least 1 year.[103] These findings have led some to suggest that mindful meditation may enhance in vivo production of melatonin and provide a complement to traditional treatments for prostate cancer. Irrespective of any direct benefits of mindul meditation on prostate cancer, Coker suggested that mindful meditation may contribute to the management of quality-of-life issues and concerns.[104]

CHINESE MEDICINE AND ACUPUNCTURE

Traditional Chinese medicine includes a variety of treatment modalities such as acupuncture, herbal remedy, and lifestyle changes. Unlike Western medicine, which labels a patient with a specific disease, Chinese medicine bases its treatment on symptoms. It believes that the human body contains an energy force called "chi."[96] Sickness is a result of an imbalance of chi or the presence of specific evils in specific organs. In acupuncture, chi flows in various pathways throughout the body. Any disruptions to these pathways may cause disease. Acupuncture corrects inadequate chi at various points near the skin through the placement of needles or the application of heat or electrical stimulation at these acupuncture points. Some believe that acupuncture stimulates the nervous system to release compounds such as opioids in the muscles, brain, and spinal cord. These compounds, in turn, change the patient's perception of symptoms and/or stimulate the release of other compounds or hormones. The National Institutes of Health issued a statement on acupuncture in 1997 that mentioned its effectiveness in relief of postoperative pain and chemotherapy-induced nausea.[105,106] Studies have also shown that acupuncture may increase interleukin levels, T lymphocytes, and natural killer cell activity in patients with cancer when compared with placebo.[107,108] Thus, patients with prostate cancer may derive benefit from acupuncture through enhancement of their immune system and pain relief.

Acupuncture for treatment of prostate cancer involves insertion of needles into several specific locations in the ear.[96] Specific areas in the ear represent the prostate. Needles may also be placed at areas in the pelvic and abdominal region to increase the immune function in the area surrounding the prostate. Needles may also be placed in the back, extremities, and the head. However, placement of these needles is not specific to the prostate. Rather, it is aimed at promoting general health.

There are virtually no studies examining the role of acupuncture in patients with prostate cancer. However, in the hands of trained acupuncturists, the side effects of acupuncture are minimal. Some adverse effects are forgotten needles, infections from needles, and pneumothorax caused by inexperienced practitioners.[96]

REFERENCES

1. Defining and describing complementary and alternative medicine. In: Panel on Definition and Description, CAM Research Methodology Conference 1995;49–57.
2. Cronan TA, Kaplan RM, Posner L, et al. Prevalence of the use of unconventional remedies for arthritis in a metropolitan community. Arthritis Rheum 1989;32:1604–7.
3. van Haselen RA, Graves N, Dahiha S. The costs of treating rheumatoid arthritis patients with complementary medicine: exploring the issue. Complement Ther Med 1999;7:217–21.
4. Berman BM, Jonas W, Swyers JP. Issues in the use of complementary/alternative medical therapies for low back pain. Phys Med Rehabil Clin North Am 1998;9:497–513.
5. Ernst E, Pittler MH. Experts' opinions on complementary/alternative therapies for low back pain. J Manipulative Physiol Ther 1999;22:87–90.
6. Garfinkel MS, Singhal A, Katz WA, et al. Yoga-based intervention for carpal tunnel syndrome: a randomized trial. JAMA 1998;280:1601–3.
7. Shlay JC, Chaloner K, Max MB, et al. Acupuncture and amitriptyline for pain due to HIV-related peripheral neuropathy: a randomized controlled trial. Terry Beirn Community Programs for Clinical Research on AIDS. JAMA 1998;280:1590–5.
8. Bensoussan A, Talley NJ, Hing M, et al. Treatment of irritable bowel syndrome with Chinese herbal medicine: a randomized controlled trial. JAMA 1998;280:1585–9.
9. Verhoef MJ, Sutherland JR, Brkich L. Use of alternative medicine by patients attending a gastroenterology clinic. Can Med Assoc J 1990;142:121–5.
10. Wilt TJ, Ishani A, Stark J, et al. Saw palmetto extracts for treatment of benign prostatic hyperplasia: a systematic review. JAMA 1998;280:1604–9.
11. Ernst E, Cassileth BR. The prevalence of complementary/alternative medicine in cancer: a systematic review. Cancer 1998;83.
12. Jacobson JS, Workman SB, Kronenberg F. Research on complementary/alternative medicine for patients with breast cancer: a review of the biomedical literature. J Clin Oncol 2000;18:668–83.
13. Lippert MC, McClain R, Boyd JC, Theodorescu D. Alternative medicine use in patients with localized prostate carcinoma treated with curative intent. Cancer 1999;86:2642–8.
14. Nam RK, Fleshner N, Rakovitch E, et al. Prevalence and patterns of the use of complementary therapies among prostate cancer patients: an epidemiological analysis. J Urol 1999; 161:1521–4.
15. Eisenberg DM, Kessler RC, Foster C, et al. Unconventional medicine in the United States. Prevalence, costs, and patterns of use. N Engl J Med 1993;328:246–52.
16. Eisenberg DM, Davis RB, Ettner SL, et al. Trends in alternative medicine use in the United States, 1990–97: results of a follow-up national survey. JAMA 1998;280:1569–75.
17. Nelson C, Woodwell D. National Ambulatory Medical Care Survey: 1993 summary. Vital Health Stat 1998;13:1–99.
18. Schappert SM. National Ambulatory Medical Care Survey: 1990 summary. Adv Data 1998:1–11.
19. Woodwell DA. National Ambulatory Medical Care Survey: 1996 summary. Adv Data 1997:1–25.
20. Woodwell DA. National Ambulatory Medical Care Survey: 1997 summary. Adv Data 1999:1–28.
21. Birmingham K, Cimons M. Alternative medicine and prostate cancer benefits from largest ever NIH increase. Nat Med 1998;4:1348.
22. Cassileth BR, Soloway M, Vogelzang NJ. Quality of life and psychosocial status in stage D prostate cancer. Qual Life Res 1992;1:323.
23. Cassileth BR. Alternative and complementary cancer treatments. Oncologist 1996;1:173–9.
24. Fair WR, Willet F, Whitore J. Lecture: back to the future—the role of complementary medicine in urology. J Urol 1999;162:411–20.
25. Lerner IJ, Kennedy BJ. The prevalence of questionable methods of cancer treatment in the United States. CA Cancer J Clin 1992;42:181–91.
26. Schwartz GG, Hulka BS. Is vitamin D deficiency a risk factor for prostate cancer? Anticancer Res 1990;10:1307–11.
27. Hanchette CL, Schwartz GG. Geographic patterns of prostate cancer mortality: evidence for a protective effect of ultraviolet radiation. Cancer 1992;70:2861–9.
28. Corder EH, Guess HA, Hulka BS. Vitamin D and prostate cancer: a prediagnostic study with stored sera. Cancer Epidemiol Biomarkers Prev 1993;2:467–72.
29. Schwartz GG. Prostate cancer and the vitamin D hypothesis. In: Jung EG, editor. Biologic effect of light. New York: Walter de Gruyter Co; 1996. p. 309–16.

30. Braun MM, Helzlsouer KJ, Hollis BW. Prostate cancer and prediagnostic levels of serum vitamin D metabolites. Cancer Causes Control 1995;6:235–9.
31. Gann PH, Ma J, Hennekens CH. Circulating vitamin D metabolites in relation to subsequent development of prostate cancer. Cancer Epidemiol Biomarkers Prev 1996;5:121–6.
32. Miller GJ, Stapleton GE, Houmiel KL. Specific receptors for vitamin D3 in human prostatic carcinoma cells. In: Karr JP, Coffey DS, Smith RG, editor. Molecular and cellular biology of prostate cancer. New York: Plenum Press; 1991. p. 253–9.
33. Miller GJ, Stapleton GE, Ferrara JA. The human prostatic adenocarcinoma cell line LnCaP expresses biologically active specific receptors for 1,25-dihydroxyvitamin D3. Cancer Res 1992;52:515–20.
34. Skowronski RJ, Peehl DM, Feldman D. Vitamin D and prostate cancer: 1,25dihydroxyvitamin D3 receptors and actions in human prostate cancer cell lines. Endocrinology 1993;132:1952–60.
35. Schwartz GG, Wang MH, Zhang M. 1,25-Dihydroxyvitamin D (calcitriol) inhibits the invasiveness of human prostate cancer cells. Cancer Epidemiol Biomarkers Prev 1997; 6:727–32.
36. Peehl DM. Vitamin D and prostate cancer risk. Eur Urol 1999;35:392–4.
37. Gross C, Stamey TA, Hancock S. Treatment of early recurrent prostate cancer with 1,25-dihydroxyvitamin D3 (calcitriol). J Urol 1998;159:2035–40.
38. Bouillon R, Okamura WH, Norman AW. Structure-function relationships in the vitamin D endocrine system. Endocrine Rev 1995;16:200–57.
39. Skowronski RJ, Peehl DM, Feldman D. Actions of vitamin D3 analogs on human prostate cancer cell lines: comparison with 1,25-dihydroxyvitamin D2. Endocrinology 1995;136:20–6.
40. Cohn W. Bioavailability of vitamin E. Eur J Clin Nutr 1997; 51:S80–5.
41. Israel K, Sanders BG, Kline K. RRR-alpha-tocopheryl succinate inhibits the proliferation of human prostatic tumor cells with defective cell cycle/differentiation pathways. Nutr Cancer 1995;24:161–9.
42. Sigounas G, Anagnostou A, Steiner M. dl-alpha-Tocopherol induces apoptosis in erythroleukemia, prostate, and breast cancer cells. Nutr Cancer 1997;28:30–5.
43. The Alpha-tocopherol, Beta Carotene Cancer Prevention Study Group. The effect of vitamin E and beta carotene on the incidence of lung cancer and other cancers in male smokers. N Engl J Med 1994;330:1029–35.
44. Heinonen OP, Albanes D, Virtamo J. Prostate cancer and supplementation with alpha-tocopherol and beta-carotene: incidence and mortality in a controlled trial. J Natl Cancer Inst 1998;90:440–6.
45. Smigel K. Vitamin E reduces prostate cancer rates in Finnish trial: U.S. considers follow-up. J Natl Cancer Inst 1998; 90:416–7.
46. Bendich A, Machlin LJ. Safety of oral intake of vitamin E. Am J Clin Nutr 1988;48:612–9.
47. Kappus H, Diplick AT. Tolerance and safety of vitamin E: a toxicological position report. Free Radic Biol Med 1992; 13:55–74.
48. Meydani SN, Meydani M, Blumberg JB. Assessment of the safety of supplementation with different amounts of vitamin E in healthy older adults. Am J Clin Nutr 1998;68:311–8.
49. Meyers DG, Maloley PA, Weeks D. Safety of antioxidant vitamins. Arch Intern Med 1996;156:925–35.
50. Clark LK, Comb GF, Turnbull BW. The nutritional prevention of cancer with selenium 1983–1993: a randomized clinical trial. JAMA 1996;276:1957–63.
51. Yoshizawa K, Willet WC, Morris SJ. Study of prediagnostic selenium level in toenails and the risk of advanced prostate cancer. J Natl Cancer Inst 1998;990:1219–24.
52. Redman C, Xu MJ, Peng Y-M. Involvement of polyamines in selenomethionine induced apoptosis and mitotic alterations in human tumor cells. Carcinogenesis 1997;18:1195–202.
53. Wilson AC, Thompson HJ, Schedin PJ. Effect of methylated forms of selenium on cell viability and the induction of DNA strand breakage. Bioochem Pharmacol 1992;43: 1137–41.
54. Nelson MA, Porterfield BW, Jacobs ET, Clark LC. Selenium and prostate cancer prevention. Sem Urol Oncol 1999; 17:91–6.
55. Katiyar SK, Mukhtar H. Tea in chemoprevention of cancer: epidemiological and experimental studies. Int J Oncol 1996;8:221–38.
56. Giovannucci E. Epidemiologic characteristics of prostate cancer. Cancer 1995;75:1766–77.
57. Kohlmeier L, Weterings KG, Steck S. Tea and cancer prevention: an evaluation of the epidemiologic literature. Nutr Cancer 1997;27:1–13.
58. Wynder EL, Rose DP, Cohen LA. Nutrition and prostate cancer: a proposal for dietary intervention. Nutr Cancer 1994;22:1–10.
59. Blot WJ, Chow WH, McLaughlin JK. Tea and cancer: a review of the epidemiologic evidence. Eur J Cancer Prev 1996;5:425–38.
60. Liao S, Umekita Y, Guo J. Growth inhibition and regression of human prostate and breast tumors in athymic mice by tea epigallocatechin gallate. Cancer Lett 1995;96:239–42.
61. Gupta S, Ahmad N, Mukhtar H. Prostate cancer prevention by green tea. Semin Urol Oncol 1999;17:70–6.
62. Messina MJ, Barnes S. The role of soy products in reducing risk of cancer. J Natl Cancer Inst 1991;83:541–6.
63. Messina MJ, Persky V, Setchell KD. Soy intake and cancer risk: a review of the in vitro and in vivo data. Nutr Cancer 1994;21:113–31.
64. Tham DM, Gardner CD, Haskell WL. Clinical review 97—potential health benefits of dietary phytoestrogens: a review of the clinical, epidemiological, and mechanistic evidence. J Clin Endocrinol Metab 1998;83:2223–35.
65. Adlercreutz H, Mazur W. Phyto-oestrogens and Western diseases. Ann Med 1997;29:95–120.
66. Knight DC, Eden JA. A review of the clinical effects of phytoestrogens. Obstet Gynecol 1996;87:897–904.
67. Tan SP, Daniel M, Lim SH. Use of soy formulae among Asian children in Singapore. Singapore Paediatr J 1997;39:191–3.
68. Aldercreutz H, Makela S, Pylkkanen L. Dietary phytoestrogens and prostate cancer. Proc Am Assoc Cancer Res 1995;36:687.
69. Hempstock J, Kavanagh JP, George N. Growth inhibition of primary human prostatic cells by phytoestrogens. J Urol 1998;159:11.
70. Peterson G, Barnes S. Genistein and biochanin-a inhibit the

growth of human prostate cancer cells but not epidermal growth factor receptor tyrosine autophosphorylation. Prostate 1993;22:335–45.

71. Akiyama T, Ogawara. Genistein, a specific inhibitor of tyrosine-specific protein kinases. J Biol Chem 1987; 262:5592–5.
72. Fotsis T, Pepper M, Adlercreutz H. Genistein, a dietary-derived inhibitor of in vitro angiogenesis. Proc Natl Acad Sci U S A 1993;90:2690–4.
73. Kyle E, Neckers L, Takimoto C. Genistein-induced apoptosis of prostate cancer cells is preceded by a specific decrease in focal adhesion kinase activity. Mol Pharmacol 1997;51:193–200.
74. Moyad M. Soy, disease prevention, and prostate cancer. Semin Urol Oncol 1999;17:97–102.
75. Boileau TW, Clinton SK, Erdman JW. Tissue lycopene concentrations and isomer patterns are affected by androgen status and dietary lycopene concentration in male F344 rats. J Nutr 2000;130:1613–8.
76. Giovannucci E. Tomatoes, tomato-based products, lycopene, and cancer: review of the epidemiologic literature. J Natl Cancer Inst 1999;91:317–31.
77. Karas M, Amir H, Fishman D. Lycopene interferes with cell cycle progression and insulin-like growth factor I signaling in mammary cancer cells. Nutr Cancer 2000;36:101–11.
78. Grant WB. An ecologic study of dietary links of prostate cancer. Altern Med Rev 1999;4:162–9.
79. Gann PH, Ma J, Giovannucci E. Lower prostate cancer risk in men with elevated plasma lycopene levels: results of a prospective analysis. Cancer Res 1999;59:1225–30.
80. Hall AK. Liarozole amplifies retinoid-induced apoptosis in human prostate cancer cells. Anticancer Drugs 1996; 7:312–20.
81. Moyad M, Pienta K, J. M. Use of PC-SPES, a commercially available supplement for prostate cancer, in a patient with hormone-naive disease. Urology 1999;54:319–24.
82. Pfeifer B, Pirani J, Hamann S. PC-SPES, a dietary supplement for the treatment of hormone-refractory prostate cancer. Br J Urol 1999;85:481–5.
83. de la Taille A, Hayek O, Buttyan R. Effects of a phytotherapeutic agent, PC-SPES, on prostate cancer: a preliminary investigation on human cell lines and patients. Br J Urol 1999;84:845–50.
84. DiPaola R, Zhang H, Lanbert G. Clinical and biologic activity of an estrogenic herbal combination (PC-SPES) in prostate cancer. N Engl J Med 1998;339:785–91.
85. Hsieh T, Chen S, Wang X. Regulation of androgen receptor and prostate specific antigen expression in the androgen-responsive human LNCaP cells by ethanolic extracts of the Chinese herbal preparation, PC-SPES. Biochem Mol Biol Int 1997;42:535–44.
86. Kubota T, Hisatake J, Hisatake Y. PC-SPES: a unique inhibitor of proliferation of prostate cancer cells in vitro and in vivo. Prostate 2000;42:163–71.
87. Small E, Frohlich M, Bok R. Prospective trial of the herbal supplement PC-SPES in patients with progressive prostate cancer. J Clin Oncol 2000;18:3595–603.
88. Gerber G. Saw palmetto for the treatment of men with lower urinary tract symptoms. J Urol 2000;163:1408–12.
89. Marks L, Partin A, Epstein J. Effects of saw palmetto herbal blend in men with symptomatic benign prostatic hyperplasia. J Urol 2000;163:1451–6.
90. Goepel M, Hecker U, Krege S, et al. Saw palmetto extracts potently and noncompetitively inhibit human alpha 1-adrenoreceptors in vitro. Prostate 1999;38:208–15.
91. Gerber G, Zagaja G, Bales G, et al. Saw palmetto in men with lower urinary tract symptoms: effects on urodynamic parameters and voiding symptoms. Urology 1998;51:1003–7.
92. Linde K, Ramirez G, Mulrow C. St. John's wort for depression: an overview and meta-analysis of randomized clinical trials. BMJ 1996;313:253–8.
93. Kerb R, Brockmoller J, Staffelt B. Single-dose and steady-state pharmacokinetics of hypericin and pseudohypericin. Antimicrob Agents Chemother 1996;40:2087–93.
94. Clark J. Psychosocial responses of the patient. In: Groenwald S, Frogge M, Goodman M, editors. Cancer nursing—principles and practice. Boston: Jones Bartlett; 1993. p. 449–67.
95. Vorbach E, Arnoldt K, Hubner W-D. Efficacy and tolerability of St. John's wort extract LI 160 versus imipramine in patients with severe depression episodes according to ICD-10. Pharmacopsychiatry 1997;30:81–5.
96. Moyad M, Hathaway S, Hai-Sha N. Traditional Chinese medicine, acupuncture, and other alternative medicines for prostate cancer: an introduction and the need for more research. Semin Urol Oncol 1999;17:103–10.
97. Gaby A. Ginkgo biloba extract: a review. Altern Med Rev 1996;1:235–42.
98. Kleijnen J, Knipschild P. Ginkgo biloba. Lancet 1992;340: 1136–9.
99. Sikora R, Sohn M, Engelke B. Randomized placebo-controlled study on the effects of oral treatment with ginkgo biloba extract in patients with erectile dysfunction. J Urol 1998;159:240.
100. Bone K. A safe herbal treatment for anxiety. Br J Phytother 1994;3:147–53.
101. Singh Y, Blumenthal M. Kava: an overview. Herbalgram 1997;39:34–54.
102. Massion A, Teas J, Herbert J. Meditation, melatonin and breast/prostate cancer: hypothesis and preliminary data. Med Hypotheses 1995;44:39–46.
103. Lissoni P, Cazzanigi M, Tancini G. Reversal of clinical resistance to LHRH analogue in metastatic prostate cancer by the pineal hormone melatonin; efficacy of LHRH analogue plus melatonin in patient progressing on LHRH analogue alone. Eur Urol 1997;31:178–81.
104. Coker K. Meditation and prostate cancer: integrating a mind/body intervention with traditional therapies. Semin Urol Oncol 1999;17:111–8.
105. NIH Consensus Development Panel on Acupuncture. JAMA 1998;280:1518–24.
106. Morey S. NIH issues consensus statement on acupuncture. Am Fam Physician 1998;57:2545–6.
107. Wu B, Zhou R, Zhou M. Effect of acupuncture on interleukin-2 level and NK cell immunoactivity of peripheral blood of malignant tumor patients. Chung Kuo Chung Hsi I Chieh Ho Tsa Chih 1994;14:537–9.
108. Yuan J, Zhou R, Zhou M. Effect of acupuncture on T-lymphocyte and its subsets from the peripheral blood of patients with malignant neoplasm. Chen Tzu Yen Chiu 1993;18:174–7.

26

Erectile Dysfunction after Treatment

RODMAN S. ROGERS, MD
SHAHRAM GHOLAMI, MD
TOM LUE, MD

Improved screening strategies have increased the detection of early-stage prostate cancer among younger and more sexually active men. As a result of prostate-specific antigen (PSA) screening beginning in the late 1980s, the incidence of new prostate cancer cases increased sharply between 1986 and 1992. Whereas the absolute incidence rate was highest in men over the age of 65, the proportional increase in new prostate cancer cases was greatest in men age 35 to 64, for whom the age-adjusted incidence rate increased by 279% between 1974 and 1991.[1] In addition, multiple sources have confirmed that prostate cancer is being detected at a lower stage since the routine use of PSA screening compared with the pre-PSA era. The National Cancer Institute–sponsored Cancer Surveillance System of the Surveillance, Epidemiology, and End Results program reported a 52% decrease in the incidence of metastatic disease between 1990 and 1994. With younger men living longer after treatment for prostate cancer, the importance of quality of life after various treatments for this disease has become increasingly important. Among patients electing therapy for prostate cancer, 45% list maintaining quality of life as a major concern guiding their choice of therapy.[2]

This chapter reviews the physiology of erectile function and pathophysiology of erectile dysfunction (ED) after treatment for prostate cancer. It also summarizes the various treatments currently used for prostate cancer, the incidence of ED in patients receiving these treatments from the contemporary literature, and the management and outcome of treatment for ED after such treatment. Oncologic therapies to be considered here are radical prostatectomy, external beam radiation therapy (XRT), brachytherapy, cryotherapy, and androgen deprivation therapy.

PHYSIOLOGY OF ERECTILE FUNCTION

Penile erection is a neurovascular event closely related to psychological status and hormonal milieu. Following arousal or sexual stimulation, penile parasympathetic nerves release neurotransmitters from the cavernous nerve terminals. Concomitant release of relaxing factors from the endothelial cells results in a relaxation of arterial and arteriolar smooth muscles, a drop in peripheral resistance, and a marked increase in arterial flow. Within the corpora cavernosa, trabecular smooth muscle relaxes, increasing compliance of the sinusoids, which facilitates filling and expansion. The sinusoidal trabeculae fill according to arterial pressure, which distends the corpora against the surrounding tunica albuginea. Venus plexuses beneath the tunica provide venous outflow channels during the flaccid state. With arterial filling of the sinusoids, these subtunical venules become compressed between the peripheral trabeculae and the tunica albuginea, resulting in almost total shutdown of venous outflow.[3,4] These events effectively trap the blood within the corpora cavernosa, and the penis changes from a dependent position to the erect state. During the full erection phase, intracavernous pressure reaches approximately 100 mm Hg. In the rigid erection phase, during masturbation or sexual intercourse, the ischiocavernosus muscles forcefully compress the base of the blood-filled corpora cavernosa (the bulbocavernosus reflex), and the penis becomes even harder. Intracavernous pressure reaches several hundred mm Hg at this time, and blood inflow and outflow temporarily cease.

Detumescence occurs when contraction of the trabecular smooth muscle reopens the venous channels. Therefore, the trapped blood drains into the systemic circulation and flaccidity returns. This cascade of events may be triggered by the cessation of erectile neurotransmitter release, the breakdown of second messengers by phosphodiesterases, or sympathetic discharge during ejaculation.

NEUROANATOMY OF ERECTILE FUNCTION

Penile flaccidity, rigidity, and ejaculation require contributions from both autonomic (sympathetic and parasympathetic) and somatic (sensory and motor) nervous systems (Figure 26–1).

Sympathetic Nerves

The sympathetic nerves to the pelvic genital organs, which contribute to ejaculation and penile detumescence, arise from the preganglionic neurons in the intermediolateral gray matter of the lower thoracic and upper lumbar segments of the spinal cord (T10–L2). The preganglionic fibers pass from the ventral roots via the white rami to the paravertebral sympathetic chain ganglia. These fibers make synaptic connection with the postganglionic neurons with cell bodies located in the preaortic plexus. Some fibers travel via the pelvic splanchnic nerves to the inferior mesenteric and hypogastric plexuses and then travel via the hypogastric nerve to the pelvic plexus. The postganglionic fibers from the preaortic plexus or hypogastric nerve enter the pelvic plexus, where they are joined by parasympathetic fibers originating from sacral pathways. Thus, the pelvic plexus is a very important site for the integration of the autonomic input to the pelvic organs.

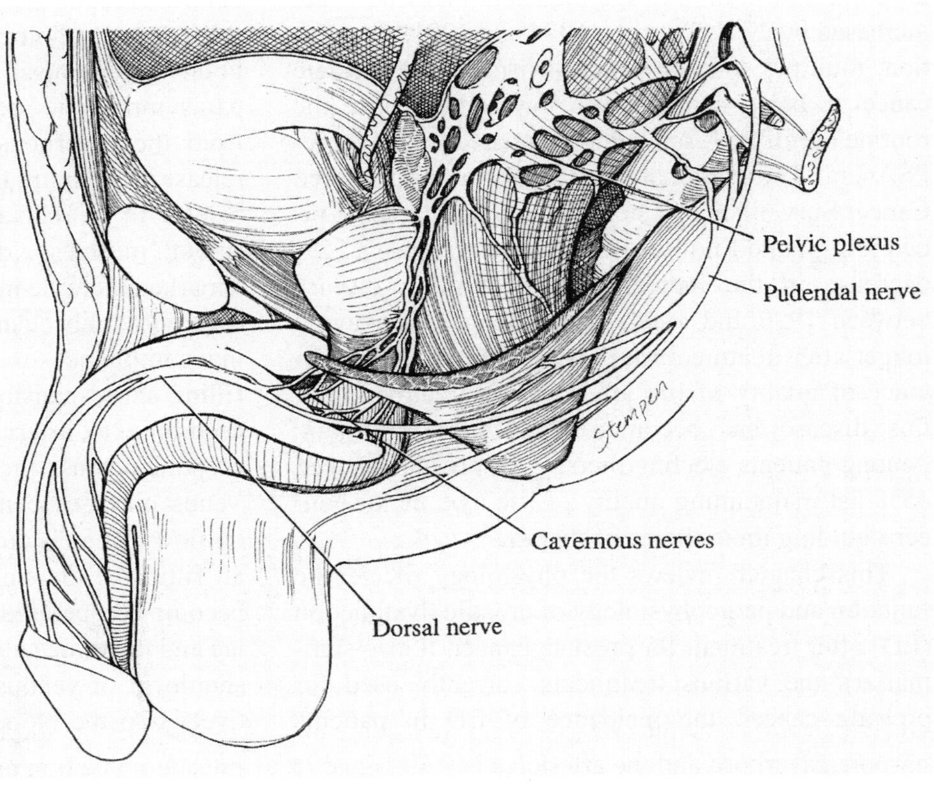

Figure 26–1. Neuroanatomy of erectile function. n = neuron; nn = nerve. (Reproduced with permission from Lue TF. Physiology of penile erection and pathophysiology of erectile dysfunction and priapism. In: Walsh PC, Retik AB, Vaughan ED Jr, Wein AJ, editors. Campbell's urology. 7th ed. Philadelphia: W.B. Saunders Co.; 1998. p. 1157–79.)

These nerve fibers enter the corpora cavernosa and travel within the trabecular erectile tissue, innervating the sinusoidal smooth muscle and vasculature.

Parasympathetic Nerves

The parasympathetic preganglionic fibers arise from S2 to S4. The sacral preganglionic nerves traveling to the pelvic plexus are termed the pelvic nerves. These form three to six distinct trunks,[5] which lie deep to the parietal pelvic fascia covering the pyriformis. After the pelvic nerves enter the presacral fascia, they join the hypogastric nerves to form the pelvic plexus. The pelvic plexus is a 4- to 5-cm curvilinear or rectangular network with stellate projections lying bilaterally in the pelvic fascia between the lower genitourinary tract and rectum.[6] The anterior margin of the plexus lies on the posterolateral aspect of the bladder and the prostate; posteriorly, it continues to the anterolateral wall of the lower rectum. The pelvic plexus provides both parasympathetic and sympathetic innervation to all of the pelvic organs: rectum, bladder, seminal vesicles, and prostate. The most caudal fibers coalesce to form the cavernous nerves, which travel along the posterolateral aspect of the seminal vesicles and prostate. They terminate in the corpora cavernosa, where they innervate the terminal arterioles and the trabecular smooth muscles responsible for the vascular events of erection and detumescence.[7]

Somatic Nerves

The paired pudendal nerves provide major somatic nerve supply to the pelvis and perineum. Originating from S2 to S4, these nerves accompany the internal pudendal vessels as they pass through Alcock's canal to innervate the striated muscles of the pelvic floor (levator ani) and the penis (ischiocavernosus and bulbocavernosus muscles). Sensory afferents from cutaneous nerve endings and receptors from the penis form the dorsal nerve. The somatic nerves are responsible for penile sensation and the rigid phase of erection.

NEUROPHYSIOLOGY OF ERECTILE FUNCTION

During penile flaccidity, smooth muscle within the corpora cavernosa and the arterioles is maintained in a semicontracted state. Three factors have been postulated to account for this: intrinsic myogenic activity,[8] adrenergic neurotransmision, and endothelium-derived contracting factors. Adrenergic nerves and adrenoceptors have been demonstrated in the trabecular smooth muscle and the cavernous and helicine arteries.[9,10] Although its role in maintaining penile flaccidity has not been definitively characterized, most researchers agree that norepinephrine is involved in the return of the penis to the flaccid state after ejaculation. The physiologic role of norepinephrine during the flaccid state may be to constrict cavernous and helicine arteries and contract trabecular smooth muscle. Several endothelium-derived contracting factors may also contribute to flaccidity. Prostaglandins E_2 and/or $F_2\alpha$ have been shown to mediate resting erectile smooth muscle in an animal model.[11] The endothelins have been shown to augment the smooth muscle contractile responses to sympathetic activity,[12] and angiotensin may play a role in modulating cavernous smooth muscle tone.[13]

During penile erection, cholinergic activity plays a dominant role via two separate mechanisms: inhibition of norepinephrine release through muscarinic receptors on adrenergic nerve terminals and stimulation of nitric oxide (NO) release from endothelial cells.[14] Nitric oxide is widely believed to be the principal neurotransmitter for penile erection.[15] Within the trabecular myocyte, NO activates a soluble guanylate cyclase that elevates intracellular levels of cyclic guanosine monophosphate (cGMP). This, in turn, stimulates the activities of cGMP-dependent protein kinases, which then phosphorylate certain proteins and ion channels, resulting in smooth muscle relaxation. Other potential neuromodulators include vasoactive intestinal polypeptide (VIP), [16] calcitonin gene–related peptide,[17] peptide histidine methionine,[18] pituitary adenylate cyclase–activating polypeptide,[19] and prostaglandins.[20] Cyclic adenosine monophosphate (cAMP) and cGMP are the second messengers involved in smooth muscle relaxation. During the return to the flaccid state, cGMP is hydrolyzed to GMP by the highly specific cGMP-binding phosphodiesterase type 5 (PDE5). The PDE5 inhibitor sildenafil acts to inhibit the hydrolysis of cGMP, thereby augmenting penile smooth muscle relaxation and erection.

PATHOPHYSIOLOGY OF ERECTILE DYSFUNCTION AFTER TREATMENT FOR PROSTATE CANCER

Erectile function is a neurovascular event modulated by psychological and hormonal status. Therefore, ED may result from impairment of one or more of the following factors: psychological, neurologic, hormonal, arterial, and cavernosal. Patients treated for prostate cancer frequently have disturbances in these factors related to the particular patient's medical history and cancer therapy. Erectile dysfunction caused by prescription pharmaceutical agents or other drugs (including tobacco and alcohol) represents a separate etiologic entity. Also, ED is associated with aging and systemic disease with a likely multifactorial etiology, as discussed below.

Psychological

As recently as 30 years ago, ED was believed to be a manifestation of some psychological problems in 90% of cases. Today, however, there is a broad consensus that, in most men, ED has both a physical and a psychological component. Brain centers controlling sexual behavior and genital erection are in the hypothalamus, limbic system, and cerebral cortex. The sacral erection centers receive either stimulatory or inhibitory input, which modulates lower nerve function. The psychological component has been hypothesized to interrupt the physiology of erection in the following ways: (1) a pathologic exaggeration of the normal suprasacral inhibition of the spinal erection center, (2) excessive sympathetic outflow resulting in failed relaxation of penile smooth muscle, and (3) inadequate release of erectile neurotransmitters. Psychological phenomena may affect sexual functioning on various conscious and subconscious levels, including the interpretation of sensory or conceived erotic input; the patient's own self-perceived functional status and sense of well-being, including anxiety level and fear of failure; the relationship with the partner; the patient's and partner's interpersonal roles; and the partner's perception of the patient's health status.

Neurologic

Lesions at any point in the central nervous system or peripheral nerves innervating the lower urinary tract may lead to ED. Parkinson's and Alzheimer's diseases, cerebrovascular accidents, and brain trauma often cause ED because of loss of libido or failure of central nervous system mechanisms initiating the erectile process. In the patient with a spinal cord injury, the degree of erectile function depends largely on the nature, location, and extent of the lesion. Psychogenic erections require intact neural pathways from the brain and spinal cord to the cavernous nerves. In a patient with an upper cord lesion, reflexogenic erection via a sacral pathway can be preserved despite the loss of psychogenic erection. Sensory input from the genitalia is essential to achieve and maintain reflexogenic erection, and this input becomes more important as the effect of psychologic stimuli abates with age. Impairment of peripheral somatic innervation to the bulbocavernosus and ischiocavernosus muscles may cause retarded ejaculation or anejaculation and failure to maintain an erection. In the majority of cases, ED following radical pelvic surgery is neurogenic in etiology. The patient's age, interval following surgery, and psychological status may also contribute.[21] During radical prostatectomy, pelvic autonomic nerves, which lie only millimeters posterolateral to the prostatic capsule, may sustain injury from transection or traction. Characteristically, this results in normal penile sensation and orgasm without penile erection. During cryosurgery for prostate cancer, the ice ball generated by supercooled transperineal probes may damage the pelvic autonomic nerves as they course by the prostate gland. Following radiation therapy, a diffuse inflammatory process results in damage to the small arterioles, and cavernous nerves undergo demyelination in the area of the radiation field. Postradiation vascular and neural damage is a variable phenomenon related to the radiation dose, intensity of the host response, and baseline level of neurovascular function in the pelvis and perineum.

Hormonal

Androgen deficiency from either hypogonadism or androgen deprivation therapy may suppress nocturnal erection and decrease sexual drive. Erection in response to visual sexual stimulation is preserved in hypogonadal men, suggesting that androgen enhances but is not essential for erection.[22] In castrated animals, a marked decrease in penile NO synthase activity, copulatory behavior, and erectile function has been reported.[23] Confirmatory studies in humans have not yet been performed, so the significance of these findings remains indeterminate. Hyperprolactinemia, whether from a pituitary adenoma or drugs, results in both reproductive and sexual dysfunction owing to the inhibition of prolactin on central dopaminergic acivity and gonadotropin-releasing hormone. Symptoms may include loss of libido, ED, galactorrhea, gynecomastia, and infertility. Following treatment for hyperprolactinemia, however, ED frequently persists, and patients may require erectogenic therapy.

Arterial

Arterial occlusive disease of the pudendal-cavernous-helicine arterial tree lowers the perfusion pressure and arterial flow to the penile sinusoidal spaces. This increases the time to maximal erection and reduces maximal penile rigidity. The most common causes of arterial insufficiency are generalized atherosclerotic disease or perineal trauma. Risk factors for generalized arterial insufficiency include hypertension, hyperlipidemia, cigarette smoking, diabetes mellitus, and pelvic irradiation.[24,25] Epidemiologic studies have confirmed a high correlation between ED and treated heart disease, treated hypertension, and a low level of high-density lipoprotein.[26] Hypertension is a well-recognized risk factor for arteriosclerosis; a prevalence of about 45% has been noted in one series of men with ED.[24] However, in hypertension, the increased blood pressure itself does not impair erectile function; rather, the associated arterial stenotic lesions are thought to be the cause. Focal stenosis of the common penile or cavernous artery is most often seen in patients who have sustained blunt pelvic or perineal trauma (eg, biking accidents) and can lead to arterial insufficiency.[24]

Cavernosal (Venogenic)

Failure to maintain a rigid erection despite adequate arterial inflow may result from inadequate occlusion of veins draining the corpora cavernosa. Veno-occlusive disease (VOD) causing ED[27] may be the result of congenital, traumatic, or degenerative causes or the result of failed smooth muscle relaxation. The diagnosis of VOD is made by documenting venous channels draining the corpora cavernosa during a pharmacologic cavernosography and by characteristic findings on infusion cavernosometry. Degenerative changes caused by Peyronie's disease, old age, diabetes, or traumatic injury (penile fracture or acquired shunts—the result of operative correction of priapism) to the tunica albuginea may lead to VOD. Anxious patients with excessive adrenergic tone[28] or patients with inadequate neurotransmitter release may have insufficient trabecular smooth muscle relaxation and also exhibit VOD. Although this phenomenon may account for rare cases of primary ED in young men, it is a common end-stage process in ED of all etiologies that results from smooth muscle atrophy. Following treatment for prostate cancer, up to 30% of patients may develop VOD in addition to neurogenic ED.

Drug Induced

Many therapeutic agents have been reported to cause ED, although the mechanism by which this effect occurs is largely unknown and in some cases may be coincidental. The sexual effect of a particular drug is typically listed with the medication side effects documented in clinical drug studies, without controlling for the occurrence of such conditions in the normal, untreated population. Drugs that modulate central neuroendocrine or local neurovascular control of penile smooth muscle have the potential to cause ED. Central neurotransmitter pathways, including 5-hydroxytryptaminergic, noradrenergic, and dopaminergic pathways involved in sexual function, may be disturbed by antipsychotics, antidepressants, and centrally acting antihypertensive drugs. Alpha-adrenergic blocking agents, such as prazosin, terazosin, and doxazosin, may cause retrograde ejaculation owing to muscular relaxation at the bladder neck and prostate. Beta-blockers may cause ED from potentiation of $\alpha 1$-adrenoceptor activity in the penis. Thiazide diuretic treatment has been reported to affect potency, but the exact mechanism is unknown. Spironolactone has been implicated in producing erectile failure, decreased libido, gynecomastia, and mastodynia. Calcium-channel blockers and α-adrenergic blockers seem to be better alternatives if patients complain of ED with other antihypertensives. Cigarette smoking may induce vasoconstriction and penile venous leakage because of its contractile effect on the cavernous smooth muscle.[29] Alcohol in small amounts improves erection and sexual drive because of its vasodilatory effect and the suppression of anxiety; however, large amounts can cause central sedation, decreased libido, and transient ED. Chronic alcoholism may result in liver dysfunction, decreased testosterone and increased estrogen levels, and alcoholic polyneuropathy, which may also affect penile nerves.[30] Cimetidine, a histamine-H_2 receptor antagonist, has been reported to suppress the libido and produce erectile failure. It is thought to act as an antiandrogen and to increase prolactin levels.[31] Other drugs known to cause ED are estrogens and drugs with antiandrogenic action, such as ketoconazole and cyproterone acetate.

AGING AND SYSTEMIC DISEASES

Multiple studies have documented a progressive decline in sexual function in "healthy" aging men. Masters and Johnson noted a number of changes, including longer latency to full erection, reduced erectile turgidity, lessened force of ejaculation and decreased ejaculatory volume, and a longer refractory period. Other changes include a reduction in penile tactile sensitivity,[32] a lower serum level of testosterone owing to hypothalamic-pituitary dysfunction,[33] and a heightened cavernous muscle tone.[28] Approximately 50% of patients with chronic diabetes mellitus have ED. In addition to the disease's effect on small vessels, it may also affect the cavernous nerve terminals and endothelial cells, resulting in deficient neurotransmitter release.[14] Chronic renal failure has frequently been associated with diminished erectile function, impaired libido, and infertility. In one study, 78% of the patients were found to have cavernous artery occlusive disease and 90% to have VOD.[34] The mechanism is probably multifactorial: depressed testosterone levels, diabetes mellitus, vascular insufficiency, multiple medications, autonomic and somatic neuropathy,[35] and psychological stress. Patients with severe pulmonary disease may fear aggravating dyspnea during sexual intercourse. Patients with exercise-induced angina, heart failure, or myocardial infarction can become impotent from anxiety, depression, or concomitant penile arterial insufficiency. Other systemic diseases such as cirrhosis of the liver, penile scleroderma, chronic debilitation, and cachexia are also known to cause ED.

INCIDENCE OF ERECTILE DYSFUNCTION IN PATIENTS AFTER TREATMENT FOR PROSTATE CANCER

Erectile dysfunction following pelvic surgery has been widely reported. Historic series document the incidence of sexual dysfunction after radical surgery for bladder or prostate cancer at over 90%. Even with simple prostatectomy for benign disease, Finkle and Prian reported an impotence rate of 29% after perineal prostatectomy and 16% after suprapubic prostatectomy.[36] Because of the close proximity of the cavernosal nerves to the prostate, ED after radical prostatectomy was a very common occurrence as recently as 20 years ago. Studying detailed anatomic dissections, Walsh and Donker pioneered the nerve-sparing technique,[5] and now up to 76% of patients undergoing radical retropubic prostatectomy and 45% with radical cystectomy are potent postoperatively.[37,38] Contemporary series describe variable potency rates based primarily on the degree of nerve preservation during surgical dissection (Table 26–1).[39–43] When the neurovascular bundle is preserved bilaterally, natural potency rates have been reported at 31 to 76%.[44] When only one neurovascular bundle is spared, natural potency rates have been reported at 13 to 56%. When a non–nerve-sparing radical prostatectomy is performed, potency rates range from 0 to 16%. Aside from the degree of nerve preservation, other factors have been associated with erectile function following radical prostatectomy. Patient age at the time of surgery is strongly associated with the return of erectile function in the postoperative period. In the series by Quinlan and colleagues, bilateral nerve preservation resulted in potency in 90% of men under 50 years, 82% in men age 50 to 60, and 69% in men age 60 to 70.[42] In contrast, only 22% of men over 70 years of age remained potent after bilateral nerve preservation at the time of radical prostatectomy. Clinical and pathologic stage and tumor volume have also been associated with postoperative potency rates in multiple series.

Table 26–1. POTENCY RATES AFTER RADICAL PROSTATECTOMY

Lead Author	N	Follow-up (yr)	Age (yr)	Nerve Preservation	% Potency
Catalona[39]	858	1.5	63	Bilateral	63
				Unilateral	47
Geary[40]	459	1.5	64	Bilateral	31
				Unilateral	13
				No preservation	1
McCammon[41]	203	3.4	64	Bilateral	45*
				Unilateral	31*
				No preservation	16*
Quinlan[42]	503		59	Bilateral	76
				Partial bilateral	64
				Unilateral	56
				No preservation	0
Drago[43]	151		64	Unilateral or bilateral†	66

The number (N) for each study represents the patients for whom potency statistics are reported.
*Represents patients with either "no difficulty" or "some difficulty" achieving erection.
†Unilateral nerve preservation performed for palpable cancer by digital rectal examination, bilateral nerve preservation performed for cancer discovered by transurethral resection, or palpably benign gland.

Following XRT, potency rates vary according to several variables. Time after XRT, pretreatment potency status, the targeting technique used, and radiation dose delivered are primary determinants of post-treatment potency (Table 26–2).[41,45–55] Radiobiologic effects on target tissues continue after the course of radiotherapy has finished, and erectile function has also been noted to change with time after treatment. In the first year after XRT, potency rates of 46 to 92% have been described. With longer follow-up, potency rates of 16 to 67% have been documented for patients 22 to 33 months after completing XRT. After 77 months, potency rates of 40 to 61% are described. The general trend is decreasing potency with time after XRT, with a plateau reached at 2 to 3 years following treatment. In the study by Turner and colleagues, potency status was examined at various intervals after XRT.[48] Although 83 men were fully potent before XRT, this number dropped to 45 (54%) men after 4 months and 20 (24%) men after 12 months. Also, men who described impaired potency before treatment were statistically significantly more likely to be rendered completely impotent at 12 months after treatment. Corroborating this temporal trend are quality of life data from the CaPSURE (Cancer of the Prostate Strategic Urologic Research Endeavor) database. Patients' quality of life after treatment for prostate cancer was evaluated with specific emphasis on domains of sexual function and bother. Litwin and colleagues found that sexual function was better immediately after XRT compared to radical prostatectomy, with both groups improving at comparable rates during the first year following treatment.[56] In the second year, however, patients treated with XRT showed a significant decline in sexual function, whereas those treated with surgery continued to improve.

Table 26–2. POTENCY RATES AFTER CONVENTIONAL EXTERNAL BEAM RADIATION THERAPY

Lead Author	N	Mo after Therapy	Age (yr)	% Potency
Hanks[45]	100	3	NS	73
Banker[46]	85	8–12	64	54
Mantz[47]	114	12	68	92
Turner[48]	182*	12	69	62
Lim[49]	46	12	NS	46
Chinn,[50] Roach[51]	113	21	75	62
Nguyen[52]	96	> 24	NS	36†
Jonler[53]	86‡	31	71	16
Crook[54]	192	33	70	65§
McCammon[41]	257	77	64	40‖
Perez[55]	210	78	NS	61

*Patients reported either having normal potency after radiation therapy or "some difficulty" with erections.
†Patients reporting full erections after external beam radiation therapy. Partial erections were reported in an additional 42%. In this series, 30% of patients reported that erections were adequate for intercourse "fairly often, usually, or always."
‡Patients who reported ability to establish a full or partial erection before external beam radiation therapy. Potency rate in this series represents patients with erections firm enough for intercourse.
§Erections "deemed satisfactory for intercourse" in previously potent patients following external beam radiation therapy.
‖Patients with either "no difficulty" or "some difficulty" achieving erection.

Advanced techniques have been developed to target the radiation beam, which may increase the dose delivered to the prostate but minimize exposure of surrounding structures. The conventional four-field box technique was used traditionally, and most of the series shown in Table 26–3 represent treatment using this standard methodology.[57–59] In the report by Nguyen and colleagues, the conventional technique was compared to conformal radiation therapy using a six-field arrangement and three-dimensional planning (3DCRT).[52] The dose delivered to the treatment isocenter was 70 Gy for the conventional treatment and 78 Gy for conformal 3DCRT. Prior to treatment, 68% of the conventional treatment group reported intercourse adequacy from “fairly often” to “always,” whereas this was reported in only 53% of the 3DCRT group. Following conventional XRT, 38% of patients reported full erections, with 27% describing intercourse adequacy as defined above. Conversely, after 3DCRT, 35% of patients reported full erections, with 31% describing intercourse adequacy. Only 14% of the 3DCRT group had tried treatments for impotence, whereas 27% of patients in the conventional XRT group had tried such treatments. Despite the poorer pretreatment erectile function in the 3DCRT group, these patients report a higher rate of full erections and intercourse adequacy compared with the conventional XRT group. Although 3DCRT appears superior to conventional RT for potency preservation, a time-dependent reduction in erectile capacity has been reported. Wilder and colleagues performed Kaplan-Meier estimates of potency preservation rates at various time points after 3DCRT.[60] Among men who were previously potent (sufficient for vaginal penetration), estimates at 1, 2, and 3 years after treatment were 100%, 83%, and 63%, respectively.

Table 26–3. POTENCY RATES AFTER INTERSTITIAL RADIATION THERAPY

Author	Age (yr)	N	Mo after Therapy	% Potency
Stock[57]	66	313*	36	79
			72	59
Sanchez-Ortiz[58]	69	81†	23	49
Wallner[59]		56‡	36	86

*Data only for those patients with either normal erectile function (score 1) or erectile function that is suboptimal but sufficient for intercourse (score 2) prior to seed implantation are included here. Potency statistics represent those with either score 1 or 2 potency following treatment.
†Data only for those patients with erectile function sufficient for vaginal intercourse before seed implantation was included. An additional 26% of men had erections firm enough for foreplay but not for penetration.
‡Data only for those patients who were “potent” prior to treatment.

Radiotherapy using implanted seeds of iodine 125 or palladium 103 (interstitial brachytherapy) has the theoretical advantage over external beam therapies in both improved radiation dosing and reduced exposure to surrounding tissues. Seeds may deliver a higher radiation dose to the prostate gland from an interstitial source implanted in the target tissue, thereby avoiding transmission through the skin and surrounding structures from an externally located radiation source. Seed implantation is also a convenient outpatient procedure, without the need for repeated treatments as in external beam therapies. Erectile function after interstitial seed implantation has been evaluated in several recent series (see Table 26–3). Evaluating only men with adequate erectile function prior to treatment, there was a general trend to worsening erectile function with time after treatment. At 36 months after seed implantation, potency rates were 79 to 86% and had decreased to 59% at 72 months posttreatment. The only large contemporary study that has used a validated quality of life questionnaire to gauge erectile function after seed implantation found a 49% potency rate at 23 months after treatment.[58]

Freezing the prostate using transperineal probes (cryotherapy) has been advocated as a primary treatment for prostate cancer and as a salvage procedure for locally recurrent disease after radiotherapy. Transrectal ultrasonographic real-time monitoring (with thermocouples at prostatic landmarks) of the freezing process is critical to ensure complete freezing while sparing surrounding structures. Despite continuous monitoring of the ice ball during the freezing phase, freezing of the cavernous nerve is common. This is most likely owing to difficulty controlling the ice ball propagation precisely and the need to completely freeze the peripheral gland for an acceptable oncologic result. To achieve complete freezing, the ice ball propagation must extend beyond the prostate capsule so that the temperature in the entire prostate achieves a sufficiently low level to attain coagulative tissue necrosis. Nerve damage from thermotrauma results in cytoplasmic crystallization and fragmentation of intracellular organelles. For this reason, it is understandable that ED following cryotherapy is common, occurring in 80 to 90% of cases reported in a small clinical series.[61]

EVALUATION AND DIAGNOSIS OF ERECTILE DYSFUNCTION AFTER TREATMENT FOR PROSTATE CANCER

Although the origin of ED after radical pelvic surgery is most likely neurogenic or vasculogenic, one should remember that erection is mediated through the coordinated interaction of the psychological, neural, hormonal, vascular, and muscular systems. Accordingly, one should adopt a multidisciplinary approach to exclude other contributory etiologic factors, especially if the patient has a history of decreased potency prior to surgery.

A detailed medical, surgical, and sexual history is important in identifying the cause. Depression secondary to the diagnosis of cancer, surgical trauma, or the creation of a stoma may contribute to the loss of libido and impotence. Physical examination should include the following: (1) breast, hair distribution, testis, thyroid (to detect an endocrine abnormality); (2) femoral and pedal pulses (for vascular insufficiency); (3) genital and perineal sensation (neurologic deficit); and (4) penile abnormalities. Recommended laboratory tests include urinalysis, complete blood count, fasting blood glucose, creatinine, lipid profile, and morning testosterone. If the testosterone level is low, a repeat study including total and free (or bioavailable) testosterone, prolactin, and luteinizing hormone values should be obtained to rule out secondary hypogonadism or prolactinoma. For neurogenic impotence, the somatic nervous system can be assessed with a relatively high degree of accuracy by measuring the latency time of the dorsal nerve and the bulbocavernous reflex; however, at the present time, the autonomic nervous system cannot be assessed directly.

Patient's Goal-Directed Evaluation and Management of Erectile Dysfunction

At our institution, diagnostic tests are planned according to the patient's goal and desired treatment (Figure 26–2).[62] All patients receive the detailed medical, psychosocial history, physical examination, and, if necessary, hormonal and laboratory test-

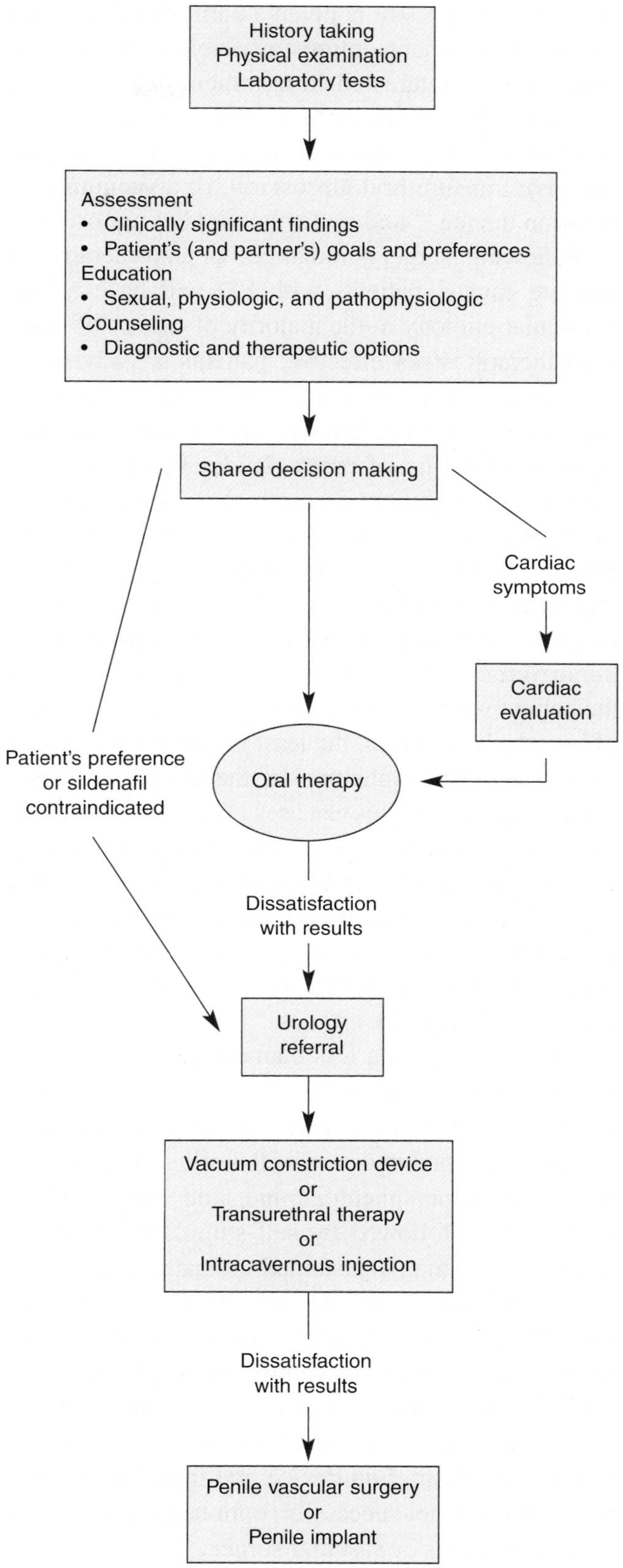

Figure 26–2. Patient's goal-directed approach to evaluation and management of erectile dysfunction.

ing. Also, the patient is given a pamphlet discussing all of the treatment options available at the current time. If he is interested in treatment and wishes to have no further workup, he is given an empiric trial of sildenafil (provided that there are no contraindications), transurethral alprostadil, or a vacuum constriction device,[63] and no further studies are ordered.

Following surgery, radiation, or cryotherapy for prostate cancer, patients with ED will have a neurovascular etiology in the majority of cases.[64] If sildenafil therapy is not effective, patients are advised to have the combined intracavernous injection and manual stimulation test (CIS test).[62] If, after intracavernous injection of 10 μg of prostaglandin E_1 or 45 mg of papaverine, the patient promptly develops a sustained rigid erection without manual genital stimulation, significant arterial or venous insufficiency is unlikely, and further vascular workup is not advised. These patients will be treated with a vacuum erection device, intracavernous injection, or transurethral therapy. If the patient wishes to have a more accurate assessment of his arterial function, the least invasive test—duplex ultrasonographic evaluation of the arterial system—will be performed. This test uses a duplex scanner with 10-MHz ultrasound and 4.5-MHz pulsed Doppler to measure the diameter and flow of the cavernous arteries before and after intracavernous injection of a vasodilator. Other authors suggest the use of Doppler waveform analysis before and after intracavernous injection to assess the arteries.

The patient with a less than adequate response to injection alone is advised to stimulate himself manually (CIS test). If the patient fails to achieve a good erection, a second injection of 0.3 mL of Trimix solution (papaverine, phentolamine, and alprostadil) is administered, followed by self-stimulation again. A good erection that is sustained indicates an adequate venous mechanism, and the patient can be a candidate for intracavernous injection therapy. If the erectile response is still poor, a vacuum constriction device is applied to see if the erection can be enhanced. If successful, the patient will be advised to use a combination of the constriction device and injection therapy; if the device is not successful, options are limited to a penile prosthesis or vascular surgery.

The vast majority of patients presenting with ED after treatment for prostate cancer have neurogenic ED and are not candidates for vascular surgery. Multiple outcome studies of penile arterial revascularization report acceptable outcomes after an isolated arterial injury. Elderly men and those with generalized vascular disease, neurologic impairment or penile scarring and trauma, are best advised against a revascularization procedure. Similarly, VOD may be diagnosed in up to 30% of men with ED of various etiologies. Recent clinical series have documented therapeutic efficacy of surgery for VOD in a select subset of patients with primary ED owing to a congenital venous leak. Because VOD is a result of atrophic penile smooth muscle, therapies directed at regeneration of smooth muscle using growth factors are conceivable. For the rare patient with prostate cancer without a neurologic defect who wishes to pursue further workup for possible vascular correction, a duplex ultrasonographic test[65] is performed to investigate the cavernous arteries. In our practice, pharmacologic cavernosometry[66] (measurement of the flow required to maintain a full erection and the rate of drop in intracavernous pressure) and cavernosography[67] (contrast study of the site of penile venous leakage) are reserved for patients with a poorly sustained erection in the presence of an adequate arterial response verified by duplex ultrasonography. Similarly, pharmacologic pudendal arteriography[68] (selective pudendal arterial study after intracavernous injection of vasodilators) will be performed only in patients who have no systemic arterial disease and are good candidates for arterial bypass surgery or angioplasty.

Patients with postoperative neurogenic impotence are ideal candidates for intracavernous pharmacotherapy. Damage to the cavernous nerves will prevent the release of neurotransmitters required to initiate the vascular events necessary for full erection. Thus, any vasoactive agents that can bypass the neurologic mechanism and produce sufficient smooth muscle relaxation of both the terminal arterioles and the sinusoids will result in erection. In patients with autonomic nerve dysfunction but normal vascular and sinusoidal systems, intracavernous injection of even a small amount of a vasoactive agent can result in a dramatic erection sustained for hours. The exact mechanism of this phenomenon is not yet clear; however, it most likely represents an impairment of the detumescence mechanism or a denervation supersensitivity response similar to that observed in the denervated bladder after bethanecol. The results have been impressive: Sidi and colleagues reported a 100% response rate in patients with purely neurogenic impotence. and in those with associated vascular insufficiency, the rate dropped to about 70%.[69]

PHARMACOLOGIC TREATMENT OF ERECTILE DYSFUNCTION

Androgen Therapy

Because of the androgen dependence of prostate cancer, androgen replacement therapy is contraindicated in patients with any evidence of residual or recurrent prostate cancer following treatment. Today, much more effective treatments are available, and testosterone therapy should be discouraged in patients whose ED is not associated with hypogonadism and in eugonadal men with any history of prostate cancer. Following radical prostatectomy, patients are followed for evidence of disease recurrence with regular clinic visits and serum PSA determinations. Although there is no outcome study evaluating recurrent cancer in patients on androgen replacement, most authorities agree that it may be appropriate only if the patient's PSA level remains undetectable 3 to 5 years after surgery.

Although androgen deficiency can certainly contribute to ED, its effect may be on central mechanisms (libido) rather than on the penile tissue itself; its overall contribution as a treatment for ED is unclear. In a recent study of eugonadal men with ED, Schiavi and colleagues showed that androgen therapy may activate sexual behavior without enhancing erectile capacity, with no effect on mood and psychological symptoms.[70] Even in hypogonadal men, androgen replacement therapy has been rather disappointing: Morales and associates reported that only 9% of patients recovered erectile function completely during oral androgen replacement.[71] The underlying cause of ED in the majority of older patients is unlikely to be androgen deficiency alone; rather, neurovascular insufficiency and smooth muscle atrophy are often concomitant. Testosterone replacement therapy may improve bone mass, muscle mass and strength, and nocturnal erections; however, if the aim of androgen replacement therapy is to restore erectile function, testosterone alone is a relatively poor choice. Oral testosterone (except testosterone undecanoate) may cause hepatotoxicity (cholestasis, hepatitis, benign and malignant tumors); thus, its use is not recommended. The long-acting injectable forms, testosterone cypionate and enanthate, are often used for replacement therapy; their recommended dosage is 200 mg intramuscularly every 2 to 3 weeks. Their major drawback is their roller-coaster effect: high activity in the first few days, with a marked decrease toward the end of the cycle. The supraphysiologic level of testosterone may increase hematocrit, depress high-density lipoproprotein cholesterol, suppress spermatogenesis, and worsen sleep apnea. Three transdermal preparations are now available, and daily application has been shown to increase serum testosterone concentrations to within the normal range in over 90% of patients. The most common adverse effects have been itching, chronic skin irritation, and allergic contact dermatitis. Regardless of the route of delivery, the dosage should be titrated in accordance with the serum level. Because of its effect on prostate growth, androgen therapy is contraindicated in patients with primary or recurrent prostate cancer or bladder neck obstruction caused by prostatic hypertrophy. Digital prostate examination should be performed and PSA values obtained to rule out prostate cancer. In patients on long-term therapy, checking the hematocrit, testosterone titer, liver function panel, lipid profile, and PSA levels every 6 months is recommended.

Oral Medications

Phosphodiesterase Inhibitor

Since its release in March 1998, the phosphodiesterase inhibitor sildenafil (Viagra) has become the drug of choice for most men with ED. This medication is a selective inhibitor of the cGMP-specific-binding phosphodiesterase type 5 (PDE 5). Following arousal and sexual stimulation, penile nerve terminals release NO at the penile smooth muscle, resulting in relaxation. As discussed previously, this occurs via cGMP-dependent protein kinase. During the return to the flaccid state, cGMP is hydrolyzed to GMP by the highly specific cGMP-binding PDE 5. Inhibition of

PDE 5 by sildenafil causes a marked elevation of cGMP levels in the glans penis, corpus cavernosum, and spongiosum, resulting in enhanced smooth muscle relaxation and therefore a better erection. In the absence of sexual stimulation, when NO and cGMP are at low basal levels, sildenafil has no appreciable effect on the penis. Because this medication augments the normal neuromuscular mechanism, its use is indicated in ED of all etiologic categories, including psychogenic, neurogenic, and vascular or combinations of these. In all, sildenafil has been evaluated in 21 randomized, double-blind, placebo-controlled trials in over 3,000 patients and in 10 open-label extension studies. These studies indicate that the number of erections and rates of penile rigidity, orgasmic function, and overall satisfaction were significantly higher with treatment.[72,73] However, sildenafil had little effect on sexual drive. Additionally, multiple studies have documented its efficacy after both surgery and radiation therapy. Following radical prostatectomy, the patient's erectile response to sildenafil is strongly related to the degree of nerve preservation, ranging from a 71 to 80% response following bilateral or unilateral nerve preservation to a 6% response following non–nerve-sparing procedures.[74–77] After treatment with conventional or 3DCRT, 67 to 74% of patients reported erectile function sufficient for intercourse using sildenafil[78,79] whereas 71 to 81% reported such a response following prostate brachytherapy.[80,81] Clinical safety data pooled from more than 3,700 patients with 1,631 patient-years of medication exposure have shown that most adverse events were mild to moderate and self-limiting in nature.[73] Common complaints included headache (16%), flushing (10%), dyspepsia (7%), nasal congestion (4%), and abnormal vision (described as a mild and transient color tinge or increased sensitivity to light; 3%). The visual effect is likely related to inhibition of PDE 6 in the retina. In clinical trials, no chronic visual impairments have been reported with sildenafil, and the incidence of visual side effects was similar in diabetic and nondiabetic patients; however, at higher doses, the incidence of adverse effects also increases two- to threefold.[82] Adverse cardiovascular events were mild and transient in the majority of cases and were similar between the sildenafil and placebo groups. For the sildenafil and placebo groups, the rates of serious cardiovascular events were 4.1 and 5.7 and the rates of myocardial infarction events were 1.7 and 1.4 (per 100 man-years of treatment).[73] However, because studies excluded patients using nitrates and those with significant concomitant medical conditions, the incidence of serious cardiovascular events may be higher in the general population. Nevertheless, it appears that sildenafil therapy is safe for most men. However, patient's cardiovascular status should be carefully assessed before treatment. Sildenafil potentiates the vasodilatory effect of nitrates, and the combination of nitrates, and sildenafil has resulted in severe systemic hypotension and 16 deaths in the United States. Therefore, nitrate use is an absolute contraindication for sildenafil therapy. The American Heart Association has published a guideline for sildenafil therapy targeted at the primary care physician.[83] Although rarely reported, patients should be warned to contact their physician if an erection lasts for more than 4 hours as more than 25 cases of prolonged erection or priapism have occurred. Caution should also be exercised in prescribing sildenafil to patients with diseases that are risk factors for priapism, such as sickle cell anemia, leukemia, or multiple myeloma.

Sildenafil is absorbed well in the fasted state, reaching maximal plasma concentrations within 30 to 120 minutes (mean 60 minutes). When sildenafil is taken with a high-fat meal, the rate of absorption is reduced, with a mean delay in T_{max} of 60 minutes. It is eliminated predominantly by hepatic metabolism (mainly cytochrome P-450 3A4), and the terminal half-life is about 4 hours. The recommended starting dose is 50 mg taken 1 hour before sexual activity, and the maximal recommended frequency is once per day. Based on effectiveness and side effects, the dose may be increased to 100 mg or decreased to 25 mg. In patients over 65, those with hepatic or renal impairment, and those taking cytochrome P-450 3A4 inhibitors (eg, erythromycin, ketoconazole, itraconazole, protease inhibitors), the lower starting dose of 25 mg should be used.

Adrenoceptor Antagonists

Yohimbine is an α_2-adrenoceptor antagonist produced from the bark of the yohim tree. It presumably acts at central adrenergic receptors in the paraventricular and medial preoptic area of the hypothalamus, areas associated with libido and penile erection. In a recent meta-analysis of seven randomized, placebo-controlled studies of yohimbine monotherapy, it was reportedly superior to placebo.[84] In several other controlled randomized studies of patients with organic ED, no significant difference from placebo was found.[85] The most frequently reported side effects include palpitation, fine tremor, elevation of blood pressure, and anxiety. As its effect is marginal, yohimbine is not recommended in patients with organic ED.

Oral phentolamine (Vasomax) has also been reported to improve erectile function.[86,87] In a clinical trial of patients with mild to moderate ED, improved erections were reported in 37% of patients receiving a 40-mg dose, 45% of those on the 80-mg dose, and 16% of patients receiving placebo. The proposed mechanism of action includes the synergistic effects of vascular dilation and blockade of systemic sympathetic tone. Side effects include headache, facial flushing, and nasal congestion. Oral phentolamine has not been approved by the US Food and Drug Administration (FDA).

Dopaminergic Agonist

Apomorphine is a potent emetic that acts on central dopaminergic (D_1/D_2) receptors. When injected subcutaneously, it induced erections in rats and humans,[88] but the side effects, notably nausea, seriously limited its clinical usefulness. A sublingual formulation (Uprima) is now in clinical trials. In one study, in patients with psychogenic or mild organic ED taking a 4-mg dose, 52% attained erection compared with 35% in the placebo group. Further, sexual intercourse was achieved in 43% of the treated group compared with 27% of the placebo group. However, nausea was reported in 17% of patients, with 4% requiring antiemetics.[88] Sublingual apomorphine has been approved in Europe but not in the United States.

Serotonergic Drugs

Trazodone is a serotonin antagonist and reuptake inhibitor used as a sedative and an antidepressant. It is associated with a rare incidence of priapism. Its effect on erection is thought to be the result of serotonergic and α-adrenolytic activity. Although trazodone alone or in combination with yohimbine has been reported to improved erectile function in some men,[89,90] its beneficial effects could not be substantiated in a double-blind, placebo-controlled, multicenter trial with a dosage of 150 mg/day.[91] Therefore, its clinical use in patients with ED is not recommended.

Transurethral Medications

Alprostadil

Prostaglandin E_1 is an endogenous unsaturated fatty acid derivative of arachidonic acid. Alprostadil is a more stable, synthetic form of prostaglandin E_1. Its initial clinical use was in the management of patent ductus arteriosus and peripheral vascular disease. Transurethral alprostadil (MUSE [medicated urethral system for erection]) is appropriate as initial therapy for organic ED, but most commonly it is the patient's second choice when sildenafil fails to produce adequate erection or is contraindicated. Two large multicenter, double-blind, placebo-controlled clinical trials conducted in the United States[89] and Europe[90] demonstrated the efficacy of MUSE in approximately 43% of patients with ED from various organic causes. The most common side effects were penile pain and urethral pain or burning. MUSE has been reported to be effective for some patients who have withdrawn from intracavernous injection therapy or in whom it has failed[92]; transurethral therapy has also been found to enhance the quality of erection produced by a vacuum constriction device.[93] The advantages of the transurethral approach include local application without requiring injection, minimal systemic effects, and the rarity of drug interactions. The major drawbacks of MUSE therapy are moderate to severe pain, low response rate, and inconsistency.[94,95] To improve the response rate, combination therapy with prazosin has been tested and has shown some additional benefit over alprostadil alone.[96] Others have investigated the use of an adjustable constriction device (Actis) placed at the base of the penis to reduce venous outflow and facilitate drug transport from the corpus spongiosum to the cavernosum. This has improved the incidence of erection adequate for sexual intercourse to around 70%.[97] The first application (usually a 500-μg dose) should be undertaken in the physician's office because of the potential complications of urethral bleeding, vasovagal reflex, hypotension, and priapism. Depending on the erectile response, the patient is instructed to increase or decrease the dosage (up to 1,000 μg or down to 250 μg). The use of a small drop of K-Y jelly at the urethral meatus facilitates insertion of the applicator.

Intracavernous Injection

Intracavernous injection was patented by de la Torre in the United States in 1978. Clinical use, however, did not begin until 1982, when Virag and colleagues first published their experience with papaverine.[98] The technique of autoinjection has since been adapted for home use, with patient acceptance after brief instruction.[99] Since the introduction of MUSE and sildenafil, intracavernous injection has become third-line therapy for most patients. In the United States, the most commonly used intracavernous drugs are alprostadil and a combination of papaverine, phentolamine, and alprostadil (Trimix).

Papaverine

Papaverine is a nonspecific phosphodiesterase inhibitor, acting to increase both cAMP and cGMP in penile erectile tissue.[100] It may also impair calcium-activated potassium and chloride currents.[101] It is metabolized in the liver, and the plasma half-life is 1 to 2 hours. Extensive experience has been gained with intracavernous injection of papaverine. The average dose ranges from 15 to 60 mg per injection. Its advantages include low cost and stability at room temperature; major disadvantages are the risk of priapism (0 to 35%) and corporal fibrosis (1 to 33%) and the occasional elevation of liver enzymes. It is rarely used alone, except in developing countries where drug cost is the main consideration.

α-Adrenergic Antagonists

Phentolamine is an α-adrenoceptor antagonist with equal affinity for α_1 and α_2 receptors. When used alone, phentolamine does not produce rigid erection[102]; however, when combined with papaverine, success rates approach 63 to 87%.[103] The most common preparation is a combination of 30-mg papaverine and 0.5- to 1-mg phentolamine. This synergistic formulation both improves erectile response and permits the use of a lower papaverine dose. As expected, it is less effective than Trimix solution (see below) and is used when patients cannot tolerate penile pain from preparations containing alprostadil. The primary side effects of phentolamine include systemic hypotension and reflex tachycardia. Its plasma half-life is approximately 30 minutes.

Alprostadil (Prostaglandin E1)

Several formulations of alprostadil have been used for intracavernous injection. The pediatric formulation Prostin VR was used first, followed by Caverject, a lyophilized powder, and Edex, which contains alprostadil in an α-cyclodextrin inclusion complex. Home injection therapy with alprostadil was reported to be safe and effective in the late 1980s.[104] It gained increasing popularity and became the first approved intracavernous agent in the United States in 1996. Clinical response was superior to that of papaverine and papaverine/phentolamine combinations, with success rates documented at more than 70%.[105,106] In addition, alprostadil has a relatively low incidence of priapism (0.35 to 4%) and fibrosis (1 to 23%).[105–109] Systemic effects are rare, presumably because of its metabolism by local prostaglandin hydroxydehydrogenase in penile tissue. The most frequent side effect is pain at the injection site or along the shaft of the penis during erection (occurring in 16.8 to 34% of patients).[105,106] The mechanism by which prostaglandin E_1 causes penile pain is via prostaglandin receptor activation, which decreases the primary afferent nociceptive threshold directly.[110] The hyperalgesic effect is more prominent in patients with partial nerve injury, such as those with diabetic neuropathy and those who have undergone radical pelvic surgery.

Vasoactive Intestinal Polypeptide

Vasoactive intestinal polypeptide is a potent smooth muscle relaxant originally isolated from the small intestine. Injection of VIP alone does not produce rigid erection[111]; when combined with phentolamine, it produces erections sufficient for sexual intercourse in up to 67% of patients.[112] Common side effects include transient facial flushing (53%), bruising (20%), pain at the injection site (11%), and truncal flushing (9%). The combination is available in several European countries but not in the United States.

Drug Combinations

The rationale for formulating drug combinations is the ability to use drugs with different mechanisms of action synergistically, permitting a much lower dosage of each to avoid side effects while improving effectiveness. Combinations such as papaverine/alprostadil,[113] ketanserin/alprostadil, and phentolamine/alprostadil[114] have been shown to be superior to alprostadil alone. The most widely used in the United States is a three-drug mixture containing variable amounts of papaverine, phentolamine, and alprostadil (Trimix), originally introduced by Bennett and colleagues.[115] The response rate to Trimix solution is reportedly as high as 90%. Although it has not been approved by the FDA, it is widely used in the United States. A six-drug combination (papaverine, ifenprodil, atropine, yohimbine, dipyridamole, and piribedil) has also been used in France, with excellent results.[98]

Clinical Aspects of Intracavernous Injection Therapy

Patients must have the first injection performed by medical personnel and receive appropriate training and education before home injection. For alprostadil, an initial dose of 2.5 μg is recommended. If the response is inadequate, increases in 2.5- to 5-μg increments can be given until a full erection is achieved or a maximum of 60 μg is reached. For other agents, one should start with a small dose (such as 7.5 mg of papaverine and 0.1 mL of drug combinations), especially in patients with nonvascular ED. The goal is to achieve an erection that is adequate for sexual intercourse but does not last for more than 1 hour, and patients must be evaluated to confirm that the erection has appropriately subsided prior to leaving the physician's office. The two major side effects of intracavernous injection in general are priapism and fibrosis (penile deviation from nodules or plaque). More powerful drugs such as Trimix are more likely to produce erection of longer duration; however, priapism is preventable through careful titration. To prevent fibrosis, we routinely instruct the patient to compress the injection site for 5 minutes (up to 10 minutes in patients on anticoagulants). Intracavernous injection therapy is contraindicated in patients with sickle cell anemia, schizophrenia or a severe psychiatric disorder, and severe venous leakage. Although the clinical response rate is quite high, the percentage of patients accepting injection therapy for chronic management of ED is much lower, even before sildenafil was introduced.[116] In long-term studies, 37.6 to 80% of patients terminated their use of injectable agents,[117,118] and many patients on injection therapy choose less invasive treatments as they become available. Interestingly, a number of patients alternate injection therapy with sildenafil or MUSE; many prefer injection in circumstances when an erection of longer duration is desired.

Recovery of Erectile Function after Prostatectomy

A prospective, randomized trial of the effect of alprostadil injection on patients after nerve-sparing radical prostatectomy was conducted on 30 patients by Montorsi and colleagues.[119] Alprostadil injections were given three times per week for 12 weeks in 15 patients, whereas another 15 patients received no treatment. When patients were evaluated 6 months after surgery, 67% of the treated group reported recovery of spontaneous erection sufficient for satisfactory sexual intercourse, compared with 20% in the observation group. The authors concluded that early postoperative alprostadil injections significantly increase the recovery rate of spontaneous erections after nerve-sparing radical retropubic prostatectomy. They postulate that programmed vasoactive injections improve cavernous oxygenation, thereby limiting the development of hypoxia-induced tissue damage. Based on this observation, we routinely encourage patients to start injection therapy shortly after recovering from radical prostatectomy.

Vacuum Erection Device

In patients who still have partial erections, a vacuum erection device is especially helpful.[63] This device is used to create a vacuum around the penis using either a hand-operated or battery-powered pump. Blood is thereby drawn into the penis to produce the erection, and then a constriction device is slipped off the device and around the base of the penis to maintain the erection. This can be left in place safely for 30 minutes, after which the constriction device is removed and flaccidity returns. After radical pelvic surgery, many patients are anxious about any invasive treatment, and this can therefore be the treatment of choice. Advantages include high efficacy, low cost, ease of use, and avoidance of drug interactions or side effects. Up to 93% of patients report satisfaction with the erection produced with the vacuum erection device, 83% report partner satisfaction, and 70% of couples report regular long-term use. Complications include penile petechiae, dusky discoloration of the glans, penile numbness, and trapping of the ejaculate.[63]

Penile Prosthesis

Prior to the introduction of the treatments listed above, the only effective treatment for patients with neurogenic impotence secondary to radical pelvic surgery was a penile prosthesis. Although the results of the initial implants were disappointing, improvements in device design have provided better and more durable semirigid and inflatable prostheses. With high degrees of acceptance and patient satisfaction, penile prostheses have remained the mainstay of therapy in patients who have failed to respond to less invasive treatments and in those with penile fibrosis.[120]

Penile prostheses have been designed in two basic types (Table 26–4), producing penile rigidity by inflation of an implanted pump or maintaining penile rigidity using a semirigid device that stays firm at all times. There are three general types of prosthesis: semirigid (malleable), hinged (mechanical), and inflatable. The malleable prostheses are made of silicone rubber with a central core of interlaced metal supports. American Medical Systems (AMS 600) and Mentor Corporation (Malleable) are the major manufacturers of these devices. Mechanical devices are also covered with silicone rubber, but the inner core is formed by interlocking rings in a column. These provide rigidity when the rings are aligned in one trajectory (ie, pointed straight) and may be bent down at other times to resemble flaccidity. The manufacturer of mechanical devices is Timm Medical (Duraphase II). The advantages of semirigid devices are that they are easy to implant, have few mechanical parts with minimal mechanical failure, and generally last longer than inflatable devices.[121,122] The major disadvantages of the semirigid devices are that the penis is never fully flaccid and lack of penile girth expansion, which makes these erections seem less natural.[123,124] These devices are challenging to conceal and are associated with a higher chance of device erosion outside the corpora cavernosa.

Table 26–4. PENILE PROSTHESES

Type	Prosthesis	Vendor
Malleable	Mentor malleable	Mentor
	Accuform	Mentor
	650	AMS
	600M	AMS
Mechanical	Dura II	Timm Medical
Inflatable		
2-piece	Ambicor	AMS
3-piece	Alpha 1 standard	Mentor
	Alpha 1 narrow-base	Mentor
	700CX	AMS
	700CXM	AMS
	700 Ultrex (3 connectors)	AMS
	700 Ultrex Plus (1 connector)	AMS

AMS = American Medical Systems.

Inflatable prostheses have been constructed in two basic designs: two-piece and three-piece prostheses. Two-piece inflatable prostheses consist of a pair of cylinders attached to a scrotal device that functions as a pump and/or fluid reservoir. Currently, one two-piece inflatable prostheses is available in the United States. American Medical Systems markets a device (AMS Ambicor) with a scrotal pump that transfers fluid from the proximal portion of the cylinders to the distal portion to provide rigidity. The prosthesis can be deflated by bending the penis at midshaft. Three-piece inflatable prostheses consist of a pair of penile cylinders, a scrotal pump, and a suprapubic reservoir. They provide better rigidity with girth expansion when inflated and a more natural appearance when flaccid. Mentor Corporation makes two three-piece inflatable prostheses (standard and narrow base), whereas American Medical Systems makes four three-piece devices: the AMS 700CX, AMS

700CXM, AMS Ultrex, and AMS Ultrex Plus prostheses (see Table 26–4). The Ultrex prostheses contain distal expansion mechanisms that can give slightly longer penile length during erection.[125]

Indicated for both ED and the coexistence of Peyronie's disease,[126,127] the three-piece inflatable implants have been the most popular, accounting for 85% of all devices implanted. These give the most natural appearance and function. About 15% of patients choose semirigid rod implants, and those with limited mental capacity or manual dexterity are encouraged to have this type of device. Because of the relative simplicity and freedom from complicated hydraulic mechanisms, the semirigid devices last longer than the inflatable prostheses. The majority of inflatable devices will have some mechanical failure or leakage and need to be replaced after 10 to 15 years.[128–131] Repair of some portion of the device may be expected in 5 to 20% of patients within the first 5 years after implantation.[132] When three-piece inflatable cylinders were compared, it was found that the girth-only expanding variety (AMS CX and Mentor Alpha 1) proved more reliable and caused fewer penile deformities than those that expanded in both length and girth (the AMS Ultrex).[125,133] Although device erosion and infection occur, with prompt intervention and appropriate management, catastrophic outcomes may be avoided with a high salvage rate. Techniques to correct these with corporoplasty have proven successful in the majority of these cases. Patient and partner satisfaction with implants has been very good, in the range of 80% or higher. A smaller penile size, lack of spontaneity, and unmet expectations regarding tactile sensitivity, arousal, and enjoyment are reported among patients who are disappointed with the result after prosthesis implantation.

Patient Selection

Men with ED who fail or reject second-line therapies and are not candidates for vascular therapy should be considered for penile prosthesis implantation (Table 26–5). Patients with ED owing to potentially reversible causes or young men with ED should be discouraged from prosthesis implantation as one cannot recover natural erectile function once a device is placed. Patient education is critical before surgery, emphasizing all conservative management options, the various implantation devices, and the expected cosmetic and functional result. The patients should be shown a representative prosthesis and receive instruction on how it works. It should be made clear that a penile prosthesis will not likely restore the full penile length achieved with the patient's natural erection. Also, the possible complications (infection, malfunction, and erosion), repair/replacement rates, and follow-up care need to be discussed in detail prior to surgery.

Table 26–5. AUTHORS' INDICATIONS AND CONTRAINDICATIONS FOR PENILE PROSTHESIS IMPLANTATION

Indications
Organic impotence—failed or unsatisfied with nonsurgical therapy
Psychogenic impotence—failed sex or psychosexual therapy, failed nonsurgical therapy
Peyronie's disease with ED and severe deformity
Contraindications
Temporary or reversible impotence
Unrealistic expectations
Convicted sex offenders

ED = erectile dysfunction.

Device Selection

In our opinion, the three-piece inflatable prosthesis most closely replicates the natural erection, and we recommend this type of prosthesis in a majority of our patients. This device allows the patient control to produce an erection as desired and return to flaccidity on command. With inflation of the three-piece device, the cylinders become harder and also grow in girth. We reserve the use of semirigid and two-piece prostheses for patients with multiple medical problems, prior extensive pelvic operations complicating placement of the reservoir, severe underlying systemic disease, very advanced age, or inability to use multicomponent devices owing to a lack of manual dexterity or understanding (Table 26–6). In patients with congenital penile curvature or Peyronie's disease, we do not use three-piece prostheses that expand in length (AMS Ultrex).[133] In patients with fibrotic corpora or with smaller penile size, we use a narrow prosthesis. Other spe-

reflexes and pudendal evoked responses in chronic haemodialysis patients. Funct Neurol 1991;6:359.
36. Finkle AL, Prian DV. Sexual potency in elderly men before and after prostatectomy. JAMA 1966;196:139.
37. Walsh PC. Radical prostatectomy, preservation of sexual function, cancer control. The controversy. Urol Clin North Am 1987;14:663.
38. Walsh PC, Mostwin JL. Radical prostatectomy and cystoprostatectomy with preservation of potency. Results using a new nerve-sparing technique. Br J Urol 1984;56:694.
39. Catalona WJ, Basler JW. Return of erections and urinary continence following nerve sparing radical retropubic prostatectomy. J Urol 1993;150:905.
40. Geary ES, Dendinger TE, Freiha FS, et al. Nerve sparing radical prostatectomy: a different view. J Urol 1995;154:145.
41. McCammon KA, Kolm P, Main B, et al. Comparative quality-of-life analysis after radical prostatectomy or external beam radiation for localized prostate cancer. Urology 1999;54:509.
42. Quinlan DM, Epstein JI, Carter BS, et al. Sexual function following radical prostatectomy: influence of preservation of neurovascular bundles. J Urol 1991;145:998.
43. Drago JR, Badalament RA, York JP, et al. Radical prostatectomy: OSU and affiliated hospitals' experience 1985–1989. Urology 1992;39:44.
44. Walsh PC, Epstein JI, Lowe FC. Potency following radical prostatectomy with wide unilateral excision of the neurovascular bundle. J Urol 1987;138:823.
45. Hanks GE. External-beam radiation therapy for clinically localized prostate cancer: patterns of care studies in the United States. NCI Monogr 1988;47:75.
46. Banker FL. The preservation of potency after external beam irradiation for prostate cancer. Int J Radiat Oncol Biol Phys 1988;15:219.
47. Mantz CA, Song P, Farhangi E, et al. Potency probability following conformal megavoltage radiotherapy using conventional doses for localized prostate cancer. Int J Radiat Oncol Biol Phys 1997;37:551.
48. Turner SL, Adams K, Bull CA, et al. Sexual dysfunction after radical radiation therapy for prostate cancer: a prospective evaluation. Urology 1999;54:124.
49. Lim AJ, Brandon AH, Fiedler J, et al. Quality of life: radical prostatectomy versus radiation therapy for prostate cancer. J Urol 1995;154:1420.
50. Chinn DM, Holland J, Crownover RL, et al. Potency following high-dose three-dimensional conformal radiotherapy and the impact of prior major urologic surgical procedures in patients treated for prostate cancer. Int J Radiat Oncol Biol Phys 1995;33:15.
51. Roach M, Chinn DM, Holland J, et al. A pilot survey of sexual function and quality of life following 3D conformal radiotherapy for clinically localized prostate cancer. Int J Radiat Oncol Biol Phys 1996;35:869.
52. Nguyen LN, Pollack A, Zagars GK. Late effects after radiotherapy for prostate cancer in a randomized dose-response study: results of a self-assessment questionnaire. Urology 1998;51:991.
53. Jonler M, Ritter MA, Brinkmann R, et al. Sequelae of definitive radiation therapy for prostate cancer localized to the pelvis. Urology 1994;44:876.
54. Crook J, Esche B, Futter N. Effect of pelvic radiotherapy for prostate cancer on bowel, bladder, and sexual function: the patient's perspective. Urology 1996;47:387.
55. Perez CA, Pilepich MV, Garcia D, et al. Definitive radiation therapy in carcinoma of the prostate localized to the pelvis: experience at the Mallinckrodt Institute of Radiology. NCI Monogr 1988;35:85.
56. Litwin MS, Flanders SC, Pasta DJ, et al. Sexual function and bother after radical prostatectomy or radiation for prostate cancer: multivariate quality-of-life analysis from CaPSURE. Cancer of the Prostate Strategic Urologic Research Endeavor. Urology 1999;54:503.
57. Stock RG, Stone NN, Iannuzzi C. Sexual potency following interactive ultrasound-guided brachytherapy for prostate cancer. Int J Radiat Oncol Biol Phys 1996;35:267.
58. Sanchez-Ortiz RF, Broderick GA, Rovner ES, et al. Erectile function and quality of life after interstitial radiation therapy for prostate cancer. Int J Impot Res 2000;12 Suppl 3:S18.
59. Wallner K, Roy J, Harrison L. Tumor control and morbidity following transperineal iodine 125 implantation for stage T1/T2 prostatic carcinoma. J Clin Oncol 1996;14:449.
60. Wilder RB, Chou RH, Ryu JK, et al. Potency preservation after three-dimensional conformal radiotherapy for prostate cancer: preliminary results. Am J Clin Oncol 2000;23:330.
61. Aboseif S, Shinohara K, Borirakchanyavat S, et al. The effect of cryosurgical ablation of the prostate on erectile function. Br J Urol 1997;80:918.
62. lue T. Impotence: a patient's goal-directed approach to treatment. World J Urol 1990;8:67.
63. Nadig PW, Ware JC, Blumoff R. Noninvasive device to produce and maintain an erection-like state. Urology 1986;27:126.
64. Zelefsky MJ, Eid JF. Elucidating the etiology of erectile dysfunction after definitive therapy for prostatic cancer. Int J Radiat Oncol Biol Phys 1998;40:129.
65. Lue TF, Hricak H, Marich KW, et al. Vasculogenic impotence evaluated by high-resolution ultrasonography and pulsed Doppler spectrum analysis. Radiology 1985;155:777.
66. Wespes E, Delcour C, Struyven J, et al. Pharmacocavernometry-cavernography in impotence. Br J Urol 1986;58:429.
67. Lue TF, Hricak H, Schmidt RA, et al. Functional evaluation of penile veins by cavernosography in papaverine-induced erection. J Urol 1986;135:479.
68. Bookstein JJ, Valji K, Parsons L, et al. Pharmacoarteriography in the evaluation of impotence. J Urol 1987;137:333.
69. Sidi AA, Cameron JS, Duffy LM, et al. Intracavernous drug-induced erections in the management of male erectile dysfunction: experience with 100 patients. J Urol 1986; 135:704.
70. Schiavi RC, White D, Mandeli J, et al. Effect of testosterone administration on sexual behavior and mood in men with erectile dysfunction. Arch Sex Behav 1997;26:231.
71. Morales A, Johnston B, Heaton JW, et al. Oral androgens in the treatment of hypogonadal impotent men. J Urol 1994;152:1115.
72. Goldstein I, Lue TF, Padma-Nathan H, et al. Oral sildenafil in the treatment of erectile dysfunction. Sildenafil Study Group. N Engl J Med 1998;338:1397.
73. Morales A, Gingell C, Collins M, et al. Clinical safety of oral

sildenafil citrate (VIAGRA) in the treatment of erectile dysfunction. Int J Impot Res 1998;10:69.
74. Feng MI, Huang S, Kaptein J, et al. Effect of sildenafil citrate on post-radical prostatectomy erectile dysfunction. J Urol 2000;164:1935.
75. Lowentritt BH, Scardino PT, Miles BJ, et al. Sildenafil citrate after radical retropubic prostatectomy. J Urol 1999;162: 1614.
76. Nehra A, Goldstein I. Sildenafil citrate (Viagra) after radical retropubic prostatectomy: con. Urology 1999;54:587.
77. Zagaja GP, Mhoon DA, Aikens JE, et al. Sildenafil in the treatment of erectile dysfunction after radical prostatectomy. Urology 2000;56:631.
78. Weber DC, Bieri S, Kurtz JM, et al. Prospective pilot study of sildenafil for treatment of postradiotherapy erectile dysfunction in patients with prostate cancer. J Clin Oncol 1999;17:3444.
79. Zelefsky MJ, McKee AB, Lee H, et al. Efficacy of oral sildenafil in patients with erectile dysfunction after radiotherapy for carcinoma of the prostate. Urology 1999;53:775.
80. Merrick GS, Butler WM, Lief JH, et al. Efficacy of sildenafil citrate in prostate brachytherapy patients with erectile dysfunction. Urology 1999;53:1112.
81. Kedia S, Zippe CD, Agarwal A, et al. Treatment of erectile dysfunction with sildenafil citrate (Viagra) after radiation therapy for prostate cancer. Urology 1999;54:308.
82. Price DE, Gingell JC, Gepi-Attee S, et al. Sildenafil: study of a novel oral treatment for erectile dysfunction in diabetic men. Diabet Med 1998;15:821.
83. Cheitlin MD, Hutter AM, Brindis RG, et al. Use of sildenafil (Viagra) in patients with cardiovascular disease. Technology and Practice Executive Committee. Circulation 1999; 99:168.
84. Ernst E, Pittler MH. Yohimbine for erectile dysfunction: a systematic review and meta-analysis of randomized clinical trials. J Urol 1998;159:433.
85. Morales A, Surridge DH, Marshall PG, et al. Nonhormonal pharmacological treatment of organic impotence. J Urol 1982;128:45.
86. Gwinup G. Oral phentolamine in nonspecific erectile insufficiency. Ann Intern Med 1988;109:162.
87. Zorgniotti AW. Experience with buccal phentolamine mesylate for impotence. Int J Impot Res 1994;6:37.
88. Heaton JP, Morales A, Adams MA, et al. Recovery of erectile function by the oral administration of apomorphine. Urology 1995;45:200.
89. Padma-Nathan H, Hellstrom WJ, Kaiser FE, et al. Treatment of men with erectile dysfunction with transurethral alprostadil. Medicated Urethral System for Erection (MUSE) Study Group. N Engl J Med 1997;336:1.
90. Williams G, Abbou CC, Amar ET, et al. Efficacy and safety of transurethral alprostadil therapy in men with erectile dysfunction. MUSE Study Group. Br J Urol 1998;81:889.
91. Meinhardt W, Schmitz PI, Kropman RF, et al. Trazodone, a double blind trial for treatment of erectile dysfunction. Int J Impot Res 1997;9:163.
92. Engel JD, McVary KT. Transurethral alprostadil as therapy for patients who withdrew from or failed prior intracavernous injection therapy. Urology 1998;51:687.
93. John H, Lehmann K, Hauri D. Intraurethral prostaglandin improves quality of vacuum erection therapy. Eur Urol 1996;29:224.
94. Porst H. Transurethral alprostadil with MUSE (medicated urethral system for erection) vs intracavernous alprostadil—a comparative study in 103 patients with erectile dysfunction. Int J Impot Res 1997;9:187.
95. Werthman P, Rajfer J. MUSE therapy: preliminary clinical observations. Urology 1997;50:809.
96. Peterson CA, Bennett AH, Hellstrom WJ, et al. Erectile response to transurethral alprostadil, prazosin and alprostadil-prazosin combinations. J Urol 1998;159:1523.
97. Lewis R. Combined use of transurethral alprostadil and an adjustable penile constriction band in men with erectile dysfunction: results from a multicenter trial. J Urol 1998; 159:237.
98. Virag R, Shoukry K, Floresco J, et al. Intracavernous self-injection of vasoactive drugs in the treatment of impotence: 8-year experience with 615 cases. J Urol 1991;145:287.
99. Zorgniotti AW, Lefleur RS. Auto-injection of the corpus cavernosum with a vasoactive drug combination for vasculogenic impotence. J Urol 1985;133:39.
100. Jeremy JY, BS, Naylor AM, et al. Effects of sildenafil, a type-5 cGMP phosphodiesterase inhibitor, and papavarine on cyclic GMP and cyclic AMP levels in the rabbit corpus cavernosum in vitro. Br J Urol 1997;79:958.
101. Brading AF, Burdyga TV, Scripnyuk ZD. The effects of papaverine on the electrical and mechanical activity of the guinea-pig ureter. J Physiol 1983;334:79.
102. Stief CG, Gall H, Scherb W, et al. Erectile response to intracavernous injection of vasoactive drugs after penile prosthesis removal. Urology 1990;36:143.
103. Fallon B. Intracavernous injection therapy for male erectile dysfunction. Urol Clin North Am 1995;22:833.
104. Stackl W, Hasun R, Marberger M. Intracavernous injection of prostaglandin E1 in impotent men. J Urol 1988;140:66.
105. Linet OI, Neff LL. Intracavernous prostaglandin E1 in erectile dysfunction. Clin Investig 1994;72:139.
106. Porst H. The rationale for prostaglandin E1 in erectile failure: a survey of worldwide experience. J Urol 1996;155:802.
107. Chew KK, Stuckey BG, Earle CM, et al. Penile fibrosis in intracavernosal prostaglandin E1 injection therapy for erectile dysfunction. Int J Impot Res 1997;9:225.
108. Canale D, Giorgi PM, Lencioni R, et al. Long-term intracavernous self-injection with prostaglandin E1 for the treatment of erectile dysfunction. Int J Androl 1996;19:28.
109. Lea AP, Bryson HM, Balfour JA. Intracavernous alprostadil. A review of its pharmacodynamic and pharmacokinetic properties and therapeutic potential in erectile dysfunction. Drugs Aging 1996;8:56.
110. Khasar SG, Ho T, Green PG, et al. Comparison of prostaglandin E1- and prostaglandin E2-induced hyperalgesia in the rat. Neuroscience 1994;62:345.
111. Kiely EA, Bloom SR, Williams G. Penile response to intracavernosal vasoactive intestinal polypeptide alone and in combination with other vasoactive agents. Br J Urol 1989; 64:191.
112. Dinsmore WW, Alderdice DK. Vasoactive intestinal polypeptide and phentolamine mesylate administered by autoinjector in the treatment of patients with erectile dysfunction resistant to other intracavernosal agents. Br J Urol 1998;81:437.

urinary incontinence may be subdivided into two varieties, stress or urge incontinence. However, the two major categories of urinary incontinence can certainly coexist.

A meaningful discussion of urinary dysfunction in this analysis must also encompass the spectrum of troublesome male lower urinary tract symptoms (LUTS). Urinary incontinence may certainly coexist with a number of LUTS—namely, urinary urgency, frequency, hesitancy, nocturia, etc. For the patient, urinary incontinence is perceived as a solitary, vexing physical complaint. For the specialist, it is the manifestation of a number of possibly concurrent lower urinary tract dysfunctions. The other major category of side effects encompasses the observed sequelae of lower urinary tract injury sustained after radiotherapy, collectively labeled as the entity radiation cystitis.

The categories of bowel dysfunction essentially parallel those of the urinary system. The symptom constellation of fecal soiling, tenesmus, and rectal pain parallels the above category of LUTS, although it is not typically categorized in this manner. Likewise, the long-term sequelae of radiation on the rectum—proctitis, hematochezia, anal stricture or stenosis, fistula formation, and bowel obstruction—also parallel the host of complications seen in radiation cystitis.

COMPLICATIONS OF PROSTATE CANCER TREATMENT

Radical Prostatectomy

Urinary Complications

Seated between the bladder neck and the rest of the male urethra, the prostate occupies an integral anatomic position within the male lower urinary tract. Therefore, it is not surprising that the quest for curative prostate cancer resection poses a significant risk to postoperative urinary sphincter function. Yet the complexity of the urinary continence mechanism remains incompletely understood.

The radical prostatectomy operation must necessarily violate this continence mechanism, but surgical techniques are being refined to better retain or reconstitute the new anatomic relationship between the bladder neck and remaining urethra. Some described techniques include bladder neck sparing, tubularized bladder neck reconstruction, and anastomotic fascial slings.[4–6]

During radical prostatectomy, the urethral conduit is securely reconstituted, but the intrinsic watertight seal may be lost. This leaves a gaping conduit, where the problem of urinary storage becomes most evident with the patient upright and active. There is an analogous condition in the female population termed "intrinsic sphincter deficiency," which is actually a subset of the broader diagnosis of stress urinary incontinence.[7] Therefore, this postprostatectomy scenario has likewise been coined "male intrinsic sphincter deficiency."[8–10] In addition, scar tissue may lead to stricture formation at the site of anastomosis.

Urinary incontinence (Table 27–1). Postprostatectomy urinary incontinence prevalence rates range widely from 2 to 31 percent.[11,12] At first glance, the disparate results would suggest that outcomes are heavily dependent on surgeon expertise. However, others would contend that outcome reporting varies in large part because of widely differing patient populations and outcome measures. Here one is well served to evaluate critically the stringency in choosing candidates for surgery (ie, preoperative cancer staging, patient age, preexisting morbidities). Likewise, the method by which continence was defined and then assessed proves equally crucial. One author may consider the term "social continence" an acceptable limit of two protective pads or less. Others may regard continence as complete dryness. Also, patient and physician perspectives of the same clinical entity may differ significantly.[3] In a prospective assessment of patients with prostate cancer, Talcott and colleagues administered patient self-report surveys regarding the side effects they experienced after various treatments.[13] At the 12-month mark within the radical prostatectomy subset, 11 percent reported significant urinary incontinence and 35 percent still routinely used protective pads.

Objective test parameters such as urodynamics testing have proven to be valuable in the assessment of postradical prostatectomy continence. Kleinhans and colleagues performed pre- and postoperative urodynamics testing of a cohort of men who had undergone radical prostatectomy.[14] They determined that at

Table 27–1. URINARY INCONTINENCE RATES AFTER RADICAL PROSTATECTOMY

	N	Follow-up (mo)	SUI (%)	Continence Definition	Total/Severe Incontinence (%)	Overall Incontinence (%)
Retropubic						
Eastham et al (1996)	581	24	5	No pads or occasional pads	4	9
Zincke et al (1994)	1,728		5	< 3 pads per day	0.8	5
Catalona et al (1999)	1,325	50	8	No pads	NA	6
Steiner et al (1991)	593	12	8	Leaks with moderate activity	0.3	8
Perineal						
Weldon (1997)	220	10	1 mild, 2 moderate, 2 severe	No daily use of pads	0	5
Ruiz-Deya (2001)	250	12	NA	≤ 1 pad per day	NA	7
Lance (2001)	190	41	NA	No leak ± pads	NA	
Laparoscopic						
Olsson (2001)	37	12	NA	No pads	NA	21.6
				Never leak		43.2
Guillonneau (2001)	133	12	NA	No pads	NA	14.5
Rassweiler (2001)	88	12	NA	No pads, no leak with stress	NA	3

NA = not available; SUI = stress urinary incontinence.

the 6-month and 1-year postoperative mark, continence was achieved in 84 percent and 97.7 percent, respectively. This conclusion seems to concur with empirical observations. Golomb and colleagues likewise performed pre- and postoperative urodynamics assessment of continence in a similar group.[15] They found that 20 percent had stress urinary incontinence, whereas 25 percent had incontinence driven by bladder storage dysfunction. This finding conflicts with conclusions from other contemporary studies, in which urodynamic assessment of the patients after prostatectomy revealed that the cause of incontinence is most commonly urethral sphincteric deficiency.[16,17]

The incidence of incontinence after radical perineal prostatectomy (RPP) is comparable to that after radical retropubic prostatectomy (RRP), with reported incidence rates ranging from 5 to 30 percent.[18–21] As with RRP, continence improves most rapidly in the first year after surgery, although it may continue to improve in the years to follow. In a prospective evaluation of 220 consecutive men who underwent RPP, Weldon and colleagues demonstrated a return of continence in 23 percent of men at 1 month, 56 percent at 3 months, and 95 percent at 10 months.[21] Advanced age was the most significant risk factor for postperineal prostatectomy incontinence in this series. Gray and colleagues sent questionnaires to 167 patients after RPP. They found that men who achieved continence did so within 2 years of surgery.[22]

Contemporary data regarding continence after laparoscopic prostatectomy have recently become available from three major centers. Whereas potential advantages of the laparoscopic approach include improved magnification and visualization during the apical dissection, the disadvantages include the loss of tactile sensation during the anastomosis as well as limitations in the range of motion associated with laparoscopic instruments during placement of anastomotic sutures. Initial incontinence rates after laparoscopic prostatectomy have ranged from 3 to 43 percent.[23–25] Certainly, these rates may improve with progression along the learning curve. However, at this time, continence outcomes after laparoscopic radical prostatectomy remain comparable to those of open surgery, despite optical improvements.

Anastomotic stricture. Reported anastomotic stricture rates after radical prostatectomy have ranged from 0.5 to 32 percent. These rates have shown some improvement in more contemporary series, likely owing to improvements in surgical technique. Surgical goals during the vesicourethral anastomosis are to create a watertight anastomosis with excellent perfusion and to achieve optimal mucosal apposition by eversion of the bladder neck. As with urinary incontinence, variations in anastomotic stricture rates may be rectal bleeding, diarrhea, and rectal ulcers to less common stricture formation, bowel obstruction, tenesmus, or fistula formation. A review of the medical literature highlights reports of significant long-term sequelae attributable to prior pelvic radiotherapy for a variety of malignancies. The examples are diverse, ranging from fecal incontinence secondary to lumbosacral plexopathy, delayed vesicocutaneous fistula, to severe hemorrhagic cystitis.[43–47]

Although hemorrhagic cystitis is a long-term sequelae in only 1 to 2 percent of the radiotherapy population, its management may be difficult and the morbidity life threatening. As with other radiation sequelae, hematuria after radiation therapy can occur years after treatment. In a review of 1,784 patients who received radiation therapy for cervical cancer, Levenback and colleagues found that the risk of hematuria increased with time, peaking at 9.6 percent at 20 years.[48] The management of hemorrhagic cystitis will be discussed in further detail in a later section. The incidence of moderate to severe hematuria after radiation therapy for prostate cancer ranges from 3 to 5 percent.[49,50]

Impact of Radiotherapy on Lower Urinary Tract Function

Radiation injury may have an insidious effect on lower urinary tract function. Over time, the deterioration of bladder storage function may adversely impact the functioning of the renal units upstream. In the most severe forms, this may lead to chronic renal insufficiency.[39]

The underlying pathophysiology of urinary incontinence and LUTS reflects impairment of the most fundamental functions of the bladder and urethra. Simply put, urinary incontinence must represent failure of the lower urinary tract to store urine, to evacuate urine, or both. Failure to store urine occurs in two scenarios: as a consequence of the bladder's inability to act as an accommodating, expanding fluid reservoir or the outlet's inability to remain sealed at the base of the reservoir.

This is a readily grasped concept but is further complicated by the reality that neither the reservoir nor the outlet is a static structure but, rather, a dynamic entity. The bladder reservoir comprises a smooth muscle wall with inherent viscoelastic properties, responsive to complex innervation and receptor profiles that remain incompletely defined. Likewise, the urethral outlet also demonstrates dynamic structural components controlled by complex innervation and influenced by a hormonal and neurotransmitter milieu. Many therapeutic interventions for prostate cancer, be it surgery or radiotherapy, threaten that balance.

Both the bladder smooth muscle and vascular endothelial cells are quite radiosensitive. Whereas acute injury to the urothelium tends to resolve, early-stage edema of both microvascular and smooth muscle compartments evolves to chronic fibrotic changes. The available experimental literature suggests that radiation injuries to the vascular endothelial cells are the source of the late bladder changes.[51] Endothelial injury leads to perivascular fibrosis. This, in turn, leads to bladder wall ischemic changes that promote fibrotic changes within the bladder smooth muscle matrix. The end result at the organ system level manifests as focal bladder ischemia, telangiectasia, and a less compliant bladder reservoir. Urodynamics assessment in the rodent model demonstrates this lasting impact of radiation on mouse bladder compliance and volume.[52]

Although this clinical impression has not been well characterized in an objective study of prostate cancer radiotherapy patients, supporting evidence comes from other radiotherapy populations. In a cohort of women with cervical cancer, Lin and colleagues used urodynamics testing to evaluate the possible effects of radical hysterectomy, pelvic radiotherapy, or both treatments on bladder function.[53] When compared to their control group, they found significant impairments of bladder storage function and urinary continence in all three subsets. The most severe dysfunction occurred in the group that had undergone extirpative surgery followed by radiotherapy. Eighty percent of the patients in this group demonstrated impaired bladder storage and 100 percent demonstrated urinary leakage with provocation. Similarly, in another cervical cancer population that had undergone pelvic radiotherapy, Zoubek and colleagues demonstrated that the deleterious effect on bladder storage function was evident as much as 30 years after treatment.

As Marks and colleagues pointed out in their review of the radiotherapy literature, urinary incontinence is not typically incorporated into radiation toxicity grading systems. Certainly, in the short-term assessment, incontinence appears to be rare. However, the above clinical series would suggest that such long-term changes leading to bladder-driven incontinence might take decades to manifest. This observation is congruent with earlier clinical impressions that the latency of urinary tract complications lags far behind that of bowel dysfunctions.[54] Certainly, if one does not recognize the phenomenon at that late stage, the association with a distant history of radiotherapy can easily be overlooked.

Conformal External Beam Radiotherapy

The radiation oncologist is faced with the dilemma that increased dose delivery to the region of the prostate tumor may improve cancer outcome but at the expense of significant, irreversible, long-term complications. Clearly, the goal is to improve the targeting of radiation delivery. Capitalizing on the advancements in three-dimensional imaging technologies and software packages, investigators have sought to "conform" radiation delivery to the irregular volume of the tumor target.[55] This technique of conformal radiotherapy allows for less radiation spillover effect on surrounding normal tissues.

The early data appeared to confirm the hypothesis that conformal radiotherapy may result in less acute toxicity when compared to the known complication rates of conventional radiotherapy.[56] More recently, a randomized clinical trial of 225 subjects in the United Kingdom compared the side-effect profiles of conformal versus conventional radiotherapy.[57] With a median follow-up of 3.6 years, the study determined that conformal techniques did not alter the incidence of bladder dysfunction but did significantly decrease the risk of late bowel complications. Although the Dearnaley and collegues' study was based on physician RTOG scoring,[57] another group sought to glean the same data from a patient-driven questionnaire. Nguyen and colleagues likewise compared the late radiation effects of conventional 70-Gy and conformal 78-Gy radiotherapy at a minimum 2-year follow-up.[58] From this format, they also concluded that the two groups experienced similar rates of urinary dysfunction; overall, 29 percent experienced persistent but mild urinary incontinence. With regard to bowel dysfunction, both treatment groups experienced an overall 10 percent incidence of fecal soiling, 27 percent experienced tenesmus, and 1 percent required antidiarrheal medication. However, the conformal technique appeared to offer a slight advantage, with a lower rate of significant changes in bowel habit.

Additionally, Dearnaley and colleagues' data demonstrated that the incidence and severity of acute side effects did not prove to be a reliable predictor of the development of late radiation side effects.[57] This is likely because short- and long-term sequelae of radiotherapy are the result of different pathophysiologic mechanisms (see acute and late effects of radiation therapy, above). Thus, Dearnaley and colleagues offered a word of caution about the current enthusiasm for conformal therapy dose-escalation trials as many sequelae may not be identified until long-term follow-up has become available. Some groups using doses up to 81 Gy report few late toxicities thus far.[33,34] Hanks and colleagues reported their 5-year outcomes after dose escalation with three-dimensional conformal radiation therapy for the treatment of prostate cancer.[34] Bowel and bladder outcomes were evaluated in 232 consecutive patients, using both a modified Late Effects on Normal Tissues Scale (LENT) for both bowel and bladder symptoms and the RTOG scale for bowel symptoms. Bladder and bowel symptoms for patients with 5-year follow-up who received 75 to 76 Gy were compared with the symptoms for patients who received any dose. Although there appeared to be slight increases in mild (LENT grade 2) bowel and bladder symptoms in patients with higher doses, severe bowel symptom rates were similar between the two groups. Therefore, the impact of three-dimensional conformal dose-escalation trials on the incidence of radiation side effects remains to be seen.

Brachytherapy

The pursuit of improved radiotherapy outcomes without significant complications led to the development of prostate brachytherapy. Like cryosurgery, this technique owes its rebirth in the 1990s to improved radiographic imaging technologies, namely transrectal ultrasonography. Preprocedure prostate volume measurements allow for the calculation of the appropriate number of radioactive seeds that will be required to fill the gland volume. Then, scopic evaluation should involve a careful evaluation of the urethra and bladder neck for bladder neck contracture or urethral stricture. Within the bladder, one can expect to see typical postradiation changes. The bladder and urethra may appear pale with areas of spidery telangiectasia, and the bladder wall may be less supple in texture but easily friable with manipulation. Similar long-term changes occur within the bowel, as characterized by radiographic imaging and endoscopy.[38,70]

Urinary incontinence may be a late manifestation of the insidious evolution of bladder storage dysfunction or urethral incompetence after radiation therapy. In this setting, the clinician must assess whether the situation involves a problem with storage, emptying, or both. This can be objectively assessed with videourodynamics testing. For the specialist, urodynamics testing offers the most objective means by which to witness the events of urinary storage and leakage. However, for the most part, this is not a feasible tool for large sample sizes and is fairly invasive testing for the patient.

Radical Prostatectomy

Evaluation of lower urinary tract symptoms after radical prostatectomy must be performed carefully, with strict attention to the potential for iatrogenic injury, particularly in the early postoperative period. Once infection has been ruled out, acute irritative symptoms should be considered part of the normal postoperative course. Should symptoms fail to resolve with anticholinergic medications, further evaluation may be warranted. Obstructive symptoms after catheter removal should alert the clinician to the possibility of urinary retention. Careful history and physical examination should elucidate this further. Although retention may be attributable to detrusor failure, the possibility of anastomotic stricture should be a consideration as well. Anastomotic strictures can present with a variety of symptoms from obstructive complaints to stress urinary incontinence. Such strictures tend to occur early in the postoperative period. In a review of 36 cases of anastomotic stricture after RRP, Park and colleagues demonstrated a mean interval to diagnosis of 4.22 months.[71] Diagnosis can be achieved with careful flexible cystoscopy.

MANAGEMENT OF BLADDER AND BOWEL SYMPTOMS AFTER PROSTATE CANCER TREATMENT

Management of Bladder Complications

Lower Urinary Tract Symptoms after Radiation

For mild irritative voiding symptoms, a combination of phenazopyridine and low-dose anticholinergic therapy is quite effective in improving bladder storage function in the short term. This is the most common clinical scenario after various forms of radiotherapy. If the acute symptoms are primarily of an obstructive nature, alpha-blockers or a rapid steroid taper may be of benefit.[72] For significant obstructive symptoms, an indwelling catheter may be placed for short-term management. Usually, postradiotherapy urethral edema or prostate swelling is the culprit. Again, some previously cited series suggest that expectant management is wiser than rushing to perform an endoscopic transurethral resection after brachytherapy or cryoablation.[60] If 2 to 4 weeks of catheter drainage do not lead to recovery of voiding function, intermittent self-catheterization is the next strategy. In most instances, persistent obstructive symptoms that arise after treatment are sufficient to make the diagnosis of obstructive uropathy. However, if the constellation of urinary symptoms overlaps with the categories of irritative symptoms or incontinence, videourodynamics testing offers the definitive characterization of the pathophysiology.

If persistent obstruction has been diagnosed, the urologist can then perform endoscopic urethral dilation or tissue resection as needed. As a consequence of any of the above prostate cancer therapies, the urethral outlet can, over time, become friable or rigid. This means that any intervention to dilate or resect urethral tissue may further compromise sphincteric function, leading to later onset of urinary incontinence.

Lower Urinary Tract Symptoms after Radical Prostatectomy

As with radiotherapy, control of irritative bladder symptoms can be achieved with a combination of phenazopyridine and low-dose anticholinergic therapy. For management of urinary retention in the early postoperative period, a 16F coudé-tipped catheter with a 5-cc balloon may be placed through a well-lubricated urethra to drain the bladder. The catheter should be left in place for 3 to 5 days to allow for bladder rest. Use of the flexible cystoscope can be of great assistance in complicated cases as the risk of injury increases with each attempt at blind catheter placement.

Bladder Storage Dysfunction

If bladder storage function has deteriorated, first-line management uses pharmacotherapy (ie, anticholinergic drugs). Repeat urodynamics assessment after a few months of maximal medical therapy should demonstrate objective improvement of the bladder pressure/volume relationship. In severe cases that do not improve with medication, surgical intervention may be indicated.

The goal of surgery in this instance is the expansion of the bladder's capacity. This may be performed by adding a large patch of isolated small intestine, known as an enterocystoplasty.[73] This technique of bladder augmentation is well accepted in the urologic arena. However, the potential short- and long-term morbidities are not inconsequential. These potential complications are well described in the urologic literature, ranging from the common prolonged ileus, chronic bowel dysfunction, to less common pelvic abscesses or bladder reservoir perforation and to the rarer but long-range concern of metaplastic transformation of the bladder-intestinal junction.[74–76]

A more contemporary alternative to this traditional bladder augmentation technique is the detrusor myectomy.[77,78] Here the goal of increasing bladder capacity is achieved by excising a large patch of scarified bladder smooth muscle. In doing so, the remaining urothelium is allowed to expand and extrude through the dome defect. In essence, the surgery intentionally creates a large bladder diverticulum.

Fortunately, most clinical presentations of bladder storage dysfunction can be satisfactorily treated with medications. However, in assessing a patient with urinary dysfunction who has any prior history of pelvic radiotherapy, it is important to entertain the notion that radiation changes may play a significant role many years later.[39]

Intrinsic Sphincteric Deficiency

This type of lower urinary tract dysfunction may be reliably characterized in the male post–prostate therapy population based on a subjective symptomatology description. Typically, the postprostatectomy patient describes episodes of leakage that occur with coughing, straining, or exertional activities. If mixed symptomatology or a concern about bladder storage dysfunction obscures the clinical picture, then videourodynamics testing is of great benefit.

For postprostectomy incontinence, a common conservative therapy has been a rigorous regimen of pelvic floor exercises. Although such therapy does no harm, in the best estimations, the regimen offers little objective improvement.[79] Videourodynamics testing of this patient population demonstrates that the external sphincter mechanism is normal and the remaining intrinsic sphincter is the zone of deficiency.[8]

Transurethral collagen injection. For mild to moderate intrinsic sphincter deficiency in women, transurethral injection of modified bovine glutaraldehyde cross-linked collagen has been quite effective.[80] The major drawback to this treatment is the limited durability of response owing to gradual breakdown and resorption of the suburethral collagen blebs. However, the same success has not translated to the male intrinsic sphincter deficiency population. Particularly in the setting of prostate cancer therapy, the resulting intrinsic sphincter deficiency is complicated by scarification of the urethral wall around the level of the anastomosis. This makes the urethral wall much less pliable for the injection of suburethral bulking agents such as collagen.

Nevertheless, a series of repeated injection sessions does offer a significant degree of improvement in the degree of stress urinary incontinence, ranging from 40 to 85 percent, with a short-term follow-up of less than 3 years.[81–83]

However, as with the female treatment population, duration of efficacy remains the problem. Currently, newer bulking agents composed of permanent materials are being clinically evaluated as possible alternatives to transurethral collagen therapy. Such agents consist of tiny beads of silicon or carbon suspended in emulsions to allow a similar mode of transurethral injection. To date, the clinical trials in the female intrinsic sphincter deficiency population show equal efficacy and the promise of longer durability.

Artificial urinary sphincter. Another commonly used treatment for male urinary incontinence is the surgical implantation of the artificial urinary sphincter prosthesis (Figure 27–1). Although most patients are not rendered completely continent, it can offer much needed improvement in the quality of life for these patients. In large series, the artificial sphincter has been shown to offer success rates as high as 83 to 86 percent.[84] This makes the efficacy of the artificial sphincter comparable to collagen injection therapy. However, the greater durability of sphincter prosthesis therapy must be weighed against a very real risk of serious complications, namely sphincter cuff erosion into the urethra, device infection, and/or device malfunction. Even in the most experienced hands, surgical revision rates range from 20 to 40 percent.[84]

Male sling. The suburethral sling has offered durable success for the treatment of intrinsic sphincter deficiency in women. In an effort to translate the same technique to male postprostatectomy incontinence, Schaeffer and colleagues have described their particular technique of placing a bulbourethral sling using a series of Goretex bolsters.[85] Their data with a mean of 22 months follow-up describe an encouraging success rate of 64 percent, even with the most difficult patients. For example, their study population included those who had undergone adjuvant radiotherapy or failed prior continence treatments. Further outcome analysis of this bulbourethral sling population revealed that a history of prior pelvic radiotherapy was associated with a much poorer success rate. Of the 12 irradiated patients in this series, only 1 (8%) achieved continence.[86]

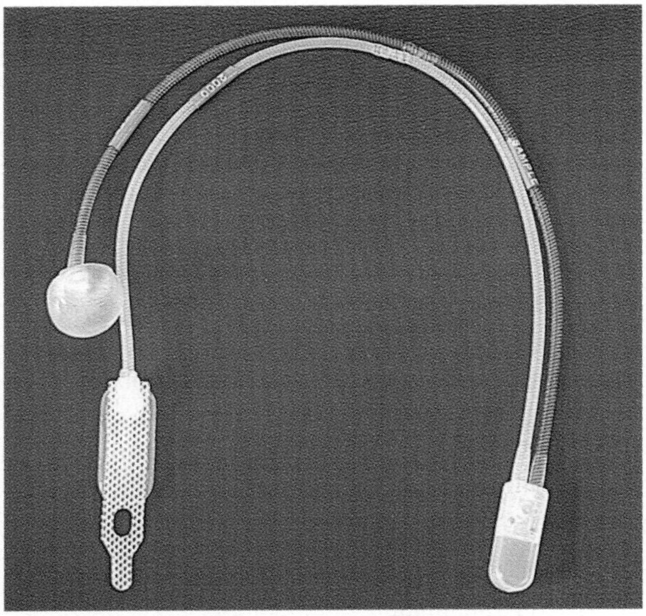

Figure 27–1. AMS 800 artificial urinary sphincter.

Postoperative urodynamics testing of the bulbourethral sling patients has likewise been valuable. Offering an objective detection of stress urinary incontinence, the findings further substantiate the reported questionnaire and retrospective chart review outcomes. Voiding pressure profiles obtained after sling placement consistently demonstrate a nonobstructive pattern.[87] The short-term data are reassuring that the sling is not merely obstructing the outlet in an effort to achieve dryness.

Anastomotic Stricture

Management of anastomotic strictures after prostate cancer therapy can be challenging. Treatment to the prostate, either extirpative or in situ, causes local scarring, which violates the bladder neck and sphincter mechanism. Attempts to aggressively dilate or incise post-treatment anastomotic strictures can result in significant urinary incontinence. Multiple treatment options have been suggested in the literature, including repeat dilations (sounds, bougies, filiforms with followers, balloons), definitive management by endoscopic incision with either electrocautery or cold knife, and expandable stent placement.

For the early postoperative bladder neck contracture, dilation with a Nephromax (Microvasive/Boston Scientific, Watertown, Massachusetts) 30F balloon dilator appears to be a good option for treatment (Figure 27–3). Using a flexible cystoscope, a wire is passed through the strictured area and into the bladder. The balloon is passed over the wire, and its proper position is confirmed fluoroscopically. The balloon is then inflated with contrast, and progress is monitored with fluoroscopy. Inflation continues until the "waist" in the strictured area disappears. A catheter is left for 2 days after the procedure. The procedure can be performed under local anesthesia. This appears to offer excellent long-term results with little risk of complications, including urinary incontinence.

Radiation-Induced Hemorrhagic Cystitis

Once the usual culprits, urinary infection and malignancy, have been ruled out, we are left with the diagnosis of hematuria induced by radiation cystitis. As described earlier, the pervasive tissue injury continues to evolve many years after the completion of radiotherapy. Sporadic episodes of severe hematuria can occur spontaneously without apparent provocation and can be quite difficult to treat. The time to its manifestation after completion of radiotherapy can also vary widely, ranging from as soon as 6 months to several years later.[88] It has been estimated that hemorrhage may occur in up to 9 percent of patients who have undergone full-dose pelvic radiotherapy.[89]

DeVries and Freiha suggested a grading scale to convey the degree of severe hematuria in such instances (Table 27–3).[90] Generally, the first line of treatment is cystoscopic clot evacuation and selective electrocauterization of bleeding points. If cautery is ineffective in controlling the degree of hematuria, the next step is intermittent or continuous bladder irrigation with various agents that coat the fragile urothelium in an effort to create a barrier. Agents such as alum, silver nitrate, sodium pentosanpolysulfate, or dilute formalin are typically used, in that order of preference.[91–94] If those methods fail, more drastic measures usually entail temporary or permanent urinary diversion, selective hypogastric arterial embolization, or even cystectomy (Table 27–4).[95]

Recent reports have revived interest in the use of hyperbaric oxygen as another promising treatment option for refractory hemorrhagic cystitis.[96–100] With this modality, the patient is placed in a treatment chamber pressurized to a range between 1.4 and 3.0 atm, while breathing 100 percent oxygen.[101] The

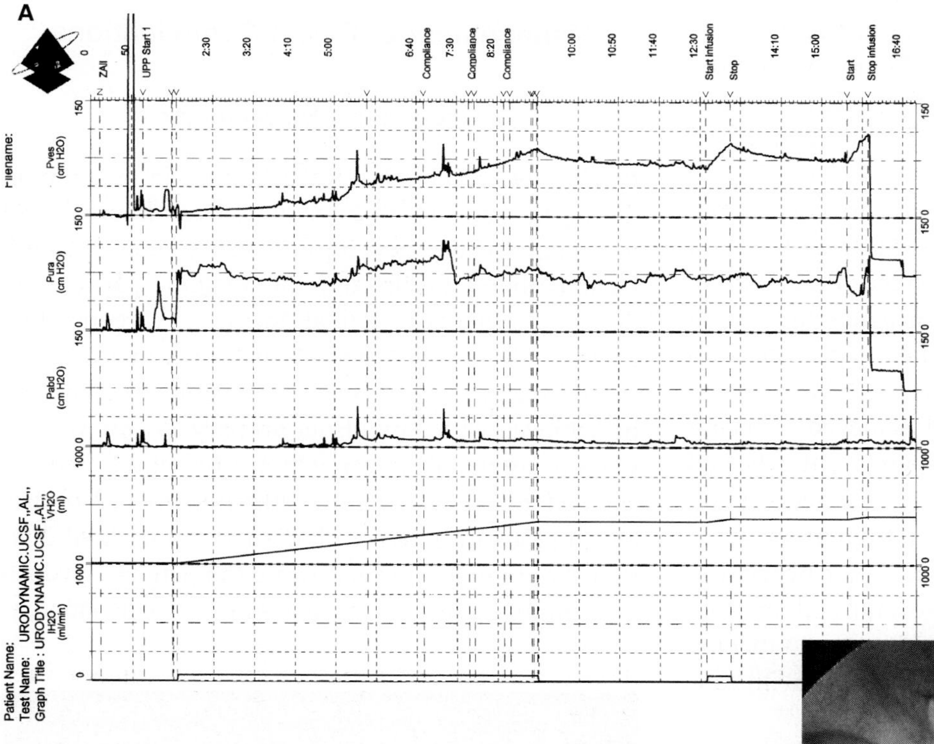

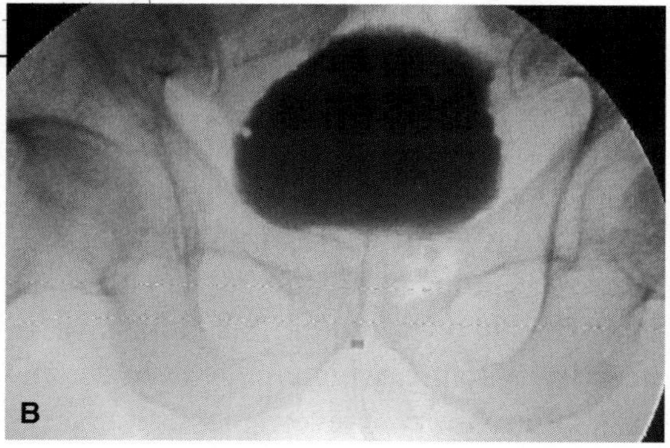

Figure 27–2. *A* and *B,* Fluorourodynamic study and voiding cystourethrogram showing noncompliant bladder with no detrusor contraction.

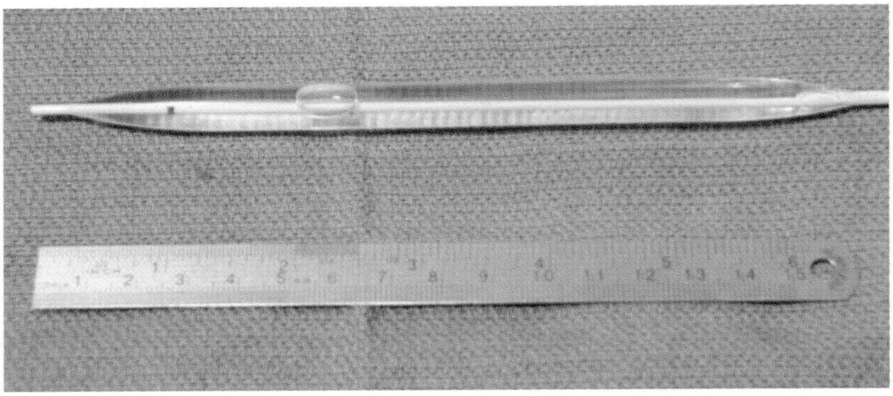

Figure 27–3. Inflated Nephromax balloon that may be used for dilation of bladder neck contracture after radical prostatectomy. Nephromax high-pressure nephrostomy balloon catheter (Microvasive/Boston Scientific, Watertown, Massachusetts).

hyperoxia milieu creates a transiently increased diffusion gradient, driving oxygen from the vascular tree into the surrounding tissues. This phenomenon acutely induces vasoconstriction, which helps to control the bladder hemorrhage. Additionally, the hyperoxia environment offers more lasting benefits with the induction of neovascularization within the chronically ischemic radiation tissues. This, in turn, leads to overall improvement in wound healing and local immune functions.

Although the acute response of refractory hematuria to this treatment is impressive, those centers with sufficient follow-up have found that the effects may be short-lived.[96,97] Del Pizzo and colleagues followed a cohort of 11 patients with moderate symptoms who were treated with hyperbaric oxygen.[96] At a median 5.1 years follow-up, only 3 had achieved a lasting response to therapy. The remaining 8 patients had subsequently required definitive surgical intervention for recurrent symptoms. Another intriguing observation regarding hematuria recurrence after hyperbaric therapy has been described by several authors. The subset of patients who are most refractory to therapy seems to demonstrate a greater association with cancer recurrence (ie, bladder or prostate).[97,98,100]

Unlike the various intravesical chemotherapy instillations described, hyperbaric oxygen therapy is a minimally invasive modality that does not adversely impact bladder structure and function. However, it does require an expensive, specialized treatment facility, which may not be readily available within proximity. Nevertheless, for severe hemorrhage unresponsive to conventional measures, hyperbaric oxygen therapy may offer life-saving control of hemorrhage and buy time for patient recovery before pursuing definitive surgical intervention.

Management of Bowel Complications

Intraoperative Bowel Injuries

Radical prostatectomy. Rectal injury is uncommon during the radical prostatectomy. Such injuries tend to occur when developing the plane between Denonvilliers' fascia and the rectum, particularly during sharp dissection at the apex. Preoperative enema will decrease the risk of local contamination should rectal injury occur. Intraoperative repair can be achieved with a two-layer primary closure with or without omental interposition. Infection can be avoided by paying careful attention to hemostasis and copious irrigation with normal saline. Anal dilation should be performed while the patient is asleep to minimize pressure on the suture line postopera-

Table 27–3. GRADING SCALE FOR THE DEGREE OF SEVERE HEMATURIA AFTER RADIOTHERAPY

Grade	Clinical Manifestation
Mild	Not producing an acute decrease in hematocrit
Moderate	Producing a decrease in hematocrit requiring transfusion of ≤ 6 U packed red blood cells
Severe	Refractory to simple irrigations; requiring tranfusion of > 6 U packed red blood cells

From DeVries and Freiha.[90]

Table 27–4. TREATMENT OPTIONS FOR HEMORRHAGIC CYSTITIS

Treatment	Technique	Mechanism of Action	Pro	Con
Formalin	Using cystosopy and general anesthesia, a cystogram is performed to rule out vesicoureteral reflux and the bladder is instilled with formalin	Hydrolizes proteins, thus coagulating mucosal and submucosal tissues	Effective No open surgery	Requires anesthesia Risk to ureters Potential for skin irritation
Alum	Using a three-way catheter, alum is instilled into the bladder with continuous bladder irrigation	Protein precipitation into the interstitial spaces causes tissue contraction and tamponade of bleeding	No anesthesia Bedside procedure Nontoxic to ureters	Encephalopathy Acidosis Potentially time consuming
Sodium pentosan sulfate	Oral or intravesical administration	A semisynthetic sulfated polysaccharide that serves as a synthetic glycosaminoglycan. Theoretically, it adheres to the bladder surface, supplementing the bladder urothelium	Ease of treatment Minimal side effects	Efficacy for hemorrhagic cystitis not well defined
Hyperbaric oxygen	Patient is placed in treatment chamber pressurized to 1.4–3.0 atm for 60–90 minutes per day, 5–7 days per week	Counters tissue ischemia of progressive endarteritis by means of hyperoxia and stimulation of angiogenesis. Acutely, it causes vasocontriction	Minimally invasive	Requires specialized treatment facility Multiple treatments required Expensive
Embolization	Using real-time fluoroscopy and percutaneous access, occlude vessel with clot, Gelfoam, coils, ethanol, or other substances	Occludes arterial blood supply of the bladder, thereby stopping bleeding	Life saving Local anesthesia Poor surgical candidates	Bladder necrosis can occur Gluteal claudication reported
Surgery	Using open surgical approach, either divert urine supravesically, perform a cystectomy, or ligate hypogastric arteries	Supravesical diversion keeps upper tracts decompressed while allowing the bladder to tamponade. Cystectomy removes hemorrhaging bladder	Definitive Life saving	Invasive Irreversible

tively. The risk of rectal injury is significantly higher (5 to 15%) during salvage prostatectomy.[102,103] Injury to the previously irradiated rectum can also be managed with primary closure, although large lacerations or patients without adequate bowel preparation may be best managed with diverting colostomy.

Unrecognized bowel injuries may lead to development of a perirectal abscess or rectourinary fistula postoperatively. Abscesses should be drained and systemic treatment with broad-spectrum antibiotics administered. Conservative management of the rectourinary fistula should be the initial course of action. This can be achieved with catheter drainage of the bladder and a low-residue diet. Should a fistula fail to improve with conservative measures, formal fistula repair may be indicated.

Laparoscopic prostatectomy. As with open radical prostatectomy, intraoperative rectal injury during laparoscopic prostatectomy is uncommon. It is important to recognize that laparoscopic prostatectomy is performed transperitoneally; therefore, infectious complications such as rectal injury may present with acute peritonitis. Guillonneau and colleagues reported rectal injuries in eight (1.41%) patients during laparoscopic radical prostatectomy. Seven of these injuries were identified and repaired intraoperatively with a one- to two-layer primary closure. One injury was recognized several days later when the patient presented with peritonitis. This was managed with laparotomy and temporary colostomy.

Radiation-Induced Acute Bowel Complications

Surprisingly little information is available regarding the management of postradiation rectal complications. The existing body of literature on the subject is plagued by two of the most common flaws of clinical studies: small patient sample sizes and therapeutic trials conducted without a placebo control arm. Without a clearly efficacious treatment option, clinicians are left to choose their own management strategies based on empiricism.

Patients usually experience a constellation of rectal symptoms, and treatment should be aimed at controlling the predominant disturbance. In the case of mild or episodic symptoms, supportive care should suffice. Antispasmodic drugs and stool softeners are the mainstay of treatment for tenesmus and mild diarrhea.

Rectal bleeding is the most concerning complication in both the acute and chronic phases, with an incidence of 6 to 8 percent among pelvic radiotherapy patients.[104,105] Certainly, in the initial assessment, other common etiologies (ie, infectious, ischemic, or toxic colitis) must be ruled out. A recent series of 109 patients treated with iodine-125 brachytherapy was assessed for the incidence and resolution rates of rectal bleeding up to 48 months postbrachytherapy.[106] Of the entire group, 19 percent experienced persistent rectal bleeding. Over the course of the follow-up interval, three subsets underwent treatments with steroid enemas, laser coagulation, or expectant management, respectively. Although their sample sizes were clearly quite small, they noted a trend toward no difference in resolution rates.

Therefore, clinical empiricism leans toward conservative management even for protracted courses of proctosigmoiditis. So, in the short term, patience and supportive measures seem quite reasonable.

Radiation-Induced Chronic Bowel Complications

Recent observations have noted a significant late-onset rectal bleeding in high-dose three-dimensional conformal radiotherapy patients. Teshima and colleagues reviewed the available data on 89 patients who developed late-onset grade 2 or grade 3 rectal bleeding complications.[105] In both subsets, the median time to presentation of bleeding did not differ significantly; 13 versus 18 months. However, as might be expected, grade 2 rectal bleeding more readily responded to conservative therapy. By multivariate analysis, they concluded that dose was the only significant variable associated with the later manifestation of rectal bleeding.

In fact, given the growing data that such serious late morbidity may result from higher radiotherapy dosing, some are advocating a change in the definition of the standard RTOG grade 3 bowel toxicity.[107] Hanlon and colleagues proposed that grade 3 rectal toxicity encompass chronic rectal bleeding, which requires at least one blood transfusion or more than two coagulation treatments. If those interventions are factored into the outcomes assessment, they argue that the incidence of grade 3/4 rectal complications would appreciably increase in contemporary outcomes reporting.

Medicated enemas. The efficacy of conservative therapy using medicated enemas appears mixed at best. The oft-cited studies involve outcomes from series of five or less patients.[108,109] Typically, the enema consists of corticosteroid, sulfasalazine, or 5-aminosalicylic acid, with the assumption being that rectal symptoms are driven by an inflammatory process. Donner argued that the underlying pathophysiology is ischemic in nature instead. Therefore, it should not be surprising that the results of treatment with anti-inflammatory agents are equivocal, if not completely ineffectual.[38]

A more promising medication for enema use is sucralfate. With a proven efficacy in the management of peptic ulcer disease, the rationale of using this drug to coat a rectal ulcer is appealing. A number of small clinical studies suggest a benefit from a repeated regimen of sucralfate enemas. In a randomized, blinded, double treatment arm trial comparing sucralfate and steroid enemas, Kochhar and colleagues demonstrated pronounced improvement in the sucralfate group (94%) versus the steroid group (53%), as confirmed by endoscopic evaluation after 4 weeks of therapy.[110] However, an important omission from this trial was the absence of a placebo control arm. As noted earlier, Wallner reported in their 48-month follow-up study that expectant management seemed as likely to achieve the same outcome as treatment intervention for rectal bleeding.[106]

Laser coagulation. However, when prolonged rectal bleeding leads to a blood transfusion requirement, some intervention is warranted. Use of a laser modality appears preferable to bipolar electrocoagulation. Because the laser energy is preferentially absorbed by the blood vessels, less trauma is inflicted on the already ischemic radiated tissues. Some groups have noted promising results using the endoscopic neodymium:yttrium-aluminum-garnet (Nd:YAG) laser or argon laser.[104,111,112] It is still unclear if one laser source is superior. However, one concern is that the Nd:YAG laser provides a greater depth of tissue coagulation: 5 mm versus 1.5 mm for the argon source. With the YAG laser's greater depth of penetration, point coagulation may lead to transmural tissue necrosis, followed by bowel perforation. Even if the coagulation depth does not traverse the bowel wall, submucosal coagulation may still theoretically pose a problem. This may exacerbate the evolving ischemic pathology of radiation injury in these tissues.

Although the short-term results are excellent, most series with sufficient follow-up report a significant recurrence of bleeding. In a sizeable series of 47 patients who underwent Nd:YAG laser therapy at the Mayo Clinic, 87 percent of the group experienced marked improvement or resolution of hematochezia.[113] However, follow-up was quite short at only 3 to 6 months. With longer follow-up, Chapuis and colleagues reported a 74 percent resolution rate, 15 percent mild recurrence, and 9 percent of patients eventually requiring operative intervention to control significant bleeding.[111] So with sufficient longitudinal follow-up, it would appear that recurrent hematochezia is likely, and repeated treatments are beneficial in achieving hemostasis.[104,112]

So when faced with significant rectal bleeding secondary to radiation proctitis, laser coagulation therapy offers a helpful temporizing measure. It can substantially decrease the blood transfusion requirement and save many patients from major surgical intervention.

Topical formalin application. For those difficult cases of hemorrhagic proctitis refractory to even laser therapy, topical application of 4 percent formalin solution has proven efficacy. This is similar to the method that has been successful in the management of hemorrhagic cystitis. Later, Rubinstein and colleagues translated the application to hemorrhagic proctitis.[114] Many report its efficacy for the treatment of hematochezia, with 75 percent success in one series and 89 percent success in another.[115,116] Some disadvantages of formalin treatment are its potential for inducing chronic anal pain and tenesmus in a minority of patients and its limitation to application within the rectum and not more proximal sources of bleeding. Chapuis and colleagues found that the combination of Nd:YAG laser coagulation followed by topical formalin application offered 89 percent of their patients substantial improvement.[111]

Surgery. Given our understanding of the evolving nature of ischemic radiation injury, major operative intervention is best avoided. Nevertheless, in the setting of suspected bowel perforation, bowel obstruction, or fistula formation, surgical repair is necessary and should not be delayed by an attempt at conservative measures.

CONCLUSION

Treatment options for men with prostate cancer are plentiful. Because controversy still persists regarding which treatment is the most efficacious for any given stage of the disease, the issue of potential treatment complications becomes that much more important.

Given such medical uncertainties, a patient's decision may be swayed by his perception of short- and long-term treatment complications. Every treatment carries its own set of significant short- and long-term side effects. This chapter focused on the acute and chronic complications of various prostate cancer treatments on lower urinary tract and bowel functions. Most complications can be managed efficiently and effectively.

REFERENCES

1. Constitution of the World Health Organization. In: World Health Organization handbook of basic documents. 5th ed. Geneva: Palais des Nations; 1952. p. 3–20.
2. Lubeck DP, Litwin MS, Henning JM, et al. Measurement of health-related quality of life in men with prostate cancer: the CaPSURE database. Qual Life Res 1997;6:385–92.
3. Litwin MS, Lubeck DP, Henning JM, et al. Differences in urologist and patient assessments of health-related quality of life in men with prostate cancer: results of the CaPSURE database. J Urol 1998;159:1988–92.
4. Licht MR, Klein EA, Tuason L, et al. Impact of bladder neck preservation during radical prostatectomy on continence and cancer control. Urology 1994;44:883–7.

5. Seaman EK, Benson MC. Improved continence with tubularized bladder neck reconstruction following radical retropubic prostatectomy. Urology 1996;47:532–5.
6. Jorion JL. Aponeurotic suspension of a vesico-urethral anastomosis after radical prostatectomy. Acta Urol Belg 1998; 66:1–4.
7. McGuire EJ. Diagnosis and treatment of intrinsic sphincter deficiency. Int J Urol 1995;2(6 Suppl 1):7–10.
8. Gudziak MR, McGuire EJ, et al. Urodynamic assessment of urethral sphincter function in post-prostatectomy incontinence. J Urol 1996;156:1131–4.
9. Ficazzola MA, Nitti VW. The etiology of post-radical prostatectomy incontinence and correlation of symptoms with urodynamic findings. J Urol 1998;160:1317–20.
10. Desautel MG, Kapoor R, et al. Sphincteric incontinence: the primary cause of post-prostatectomy incontinence in patients with prostate cancer. Neurourol Urodyn 1997;16: 153–60.
11. Catalona WJ, Bigg SW. Nerve-sparing radical prostatectomy: evaluation of results after 250 patients. J Urol 1990;143: 538–44.
12. Fowler FJ Jr, Barry MJ, Lu-Yao G, et al. Patient-reported complications and follow-up treatment after radical prostatectomy. The National Medicare experience: 1988–1990. Urology 1993;42:622–9.
13. Talcott JA, Rieker P, et al. Patient-reported symptoms after primary therapy for early prostate cancer: results of a prospective cohort study. J Clin Oncol 1998;16:275–83.
14. Kleinhans B, Gerharz E, et al. Chnages of urodynamic findings after radical prostatectomy. Eur Urol 1999;35:217.
15. Golomb J, Dotan Z, et al. Can preoperative urodynamic examination allow us to predict the risk of incontinence after radical prostatectomy? Prog Urol 1999;9:288–91.
16. Gudziak MR, McGuire EJ, et al. Urodynamic assessment of urethral sphincter function in post-prostatectomy incontinence. J Urol 1996;156:1131–4.
17. Presti JC Jr, Schmidt RA, Narayan PA, et al. Pathophysiology of urinary incontinence after radical prostatectomy. J Urol 1990;143:975–8.
18. Lance RS, Freidrichs PA, Kane C, et al. A comparison of radical retropubic with perineal prostatectomy for localized prostate cancer within the Uniformed Services Urology Research Group. BJU Int 2001;87:61–5.
19. Bishoff JT, Motley G, Optenberg SA, et al. Incidence of fecal and urinary incontinence following radical perineal and retropubic prostatectomy in a national population. J Urol 1998;160:454–8.
20. Ruiz-Deya G, Davis R, Srivastay SK, et al. Outpatient radical prostatectomy: impact of standard perineal approach on patient outcome. J Urol 2001;166:581–6.
21. Weldon VE, Tavel FR, Neuwirth H. Continence, potency and morbidity after radical perineal prostatectomy. J Urol 1997;158:1470–5.
22. Gray M, Petroni GR, Theodorescu D. Urinary function after radical prostatectomy: a comparison of the retropubic and perineal approaches. Urology 1999;53:881–90; discussion 890–1.
23. Olsson LE, Salomon L, Nadu A, et al. Prospective patient reported continence after laparoscopic radical prostatectomy. Urology 2001;58:570–2.
24. Guillonneau B, Cathelineau X, Doublet J, Vallancien G. Laparoscopic radical prostatectomy: the lessons learned. J Endourol 2001;15:441–5.
25. Rassweiler J, Sentker L, Seemann O, et al. Laparoscopic radical prostatectomy with the Heilbronn technique: an analysis of the first 180 cases. J Urol 2001;166:2101–8.
26. Surya BV, Provet J, Johanson KE, Brown J. Anastomotic strictures following radical prostatectomy: risk factors and management. J Urol 1990;143:755–8.
27. Tomschi W, Suster G, Holtl W. Bladder neck strictures after radical retropubic prostatectomy: still an unsolved problem. Br J Urol 1998;81:823.
28. Ramon J, Rossignol G, Leandri P, et al. Morbidity of radical retropubic prostatectomy following previous prostate resection. J Surg Oncol 1994;55:14.
29. Dalton DP, Schaeffer AJ, Garnett JE, et al. Radiographic assessment of the vesicourethral anastomosis directing early decatheterization following nerve-sparing radical retropubic prostatectomy. J Urol 1989;141:79.
30. Lerner SE, Blute ML, Lieber MM, et al. Morbidity of contemporary radical retropubic prostatectomy for localized prostate cancer. Oncology 1995;9:379–82.
31. Viville C. Rectal injuries in radical prostatectomies for cancer. Survey of the ANFUC (Association National de Formation Urologique Continue) 1994. J Urol (Paris) 1995;101:65–8.
32. Lassen PM, Kearse WS Jr. Rectal injuries during radical perineal prostatectomy. Urology 1995;45:266.
33. Zelefsky MJ, Leibel SA, Gaudin PB, et al. Dose escalation with three-dimensional conformal radiation therapy affects the outcome in prostate cancer. Int J Radiat Oncol Biol Phys 1998;41:491–500.
34. Hanks GE, Hanlon AL, Schultheiss TE, et al. Dose escalation with 3D conformal treatment: five year outcomes, treatment optimization, and future directions. Int J Radiat Oncol Biol Phys 1998;41:501–10.
35. Garnick MB. Prostate cancer: screening, diagnosis and management. Ann Intern Med 1993;118:804–18.
36. Crook J, Esche B, et al. Effect of pelvic radiotherapy for prostate cancer on bowel, bladder, and sexual function: the patient's perspective. Urology 1996;47:387–94.
37. Catalona WJ. Management of cancer of the prostate. N Engl J Med 1994;331:966–1004.
38. Donner CS. Pathophysiology and therapy of chronic radiation-induced injury to the colon. Dig Dis 1998;16:253–61.
39. Zoubek J, McGuire EJ, Noll F, DeLancey JO. The late occurrence of urinary tract damage in patients successfully treated by radiotherapy for cervical carcinoma. J Urol 1989;141:1347–9.
40. Pilepich MV, Asbell SO, Krall JM, et al. Correlation of radiotherapeutic parameters and treatment related morbidity—analysis of RTOG study 77-06. Int J Radiat Oncol Biol Phys 1987;13:1007.
41. Lawton CA, Won M, Pilepich MV, et al. Long-term treatment sequelae following external beam irradiation for adenocarcinoma of the prostate: analysis of RTOG studies 7506 and 7706. Int J Radiat Oncol Biol Phys 1991;21:935–9.
42. Cho KH, Lee CKK, Levitt SH. Proctitis after conventional external radiation therapy for prostate cancer: importance of minimizing posterior rectal dose. Radiology 1995;195: 699–703.

43. Iglicki F, Coffin B, et al. Fecal incontinence after pelvic radiotherapy: evidences for a lubosacral plexopathy. Report of a case. Dis Colon Rectum 1996;39:465–7.
44. Lau KO, Cheng C. A case report—delayed vesicocutaneous fistula after radiation therapy for advanced vulvar cancer. Ann Acad Med Singapore 1998;27:705–6.
45. Bevers RF, Bakker DJ, et al. Hyperbaric oxygen treatment for haemorrhagic radiation cystitis. Lancet 1995;346:803–5.
46. Ferrer Puchol MD, Borrel Palanca A, et al. Severe hematuria caused by radiation cystitis. Selective percutaneous embolization as an alternative therapy. Actas Urol Esp 1998;22:519–23.
47. Mathews R, Rajan N, et al. Hyperbaric oxygen therapy for radiation-induced hemorrhagic cystitis. J Urol 1999;161:435–7.
48. Levenback C, Eifel PJ, Burke TW, et al. Hemorrhagic cystitis following radiotherapy for stage Ib cancer of the cervix. Gynecol Oncol 1994;55:206–10.
49. Presti JC Jr, Marks LB, Carroll PR. Radiation injury to the bladder: characteristics and management. In: McAninch JW, editor. Traumatic and reconstructive urology. Philadelphia: WB Saunders; 1996.
50. Amdur RJ, Parsons LT, Fitzgerald LT, et al. Adenocarcinoma of the prostate treated with external-beam radiation therapy: 5-year minimum follow-up. Radiother Oncol 1990;18:235–46.
51. Marks LB, Carroll PR, Dugan TC, et al. The response of the urinary bladder, urethra, and ureter to radiation and chemotherapy. Int J Radiat Oncol Biol Phys 1995;31:1257.
52. Lundbeck F, Ulso N, Overgaard J. Cystometric ealuation of early and late irradiation damage to the mouse urinary bladder. Radiother Oncol 1989;15:383–92.
53. Lin HH, Sheu BC, et al. Abnormal urodynamic findings after radical hysterectomy or pelvic irradiation for cervical cancer. Int J Gyn Obstet 1998;63:169–74.
54. Perez CA, Breaux S, Bedwinek JM, et al. Radiation therapy alone in the treatment of carcinoma of the uterine cervix. II. Analysis of complications. Cancer 1984;54:235–46.
55. Fuks Z, Horwich A. Clinical and technical aspects of conformal therapy. Radiother Oncol 1993;29:219–20.
56. Hanks GE, Schultheiss TE, Hunt MA, et al. Factors influencing incidence of acute grade 2 morbidity in conformal and standard radiation treatment of prostate cancer. Int J Radiat Oncol Biol Phys 1995;31:25–9.
57. Dearnaley DP, Khoo VS, Norman AR, et al. Comparison of radiation side-effects of conformal and conventional radiotherapy in prostate cancer: a randomised trial. Lancet 1999;353:267–72.
58. Nguyen LN, Pollack A, et al. Late effects after radiotherapy for prostate cancer in a randomized dose-response study: results of a self-assessment questionnaire. Urology 1998;51:991–7.
59. D'Amico AV, Coleman CN. Role of interstitial radiotherapy in the management of clinically organ-confined prostate cancer: the jury is still out. J Clin Oncol 1996;14:304–15.
60. Gelblum DY, Potters L, Ashley R, et al. Urinary morbidity following ultrasound-guided transperineal prostate seed implantation. Int J Radiat Oncol Biol Phys 1999;45:59–67.
61. Gelblum DY, Potters L. Rectal complications associated with transperineal interstitial brachytherapy for prostate cancer. Int J Radiat Oncol Biol Phys 2000;48:119–24.
62. Onik GM, Cohen JK, Reyes GD, et al. Transrectal ultrasound guided percutaneous radical cryosurgical ablation of the prostate. Cancer 1993;7:1292–9.
63. Badalament RA, Bahn DK, Kim H, et al. Patient-reported complications after cryoablation therapy for prostate cancer. Urology 1999;54:295–300.
64. Cohen JK, Rooker GM, et al. Cryosurgical ablation of the prostate: treatment alternative for localized prostate cancer. Cancer Treat Res 1996;88:167–86.
65. Derakhshani P, Neubauer S, et al. Cryoablation of localized prostate cancer. Experience in 48 cases, PSA and biopsy results. Eur Urol 1998;34:181–7.
66. Saliken JC, Donnelly BJ, et al. Outcomes and safety of transrectal US-guided percutaneous cryotherapy for localized prostate cancer. J Vasc Interv Radiol 1999;10(2 Pt 1):199–208.
67. Cespedes FD, Pisters LL, et al. Long-term followup of incontinence and obstruction after salvage cryosurgical ablation of the prostate: results in 143 patients. J Urol 1997;157:237–40.
68. Cox RL, Crawford ED. Complications of cryosurgical ablation of the prostate to treat localized adenocarcinoma of the prostate. Urology 1995;45:932–5.
69. De la Taille A, Hayek O, et al. Salvage cryotherapy for recurrent prostate cancer after radiation therapy: the Columbia experience. Urology 2000;55:79–84.
70. Capps GW, Fulcher AS, et al. Imaging features of radiation-induced changes in the abdomen. Radiographics 1997;17:1455–73.
71. Park R, Martin S, Goldberg J, Lepor H. Anastomotic strictures following radical prostatectomy: insights into incidence, effectiveness of intervention, effect on continence, and factors predisposing to occurrence. Urology 2001;57:742–6.
72. Speight JL, Shinohara K, Pickett B, et al. Prostate volume change after radioactive seed implantation: possible benefit of improved dose volume histogram with peroperative steroid. Int J Radiat Oncol Biol Phys 2000;48:1461–7.
73. Flood HD, Malhotra SJ, et al. Long-term results and complications using augmentation cystoplasty in reconstructive urology. Neurourol Urodyn 1995;14:297–309.
74. Herschorn S, Hewitt RJ. Patient perspective of long-term outcome of augmentation cystoplasty for neurogenic bladder. Urology 1998;52:672–8.
75. Rogers CJ, Barber DB, et al. Spontaneous bladder perforation in paraplegia as a late complication of augmentation enterocystoplasty: case report. Arch Phys Med Rehabil 1996;77:1198–200.
76. Barrington JW, Fulford S, et al. Tumors in bladder remnant after augmentation enterocystoplasty. J Urol 1997;157:482–5.
77. Leng WW, Blalock HJ, et al. Enterocystoplasty or detrusor myectomy? Comparison of indications and outcomes for bladder augmentation. J Urol 1999;161:758–63.
78. Stohrer M, Gocpel M, et al. Detrusor myectomy (autoaugmentation) in the treatment of hyperreflexive low compliance bladder. Urologe Q 1999;38:30–7.
79. Burgio KL. Behavioral therapy: practical approach to urinary incontinence. Contemp Urol 1994;6:24–36.
80. Cross CA, English SF, Cespedes RD, et al. A followup on transurethral collagen injection therapy for urinary incontinence. J Urol 1998;159:106.

81. Aboseif SR, O'Connell HE, Usui A, et al. Collagen injection for intrinsic sphincteric deficiency in men. J Urol 1996; 155:10–3.
82. Elsergany R, Ghoniem GM. Collagen injection for intrinsic sphincteric deficiency in men: a reasonable option in selected patients. J Urol 1998;159:1504–6.
83. Griebling TL, Kreder KJ Jr, Williams RD. Transurethral collagen in injection for treatment of postprostatectomy urinary incontinence in men. Urology 1997;49:907–12.
84. Leibovich BC, Barrett DM. Use of the artificial urinary sphincter in men and women. World J Urol 1997;15: 316–9.
85. Schaeffer AJ, Clemens JQ, Ferrari M, Stamey TA. The male bulbourethral sling procedure for post-radical prostatectomy incontinence. J Urol 1998;159:1510–5.
86. Clemens JQ, Bushman W, Schaeffer AJ. Questionnaire-based results of the bulbourethral sling procedure. J Urol 1999; 162:1972–6.
87. Clemens JQ, Bushman W, Schaeffer AJ. Urodynamic analysis of the bulbourethral sling procedure. J Urol 1999;162: 1977–81.
88. Dean RJ, Lytton B. Urologic complications of pelvic irradiation. J Urol 1978;119:64.
89. Ram MD. Complications of radiotherapy for carcinoma of the bladder. Proc R Soc Med 1970;63:93.
90. DeVries CR, Freiha FS. Hemorrhagic cystitis: a review. J Urol 1990;143:1.
91. Mukamel
92. Kumar APM, Wren ELJ, Jayalakshmamma B, et al. Silver nitrate irrigation to control bladder hemorrhage in children receiving cancer therapy. J Urol 1976;116:85.
93. Parsons CL. Successful management of radiation cystitis with sodium pentosanpolysulfate. J Urol 1986;136:813.
94. Shrom SH, Donaldson MH, Duckett JW, et al. Formalin treatment for intractable hemorrhagic cystitis. A review of the literature with 16 additional cases. Cancer 1976;38:1785.
95. Kranc DM, Levine LA. Hemorrhagic cystitis. AUA Update Series 1992;11:241.
96. Del Pizzo JJD, Chew BH, Jacobs SC, et al. Treatment of radiation-induced hemorrhagic cystitis with hyperbaric oxygen: long-term followup. J Urol 1998;160:731.
97. Weiss JP, Mattei DM, Neville EC, et al. Primary treatment of radiation-induced hemorrhagic cystitis with hyperbaric oxygen: 10-year experience. J Urol 1994;151:1514.
98. Norkool DM, Hampson NB, Gibbons RP, et al. Hyperbaric oxygen therapy for radiation-induced hemorrhagic cystitis. J Urol 1993;150:332.
99. Schoenrock GJ, Cianci P. Treatment of radiation cystitis with hyperbaric oxygen. Urology 1986;27:271.
100. Rijkmans BG, Bakker DJ, Dabhoiwala NF, et al. Successful treatment of radiation cystitis with hyperbaric oxygen. Eur Urol 1989;16:354.
101. Thom TR. Hyperbaric oxygen therapy: a committee report. Bethesda (MD): Undersea and Hyperbaric Medicine Society; 1992.
102. Zincke H. Radical prostatectomy and exenterative procedures for local failure after radiotherapy with curative intent: comparison of outcomes. J Urol 1992;147:894–9.
103. Rogers E, Ohori M, Kassabian VS, et al. Salvage radical prostatectomy: outcome measured by serum prostate specific antigen levels. J Urol 1995;153:104–10.
104. Silva RA, Correia AJ, et al. Argon plasma coagulation therapy for hemorrhagic radiation proctosigmoiditis. Gastrointest Endosc 1999;50:221–4.
105. Teshima T, Hanks GE, et al. Rectal bleeding after conformal 3D treatment of prostate cancer: time to occurrence, response to treatment and duration of morbidity. Int J Radiat Oncol Biol Phys 1997;39:77–83.
106. Hu K, Wallner K. Clinical course of rectal bleeding following I-125 prostate brachytherapy. Int J Radiat Oncol Biol Phys 1998;41:263–5.
107. Hanlon AL, Schultheiss TE, et al. Chronic rectal bleeding after high-dose conformal treatment of prostate cancer warrants modification of existing morbidity scales. Int J Radiat Oncol Biol Physics 1997;38:59–63.
108. Goldstein F, Khoury J, Thornton JJ. Treatment of chronic radiation enteritis and colitis with salicylazosulfapyridine and systemic corticosteroids. Am J Gastroenterol 1976;65: 201–8.
109. Baum CA, Biddle WL, Miner PB. Failure of 5-aminosalicylic acid enemas to improve chronic radiation proctitis. Dig Dis Sci 1989;32:758–60.
110. Kochhar R, Patel F, Dhar A, et al. Radiation-induced proctosigmoiditis: prospective, randomized, double-blind controlled trial of oral sulfasalazine plus rectal steroids versus rectal sucralfate. Dig Dis Sci 1991;36:103–7.
111. Chapuis P, Dent O, et al. The development of a treatment protocol for patients with chronic radiation-induced rectal bleeding. Aust N Z J Surg 1996;66:680–5.
112. Taylor JG, DiSario JA, Buchi KN. Argon laser therapy for hemorrhagic radiation proctitis: long-term results. Gastrointest Endosc 1993;39:641–4.
113. O'Connor JJ. Argon laser treatment of radiation proctitis. Arch Surg 1989;124:749.
114. Rubinstein E, Ibsen T, Rasmussen RB, et al. Formalin treatment of radiation-induced hemorrhagic proctitis. Am J Gastroenterol 1986;81:44–5.
115. Saclarides TJ, King DG, et al. Formalin instillation for refractory radiation-induced hemorrhagic proctitis. Report of 16 patients. Dis Colon Rectum 1996;39:196–9.
116. Yegappan M, Ho YH, et al. The surgical management of colorectal complications from irradiation for carcinoma of the cervix. Ann Acad Med Singapore 1998;27:627–30.

28

Palliative Care

DAVID M. REESE, MD

Many patients with advanced prostate cancer have bone pain or functional impairments that adversely affect quality of life, and provision of appropriate supportive care is an integral component of their clinical management. Although palliative medicine is becoming more established as a separate discipline within oncology (especially in the United Kingdom, Canada, and Australia), most supportive care for patients with advanced prostate cancer continues to be delivered by physicians without specific training in the field. Since palliative care is defined by the World Health Organization (WHO) as the "active total care of patients whose disease is not responsive to curative treatment," the medical oncologist, urologist, or radiation therapist must be proficient in the delivery of broad-based supportive care, including relief of physical symptoms and psychosocial support.[1]

DISEASE-RELATED SYMPTOMS: THE SCOPE OF THE PROBLEM

Despite its prevalence in the population, specific information regarding morbidity and quality of life in patients with advanced prostate cancer is relatively scarce, and appropriate longitudinal studies using validated instruments have only recently been initiated. However, several older surveys do suggest a high prevalence of symptoms and functional disturbances in patients with advanced prostate cancer. In one study of 172 patients and their spouses or partners, fatigue, urinary symptoms, and pain were very common.[2] In addition, neuropsychological symptoms such as depression, anxiety, and irritability were also common in both patients and partners and were associated with poor quality of life. Other surveys of patients with hormone-refractory prostate cancer also found pain, fatigue, excessive worrying, drowsiness, sadness, sleep disturbance, and nervousness to be present in more than half of all patients.[3,4] These data confirm the widely held clinical view that disease-related symptoms that adversely affect quality of life are very prevalent in patients with advanced prostate cancer.

Recently, there has been a surge of interest in developing methodologies to measure quality of life that are specific to prostate cancer. Generic health-related quality-of-life survey instruments, which may be helpful in the development of global health policy or the distribution of resources, are generally poor measures of functionality in patients with prostate cancer.[5] More specific instruments have therefore been developed, but these often focus on particular domains of illness such as pain or sexual function and thus may not encompass all relevant aspects of the disease process. Nevertheless, at least nine prostate cancer–specific surveys have been used to measure health-related quality of life in patients with prostate cancer, focusing on aspects of the disease and its treatment such as urinary, sexual, and bowel function; physical function; psychological function; and disease-related pain.[6] However, no single instrument has been developed that is applicable to patients across the spectrum of disease, and this must be a top priority for future quality-of-life research. In addition, standardization of instruments will be critical for these methodologies to generate data that can be used to guide patient management and inform policy decisions.

The remainder of this chapter is devoted to a review of management strategies for specific symptoms commonly encountered in the patient with advanced prostate cancer.

BONE PAIN

Pain from osseous metastases is one of the most common symptoms reported among men with advanced prostate cancer and is typically present in 60 to 70% of patients.[7] In assessing the patient with prostate cancer who has pain, it is essential to obtain a relevant pain history, including location, duration, and type of pain, as well as the effectiveness of analgesic maneuvers. Many clinicians find that having patients rank the pain on a scale of 1 to 10 and using a visual analogue scale (VAS) in which the patient marks the level of pain on a line 10 cm in length are useful ways of quantifying the degree of cancer pain a patient is experiencing. In fact, use of VAS instruments has become common in clinical trials investigating new therapies for the treatment of hormone-refractory prostate cancer.

One practical guideline for management of cancer pain is the WHO analgesic ladder.[1] This approach suggests starting with a nonopioid (with or without an adjuvant) for mild pain initially, followed by an opioid plus a nonopioid (with or without an adjuvant) for moderate pain. For patients with severe pain, opioids with or without nonopioids are recommended.

The use of nonsteroidal anti-inflammatory drugs (NSAIDs) may be useful in treating osseous pain since much of the discomfort may result from periosteal irritation in the bone. The choice of NSAID may not be particularly important, and a period of trial and error may be necessary. Evaluating the cost, side-effect profiles, and efficacies of the various NSAIDs should be individualized. Glucocorticoids, in addition to any antitumor effect, also serve as potent anti-inflammatory agents and can alleviate bone pain.[8] In general, we prescribe steroids for patients with symptomatic hormone-refractory prostate cancer not receiving other anticancer therapy, although the use of both steroids and NSAIDs should be avoided given the potential for enhanced gastrointestinal toxicity.

For patients with significant bone pain despite the use of adequate analgesics, the use of either local or systemic radiation therapy may be appropriate. In particular, radiotherapy may prevent some complications of bony metastasis, including spinal cord compression and pathologic fractures.

External beam radiotherapy (EBRT) is generally effective and well tolerated when directed at specific sites of bony metastasis. The optimal doses and fractionation schedule for palliative EBRT are not certain, although most programs provide total treatment doses of 20 to 40 Gy given over 5 to 20 treatment fractions. External beam radiotherapy can be expected to result in pain relief in approximately 80% of patients, with 40% experiencing complete pain relief at the treated site.[9] The side effects of EBRT depend on the site being treated and the degree of exposure of normal tissue. For example, esophagitis may result when the cervical or upper thoracic spine is irradiated, whereas diarrhea is not infrequent during or following pelvic radiation. The use of conformal radiotherapy techniques, which are increasing in availability, may minimize the side effects of EBRT.

Patients with widespread, uncontrolled bony pain may be candidates for radioisotope therapy. Strontium 89 has been the most widely investigated compound, although a number of radioisotopes are now used to treat painful bony metastases (Table 28–1). All of these agents are used because they are preferentially incorporated into bone, although their half-lives and actual distribution within the bony matrix may differ substantially.

Strontium 89 is a radioisotope that is chemically similar to calcium and thus accumulates in bone. It does tend to accumulate to a greater degree at sites of bony metastasis when compared with normal bone tissue, and, in fact, the concentration of strontium 89 is up to five times as high in metastatic deposits.[10] A large number of clinical trials have been performed

Table 28–1. RADIOISOTOPE THERAPY OF PAINFUL BONE METASTASES

Commonly used agents
Strontium 89
Samarium 153
Other agents
Phosphorus 32
Iodine 131
Tin 117m
Rhenium 186
Yttrium 90

using strontium 89, either alone or in combination with local EBRT. In general, the most comprehensive studies report improvements in pain in 50 to 80% of treated patients.[11–15] Strontium 89 therapy is usually well tolerated, although, in our experience, it often results in prolonged or persistent myelosupression, particularly thrombocytopenia. Thus, we usually reserve use of this agent for patients with severe pain who are not candidates for aggressive systemic treatment such as chemotherapy. Use of strontium 89 may also be associated with pain flare at the sites of metastasis, and if this occurs, use of concomitant EBRT is usually effective in controlling pain.

Samarium 153 has also been approved by the US Food and Drug Administration for the treatment of painful bony metastases, and clinical response rates are comparable with those obtained with strontium 89.[16] Because it has a physical half-life of 1.9 days (compared with 50.5 days for strontium 89), it has been hoped that samarium 153 would induce less significant and permanent myelosuppression than strontium. However, in our experience, significant cytopenias are often observed after the use of samarium 153, and we also use this agent only if patients will not be receiving additional cytotoxic therapy. Older isotopes, including phosphorus 32 and iodine 131, should not be used because they do not selectively accumulate at the sites of bony metastasis. More recently developed isotopes such as rhenium 186 and tin 117m have been primarily used in investigational settings, and their ultimate clinical utility remains to be determined.[17]

Bisphosphonates, which inhibit osteoclast activity, may also play a role in the treatment of bony metastases. Pamidronate has reduced skeletal complications and bone pain when used in patients with multiple myeloma and metastatic breast cancer,[18,19] and preliminary results suggest that it may be effective in prostate cancer.[20,21] Further investigation of this compound is ongoing. Clodronate, available in both intravenous and oral forms, has been reported to reduce the incidence of skeletal metastases in breast cancer when used as part of adjuvant therapy.[22] A pilot study in 27 patients with metastatic prostate cancer reported pain relief in 37% of patients.[23] The further investigation of bisphosphonates as both adjuvant pain medications and in the prevention or progression of bony metastases is a high priority in prostate cancer clinical research.

The judicious use of analgesics, targeted radiation therapy, and perhaps adjunctive medications such as bisphosphonates should result in adequate control of bone pain in the vast majority of patients with advanced prostate cancer. For the rare patient with uncontrolled pain despite the above measures, referral to a pain management clinic is appropriate.

FATIGUE, ANEMIA, AND ANOREXIA

Fatigue is one of the most common symptoms present in patients with advanced prostate cancer and is usually reported in more than 70% of patients.[2–4] In prostate cancer, fatigue may be attributable to many causes, including anemia, increased catabolism associated with tumor metabolism, side effects of treatment such as chemotherapy or radiation therapy, and effects associated with androgen deprivation or the use of drugs such as opiates.[5] Despite its prevalence, the treatment of fatigue in patients with prostate cancer is often frustrating. To best address fatigue in this patient population, a thorough assessment of potentially contributing factors is essential.

Anemia is one correctable cause of fatigue in patients with prostate cancer. Anemia is common in patients receiving combined androgen blockade (CAB), and up to 75% of patients on CAB will experience some degree of anemia.[24,25] Transfusion of packed red blood cells will rapidly correct anemia in patients who have significant symptoms, but a preferable long-term alternative is the use of recombinant erythropoietin. Subcutaneous administration of erythropoietin, in addition to effectively raising hemoglobin levels, has been found to increase overall quality of life, energy level, and activity level in patients with cancer treated with chemotherapy.[26] In studies specifically examining the effects of erythropoietin in patients with prostate cancer, use of the growth factor has been associated with correction of anemia and improvement in fatigue.[24,27] New weekly schedules of administration make delivery of erythropoietin quite simple.[28] Although erythropoietin therapy is expensive, its long-term use in patients with cancer may actually be cost effective when compared to periodic blood transfusion.[29]

Another contributing factor in the development of fatigue in patients with prostate cancer is anorexia with possible associated weight loss. Anorexia-cachexia in patients with cancer is a complex physiologic phenomenon that is incompletely understood, although diversion of calories from host tissues to tumor and production of specific cachexia-inducing factors such as cytokines and neuropeptides both likely play a role.[30–33] Although treatment of anorexia-cachexia with parenteral nutrition does not improve survival in patients with cancer, the use of progestational drugs can stimulate appetite, increase food intake and weight, and improve energy level. A number of randomized, placebo-controlled trials have demonstrated that megestrol acetate is effective in patients with advanced cancer,[32,34–36] and we recommend a trial of megestrol acetate in doses of 160 to 800 mg/day in patients with significant anorexia or weight loss. Megestrol acetate also has modest antitumor effects in patients with hormone-refractory prostate cancer,[37] although prolonged use of the agent may lead to paradoxical effects as an androgen-receptor agonist, and, occasionally, withdrawal of the drug is associated with prostate-specific antigen declines and/or objective disease regression.[38] Further elucidation of the neurochemical pathways responsible for inducing anorexia and cachexia will be required, and, eventually, use of newer agents such as serotonergic blockers or thalidomide may prove efficacious.[39,40]

URINARY SYMPTOMS

Urinary symptoms such as incontinence, obstruction, dysuria, and hematuria are not infrequent in patients with advanced prostate cancer. Urinary symptoms usually develop owing to local tumor extension or ureteral obstruction from extensive retroperitoneal adenopathy. Frequent monitoring of renal function in patients with known regional adenopathy or local tumor recurrence is essential.

The treatment of urinary symptoms should be targeted at the underlying cause of the problem. For patients with obstruction, the use of cystoscopically placed stents or percutaneous nephrostomy tubes may be necessary to ensure adequate renal drainage. On occasion, transurethral resection of the prostate (TURP) can relieve distal obstruction owing to locally invasive tumor, although, in this setting, the procedure does have the risk of inducing or worsening incontinence. Cystoscopy or TURP may also help to control hematuria if a site of bleeding amenable to surgical intervention is identified. Patients with significant ongoing blood loss may require placement of a three-way urinary catheter for the purpose of continuous bladder irrigation. In all cases, careful attention to functional outcome is required since decrements in urinary function are a common cause of declines in quality of life in patients with advanced prostate cancer.

PSYCHOLOGICAL SYMPTOMS

Impairments in psychological well-being and function are common in patients with advanced cancer. Close to half of all patients with cancer may have a diagnosable psychiatric disorder, usually an adjustment disorder with depression.[41] In fact, it is estimated that 20 to 25% of patients with advanced cancer suffer from depression severe enough to impair function and warrant treatment with antidepressant drugs.[42] In addition, depression in patients with cancer may be associated with particularly poor quality of life and may indeed correlate with lower long-term survival.

Despite its prevalence and clinical significance, depression in the patient with cancer may be difficult to diagnose since many of the neurovegetative symptoms associated with depression may also be secondary to the underlying malignancy itself.[43] Thus, careful questioning of the patient with advanced prostate cancer with regard to psychological well-being is essential, especially since effective pharmacologic interventions are available. Use of tricyclic antidepressants, selective serotonin reuptake inhibitors (SSRIs), and, occasionally, stimulants may all play a role in the treatment of the depressed patient with prostate cancer.[5] The SSRIs, in particular, may be useful in elderly patients given the favorable side-effect profile. In patients with severe depression or suicidal ideation, immediate referral to a psychiatrist is appropriate.

CONCLUSIONS

Provision of adequate supportive care to patients with advanced prostate cancer remains a major challenge. Careful attention to the patient's symptomatology, with targeted interventions, may result in improvements in quality of life equivalent or superior to the treatment of the cancer itself, and a continuous reassessment of a patient's palliative care needs is essential for the involved physician. Further research advances, in particular in identifying the most important determinants of quality of life in patients with advanced prostate cancer, will be required to improve functional well-being in this population.

REFERENCES

1. World Health Organization. Cancer pain and palliative care. Geneva: World Health Organization; 1990. Technical report series 804.
2. Kornblith AB, Herr HW, Ofman US, et al. Quality of life of patients with prostate cancer and their spouses: the value of a data base in clinical practice. Cancer 1994;73:2791.
3. Portenoy RK, Thaler HT, Kornblith AB, et al. Symptom prevalence, characteristics, and distress in a cancer population. Qual Life Res 1994;3:183.
4. Fossa SD, Aaronson NK, Newling D, et al. Quality of life and treatment of hormone resistant metastatic prostatic cancer. The EORTC Genito-Urinary Group. Eur J Cancer 1990;26:1133.
5. Esper P, Redman BG. Supportive care, pain management, and quality of life in advanced prostate cancer. Urol Clin North Am 1999;26:375–89.
6. Sommers SD, Ramsey SD. A review of quality-of-life evaluations in prostate cancer. Pharmacoeconomics 1999;16:127–40.
7. Akakura K, Akimoto S, Shimazaki J. Pain caused by bone metastases in endocrine therapy-refractory prostate cancer. J Cancer Res Clin Oncol 1996;122:633–7.
8. Tannock I, Gospodarowics M, Meakin W, et al. Treatment of metastatic prostate cancer with low-dose prednisone: evaluation of pain and quality of life as prognostic indices of response. J Clin Oncol 1989;7:590–7.
9. Friedland J. Local and systemic radiation for palliation of metastatic disease. Urol Clin North Am 1999;26:391–402.
10. Robinson R, Blake GM, Preston DF, et al. Strontium-89: treatment results and kinetics in patients with painful metastatic prostate and breast cancer in bone. Radiographics 1989;9:271–81.
11. Laing AH, Ackery DM, Bayly RJ, et al. Strontium-89 chloride for pain palliation in prostatic skeletal malignancy. Br J Radiol 1991;64:816–22.
12. Haesner M, Buchali K, Pink V, Lips H. Efficacy of ^{89}Sr therapy in 200 patients with bone metastases of a prostatic carcinoma. Nuklearmedizin 1992;31:48–52.
13. Robinson RG, Preston DF, Baxter KG, et al. Clinical experience with strontium-89 in prostatic and breast cancer patients. Semin Oncol 1993;20 Suppl 3:44–8.
14. Porter AT. The use of strontium-89 in metastatic cancer: US and UK experience. Oncology 1994;8:24–9.
15. Quilty PM, Kirk D, Bolger JJ, et al. A comparison of the palliative effects of strontium-89 and external beam radiotherapy in metastatic prostate cancer. Radiother Oncol 1994;31:33–40.
16. Lamb HM, Faulds D. Samarium 153Sm lexidronam. Drugs Aging 1997;11:413–8.
17. Maxon HR, Thomas SR, Hertzberg VS, et al. Rhenium-186 hydorxyethylidene diphosphosphonate for the treatment of painful osseous metastases. Semin Nucl Med 1992;23:33–40.
18. Berenson JR, Lichtenstein A, Porter L, et al. Efficacy of pamidronate in reducing skeletal events in patients with advanced multiple myeloma. Myeloma Aredia Study Group. N Engl J Med 1996;334:488–93.
19. Hortobagyi GN, Theriault RL, Porter L, et al. Efficacy of pamidronate in reducing skeletal complications in patients with breast cancer and lytic bone metastases. N Engl J Med 1996;335:1785–91.
20. Lipton A, Glover D, Harvey H, et al. Pamidronate in the treatment of bone metastases: results of 2 dose-ranging trials in patients with breast or prostate cancer. Ann Oncol 1994;5 Suppl 7:s31–5.
21. Clarke NW, McClure J, George NJR. Effect of disodium pamidronate in metastatic prostate cancer. Eur J Cancer 1991;27 Suppl 2:117.
22. Diel IJ, Solomayer EF, Costa SD, et al. Reduction of new metastases in breast cancer with adjuvant clodronate treatment. N Engl J Med 1998;339:357–63.
23. Cresswell SM, English PJ, Hall RR, et al. Pain relief and quality of life assessment following intravenous and oral clodronate in hormone-escaped metastatic prostate cancer. Br J Urol 1995;76:360–5.
24. Strum SB, McDermed JE, Scholz MC, et al. Anaemia associated with androgen deprivation in patients with prostate cancer receiving combined androgen blockade. Br J Urol 1997;79:933–41.
25. Asbell SO, Leon SA, Tester WJ, et al. Development of anemia and recovery in prostate cancer patients treated with combined androgen blockade and radiotherapy. Prostate 1996;29:243–8.
26. Glaspy J, Bukowski R, Steinberg D, et al. Impact of therapy with epoetin alfa on clinical outcomes in patients with nonmyeloid malignancies during cancer chemotherapy in community oncology practice. Procrit Study Group. J Clin Oncol 1997;15:1218–34.
27. Beshara S, Letocha H, Linde T, et al. Anemia associated with advanced prostatic adenocarcinoma: effects of recombinant human erythropoietin. Prostate 1997;31:153–60.
28. Tsukuda M, Yuyama S, Kohno H, et al. Effectiveness of weekly subcutaneous recombinant human erythropoietin administration for chemotherapy-induced anemia. Biotherapy 1998;11:21–5.
29. Glaspy JA. Economic outcomes associated with the use of hematopoietic growth factors. Oncology 1995;9 Suppl 11:93–105.
30. Beck S, Mulligan H, Tisdale M. Lipolytic factors associated with murine and human cancer cachexia. J Natl Cancer Inst 1990;82:1922–6.
31. Mahony S, Beck S, Tisdale M. Comparison of weight loss induced by recombinant tumor necrosis factor with that

produced by a cachexia-inducing tumor. Br J Cancer 1988;57:385–9.

32. Body JJ. The syndrome of anorexia-cachexia. Curr Opin Oncol 1999;11:255–60.
33. Inui A. Cancer anorexia-cachexia syndrome: are neuropeptides the key? Cancer Res 1999;59:4493–501.
34. Bruera E, MacMillan K, Hanson J, et al. A controlled trial of megestrol acetate on appetite, caloric intake, nutritional status, and other symptoms in patients with advanced cancer. Cancer 1990;66:1279–82.
35. Loprinzi CL, Ellison NM, Schaid J, et al. A controlled trial of megestrol acetate treatment of cancer anorexia and cachexia. J Natl Cancer Inst 1990;82:1127–32.
36. Loprinzi CL, Michalak JC, Schaid DJ, et al. Phase III evaluation of four doses of megestrol acetate as therapy for patients with anorexia and/or cachexia. J Clin Oncol 1993;11:762.
37. Reese DM, Small EJ. Secondary hormonal manipulations in hormone refractory prostate cancer. Urol Clin North Am 1999;26:311–21.
38. Dawson NA, McLeod DG. Dramatic PSA decline in response to discontinuation of megestrol acetate in advanced prostate cancer. J Urol 1995;153:1946–7.
39. Edelman MJ, Gandar DR, Meyers FJ, et al. Serotonergic blockade in the treatment of the cancer anorexia-chachexia syndrome. Cancer 1999;86:684–8.
40. Bruera E, Neumann CM, Pituskin E, et al. Thalidomide in patients with cachexia due to terminal cancer: preliminary report. Ann Oncol 1999;10:857–9.
41. Spiegel D. Cancer and depression. Br J Psych 1996; Suppl:109–16.
42. Bottomley A. Depression in cancer patients: a literature review. Eur J Cancer Care 1998;7:181–91.
43. McDaniel JS, Musselman DL, Porter MR, et al. Depression in patients with cancer: diagnosis, biology, and treatment. Arch Gen Psychiatry 1995;52:89–99.

Index

Page numbers followed by f indicate figure; those followed by t indicate table.